Medical Transcription

Techniques, Technologies, and Editing Skills

Third Edition

Alice G. Ettinger RN, MSN, CPNP
Blanche Ettinger, EdD

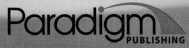

Paradigm PUBLISHING

St. Paul • Los Angeles • Indianapolis

Acquisitions Editor: Alison Brown Cerier
Senior Developmental Editor: Christine Hurney
Production Editor: Bob Dreas
Cover and Text Designer: Jaana Bykonich

Production Specialists: Jaana Bykonich, Charles Sawyer
Copy Editor: Kristin Wall
Proofreader: Laura Nelson
Indexer: Terry Casey

Photo Credits: p. 4, © H Armstrong Roberts/ Retrofile /Getty Images; p. 7 © AP IMAGES; p. 8, left, © Terri Miller / E-Visual Communications, Inc.; p. 8, right, © Terri Miller / E-Visual Communications, Inc.; p. 27, © Terri Miller / E-Visual Communications, Inc.; p. 34, © ER Productions/CORBIS; p. 37, Image courtesy of HTH Engineering; p. 41, © Bill Wolfe / Shutterstock.com; p. 42 ,© Chris Fredriksson / Alamy; p. 62, © InstinctDesign / Shutterstock.com; p. 169, lower left, © Germán Ariel Berra / Shutterstock.com; p. 169, upper right, Cameron Swinton / Shutterstock.com; p. 169, lower right © Johanna Goodyear / Shutterstock.com p. 170, Custom Medical Stock Photo; p. 192, © K Chelette / Shutterstock.com; p. 217 © Kmitu / Shutterstock.com; p. 362, © Michael English/Custom Medical Stock Photo

Text ISBN 978-0-76383-106-6
Text with Dictations and Templates CD ISBN 978-0-76383-109-7
© 2009 by Paradigm Publishing, Inc.
875 Montreal Way
St. Paul, MN 55102
E-mail: educate@emcp.com
Web site: www.emcp.com

16 15 14 13 12 11 10   4 5 6 7 8 9 10

Brief Contents

Contents

To the Student

Congratulations on choosing the dynamic field of medical transcription! Medical transcriptionists translate a healthcare provider's oral dictations into a written medical record. Medical transcriptionists today are valued for their expertise in medical language and healthcare documentation. As a transcriptionist, you will help produce the accurate records that are essential for effective medical care. The reports you transcribe will be used to obtain the appropriate reimbursement for medical services and will serve as a legal record.

This textbook has been designed to help students like you develop the skills and knowledge of an entry-level professional. You will build speed and accuracy by working with reports that begin at the easiest level and become gradually more challenging.

You will also develop expertise in medical language, editing, and the necessary computer and transcription technology. This textbook emphasizes these three core skills, which are fundamental to a successful career in medical transcription. You will learn about fourteen medical specialties, with an emphasis on the medical terminology that healthcare providers use. Exercises will help to develop your skills in editing and proofreading, which are important for accuracy and consistency of style. You will also learn about technologies used in medical transcription and start making these tools work for you.

The intensive but practical approach of this textbook will prepare you well for your career. You will be ready for your role in supporting the safety of patients and helping them receive high-quality care as you begin your career as a vital member of the healthcare team.

How This Text Is Organized

Medical Transcription: Techniques, Technologies, and Editing Skills, Third Edition has two parts. Part 1 introduces the core skills necessary for the transcriptionist and Part 2 provides background and practice in transcribing for fourteen medical specialties.

Part 1: Preparing to Transcribe

The four chapters in Part 1 introduce the field of medical transcription. Chapter 1 explains the role of the transcriptionist in the healthcare team, highlights the professional principles of transcription work, and introduces the skills needed to transcribe efficiently and effectively. The chapter also presents the kinds of medical reports that will be transcribed throughout the course.

Chapter 2 describes the technologies that transcriptionists use in their work. You will learn the functions of the basic transcription tools, including the foot pedal and headset, transcription software, and your computer. You will also learn about the productivity tools that transcriptionists find invaluable, including templates, macros, and text expanders.

Chapter 3 is a review of basic medical terminology, including word parts, basic anatomy, and diagnostic terms. You will continue to build your knowledge of medical terminology throughout the book.

Chapter 4 introduces the editing rules that guide medical transcriptionists. It covers style, format, grammar, and punctuation. There are exercises throughout this chapter, which will also be a helpful resource as you transcribe reports in the specialty chapters in Part 2.

Part 2: Transcribing for the Specialties

Part 2 is about transcribing for fourteen major medical specialties. Each chapter begins with an introduction to the specialty, including related anatomy, diagnostic procedures, diseases, and conditions. This background and context will help you recognize and understand what you hear in the dictations.

A Terms Bank lists key terminology for each medical specialty. Pronunciations and brief definitions will help you build your knowledge of words within the specialty and other words that are found in the chapter's exercises and transcription work.

The next section of each specialty chapter is called Building Language Skills. The exercises in this section will develop your skills in spelling, recognizing alike words (either words that sound alike or are the same or similar in spelling), word choices, word parts, and proofreading. An exercise called Thinking Like a Professional presents a common workplace challenge and asks "What should you do?"

Each specialty chapter ends with the section called Building Transcription Skills. You will begin by learning about the sections and the formatting of a particular medical report. You will then transcribe, edit, and correct a series of reports using audio dictation files found on the Dictations and Templates CD.

A tool called a Performance Comparison Chart will help you identify and track patterns in transcription errors. This will help you see where you are improving and where you need more work. Do you need to work harder on terminology, listening, proofreading, or editing? Your instructor may ask you use this form to document your errors on some of the transcribed reports. You will find the form on the CD that accompanies this textbook.

For each type of report, you can start with an electronic template that contains standard headings and formatting. Professional transcriptionists use such templates to help ensure consistency and make it easier to access information in the medical record. Appendix A lists the standard report headings in the templates and provides examples of the type of information found under those headings.

Appendix B explains how to use the templates provided on your CD.

In Appendix C, you will have an opportunity to try a form of transcription work that is increasingly common: editing speech-recognized text. You will edit and format a text file that was produced by a speech recognition software program, while listening to the original, authentic dictation. You can practice your editing skills while learning about this new methodology in medical transcription.

Appendix D provides a job simulation to help you evaluate your job readiness. The corresponding transcription files are available on the Dictations and Templates CD. Appendix E provides tips for job searching and developing a résumé.

Student Resources

A Dictations and Templates CD is included with each copy of *Medical Transcription*. This CD includes:
- The dictation files in MP3 format
- Electronic medical report templates
- Dictation files and drafts for the speech recognition exercises in Appendix C
- Performance Comparison Chart

The CD can be played on any personal computer (at school or home), as long as you have a disc drive. To transcribe the files, you will use a foot pedal, transcription software, and a headset. Some schools may provide these tools to their students as part of the course materials. If you need these items, you can purchase a set at a special price, for use at either school or home. Go to this text's Internet Resource Center at www.emcp.net/MedTrans3e for a link to www.startstop.com/emcp. There, you can order a foot pedal, headset, and a fully functioning student version of the Start and Stop transcription software at a reduced price using the discount code paradigm1.

The text's Internet Resource Center also provides a variety of reference material, including an electronic version of the Terms Banks, study tips, ergonomic workstation check lists, tips for communicating online, and tutorials about file management and Windows.

To the Instructor

Medical Transcription: Techniques, Technologies, and Editing Skills, Third Edition provides introductory training for working in the field of medical transcription. *Medical Transcription* is presented in the context of fourteen medical specialties. The text is supported with approximately 8 hours of dictations of increasing difficulty. Conservatively, this translates into approximately 100 hours of student transcription, proofreading, and editing work. The text's exercises and transcription work integrate medical terminology, anatomy, and disease processes into the transcription course.

This textbook aligns with the model curriculum of the Association for Healthcare Document Integrity (AHDI). A curriculum map of the text to the COMPRO model curriculum is available on the publisher's Web site. The book follows the guidelines in *The Book of Style of Medical Transcription, Third Edition*. The text also conforms with standards set by The Joint Commission and ASTM International.

This third edition of *Medical Transcription* features:

- New chapter on medical transcription and technology
- Document templates for the transcription exercises (on the student CD, and explained in the new Appendix B)
- New chapter exercises, Thinking Like a Professional, to help students develop critical thinking and problem-solving skills
- New speech recognition exercises (Appendix C) in which students edit draft text output by speech recognition software while listening to the corresponding authentic dictations (available on the Dictations and Templates CD)
- More transcription tips to help students think critically about formatting and editing issues when transcribing the reports
- Foot pedal and player software packaging options for institutional or student purchase
- A Web-based document checker option that will download MP3 files and document templates and will collect, correct, and score transcribed reports
- Updated medical information and style guidelines

Students are encouraged to document the errors made in typing the chapter's model report and at least three of the transcribed reports using the Performance Comparison Chart. This chart will help students identify, categorize, and track patterns in transcription errors and is a simple way of examining and evaluating language skills, knowledge of terminology, listening ability, proofreading competency, editing power, and concentration. By using this tool, students will eventually internalize the quality standards by which transcription work will be judged in the workplace. An electronic template of this form is available on the Dictations and Templates CD.

Instructor support for this text is provided in print and electronic formats. The printed Instructor's Guide is delivered as loose, hole-punched sheets to place in a three-ring binder. This format makes it easy to pull out a model answer for your reference, or to customize the materials for your own needs. The instructors' resources include:

- Course planning resources including syllabus suggestions and course objectives
- PowerPoint slides
- Answers for the exercises
- Model transcribed reports
- Chapter assessments and examinations
- Grading sheets

The Instructor Resources CD included with each Instructor's Guide contains answer keys for all of the text's exercises as well as live Word file model answers for the 114 transcribed reports. For each specialty chapter there is also an assessment, which includes a medical terminology written test and a dictated report. In addition, there is a midterm exam covering Chapters 1–9 and a final exam covering Chapters 10–16. A midterm dictation and six final exam dictations are also available. Assessment dictations are not available on the student CD.

You can evaluate and grade student transcriptions on printouts or can use Word's compare feature to identify many types of errors. Instructions on using the compare tool are provided.

For programs using Microsoft Word 2007, a Web-based document checker is available for evaluating transcription work. Using the SNAP document checker software, students can download document templates, transcribe the dictation files offline, and upload their transcribed reports for automatic grading and evaluation.

Acknowledgements

The authors would like to thank the following reviewers for their expert advice and opinions, which guided the planning for the new edition:

Margaret Medford Bridges
Weatherford College
Weatherford, Texas

Laura Bryan, CMT, FAAMT
Mesquite, Texas

Lisa Cantrell, MEd
Elizabethtown Community and Technical College
Elizabethtown, Kentucky

Cathy Davis-Johnson, BS, MS
Middle Georgia Technical College
Warner Robins, Georgia

Piper Hamlin, BS
Lane Community College
Eugene, Oregon

Sharon Horton, RHIT
Wallace State Community College
Hanceville, Alabama

April Howell, MBA, BS
Shasta College
Redding, California

Cathy Kelley-Arney, CMA, MLTC, BSHS
National College of Business and Technology
Bluefield, Virginia

Crystal L. Kitchens, BS, MS, CMT
Richland Community College
Decatur, Illinois

Helen Littrell
Klamath Falls, Oregon

Donna L. Maher, MS, RD
Renton Technical College
Renton, Washington

Lea M. Sims, CMT, FAAMT
Director of Communications and Publications
Association for Healthcare Documentation Integrity
Jacksonville, Florida

Paula L. Stoltz, CMT, FAAMT
Medical Transcription Education Center, Inc.
Fairlawn, Ohio

Monique L. Williams, MSA, CCRP
Southwest Tennessee Community College
Memphis, Tennessee

The authors and editorial staff would like to make special acknowledgement of the specific contributions of a few of the individuals listed above. We thank Laura Bryan for her work in providing technology-related content and advice. We especially recognize her contributions to Chapters 1 and 2, as well as her work with developing this edition's report templates and Appendixes A and B.

We thank Kristin Wall, who applied her editing experience and detailed knowledge of *The Book of Style for Medical Transcription, Third Edition* to the copyediting of the text and corresponding report answer keys. We appreciate the care and dedication she showed in her work.

Lea Sims reviewed and helped update the content of Chapter 4 to make sure it conformed to the style recommendations and preferences defined in *The Book of Style for Medical Transcription*.

Piper Hamlin helped develop the speech recognition activities found in Appendix C. As speech recognition technology advances, it will be important for medical transcriptionists to be able to edit draft text, and Piper's contributions have provided an excellent opportunity for developing these skills. We also thank the physicians at St. Peter's University Hospital in New Brunswick, New Jersey, for their samples of authentic dictation contributed for these activities.

Part One

Preparing to Transcribe

An Introduction to Medical Transcription

Medical transcription is one of many growing professions in health care. It offers many challenges as well as flexible career paths. This specialty is particularly suited to individuals who like to work independently, learn continuously, are detailed-oriented, and strive to produce an accurate product.

Objectives

» Examine the overall job environment, types of careers, and future opportunities in the field of medical transcription.

» Study the job expectations and performance standards required by the industry.

» Assess readiness for a career in medical transcription by examining personal aptitude and attributes.

» Ensure accurate interpretation and documentation of clinical information through the use of references and resources.

» Describe the purpose and types of information contained in the most common types of reports transcribed.

» Understand the issues and importance of record confidentiality.

Overview of the Profession

The word *transcription* is created from two combining forms: *trans* and *scriba*. The prefix *trans* means across, beyond, through, so as to change; *scriba* means official writer. From this definition comes the meaning for transcription: to change the spoken word to the written word.

Transcription had its beginnings in early times when few people could read or write, and scribes were hired to copy and interpret the spoken word. Their job was considered important since they frequently transcribed legal and sacred orations into written documents that became the rules and principles by which the society governed its members. Their work provides us with a rich heritage of historical records that portrayed life in their era.

The specialty of medical transcription had its beginnings in the early 1900s when medical stenographers became scribes for physicians who originally had maintained all of their own records. These medical stenographers helped lighten the load for busy physicians by manually documenting all of their patient interactions. Because the technology we have today was not available, medical stenographers frequently had to follow physicians during rounds, frantically trying to hear and record every word for medical record documentation.

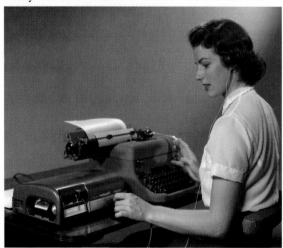

As was true for the medical transcriptionist in the 1950s, today's medical transcriptionist (MT), must strive for speed and accuracy when transcribing reports. Fortunately, MTs today benefit from advanced technology to facilitate medical documentation.

The career of medical transcription evolved with the development of dictating equipment during World War I. Physicians were able to dictate their findings, modes of treatment, and medical reports for transcription without face-to-face contact. With today's current technology, a medical transcriptionist (MT) may never have face-to-face contact with any dictators. The vast majority of dictation is created by physicians (medical doctors and doctors of osteopathy), but you may also encounter dictation from physician assistants, nurses, physical therapists, dentists, and other professionals who provide direct patient care. For this reason, you may see dictators referred to as "practitioners" or "providers" or less commonly as "authors" or "originators." From local neighborhood hospitals and clinics to major medical centers and research facilities, providers rely on medical transcriptionists to create accurate documentation for their patient records. Thus, the MT serves as a vital link between the caregiver and the patient.

The Medical Transcriptionist as a Member of the Healthcare Team

As an MT, you have an important role as a member of the healthcare team. According to the Association for Healthcare Documentation Integrity (AHDI)—formerly the American Association for Medical Transcription (AAMT)—the professional organization for medical transcriptionists, an MT is ". . .a medical language specialist who transcribes and interprets dictation by physicians and other healthcare providers regarding patient assessment, workup, therapeutic procedures, clinical course, diagnosis, prognosis, etc., in order to document patient care and facilitate delivery of healthcare services." In essence, MTs transfer the physician's spoken words via analog recording or digital dictation systems into typewritten, computerized, legal documents. These documents describe the historical and factual data about events leading up to and surrounding patient care and treatment, the outcome of the illness or condition, and the details surrounding release from the hospital.

Some of the most commonly transcribed medical documents include office notes, history and physical examinations, consultations, operative reports, correspondence, pathology reports, discharge summaries, and radiology reports. Because these documents become the foundation for a patient's healthcare record, the medical transcriptionist's main responsibility is to produce impeccably accurate reports. A medical transcriptionist also may be responsible for record maintenance, i.e., keeping logs of daily work, printing, charting, or delivering medical reports; training; providing administrative support; and evaluating equipment.

MTs also have a critical role in patient safety and risk management. Risk management in a medical setting involves the identification of issues which could lead to harm, defamation, or litigation. Medical providers often work under stressful and harried conditions and at times misspeak while dictating. Transcriptionists provide a safety net to catch discrepancies or possible errors within the document and then call them to the attention of the provider. Paying close attention and applying critical thinking to the transcription process protects the patient by averting potential mistakes caused by dictation errors. Comments made in the course of dictation that may be inflammatory or slanderous should be called to the attention of the facility's risk manager.

The Transcription Process

The transcription process (see Figure 1.1) actually begins with a patient's visit to the healthcare provider, often referred to as a "patient encounter." The healthcare providers must document the encounter, recording their impressions, plans, and any care provided. Physicians and nurses typically make handwritten notes during the course of the patient's visit, but the details of the encounter should be organized and summarized in a format that is easy to read and easily shared among other caregivers. Recording pertinent information about the encounter that can be referenced during the patient's subsequent visits or shared with other healthcare providers contributes to continuity of care. Most physicians prefer to generate a report by dictating their findings, impression, and plan of care. There are several types of devices used to record dictation, the most common being handheld recorders and telephone-enabled dictation

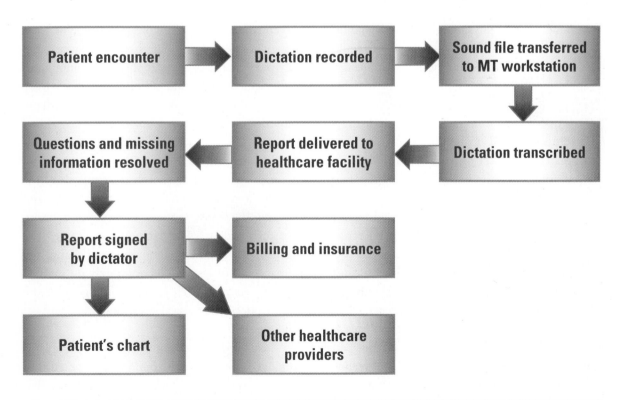

Figure 1.1 The Transcription Process

servers. After recording, the audio file is then transferred to the medical transcriptionist's workstation. The MT plays back the dictation while keying the information into a word processor. The completed transcript is returned to the hospital or clinic to be "authenticated" (i.e., signed) by the dictator and filed in the patient's chart (either in electronic or in hard copy form). Copies of the report may also be forwarded to other healthcare providers as well as the billing and coding department. Because quality patient care depends on timely communication between the various members of the healthcare team, it is important that reports be dictated, transcribed, and returned for authentication as soon as possible—sometimes in as little as two hours. In addition, many insurance companies require transcribed reports to justify billing or for pre-approval of planned procedures. These requirements further emphasize the need to complete the dictation-transcription process promptly.

There is still a wide variety of methods for recording dictation and delivering the recorded sound file to the transcriptionist. The exact steps depend on the method used to record the dictation. Traditionally, physicians have used hand-held cassette recorders. Use of cassette tapes requires the dictator and the transcriptionist to be geographically close to one another in order to deliver the tapes directly to the MT. The transcriptionist who works from a home office picks up the tapes and returns printed documents transcribed from the previous day's set of tapes. Cassette tapes are played using a desktop transcriber and a foot pedal to stop and start the dictation.

Cassette recorders are gradually being replaced with digital hand-held recorders. Digital recorders create sound files that can be managed using personal computers. These electronic files can be transferred over networks (including the Internet), and therefore do not require the transcriptionist to pick up cassettes. Electronic (digital) files are played using computer software and a foot pedal attached to the computer. Since Internet technology has become more prevalent, many transcriptionists take advantage of electronic methods to receive dictation and return transcribed documents (referred to as digital transcription). The MT no longer needs to be located in close proximity to the dictator, making it possible for an MT in California to transcribe for a physician who practices medicine in New York City. The Internet has removed all geographical boundaries in transcription, creating a global transcription market.

While individual physicians may use hand-held recorders in their private practices, hospitals, on the other hand, often use large, computerized dictation equipment capable of recording hundreds of files at a time. Physicians use dictate stations that are "hard wired" to the dictation equipment or they may use telephone lines to connect to the dictation equipment. Transcriptionists access dictation files using equipment specifically designed to retrieve the sound files, such as transcribing stations connected directly to the dictation equipment, C-phones, which use telephone lines to connect to the dictation equipment, or computer interfaces. Often, hospitals use integrated systems that include file management and word processing software.

Speech Recognition

Speech recognition (SR) software analyzes speech and converts the spoken word into text. The technology has been developing over many years, and only recently has become sophisticated enough to produce medical documents with enough accuracy to make the technology cost-effective, as many transcriptionists can transcribe a report faster than extensively editing a highly inaccurate report created by speech recognition. Once perceived as a threat to an MT's job, speech recognition is now seen as a tool for enhancing productivity and relieving the transcriptionist of hours of continuous keyboarding. This technology changes the mechanics of an MT's job but does not change the primary role of assuring an accurately transcribed medical report. Speech recognition highlights the transcriptionist's medical knowledge and critical thinking skills.

When speech recognition technology is employed, the recorded sound file is routed to a speech recognition engine (software program) that converts digital sound patterns into text. The transcriptionist receives the sound file along with the text file to be edited. Once edited, the transcribed report is returned to the healthcare facility for signature and charting.

Changes in Medical Transcription

With the rapid growth in healthcare industries, employment in the medical transcription profession is expected to grow at a faster rate than the average for other industries. There has been a steady rise in the demand for medical transcription due to changes in documentation requirements. Whereas many healthcare professionals previously maintained hand-written records, third-party payers such as Medicare and private insurance companies now require legible, type-written documentation to support claims submitted for payment.

The increased demand for knowledgeable medical transcriptionists is also due to increased specialization in medical treatment and technological advances in the diagnosis and treatment of disease. Many specialty areas in health care are providing job opportunities for qualified individuals. The demand for medical transcriptionists is also expected to increase because of the increasing medical needs of the aging population. While the demand for transcriptionists will continue to rise, the methods of actually performing transcription may become more diverse. With the advancement of speech recognition technology as well as the emerging electronic health record, there will be a need for medical transcriptionists skilled in reviewing and editing electronically created records. With an educational foundation in the language of medicine, anatomy, pharmacology, and diseases, medical transcriptionists will be well positioned to work within the emerging electronic healthcare environment.

The globalization of the workforce and advances in technology are also impacting the field of medical transcription. The number of skilled medical transcriptionists has not kept pace with the rise in work volume, and the gap in the workforce has caused a significant amount of work to be transcribed offshore in countries such as India and the Philippines. There has also been a shift toward productivity-enhancing technologies such as speech recognition. Documents produced offshore and those created by speech recognition require proofing and editing to assure the high levels of accuracy needed in a medical report, so a growing number of transcriptionists work as editors, as opposed to transcribing in the traditional sense of listening and typing. It is anticipated that the depth of knowledge required to perform medical documentation tasks in the future will increase, while the need for fast typing skills may actually decrease.

The emerging electronic health record (EHR) is going to have profound effects on the entire medical community. Instead of physicians maintaining paper records within their individual offices, the goal of the EHR initiative is to create paperless records that are accessible to all healthcare providers through computerized networks. The EHR is creating new methods for documenting patient care, but the core knowledge you gain as a medical transcriptionist combined with your computer skills will enable you to evolve into new roles and remain a vital part of the medical community. Someday, you may refer to yourself as a medical record editor or even a medical documentation specialist.

Employment Opportunities

Medical transcription is a field with many possibilities and areas for advancement. As a professional, multi-skilled medical worker, the medical transcriptionist can choose from a variety of employment options. You can work in the transcription department or medical records section of a hospital or

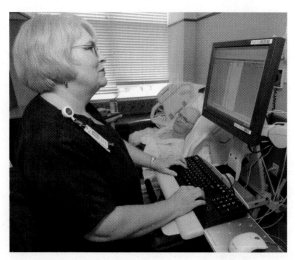

An electronic health record (EHR) allows healthcare providers to access a patient's record through a secure, computerized network.

clinic; or you can work in a radiology, pathology, or emergency department. You might also find employment in a physician's office, professional medical group practice, outpatient clinic, rehabilitation center, psychiatric hospital, insurance company, medical research center, or a medical school. Many transcriptionists choose to work for a medical transcription service and perform transcription from a home office. Medical transcriptionists can work within a specific medical specialty such as cardiology or neurology, or work in a hospital setting and learn many different areas of medicine.

More and more, transcriptionists are working from their homes, and often this is a motivating factor for pursuing a career in medical transcription. It is important to realize that this is a demanding field requiring concentration, attention to detail, and strict adherence to deadlines. All MTs, but especially those who work from their home offices, must be self-disciplined, organized, and have good time-management skills. Arrangements should be made for children in the home while working to eliminate constant distractions and interruptions that cause errors and delay the timely return of important patient care documentation. Consideration should also be given for appropriate work space that complies with security and privacy rules.

In addition to having a wide choice in work environments, medical transcriptionists have several career options. You may opt to become independent and work at home using your own equipment, including a computer, dictation system, and Internet communications. You may choose to become an instructor, proofreader, or editor. You can also continue your education to pursue a management or leadership role. You may even want to establish your own company and employ other medical transcriptionists. Whatever route you take, here is some important advice: *The more knowledge and skills you acquire relevant to the medical field, the greater your opportunities.* Medical transcription is more than listening to someone's voice and typing what you hear. You have to acquire a great deal of knowledge and experience to do the job well. Recognizing the important role medical transcriptionists play in patient care and understanding all of the duties that the job entails will help you get a good start in the field.

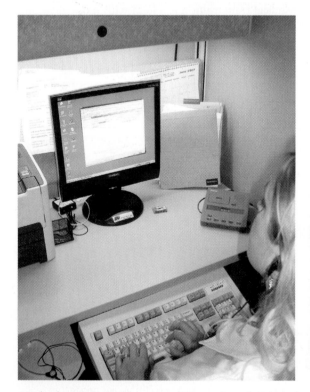 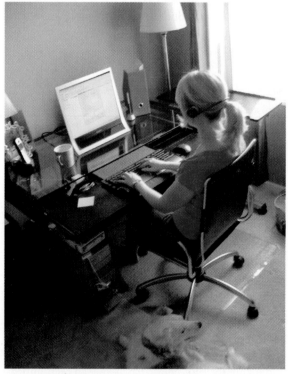

Medical transcriptionists can work in a variety of settings, from a hospital's transcription department to a home office.

Personal Attributes of the Medical Transcriptionist

Successful medical transcriptionists share certain traits that allow them to fulfill their duties. Attributes include accountability on the job, the ability to get along with diverse individuals, flexibility, and a willingness to assume responsibility when necessary. Table 1.1 lists the common traits of medical transcriptionists. Many of these attributes relate to skills that you can develop even if you do not have them now.

In addition to the attributes listed in Table 1.1, job advertisements for medical transcriptionists might request the following attributes for their applicants:

- Acute-care medical transcription experience
- Familiarity with a specific specialty such as radiology

Table 1.1

Traits of Medical Transcriptionists

A special interest in medical language and a fascination with the medical profession

Exceptional listening skills

Above-average keyboarding skills

Good memory retention

Accurate spelling skills

A thorough knowledge of English language and grammar rules

An investigative mind

A commitment to quality performance and accuracy in all tasks

Self-discipline and an independent nature

An attention for details

A dedication to professional development and an enthusiastic commitment to learning

An ability and willingness to ask questions when uncertain of the situation

A long attention span

- Excellent organizational skills
- "Can-do" attitude
- Self-starter
- Proficiency and ease with computers

Required Knowledge and Skills

Medical transcription requires practical, detailed knowledge of many aspects of health care and healthcare records as well as keyboarding and listening skills. The keyboarding skill required for many positions is at least 50 words per minute. Many jobs require 60 words per minute or more. Some experienced transcriptionists transcribe 78-90 words per minute. Familiarity with a variety of reports, including emergency room visits, chart summaries, surgical procedures, and diagnostic imaging studies, is necessary. To produce accurately transcribed documents, the transcriptionist must know the language of medicine, including terms related to anatomy and physiology, diagnostic procedures and treatment, medical jargon, and abbreviations.

Medical transcriptionists require skills shown in Table 1.2. While on the job, the transcriptionist continues to learn and improve skills, acquires new knowledge of ways of improving patient care, and takes pride in a job well done.

Table 1.2

Medical Transcriptionist Job Skills

Working knowledge of medical terminology

An understanding of anatomy, physiology, and disease processes

Familiarity with pharmacology and laboratory tests

Knowledge of medical transcription practices and guidelines

Proficiency in English grammar, usage, and punctuation

Proficiency in Microsoft Windows and Microsoft Word

Ability to use transcription equipment

Ability to use a wide range of references

An understanding of medical, legal, and ethical issues related to confidentiality

Professional Principles of Transcription

Throughout this text you will be learning and developing the skills involved in high-quality transcription. These skills include recognizing and understanding medical terminology, proofreading and editing for correct word usage and the mechanics of punctuation and capitalization, and keying medical reports in the correct format and style. As you develop your abilities, keep in mind the cardinal goals shared by the best professional medical transcriptionists: accuracy, speed, confidentiality, and ethical behavior.

Increase Speed While Striving for Accuracy

To be successful in transcription, you will need to have high-level keyboarding skills. During your course of study, try to steadily increase your speed. This depends on the integration of two separate skills: (a) keyboarding ability and (b) application of your growing knowledge base. A medical transcriptionist can only key as fast as the dictated word can be heard, researched, spelled correctly, and fit into context. Your instructor may establish speed criteria for you to meet as you complete this beginning course. Having realistic goals that approximate industry standards can help you focus, evaluate your progress, and improve.

Unless your document is accurate, a fast typing speed is useless. A medical transcriptionist should always strive for accuracy first and then work toward speed. Learn from your mistakes, ask for help, and apply your own creativity and curiosity as you research answers to questions. Remember that each dictated report becomes a legal document as well as a medical record on which the care and treatment of the patient is based. Because records play such an important role in patient care communication, it is important to correct any errors identified after the report has been transcribed. Each employer has specific procedures and guidelines to correct, change, or add information.

Certification

In the area of medical transcription, according to the *Occupational Outlook Handbook,* opportunities would be best for those who earn an associate degree or who achieve certification from the Association for Healthcare Documentation Integrity (AHDI). In the United States, professional associations fulfill an important role in setting standards of practice and administering certification programs. These programs are honored by most organizations because the standards are established by individuals who are experts in that particular field and have the highest level of practical knowledge. The main purpose of certification is to protect the health, safety, and welfare of the public. In addition, setting uniform standards helps educators prepare their students for entry-level work and enables employers to select qualified persons for the job. Being able to demonstrate that you meet or exceed certain standards increases your employment opportunities.

AHDI offers two levels of certification for medical transcriptionists that correspond to the AHDI's Professional Level 1 and Level 2 job descriptions for medical transcriptionists. (See the AHDI Web site at www.ahdiOnline.org for the complete Level 1, 2, and 3 job descriptions.) Recent graduates of a medical transcription program can take the Registered Medical Transcriptionist (RMT) examination. This exam, which does not require work experience, tests for fundamental knowledge in the areas of medical terminology, anatomy, physiology, disease processes, pharmacology, laboratory, diagnostic procedures, and medicolegal issues. Obtaining the RMT credential will be an important step in establishing your commitment to professionalism and continuing education as well as making it easier to land your first job. The Certified Medical Transcriptionist (CMT) examination requires a minimum of two years of multispecialty transcription experience. This second-level exam covers the same content areas as the RMT but tests for more in-depth knowledge and critical thinking skills. Obtaining this credential signifies your ongoing commitment to excellence, continuing education, and professional development.

Ethical Guidelines

When working in a medical environment, employees must maintain ethical standards in accordance with the law. Ethics relate to moral action and a personal code of conduct, and individuals are expected to conform to professional standards of personal integrity. Behaving ethically means conducting oneself in a manner that will bring dignity and honor to one's profession and person. It means that no matter what is happening in your personal life, you remain objective and expend your best effort with each report. It also means that you respect the dignity of patients and provide considerate care and communication through your work habits so as not to cause a patient harm.

AHDI has established a code of ethics for members of the association as well as those who hold the RMT or CMT credential. The code states:

Medical transcriptionists are vigilant advocates for quality patient documentation and adhere to the highest privacy and security provisions. We uphold moral and legal rights of patients, safeguard patient privacy, and collaborate with care providers to ensure patient safety, public health, and quality of care to the fullest extent possible, through the practice of medical transcription.

A complete copy of the AHDI's Code of Ethics is available on the AHDI Web site.

Professional Development

The medical profession is ever-changing. New terminology, treatments, procedures, equipment, and medications are implemented at an amazing pace. This dynamic environment requires all healthcare professionals to continue their education throughout their career. Professional development involves

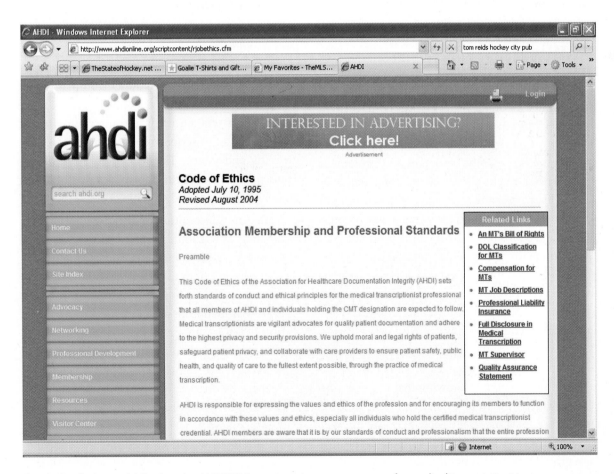

The Code of Ethics published on the AHDI Web site is an important resource for medical transcriptionists.

continuing education in the practical aspects of one's chosen field as well as cultivating leadership, management, interpersonal, and communication skills. One of the most important functions of a professional association is to provide opportunities for professional development and networking with colleagues and industry vendors (those companies that supply products and services that you use in your day-to-day work). Given the complexity and anticipated evolution of the electronic health record, MTs are well advised to join one or more of the professional associations involved in healthcare documentation and remain up-to-date with changes in medicine and technology. Classes in all subject areas are easily accessible online through private educational companies and community colleges. Continuing education articles are published monthly in trade magazines, and professional organizations offer seminars, symposia, conventions, journals, and various online formats for continued learning.

Basic Transcription Skills

If you are not familiar with the process of medical transcription, deciding where to begin can feel a bit overwhelming. As with learning any new skill, it is helpful to begin by familiarizing yourself with the steps in the process, the resources and equipment you will need, and how you will use those materials. As you learn, be patient and give yourself time to become comfortable with this unique way of interpreting and communicating medical information.

As you learn to transcribe medical documents, you will be integrating several skills: critical thinking, correct use of medical terminology, English grammar and punctuation, listening, and keyboarding. Initially, you may experience some frustration dealing with the challenges of this demanding area of study. But these challenges should be balanced with the satisfaction of knowing that you will one day play a critical role in an important area of health care. As a medical transcriptionist, you will provide essential services and support to healthcare providers who count on you to communicate medical information accurately and promptly. You become a partner in the vital area of documenting people's health care. For this reason, it is very important that you check your work with careful proofreading and editing.

Steps for transcribing medical documents are outlined in Table 1.3. As you review the steps, create a mental picture of each one to help you learn the entire sequence. Specific information on using transcription equipment will be provided in Chapter 2.

Understanding the basic process of transcribing is just the start of becoming an effective MT. True skills are developed and demonstrated in the editing and proofreading processes. Editing involves slight modifications to words, punctuation, or sentence structure in order to clarify the dictator's intended meaning. Proofreading, on the other hand, corrects keyboarding and transcription errors.

Editing for Clarity

When we speak, our tone, inflection, and pauses lend meaning to our words. Written communication lacks the auditory clues that make the meaning more clear, especially when sentences run together and phrases are misplaced. For this reason, there are instances when a medical transcriptionist will need to edit a transcribed report in order to clarify meaning and intent. *The Book of Style for Medical Transcription, Third Edition,* provides the following guidelines for editing dictated reports:

> Verbatim transcription of dictation is seldom possible. MTs should prepare reports that are as correct, clear, consistent, and complete as can be reasonably expected, without imposing their personal style on those reports. Editing is inappropriate in medical transcription when it alters information without the editor's being certain of the appropriateness or accuracy of the change, when it second-guesses the originator, when it deletes appropriate and/or essential information, and when it tampers with the originator's style. Edit grammar, punctuation, spelling, and similar dictation errors as necessary to achieve clear

Table 1.3

Steps to Follow When Transcribing a Report

1. Place all of the information and materials you will need at your workstation, including reference materials.

2. Plug the headset into the computer's headset port (often color-coded red and marked with a headset icon). Adjust the headset and earphones so that they rest comfortably over or in your ear (depending on headset style).

3. Position the foot control in the desired location and make sure it is connected to the appropriate port on your computer—usually the USB port.

4. Turn on your computer.

5. Open the transcription software that plays back the dictation and locate the appropriate dictation file.

6. Start your word processing program and open a new document or the appropriate report template that corresponds to the report being dictated.

7. Test the foot pedal and adjust the volume and speed controls as necessary.

8. Listen carefully for the report type to be dictated as well as the patient's name and the date.

9. Transcribe the dictation, using the process of "listen, stop, and key." Press the foot pedal and listen to a single sentence or phrase (whatever number of words you can mentally retain and repeat to yourself), lift your foot off the pedal to pause the playback, and then key the words. Use your reference materials to help you identify unfamiliar words. Leave blank spaces for words you cannot hear or do not understand.

10. Review the transcribed report again using critical thinking skills. Is each sentence constructed properly? Are there any discrepancies in right/left, he/she? Does the diagnosis fit with the findings? For example, does the x-ray report indicate a fracture, yet the diagnosis is "ankle sprain"? Are there any inconsistencies such as a prostatectomy performed on a female patient? Confirm that the dictation was heard correctly and mark any areas that need the dictator's attention.

11. Carefully proofread the document for keying errors, misspelled words, missing or misplaced punctuation, and incorrect format. Use the print preview feature of your word processor (if available) to view the document as it will print. Check the page margins, page breaks, and proper use of headers and footers.

communication. Likewise, edit slang words and phrases, incorrect terms, incomplete phrases, English or medical inconsistencies, and inaccurate phrasing of laboratory data.

Follow these simple rules for editing:

- Add punctuation if not dictated; and correct punctuation that is dictated incorrectly.
- Make a word singular or plural if it is dictated incorrectly.
- Correct subject-verb agreement if dictated incorrectly.
- Choose one tense when the dictator uses different tenses throughout the document unless the dictator is distinguishing between past and present events.
- Correct improper use of the articles *a* and *an* so that words beginning with a vowel or vowel sound are preceded with *an*.
- Correct misplaced prepositional phrases (e.g., "The patient's father died when he was two years old" would correct to "The father died when the patient was two years old").

Remember, the goal of the transcriptionist is to ensure that the final transcribed report accurately reflects the intentions of the dictator and that the meaning of the document is clear for the reader.

Proofreading for Accuracy

All transcriptionists develop successful methods to proofread their work. As you gain experience in the field, you will determine your own particular approach. You should always proofread as you key and then again after you have transcribed the document. Replay the audio while reading the keyed document on the screen, keeping in mind the following bulleted points:

- Evaluate punctuation. Are commas, semi-colons, and colons used correctly?
- Evaluate spelling. Check your document using the spell-check feature and review for sound-alike words such as their/there, here/hear, right/write, sight/site, effect/affect. Refer to an English or a medical dictionary to confirm the meaning of sound-alike words to be sure you have applied the correct spelling.
- Evaluate possible keying errors. Pay particular attention to numbers, checking for dropped numbers or misplaced decimals (e.g., 4-year-old instead of 44-year-old or 15g instead of 1.5g).
- Evaluate layout. Use the Print Layout View feature to display an entire page of your document. Is the format correct and consistent throughout? Are page breaks appropriate so that there are no widows or orphans or stranded signature lines? Have you filled in all blank spaces?

Dealing with Jargon and Clipped Sentences

Individual dictation styles vary from very formal to informal. Dictators use recurring phrases and terms that reflect their own speech patterns, culture, and geographic area. Many commonly used medical phrases are treated as if they are sentences. It is acceptable to use clipped sentences or fragments in portions of the medical report if they have been dictated that way. This typically applies to the Physical Examination, Review of Systems, and Laboratory Data sections. For example, the physical exam may include sentence fragments such as "No clubbing, cyanosis, or edema. Pulses 2+ and equal." Likewise, many dictators do not dictate the subject of a sentence when the subject is the patient. For example, instead of dictating, *"The patient complains of…"*, the dictator will drop the subject and state, *"Complains of…"* If you make a complete sentence from a fragment, be sure the sentence makes sense and that the original meaning or intent has not been changed. Be consistent with a particular style throughout the report. As you gain experience, you will become familiar with styles of dictation and medical jargon. It is important to adhere to departmental style guidelines as well as provider preference when determining acceptable sentence structure.

Transcribing Different Styles

There are many styles of medical writing. Many caregivers will use a formal style for correspondence and consultation notes, which are typically read by their colleagues, but then use an informal style with incomplete sentences and loosely followed formats for progress notes that are only seen by that physician and the physician's staff. Style guides define the appropriate use of numbers (Arabic, Roman, or spelled out), capitalization, sentence spacing, abbreviations and short forms, date formats, symbols, and other elements of written communication.

Professional journals establish style guides, or style sheets, that must be followed when submitting an article for publication. If you transcribe an article to be submitted to a professional journal, be sure to reference the appropriate style guide, which will be available on the publication's Web site. You may also find it helpful to borrow a copy of the journal from the dictator or from the library.

Hospitals and large medical centers typically have their own style guide, and providers in private practice may have individual preferences, so it is important that you follow the direction of the person for whom you work. If specific guidance is not given, use industry-standard style guides such as *The Book of Style for Medical Transcription* and the *American Medical Association Manual of Style*. You must be flexible, especially if you transcribe for several different dictators who have their own preferences. Most of all, be consistent within each document that you transcribe.

Understanding Dictator Accents

The percentage of medical providers who have been educated in other countries and who speak English as a second language (ESL) continues to rise. These providers, who may have accents or difficulty with English grammar, present unique challenges for the MT. It is important to understand differences in language and speech patterns in order to accurately transcribe reports and to be able to communicate with the dictator regarding unknown or confusing terminology.

Problems encountered with ESL dictators include substitution of sounds (e.g., the "t" sound replaced with a "d" sound), stress on the wrong syllable, incorrect sentence structure, and/or incorrect use of gender pronouns such as "he" and "she." Typically, these dictators will construct sentences in the same manner as their native language. English sentences generally begin with the subject whereas other languages place the subject at the end of the sentence. Spanish places the adjective after the noun, as opposed to English which places the adjective before the noun it describes.

As a general rule, do not second-guess the non-native English speaking dictator. Try to retain the basic style that is dictated, but edit for obvious errors as noted above. Here are some helpful suggestions:

- Request copies of previously transcribed reports and study them. Note phrases that are used often and look for patterns in sentence structure.
- Listen to the dictation once from beginning to end, transcribing all of the words you can without stopping or replaying the tape.
- Key a symbol, such as an asterisk or ampersand, for every word, phrase, or sentence that you cannot decipher.
- Go through the audio a second time using contextual clues to help fill in the blanks. Use words that you have already transcribed to note patterns of pronunciation, such as the letter *e* being pronounced as a long *a* or missing consonant sounds at the end of words.

Although some dictators are initially difficult to understand, once you decipher their particular speech anomalies, you will be able to transcribe them with surprising accuracy.

Reference Skills

Medical language is vast and ever-changing, and dictation often presents the transcriptionist with unfamiliar terminology. Fortunately, transcriptionists have many reference tools available for identifying and applying the correct terminology. Using references effectively is paramount to producing an accurate and complete document. There are several techniques to help you with unfamiliar words, improve accuracy, and reduce the number of blanks and questions in your transcribed reports. Selecting the appropriate reference and searching for terms, phrases, equipment, and medications are skills that improve with experience. The knowledge that you acquire through this text will lay the foundation for your research skills, and you will continue to hone those skills as you continue your career.

Searching for Terms

There are basically two types of word searches. The first is to locate the correct spelling or confirm the meaning of a word that you have heard clearly. The second type of search is to decipher a word or phrase that is unfamiliar or difficult to understand. Use the reference materials described on the following pages along with the tips described below to help you produce complete and accurate reports:

- It is easy to misinterpret a sound because many letters sound the same. Table 1.4 provides tips for discerning similar sounds. For example, the letter pairs *a* and *h*; *m* and *n*; *b* and *v*; *b* and *d*; and *f* and *s* cannot be distinguished, especially when the word or abbreviation is unfamiliar in the first place. Refer to Table 1.5 for other sounds that sound the same.
- Whole syllables, not just single letters, are sometimes confused. Table 1.5 provides some alternative spellings for some hard-to-discern word beginnings and endings. Syllables that begin a word are shown with a hyphen at the end. Syllables that end a word are shown with a hyphen before them.
- Anatomy illustrations can be useful for locating terms that have been mumbled or partially obscured by background noise. For example, if you know that the dictator is talking about a muscle in the face but you cannot hear the first sound in the word, looking at the figure reference may help you identify the name of the muscle dictated.
- If unable to decipher the word or phrase after two or three attempts, leave a blank (five underscore characters) in place of the missing word or phrase and continue to transcribe the

remainder of the report. It is possible the word or phrase may be repeated more clearly later in the dictation.

- For the most difficult words or phrases, read the entire report and then use the surrounding context to consider what might reasonably fit into the sentence at that point—a noun, a verb, an instrument, a medication, or possibly an abbreviation, or a number? Use your knowledge of combining forms and root words to begin your search based on the context. For example, if the context is a muscle, begin your search with "myo" as opposed to "mio."

Table 1.4

Tips for Discerning Similar Sounds in Dictation

If you hear ...	Consider ...	Examples
c	k and g	Kufs disease, guanine
f	ph	phacocyst, farnesol
i (short *i* as the first or second sound)	e, a, and y	enalapril, yttrium, Restoril
y	j	Jungian analysis
k	c, ch	kaliuresis, chiasm
m	n	nodal, naproxen
n	m, pn, gn, mn, kn, cn	nacreous, macrocyte, pneumonia, gnathic, mnemic, knismogenic, cnemis
s	z, c, ps	zymoscope, ciliary, pseudopsia
t	b, p, pt, ct, v	popliteal, ptosis, vinculum
z	x	Xylocaine, Xanax, xanthiuria, Zaglas ligament

Table 1.5

Tips for Discerning Word Parts in Dictation

If you hear ...	Consider ...
-able	-ible
-air	-are, -aer
-ance	-ence
-ant	-ent
ante-	anti-
-cer	-cre
-cks, -gz	-x
dis-	dys-
-ei	-ie
-ere	-ear, -eir, -ier
fizz-	phys-
hyper-	hypo-
inter-	intra-
-is	-us, -ace, -ice
-le	-tle, -el, -al
ny-	gn-, n-
para-	peri-, pero-
per-	par-, pir-, por-, pur-, pre-, pro-, pru-, pyr-
peri-	para-, pero-
pre-	per-, pra-, pri-, pro-, pru-
si-	psi-, ci-
super-	supra-
-tion	-sion, -cion, -cean, -cian
-tious	-seous, -scious
-ture	-teur
we-	whe-
wi-	whi-
zi-	xy-

- Listen again to the sounds on either side of the blank and change the way you are dividing the syllables into words. For example, what sounds like "history oseal" might be "hysterocele."
- Consider that the word is actually an instruction from the dictator to the transcriptionist and not a medical term. Examples such as "go back to HPI" or "disregard that" can be confusing. Dictated punctuation often trips up the MT, especially the common phrase "period paragraph," signifying the end of the paragraph, or the phrase "full stop," indicating the end of a sentence.
- Searching for drug names can be aided by using contextual clues. Review the list of diagnoses or reported medical problems and consider medications that are used to treat those problems. Drug references typically list medications by indication, providing a "reverse lookup" method. Another helpful tool is a list of sound-alike drug names sometimes included in an appendix. Also, use the drug's indication as a clue to possible spelling patterns, as in the cholesterol-lowering medication WelChol. As always, make sure the drug indication fits the context. No matter how well it matches what you hear, it is not reasonable to type a drug used for prostatic hypertrophy in a report of a 5-year-old.
- Many medical terms sound alike (e.g., arthrectomy and atherectomy; dysphagia and dysphasia). Use a medical dictionary to make sure the term you transcribe fits the context.

Using Transcription References

As a medical transcriptionist, it is important that you maintain an up-to-date reference library. Medical language is constantly changing and new terms, procedures, medications, and names of equipment are added to the medical lexicon daily. You will want to keep up with current editions, as later editions of resource books may have a significant number of new entries.

Although the list of available books is enormous, experienced MTs generally agree that only a few are essential for the beginning transcriptionist. The following references are must-have books that provide general information on medical terminology, language, style, drug names, and technical terms. As you encounter new specialties in your work, you will want to add specialty-specific books to your collection—for example, OB/GYN (obstetrics/gynecology), neurology, radiology, and oncology.

Medical Dictionary   A medical dictionary is the medical transcriptionist's primary reference, providing an alphabetical listing of terms and their definitions, pronunciation keys, and word origin information. Take time to explore your dictionary, especially the appendices in the back and user's guide in the front. Medical dictionaries are also available in electronic form, which allow you to search for terms in many ways that are not possible with printed references. Techniques for searching electronic references will be described later in this chapter.

Medical Glossary   A medical glossary is similar to a dictionary, but may also include an explanation of current use or examples of usage. Glossaries are updated more often than dictionaries and thus contain newer or trendier terms. Criteria for new glossary entries are not as strict as new entries to a dictionary, so emerging terms may be included and less common words removed. An exceptionally useful glossary for medical transcription is *Vera Pyle's Current Medical Terminology*. This reference also contains entries according to phonetic spelling for terms that might not be found otherwise—such as *cabbage*, which is actually written CABG (coronary artery bypass graft).

Drug Book   Medication names can be among the most challenging terms to research, so an up-to-date, high-quality pharmaceutical reference is a must-have resource for all medical transcriptionists. Drug references list drug names with their proper capitalization, indications, use, usual dosage and dosage forms, as well as cross-references by class and indication. Your drug book will get the most wear and tear. As an added feature, drug references often contain a list of laboratory values (reference ranges), abbreviations commonly used in medication orders, chemotherapy regimens, and a list of sound-alike drug names.

Medical Style Guide   A medical style guide provides information on report formats and the use of abbreviations, numbers, capitalization, and punctuation. The standard guide is *The Book of Style for Medical Transcription, Third Edition,* published by the Association for Healthcare Documentation Integrity; however, there are several other style books available. On the job, check with your employer and/or dictator for a specific reference. Transcription work in this text will closely follow *The Book of Style for Medical Transcription, Third Edition.*

Medical Word Book and Medical Phrase Index   Word and phrase books are very popular with medical transcriptionists. These books are published by specialty (e.g., cardiology, neurology, and orthopedics) and list specific words and phrases that are used in the given area of practice. These books are also referred to as medical spellers. They differ from dictionaries in that word books do not contain definitions or pronunciations. Words are listed alphabetically as well as by categories and phrases, which can be extremely useful for locating a particular disease or joint, for example, or when you hear only one or two words of a phrase. If you do not find the word or phrase in one medical speller, try another. Reference books for medical equipment words and books of medical phrases have many of the same categories, but a specific suture, for example, may only be listed in one of them. Since spellers do not contain definitions, you must always verify the meaning of the word in a medical dictionary to make sure the word fits within the context of your report.

Medical Equipment and Surgical Word Books   Medical equipment and surgical word books are like medical spellers. They list specific equipment names—especially trade names (e.g., McLean clamp)—and surgical terminology that you will not likely find elsewhere (e.g., Lempert incision).

Abbreviations and Acronyms Reference   This type of reference indexes abbreviations and acronyms with their fully expanded meaning, although it will typically not contain definitions of the words represented by the abbreviation. Dictators use many abbreviations, so it is important that you have a good resource for verification. Never assume that you have heard an abbreviation correctly. Always look up the abbreviation to make sure it is correct and that it fits into the context of what you are transcribing. Spoken letters are extremely difficult, if not impossible, to discriminate, which is why the police and military use a phonetic alphabet (alpha, bravo, Charlie). If you cannot decipher a word or phrase but can understand some of the syllables, check to see if it is an acronym or abbreviation. For example, the abbreviation GERD (gastroesophageal reflux disease) is often dictated as the word "gurd."

Laboratory Word Book   Laboratory references are useful for researching diagnostic test names, indications, specimen type (blood, urine, stool), and reference ranges (normal values). This type of reference may also contain a list of eponymic diseases and syndromes, scientific notations, symbols, a periodic table of elements, weights and measures, and conversion charts.

Eponym Book   Eponyms are names of diseases, procedures, tests, or pieces of equipment derived from an individual's name, such as Homans sign and Parkinson disease. Many eponyms are included in medical dictionaries and spellers, but you may also find it useful to have these terms in a separate reference. Although most providers still dictate eponyms in the possessive form, style guides, including the *AMA Manual of Style* and *The Book of Style for Medical Transcription* recommend dropping the *'s* (e.g., Tinel sign *not* Tinel's sign).

English Dictionary and Other Nonmedical References   The importance of having and using an unabridged English dictionary cannot be emphasized enough. It is just as important to use the correct English word as it is to apply the correct medical terminology. Homonyms are especially problematic and care should be taken to apply the correct spelling for the given context. A quick search of the Internet for "commonly confused words" is a worthwhile exercise (and may reveal quite a few surprises). Also consider that medical providers, being highly educated, have extensive vocabularies and often dictate uncommon English words or expressions borrowed from other languages. When researching a new or difficult term, do not assume it is medical, as you may very well find the word in *Merriam-Webster's*.

Additional nonmedical resources that provide essential information include:

- *The Gregg Reference Manual, 10th Edition*, a manual of style, grammar, usage and format for business and publications
- Position papers published by the Association for Healthcare Documentation Integrity (www.ahdiOnline.org)

Using Electronic References

Electronic references are dictionaries, medical spellers, and drug references stored in a digital format that install onto your hard drive. The Internet is also an electronic reference. References stored in electronic form can be searched in ways not offered by traditionally bound materials, making it much easier to find unfamiliar words. Electronic references can be searched using a few letters within the word, at the end of the word, or within the definition. Dictionaries often include pronunciation files so you can hear the word pronounced correctly. Cross-references are linked so you can move to a related entry with a single mouse click. Using electronic references can actually increase your efficiency and accuracy by greatly reducing the time you spend searching for terms and definitions. Electronic references are sold on CDs, and therefore require very little shelf space, which makes them perfect for small office spaces. Not all transcription references can be purchased electronically, but the selection is increasing steadily.

The key to using electronic references is to make them easily accessible while you are transcribing. Create shortcuts on the desktop, the QuickLaunch bar, or on the Start menu for accessing your references so that you can open them with minimal keystrokes. Learn the shortcut keys used within each program so that you can open the reference, locate needed information, and return to your working document without taking your hands off the keyboard. You will find that with practice you can easily look up a definition and return to your document in less than 30 seconds. Knowing that you can verify information quickly and easily will prevent you from "guessing" or putting off that critical confirmation step that assures an accurate report.

An electronic reference includes an index, which is the list of entries presented alphabetically, as you would expect to see them listed in a book. Scroll up and down through the index in the same way you would glance through entries in your dictionary or medical speller. Select the entry to display the definition or other information associated with the entry. You can also type the first few letters of the word into the text box to move directly to that entry. To search with partial information, select the Search tab (search mode). Use the following universal search characters and methods to locate information:

- Use an asterisk (*) to represent characters or numbers that are unknown (none, one, or unlimited characters). For example, you hear a beginning *m* sound, a *g* in the middle and *n* at the end. Type the following into the search box: *m*g*n*. Sample results for this search would include malpighian, megacolon, and methyl green. To search using the end of the word, type an asterisk plus the ending sound. For example, type **pian* to find words such as pian, fallopian, and cyclopian. Select words from the list of results to view the definition or other information contained within that entry.
- Use a question mark (?) to represent a single unknown character or number. Results for a search using *h?t* would include hat, hit, hot, hut, and HST.
- To search for words related to a concept, search the reference by definition or subentry. For example, for words related to the concept of pain, change the search mode to search within the definition. Type *pain* in the search box. Sample search results would include anesthetic, angina, and causalgia.

Online Resources

The Internet is a significant source of information, but one must evaluate the information very carefully and then confirm the information with a trusted source before incorporating it into a document. To search for information on the Internet, use a search engine such as Google, Yahoo!, or MSN Search. These engines constantly scan the World Wide Web and index every page that has been posted on the Web. When you search for a word or phrase, the engine will present a list of Web pages contained in the engine's index that contain the word(s) in your search.

The search engine Google (www.google.com) is one of the most popular search engines. Read more about how to utilize the many features available on Google by clicking Help at the bottom of the Google home page. Google image searches can be especially useful, too.

To perform an Internet search, open the search engine's home page, and then type one or several keywords into the search box. Adding several words to your search may make the search results more meaningful. For example, searching for *brace* would return millions of search results. Add words from the context of the report to narrow the results, such as *brace leg fracture*. Place quotation marks around phrases such as *"left ventricular hypertrophy."* You can also combine search techniques (quotation marks and search characters) like this: *"* splint" greenstick fracture.*

The search engine does not discriminate or evaluate the information for accuracy or spelling; the user must do that. Never extract information from a public discussion forum, a doctor's personal Web site, or patient support organizations. These sites are notorious for typos and misinformation. A popular site among transcriptionists is MedlinePlus

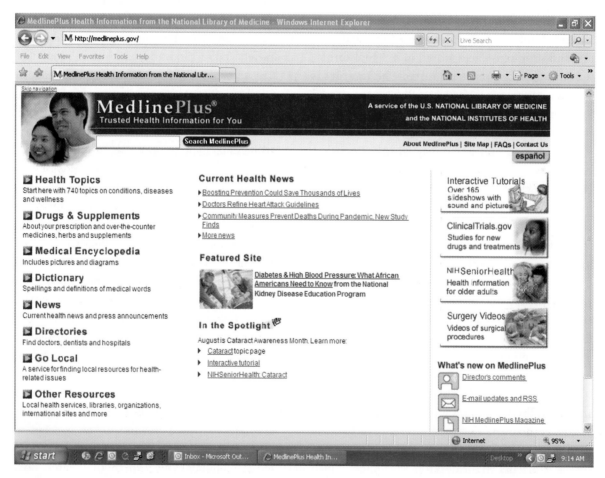

MedlinePlus at medlineplus.gov is an excellent Web site published by the National Institutes of Health. It provides access to a medical encyclopedia, dictionary, and other information valuable to the medical transcriptionist.

(www.medlineplus.gov). Other trustworthy sources of information on the Internet (for medical purposes) include sites managed by research hospitals or university hospitals. For products, equipment, and drug names, use the manufacturer's Web site.

The following Web sites may be especially useful:

- Association for Healthcare Documentation Integrity (AHDI): www.ahdionline.org
- American Health Information Management Association (AHIMA): www.ahima.org
- Medical Transcription Industry Association (MTIA): www.mtia.com
- American Cancer Society (ACS): www.cancer.org
- American Medical Association (AMA): www.ama-assn.org
- OneLook online dictionary collection: www.onelook.com
- MedlinePlus, a service of the national Library of Medicine: www.medlineplus.gov
- Rx List, a searchable pharmaceutical database: www.rxlist.com
- FDA database for newly approved drugs and devices: www.fda.gov/search/databases.html
- *Advance for Healthcare Professionals*, a trade magazine and Web site: www.advanceforhim.com
- *For The Record*, a trade magazine and Web site: www.fortherecordmag.com

Medical transcriptionists have created a lively and mutually supportive online community where you can find others who have similar interests and questions. For example, within a chat forum, a medical transcriptionist may pose a question about the use of hyphens. Or, someone else might ask for help finding the spelling of certain terms or physicians' names. Over the Internet, you can get advice and information from hundreds of working medical transcriptionists quickly and easily. Be careful, however, not to assume the information is correct. Information shared with you over the Internet or gleaned from a Web site should always be confirmed with a reputable source. The following are online forums where MTs gather:

- Professional Practices Network (AHDI): www.ahdiOnline.org/forum
- Medical Transcription Daily: www.mtdaily.com
- MTChat: www.mtchat.com

Medical Records

A medical record is a permanent compilation of written documents that provide information and insight into a patient's life and health history. Many healthcare professionals contribute reports and information to this record. Since patient care is multidisciplinary, and order and organization are important in communication, the healthcare industry has developed specific policies, procedures, and guidelines that determine how medical records are organized.

Standard-Setting Organizations

Four major medical organizations have developed standards for preparing and managing medical records.

- The Association for Healthcare Documentation Integrity (AHDI) is a nonprofit professional association for medical transcriptionists, MT students, and others who have an interest in healthcare documentation. AHDI administers a certification exam and publishes a medical report style guide as well as a journal for members.
- The Joint Commission (formerly Joint Commission on Accreditation of Healthcare Organizations) is a nongovernmental agency that offers a voluntary healthcare accreditation process for hospitals. Part of the accreditation process requires compliance with The Joint Commission's standards for the kinds of information entered into the medical record, the completeness of medical reports, abbreviation systems, and turnaround times for report dictation and transcription.
- The American Medical Association (AMA) is the professional organization for physicians that has developed several medicolegal forms, which hospitals use regularly, including a variety of patient consent forms.

- The American Health Information Management Association (AHIMA) is an association for coders and health information managers and administrators. AHIMA makes broad guidelines for the development and distribution of patients' medical record information, including positions on the patient's right of access.

Other organizations involved in standard setting for healthcare documentation include the following:

- The National Committee for Quality Assurance (NCQA) is a nonprofit association that makes recommendations for improving healthcare.
- Health Level Seven (HL7) is the organization that sets standards for interoperability of electronic health data. The importance of this organization's work is increasing as the United States (and many other countries around the world) moves toward an electronic health record, which will allow health data to be exchanged between medical providers and hospital systems nationwide.
- ASTM International is the organization that sets standards for materials and processes. ASTM includes committees that focus on medical processes and materials, including dictation and transcription of medical records.
- The Centers for Medicaid & Medicare Services (CMS) is the administrator of the medical entitlement programs for the elderly, disabled, and children. The CMS establishes requirements for proper reimbursement, including information that must be contained in the medical record.

Problem-Oriented Medical Record

In the 1960s, the healthcare industry developed a record-keeping method to standardize information and make it quickly accessible to all practitioners. The problem-oriented medical record (POMR) is a method of record-keeping centered on the patient's specific health problems. This system provides a logical, systematic analysis of the relevant data. For team members, it allows effective communication that focuses on a problem list, or statements of the patient's health-related problems, as addressed by various healthcare disciplines. Additions to the list may be made by any healthcare professional.

The POMR system divides the medical record into four main sections: the database, the problem list, the plan, and the progress notes.

The database is the section of the chart where all information about the patient's history and current health status is recorded and continuously updated. The database contains input from many sources and includes past and current physical examination results, x-ray and test data, social and occupational histories, and any other information about the patient.

The database contains the history and physical (H&P), a two-part report documenting the patient's medical history and the findings of a complete physical examination. Hospitals require an H&P to be performed for each patient within a few hours of admission, and physicians may not be allowed to perform surgical or diagnostic procedures unless a record of the current H&P is included in the patient's chart.

The problem list is a numbered list of the patient's problems, which may include a specific diagnosis, a symptom, an abnormal test result, or other health problem. The problem list serves as a basis for the plan of care and includes areas for observation, diagnosis, treatment and/or management, and patient and family education. All problems are identified from physiologic, psychosocial, economic, occupational, and other standpoints. Usually each problem is assigned a number to simplify charting.

The plan is a description of actions to be taken to address the various active items on the problem list. A separate plan is noted for each identified problem. Plans include a notation of who might carry out each plan and traditionally includes the areas of diagnosis, treatment, and patient education.

The progress notes section contains documentation of observations, assessments, care plans, orders, and other relevant information for all members of the healthcare team. Placing all progress notes in one section of the chart provides easy access for anyone providing care to the patient and encourages coordination of care through effective communication.

SOAP Note Format A key component of the POMR is the SOAP note. The SOAP note format is a standard format for arranging information in a medical report and is commonly applied to chart notes and progress notes, both part of the POMR system. Caregivers use the letters S, O, A, and P to identify the following parts of the document:

- **S**ubjective—the patient's description of the problem
- **O**bjective—information observed during the physical exam as well as laboratory or x-ray data
- **A**ssessment—an evaluation of the information gathered to produce a diagnosis
- **P**lan—the details of what will be done to address the diagnosis and related problems

Narrative-Style Charting An alternative to the POMR is the traditional narrative-style chart. In this method, information is organized according to its source (e.g., physicians, nurses, and therapists). Because data are not grouped by type-specific information in these charts, quick retrieval of information may be difficult and documents may contain repetition.

Medical Report Formats

Individual medical reports appear in standard formats to help medical professionals organize and access information about a patient. These standard formats give the medical transcriptionist a tool for easy keying of a concise record that allows rapid scanning and quick retrieval of information by any member of the healthcare team.

Each chapter of this text features one of the medical document types described and presents models based on AHDI's, ASTM's, and The Joint Commission's style, format, and content guidelines for transcribing that document as well as expected turn-around-times (time allowed to complete the transcription). Follow these guidelines to learn the generally accepted report formats. When you are on the job, however, consider the guidelines a starting point. In all cases, it is the dictator of the report who has the final word on style. Medical transcriptionists must follow their employers' specific style preferences. Appendix A provides a list of headings found in each report type transcribed for this text and describes the type of information found under each heading.

Chart Note Chart notes, also called progress notes or office notes, are brief reports that document the findings from each examination of the patient. The chart note is featured in Chapter 5 in the SOAP note format.

Consultation Request, Report, or Letter The consultation request, report, or letter documents the findings of a specialist who is asked to see the patient of an attending physician to offer a second (or expert) opinion. See Chapter 6 for an illustration and explanation of the consultation letter.

Operative Report The operative report describes a surgical or other invasive procedure. Whenever a surgical procedure is done in a hospital, outpatient center, or clinic, an operative report should be recorded in the medical record. The operative report is illustrated and discussed in Chapter 7.

Discharge Summary The discharge summary describes the reason a patient was admitted to the hospital, a short history, and a sequential listing of events and treatment that occurred during the patient's hospitalization, and a final diagnosis(es) upon release from the hospital. See Chapter 8 for an illustration and discussion of the discharge summary.

Radiology Report Radiology reports describe findings and interpretations from x-rays or special diagnostic studies performed in a radiology department. They list a radiologic diagnosis by the radiologist who reviews the films or test results. The radiology report is featured in Chapter 9.

Pathology Report The pathology report describes disease-related findings from a sample of tissue that has been examined by a pathologist, a specialist in laboratory medicine. This report is illustrated and explained in Chapter 10.

History and Physical   When a patient enters a healthcare system, the healthcare provider generates a comprehensive document called a history and physical (H&P), which becomes the foundation for the medical record. This two-part report documents the patient's medical history, the immediate problem that prompted the patient to seek help, a social and family history, and the findings of a complete physical exam. The primary purpose of the history and physical is to help the provider determine the diagnosis(es)—the basis for the patient's care and their treatment.

For the history portion (called *subjective* information since it is supplied by the patient), the examiner interviews the patient, asking first for the reason that prompted the visit (also called the *chief complaint*). This is followed by questions about childhood illnesses and all previous diseases, surgical procedures, allergies, and current medications and immunizations. Also included are questions about parents' and siblings' state of health. Finally, the physician asks the patient questions about all the body systems in a cephalocaudal (head-to-tail) order.

The second part of the report is the complete physical examination (called *objective* information because the physician observes it), which also is conducted in cephalocaudal order. Other objective information includes vital statistics and general appearance.

Finally, at the end of the report is the physician's impression or diagnosis and a plan of care. Figure 1.2 displays a sample history and physical report. This report will be studied in greater detail in Chapter 12.

Autopsy Report   The autopsy report is also a pathology report that is requested by the attending physician or a coroner to determine a patient's cause of death. Also called a postmortem, this report is featured in Chapter 16.

Components of Hospital Charts

The hospital chart is composed of several types of reports, notes, and documents. Each hospital medical chart provides information for one admission for one individual patient. Table 1.6 provides a list of the basic components that may be contained in the chart of an inpatient. The discussion that follows further details information about the contents of these individual reports.

Medicolegal Issues

As a member of the health information management team, you should be aware of how medical records are used and the laws and guidelines which govern them.

Medical records are used to provide:
- A means of communication for patient treatment and care
- Justification for insurance and compensation purposes
- A means to support research and education, monitoring medical treatments that are successful and those that need improvement
- Statistics for planning how to best use future resources
- Objective documentation of care or evidence to protect the legal interests of the hospital, physician, and the patient in a court of law

Although each hospital or physician establishes specific rules and procedures regarding medical records, there are general guidelines for handling patient information. These rules have been developed in the courts through years of litigation.

Confidentiality   Maintaining confidentiality is a legal requirement when working in the healthcare profession. MTs have a moral responsibility to keep all patient information confidential. MTs must protect the privacy of patients by not discussing patient information with anyone and by making sure that only those people authorized to see a patient's record have access to it. Although medical transcriptionists have always been cognizant of patient privacy, in recent years the federal government has enacted laws and guidelines that govern the way medical information is used, stored, and discarded. These rules are established by the Health Insurance Portability and Accountability Act (HIPAA). The complete HIPAA document is very extensive, covering all aspects of the patient's information; only parts of the enactment

PATIENT NAME: Raymond Cheever
MR #:   93-22-17
PHYSICIAN: Harry Washington, MD
DATE: 07/10/20XX

CHIEF COMPLAINT
Severe pain in the left hip.

HISTORY OF PRESENT ILLNESS
The patient is a 57-year-old white male who is admitted from the emergency department with
hypertension, hyperglycemia, and greater trochanteric bursitis. The patient has been under treatment
for greater trochanteric bursitis with Lortab and Naprosyn. He returns today because of increasing left
hip pain. In the emergency room, he was noted to be significantly hypertensive and hyperglycemic. He is
unaware of having a history of either.

PAST MEDICAL HISTORY
Negative.

SURGICAL HISTORY
Tonsils and adenoids removed in early childhood.

SOCIAL HISTORY
The patient does not smoke at present. He stopped smoking 6-7 years ago; he smoked an average of a
pack per day for many years. He denies ethanol use. He is married. He has 2 children who are alive and
in good health. He works as a plant manager for a chemical company.

FAMILY HISTORY
His mother is alive and in good health. His father is deceased secondary to complications of black lung
and asthma. He has 2 brothers and 1 sister. He thinks his sister has a history of hypertension.

ALLERGIES
No known allergies.

CURRENT MEDICATIONS
1. Lortab 7.5 mg daily.
2. Naprosyn 375 mg daily.

REVIEW OF SYSTEMS
A full review of systems was negative. He states that his weight has been stable in the past year. He
denies polyuria, polydipsia, or polyphagia.

PHYSICAL EXAMINATION
GENERAL: Well-developed, well-nourished male in no acute distress.
VITAL SIGNS: Blood pressure 200/104. Repeat, after rest and pain medication, was 170/96. The pulse
was 72. Respiratory rate was 18 and labored. Patient refused to be weighed at this time because of pain.

(continued)

Figure 1.2   Example of a History and Physical Report

HISTORY AND PHYSICAL
PATIENT NAME: Raymond Cheever
MR #: 93-22-17
DATE: 07/10/20XX
Page 2

HEENT: Pupils were somewhat constricted, but fundi were visualized minimally. No hypertensive retinopathy, exudates, hemorrhages, or papilledema was noted. Oral examination revealed no ulcerations, erosions, or masses.
NECK: Supple, without lymphadenopathy. The carotid upstrokes were brisk and equal bilaterally, without bruits. Thyroid nonpalpable.
THORAX AND LUNGS: Chest was clear to auscultation in all fields.
CARDIOVASCULAR: Regular rate and rhythm, without murmurs, thrill, gallop, or click.
ABDOMEN: Nontender, nondistended, without masses, organomegaly, guarding, tenderness, or rebound.
EXTREMITIES: No clubbing, cyanosis, or edema. Peripheral pulses were intact, with good upstrokes. Palpation of the left hip did reveal tenderness, although the patient did report it was much improved after analgesia.

LABORATORY DATA
Review of the Chem-7 revealed a blood sugar of 201. His urinalysis revealed greater than 1000 glucose. CBC revealed a hemoglobin of 16.3 and a hematocrit of 50, white count was 14.7, platelets were 291,000; differential was essentially within normal limits.

IMPRESSION
1. Marked hypertension.
2. Asymptomatic hyperglycemia with glycosuria.
3. Left greater trochanteric bursitis.

PLAN
1. Admit.
2. Orthopedic consultation.
3. Endocrinology consultation.
4. Cardiology consultation.

_____

Harry Washington, MD

HW/XX
D: 07/10/20XX
T: 07/11/20XX

Figure 1.2   Example of a History and Physical Report (Continued)

Table 1.6

Components of an Inpatient Chart

Component	Contents
Summary sheet (face sheet)	Contains patient demographics and authorization for treatment. If the patient was admitted from the emergency department (ED), the emergency department report may be found here or within the History and Physical section.
History and physical	May include the emergency department report. Includes admission intake information.
Physician orders	Includes instructions to the healthcare team for the patient's treatment and care.
Diagnostic report	May include the following, or they may be listed separately. • Laboratory and delivery report • Radiology report • Electrocardiogram/ echocardiogram • Pathology report
Operative report	Includes a separate report for the recovery room record.
Progress notes (chart notes, office notes)	May include the following, or they may be listed separately. • Nurse notes • Social service notes
Consultation request or letter	No additional contents unless a consultation was needed.
Discharge summary	No additional contents until discharge.
Autopsy report	May include lab reports.

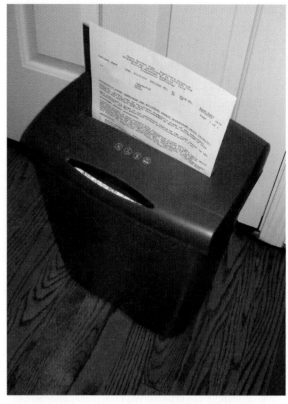

Medical transcriptionists should shred documents that contain private patient information before discarding.

are relevant to transcription. Specific guidelines that apply to MTs and medical transcription service owners are available to members of AHDI. Another useful reference for medical transcriptionists is *Stedman's Guide to the HIPAA Privacy Rule* by Kathy Rockel, CMT, FAAMT. Failure to comply with HIPAA guidelines can result in considerable fines. The following list outlines very basic guidelines for assuring the privacy and confidentiality of patient reports:

- Be careful when faxing or delivering reports so that they are not routed to the wrong fax number or the wrong medical office. Use cover sheets with all fax transmissions.
- Make sure that your computer screen cannot be viewed by others around you. Maintain passwords on your computer to prevent others from accessing your transcription files. Other security issues related to your computer will be discussed in Chapter 2.
- No identifying information on a patient should leave a medical transcriptionist's place of employment. The patient's authorization must be received for disclosure of any information to a third party, including the patient's insurance company. A release form must specify the information to be released, to whom, and the purpose.
- Do not store patient records in your home or office. An MT is not responsible for archiving

patient records, so transcribed reports should be destroyed after billing and business processes have been completed. Any printed documents containing patient information should be shredded thoroughly before discarding.

- Maintaining patient privacy also means that the medical transcriptionists should access chart information only as necessary to provide for the accuracy of the document being transcribed.
- Never discuss a patient's record with friends or family, and do not discuss patient information with the patient's family.

As an added measure to protect patient privacy, many healthcare facilities avoid using the patient's name within the body of the report. This is especially important if the facility aggregates information from transcribed reports for research and/or statistical purposes. When the patient's name is dictated within the body of the report, the name is replaced with "patient" or "the patient." This guideline has been followed in the transcription exercises included with each specialty chapter in this book. When transcribing the reports for the patient studies, type the patient's name on the designated line at the top of each page, but within the body of the report, replace the patient's actual name with "patient" or "the patient" as appropriate.

Check your hospital or workplace policy for complete confidentiality guidelines. Your employer may require you to sign a confidentiality agreement. Violation may result in termination or prosecution. Even if you work from home, you are bound by the principles of confidentiality.

Retention   The period of retention of medical records is governed by state and local laws. It is typically seven to ten years for original records. Some institutions keep their records indefinitely.

Ownership of Document and Content   Medical records that are created in a healthcare facility are considered to belong to that particular facility, as the facility owns the paper on which the record is written. However, the patient owns the information contained in the record. Access to the record is regulated by federal and individual state laws.

Release of Information   Medical transcriptionists should not release information related to patient care; however, there are some instances where release of information can be accomplished legally. All requests should be processed according to the institution's release-of-information guidelines, with the emphasis on confidentiality. There can be no disclosure to any unauthorized person. If there is any doubt whatsoever about releasing information, the medical transcriptionist should not release the information but rather should refer the request to the proper authority. Security of patient records, both computer records and paper records, is very important.

Medicolegal issues that relate to medical records vary from state to state. On the job, you will need to familiarize yourself with the policy manual or office procedure manual detailing your employer's rules for the release of information. If you have questions, consult your supervisor, your employer, or your employer's legal consultant.

Medicolegal Terms   Table 1.7 lists some important legal terms with which a medical transcriptionist should become familiar.

Try Transcription

This chapter, and each chapter in Part 2 of this text starting with Chapter 5, contains a series of dictated reports to be transcribed. These transcription exercises come from actual patient documents, and the recordings are designed to simulate authentic dictation. By transcribing these reports following the steps outlined in Table 1.3, you will develop your transcribing, editing, and language skills. Begin your career as a medical transcriptionist by transcribing the following reports. The dictation files are available in the folder for Chapter 1 on the Dictations and Templates CD that accompanies this text.

Table 1.7

Important Legal Terms

Term	Definition	Term	Definition
Authentication (electronic signature)	A signature or electronic notation indicating that the document has been reviewed and accepted by the author (dictator).	Protected health information (PHI)	Any information gathered in the course of a patient's care that can reasonably be used to identify that individual.
Breach of confidential communication	The unauthorized release of patient information.	Right of privacy	The right to be let alone and free from unwarranted publicity and to withhold personal information from public scrutiny if so desired.
Defamation	Slander or libel.	Risk management	Identifying problems for the purpose of forestalling or preventing injury.
Independent contractor	An individual who is hired to complete a specific task but is not under the control of the person contracting the work and thus does not have the same rights as an employee.	Slander	A witnessed statement that damages a reputation or subjects a person to ridicule.
Informed consent	Permission to perform a procedure after full disclosure of the risks and benefits of the procedure.	Standard of care	An established protocol or reasonable course of action that a prudent person would follow to provide care and providing less than this standard is considered negligence.
Invasion of the right of privacy	Needless investigation into another's personal affairs where there is no valid reason to do so, in a way to cause public embarrassment or humiliation to that person.	Statutory employee	An employee that might otherwise be considered an independent contractor, but for the purposes of federal income tax, is considered an employee.
Libel	A written statement or graphic portrayal made or given to a third party that damages a reputation or subjects a person to ridicule.	Subpoena	A writ commanding a specified person to appear in court or else serve a penalty for failure to appear. A subpoena of medical records must be honored because it is a legal document.
Malpractice	Improper or unethical conduct or care by a healthcare practitioner.		
Nonprivileged information	This type of information can be disclosed without the patient's permission and usually relates to admission/discharge, treatment dates, name and address of the patient, and name of the individual who accompanied the patient to the hospital or physician's office.	*Subpoena duces tecum*	A writ commanding a person to produce in court certain specified documents or evidence; Latin meaning "in his possession."
Privileged communication	Information that may be disclosed only with the patient's permission.	Writ	A written order issued by a court or judicial officer commanding a specified person to perform or refrain from performing a specified act.
Privileged information	Any and all information that can only be disclosed with the patient's permission.		

Transcription Practice 1.A

This letter explains the employee healthcare program provided by the Marathon Health Services company.

REPORT 1.1 Letter

Use dictation file Report0101.mp3. Save the transcribed document as XXReport01.01, using your initials in place of the *XX* in the file name.

Preferred format will vary by agency, but AHDI prefers block format. See Figure 6.2 on page 184 for an example of a letter in block format. Set the document's margin at 1 inch.

Transcription Practice 1.B

A position as an administrative medical assistant is open at River Oak Medical Center. Ms. Anita Brooks, a graduate of Winthrop College, is being recommended by Mr. Peter Harris, Director of Placement.

REPORT 1.2 Letter

Use dictation file Report0102.mp3. Save the transcribed document as XXReport01.02, using your initials in place of *XX* in the file name.

Inside addresses will be spelled out by dictator.

CPT codes are used in medical billing.

Check the spelling of the various disciplines used in the dictation.

Listen for these names:
Harley Association
Winthrop College

Transcription Practice 1.C

The Ohio Healthcare Treatment Center, the Women's Club of Danbury, and Springfield Hospital have joined forces to offer health-related seminars. Residents of the community are invited to attend. No entrance fee is required; however, individuals interested in attending must register in advance.

REPORT 1.3 Announcement

Use dictation file Report0103.mp3. Save the transcribed document as XXReport01.03 using your initials in place of the *XX* in the file name.

Leave four blank lines after the dateline to personalize the letter, if desired.

Madeline Delroy, a medical assistant, is the dictator.

Health care is one word when used as a compound modifier and two words when used as a noun.

Use the spell-check feature of your word processor and carefully proofread the document for sentence structure, transcripted meaning, capitalization, and punctuation.

Transcription Practice 1.D

Changes are occurring in conventional medicine and alternative therapies are being used by a large percentage of the population. Facilities that use conventional medicine are now starting to evaluate alternative therapies. This informational report cites a number of approaches being used for health care.

REPORT 1.4 Informational Report

Use dictation file Report0104.mp3. Save the transcribed document as XXReport01.04 using your initials in place of the *XX* in the file name.

Use solid caps when keying side headings.

Leave a line space before and after a side heading.

Check the meaning of terms with which you may not be familiar.
    alternative therapies
    comprehensive
    concerted
    holistic
    impacting
    self-hypnotic
    vertebrae
    vital signs

There is one misuse of the word *which* in this report. It should be replaced with the word *that*.

Two

Medical Transcription and Technology

Technology has impacted every aspect of the field of medical transcription. From the advances in medical treatment, which add to the ever-expanding vocabulary, to the advances in personal computers and the Internet, which have made transcription a mobile, global profession, understanding and using technology to its best advantage has become an integral part of a transcriptionist's job.

Objectives

» Compare and contrast analog and digital equipment used in medical transcription.

» Understand basic computer terminology, maintenance, and word processing skills.

» Use keyboarding techniques and shortcut keys.

» Use email to communicate effectively.

» Understand guidelines for computer security and patient confidentiality.

» Explain how speech recognition technology affects medical transcription.

» Describe tools that increase a transcriptionist's productivity and accuracy.

» Apply ergonomic principles.

Transcription Tools

Medical transcription requires the integration of three distinct skill sets: auditory discrimination, language, and computer competency. One must be able to operate the equipment used to play the audio files as well as the equipment used to create the written document. This chapter will introduce you to the various types of hardware and software you are likely to encounter in the workplace.

For many years, a cassette tape recorder, desktop transcriber, and typewriter were the primary tools of the trade, but modern transcription uses digital recording devices as well as various software programs to complete the transcription process.

Digital Recorders

Digital dictation and transcription equipment does not use cassette tapes (analog technology) but instead captures the voice on digital media (hard disks or memory cards). One of the most common methods for capturing dictation uses sophisticated voice servers (computers) with integrated telephone lines that allow dictators to record dictation using a standard telephone. The dictator dials a specified phone number, which is answered by a computer. The dictator uses the phone to key in a unique dictator identification number. The dictator may also key in patient identification numbers and specify a work type (i.e., report type) to be dictated. Computerized voice servers, used by hospitals and large transcription services, are capable of handling many phone lines at one time and can record hundreds of dictation files per day.

Dictators may also use a digital handheld recorder that is small enough to fit in a pocket, allowing them to dictate anytime, anywhere. These recorders use flash memory cards (like a digital camera) to store the dictation. The sound quality and clarity of digital files are very good and a vast improvement over cassette tapes.

After recording, digital files created on a handheld recorder are transferred from the recorder's memory card to a computer. Files created by a computer-based recording system are already on a computer. Digital files created by either method can be transferred to the transcriptionist's workstation using a network or Internet connection. In fact, digital audio files can be manipulated the same way as other computer files—they can be moved, copied, renamed, deleted, transferred across a network or Internet connection, or attached to email. Audio files may also be burned to a CD and played on a computer equipped with a CD or DVD drive.

Transcription Software

The transcriptionist transcribes the digital audio file using transcription software, a foot pedal, a

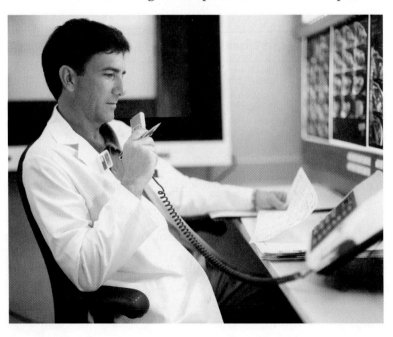

A dictation file can be created by a healthcare provider by calling into a computerized voice server. Dictation files remain private through the use of identification numbers and pass codes.

headset, and a word processor. Transcription software allows the transcriptionist to adjust the speed and volume of the audio file as well as control the playback using a foot pedal or keyboard commands. Transcription software includes an adjustable auto-rewind feature that automatically backs up one or two seconds each time the play button is released. This helps prevent words from being missed while stopping and starting the playback.

There are many brands of transcription software available. Products with very basic features can be downloaded from the Internet free of charge. Name-brand digital recorders may also include transcription software. When evaluating transcription software, it is important to match compatible file formats with the format created by the dictation equipment. The most common file formats include .wav, .mp3, and .dss. Some software brands integrate file transfer software to assist in downloading (moving files toward you) and uploading (moving files away from you). Many transcription services and hospitals use transcription platforms that integrate file management, transcription software, and word processing.

Speech Recognition Software

Speech recognition (SR) technology is slowly finding its place in medical transcription. Originally, the technology was predicted to completely replace the transcriptionist. However, the limitations of the technology have been realized and now it is marketed as a productivity tool for transcriptionists. The technology is not yet accurate enough to replace the transcriptionist, so all transcripts created by speech recognition software must be thoroughly reviewed by a medical transcriptionist. Not all dictation can be processed using speech recognition because many dictators speak too fast, do not articulate, or repeat or correct themselves too often. Large hospitals and transcription services

are integrating this technology into their workflow to assist transcriptionists in transcribing more dictation files in less time.

Speech recognition software is categorized as front-end or back-end. Front-end systems convert the text as it is dictated. The dictator speaks into a microphone attached to the computer and edits the text as it appears on the computer's display. As the user edits the text, the software "learns" and adapts to the user's speech patterns, making the recognition software more accurate the longer it is used. Front-end systems are most commonly used by radiologists (doctors who interpret various x-ray studies). Their unique workflow, which is restricted mostly to a reading station, is amenable to front-end speech recognition technology, whereas most physicians who are constantly moving between exam rooms and hospital rooms choose not to use front-end systems.

Back-end systems work in the background so-to-speak. The dictator records a medical report using a digital recording system. After the recording is complete, the audio file is processed by a speech-recognition engine, which converts the audio to text. It may be processed further to add formatting and punctuation. The transcriptionist is presented with a transcribed document file along with the corresponding voice file. As the voice file is played, the cursor on the screen highlights the corresponding words in the document and the transcriptionist corrects any errors found. Corrected transcripts are sent back through the SR engine to be analyzed in light of the changes, allowing the engine to "learn" and become more accurate. Speech recognition engines and formatting software are expensive and are typically used by large transcription services and hospitals.

Proofreading SR files requires extraordinary attention to detail and continuous critical thinking. The speech recognition software will not insert

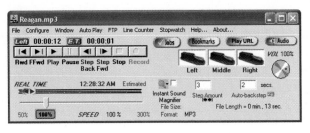

Transcription software allows the transcriptionist to play a digital recording while keying into a word processing file. The software can control the playback of the recording through keyboard controls or a foot pedal.

incorrectly spelled words, but it *will* insert sound-alike words and nonsensical phrases. It is easy to be deceived when listening to the audio and reading the report simultaneously, because the sounds that you hear will match the text but not necessarily the intended meaning. The editor must constantly evaluate the context and meaning so as not to be fooled by what is heard and seen. For example, the doctor may have dictated "anovulatory patient" and the recognition software might transcribe the phrase as "an ovulatory patient." Although these phrases appear almost identical, they are opposite in meaning! A transcriptionist with a working knowledge of medical terminology, disease processes, and the subtleties of language will recognize the error and correct the text to match the *intended* meaning.

The proofreading exercises throughout this text allow you to concentrate on meaning and language usage, which is indispensable when producing quality documents generated from speech recognition technology. In addition, Appendix C provides exercises that require you to correct text output by speech recognition software.

Foot Pedal

The foot pedal, also called a foot control, attaches directly to the computer and allows the transcriptionist to control the audio file without taking his or her hands off the keyboard. Pressing the play button on the foot pedal causes the transcription software to play; releasing the pedal stops the playback. Foot pedals may have two or three foot positions, or buttons, corresponding to play, rewind, and fast forward. With most contemporary models, the play button is in the center; fast forward is on the right; and rewind is on the left. The left and right can be programmed differently depending on the transcriptionist's preference. Computer foot pedals attach to the computer by way of a serial port (9 pins), a game port (15 pins), or a USB connection. The foot pedal connection type is determined by the transcription software. Although they look nearly identical, foot pedals designed for analog transcribe stations will not work on a computer (and vice versa) because the connectors are not interchangeable.

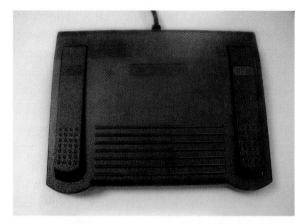

A foot pedal allows a transcriptionist to control the playback of a digital dictation file without removing his or her hands from the keyboard.

Headset

The headset is an important tool for assuring good auditory acuity. The headset has two earphones, or earpieces, attached to a cord that plugs directly into the computer. The earphones sit comfortably in or over each ear and are connected with a lightweight band that rests below the chin. Headsets are important for maximizing clarity and for privacy. Most headsets connect to the computer using a standard 3.5 mm plug. Desktop speakers are not ideal for transcription because they significantly decrease auditory discrimination. Accurate transcription depends on hearing every single syllable! In addition, desktop speakers are not appropriate for use if the dictation files can be overheard by others. It is important to protect patient privacy.

Headsets are available with a variety of earpiece styles. Some earpieces, called buds, fit into the external ear canal. You will also find speaker-style earpieces that rest just outside the ear canal as well as over-the-ear styles that cover the entire ear. Whichever style you select, you may find that it takes some time to adapt to wearing a headset for several hours at a time. Before you start to play a recording, adjust the volume to a comfortable level.

Analog Dictation

For many years, cassette tape recorders were the main dictation tool used by physicians in their private practice. Although many physicians still use cassette recorders, the industry is moving away

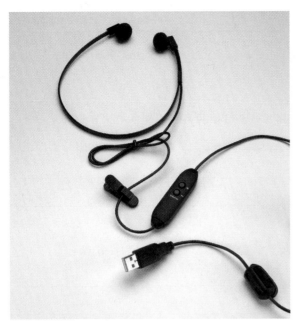

It is important to use a headset that is comfortable and provides high-quality playback of dictation recordings.

Table 2.1

Analog Transcriber Features and Functions

Feature	Function
Index Counters	Some transcribers have an index counter that measures the length of dictation on a cassette. This is a useful tool for finding a specific dictation or for noting a point in a dictation to which you can return.
Auto Playback/ Auto Rewind	This feature causes the tape to back up a specified amount of time (usually 1–2 seconds) each time you lift your foot off the foot pedal. This prevents words and phrases from being inadvertently missed as you stop and start.
Speed Control	This feature allows you to increase or decrease the playback speed to adjust for the dictation speed and your transcription speed.
Tone	This feature mutes or accentuates consonants (treble/bass) for nasal tones or a stuttering style of dictation.
Erase	This feature allows you to clear or erase tapes. Be careful with this button to make sure you do not erase dictation before it is transcribed.

from this outmoded technology. Analog cassette recorders come in two styles: a desktop recorder with a microphone or a portable, hand-held style with a microphone built in. The cassette tapes come in three sizes: standard, microcassette, and mini. The transcriptionist listens to the audio recording using a desktop transcriber, also called a transcribe station, which plays the corresponding cassette size. (Most transcribers will only play one tape size.) The transcriber allows the transcriptionist to control the speed of the playback as well as start and stop the playback using a foot pedal. Features found on most transcribers are listed in Table 2.1.

Exercise 2.1   Tools of the Trade

Describe four essential tools that a medical transcriptionist uses to transcribe audio files.

_____

_____

_____

_____

In the future, more and more transcriptionists will edit reports that the computer "transcribed" from voice input.

1. How would this scenario change your job as a medical language specialist?

   _____

   _____

   _____

2. How would your job remain the same?

   _____

   _____

   _____

Exercise 2.3   **Fix This**

The paragraph that follows was dictated and transcribed using speech recognition software. Edit it by making corrections to punctuation and the context and key it. Save the document as XXExercise02.03, using your initials in place of the *XX* in the file name.

HISTORY OF PRESENT ILLNESS

The patient is a 40 year old mail admitted to Riverside medical center for treatment of deep vein thrombophlebitis in his left lower extremity. The patience has always been healthy, has never been hospitalized, and has had no medical problems until recently. About 6 weeks ago, he developed a superficial thrombophlebitis of the left low extremity. He was treated for this without incident and scenes to improve. About 1 week ago, he was trying to get back into shape and started working out on a treadmill. He noted some discomfort in his left calf, which she had attributed to muscle pain and continued his exercise. All over the past 24 hours, the left of lower extremity has become more painful and swollen. He was seen by doctor Winston at the Riverside medical center and a Doppler ultrasound was performed demonstrating clear evidence of deep venous thrombosis. He is now admitted for treatment of that condition. He has not had any undue shortness of breath, nor has he had any polyp petitions, cough, or chest pain. The notes that he usually runs a rapid Paul's in the range of 80 or 90.

Personal Computers

Modern medical transcription relies heavily on personal computers. Knowing how to operate a personal computer (PC) will increase your efficiency and productivity, resulting in higher income potential and significantly less on-the-job frustration. Operating a computer correctly will also protect the privacy and security of the patients you serve. Technology is never stagnant, and as an important part of the healthcare team, a desire for continuous learning will serve you well.

Most software programs use the same standards or conventions, so you can apply what you know about one program to many other programs. Instead of memorizing hundreds of minute details, concentrate on the fundamental concepts that all programs share and look for repeating patterns.

Introduction to Windows

The operating system controls and coordinates all other parts of the computer while applications (also called programs) perform specific functions such as word processing. The most widely used operating system is sold by Microsoft Corporation under the trade name Windows. The current version is Windows Vista, which supersedes Windows XP.

The majority of transcription software, as well as word processing programs, are designed to run on "PCs," a reference to personal computers running the Windows Operating System (as opposed to Apple brand computers referred to as "Macs"), so you will want to become proficient in the use of computers that use Windows Vista and/or the preceding version, XP. The hallmark of the Windows Operating System is the graphical user interface (GUI), which allows computer files and commands to be represented by pictures (icons), eliminating the need to understand complicated computer language. Icons can represent any type of object such as an application, a folder, a file, or a specific command (e.g., Bold, Align left, Print). In addition, the act of *moving icons* across the computer screen (called dragging) emulates commands such as Move, Copy, Attach, Create shortcut, and Delete.

Table 2.2 describes fundamental elements and concepts used by Windows. Understanding these basic terms will help you understand computer reference books and will also help you communicate more effectively with technical support personnel. Use this list as a basis for further independent study. Figure 2.1 shows a Windows Vista Explorer window (also referred to as Computer or My Computer in Windows XP)

The Monitor, Mouse, and Keyboard

The monitor, mouse, and keyboard are integral components of a personal computer. The monitor is an output device that allows the user to interact directly with the computer in conjunction with the mouse and keyboard. The mouse and keyboard are called input devices. They provide a method for the user to interact directly with the computer in order to give commands and type text.

Monitor Monitors, which display the information on your computer, come in a range of sizes and types. Cathode ray tube (CRT) monitors are falling out of use, mostly because they are bulky, consume a lot of desk space, and generate heat. Flat-panel monitors run cooler, consume less energy, and take up far less space. Larger monitors, such as 17- or 19-inch displays, provide a larger viewing area, allowing the user to increase the "zoom" setting within their word processor. Larger zoom settings, such as 120% to 150%, increase the size of the text as it is displayed on the monitor, thereby decreasing eyestrain. This is especially important for a professional transcriptionist. The Zoom setting can be found on the View tab (or menu) of your word processor.

Mouse A computer mouse has two buttons that sit at the upper left and right corners (left button and right button) and a scroll wheel that sits on top of the mouse between the two buttons. Pressing the buttons is called "clicking" because of the characteristic clicking sound when the buttons are pushed. The wheel on top is used to move up and down a computer screen in a smooth, even motion called scrolling. The mouse is an integral part of the graphical

Table 2.2

Windows Terminology

Term	Definition
Desktop	The first screen that is displayed after a full startup of your computer.
Dialog box	A collection of commands displayed within a window that allows you to change settings and options.
Display (noun)	The image seen on the computer monitor.
Display (verb)	To make an object visible.
Exit (✗)	The command to close (put away) a file or exit an application. Once closed, a file or application will no longer have a button on the Taskbar.
Folder	An electronic version of a manilla file folder used to sort and organize computer files.
Icons	Visual representations of computer files and commands.
Maximize (☐)	The command that enlarges the window to the largest possible size, usually the size of your monitor's screen. If a window has been maximized, it can be restored to a smaller window size using the Restore command (⧉).
Menu bar	A horizontal list of drop-down menus located beneath the Title bar.
Minimize (▬)	The command that hides the window but does not close or exit the window. The file can be made active again by clicking the corresponding button on the Taskbar.
Notification Area	Area in the lower right corner of the computer screen that shows the current time and contains icons for programs or processes that run continuously such as virus scanners, network connections, and email monitors. Alerts and notifications also appear in this area as "bubbles."
Select	To choose or single-out an item on the computer display in order to carry out a command on that item. The most common way to select an item is to move the mouse pointer over the item and click the left mouse button.
Shortcut icons	A special type of icon that opens files or folders when clicked. Shortcut icons have a small curved arrow in the lower left corner to indicate they represent shortcuts to access the item, not the *actual* file, folder, or application.

Term	Definition
Shortcut menus	A list of commonly used commands that appears when an object such as text, an icon, or a file name is clicked using the right mouse button.
Start Button	The button displayed in the lower left corner of the desktop that opens the Start Menu.
Start Menu	A list of computer programs, utilities, and folders stored on your computer. Click items on the menu to open.
Taskbar	The horizontal bar that rests along the lower edge of the computer screen that displays buttons for each program that is currently in use.
Title bar	The uppermost edge of a window that displays the name or contents of the window and also contains the window-control commands for closing and minimizing (hiding) the window.
Toolbars and ribbons	A collection of commands grouped by task and arranged horizontally.
View	An important concept that relates to the way information is displayed. Information stored on a computer can be displayed in many different ways depending on how you want to use that information. *The information itself is not changed or deleted*, it is just presented to the user in ways that hide distracting data or accentuate needed data. Look for the View command on menus and ribbons.
Window	The cardinal concept that gives Windows (with a capital W) its name. A window (with a lowercase w) is a rectangular space that visually separates individual applications and other types of work spaces on your computer's display.
Windows Explorer	Windows' main tool for managing the files and folders on your computer. To open Explorer, click the Start button and click *Computer* (*My Computer* in Windows XP).

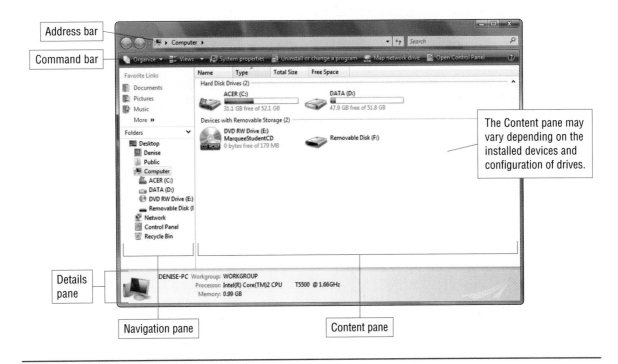

Address bar

Command bar

The Content pane may vary depending on the installed devices and configuration of drives.

Details pane

Navigation pane

Content pane

Figure 2.1   Windows Vista Explorer

interface because it can point to any position on the screen without having to follow horizontal or vertical paths like the arrow keys on the keyboard.

Selecting an item (left click) and then clicking the *right* mouse button will reveal a shortcut menu with a list of commands. The right-click menus, also called shortcut menus, change depending on the item that is selected so that no matter what item you select, you will see the most commonly used commands for that item. Usually, the fastest way to complete a specific computer task using the mouse is to locate the item you want to work with, right-click, and then choose a command from the menu.

In addition to selecting and clicking, there are other mouse techniques that are important to learn.

- **Drag:** A mouse technique for moving items to a different place on the display. Point to an object on the screen, press *and hold* the left mouse button while moving the pointer to a new location. Release the mouse button when the object is in the new location. Use this technique for arranging icons on your desktop, rearranging windows, and moving text within a document.
- **Drag and drop:** A mouse technique for moving or copying files, folders and text. For example, you may want to move a file from one folder

to another. To do this using the mouse, select the file to be moved, hold down the left mouse button, and drag the file toward the other folder. Continue holding the mouse button and hover the pointer over the folder and then release the mouse button.

- **Double click:** Clicking the left mouse button two times in rapid succession. This mouse technique typically opens the selected file or application. If there is a delay between clicks, Windows will interpret two separate clicks and you will get a different result.

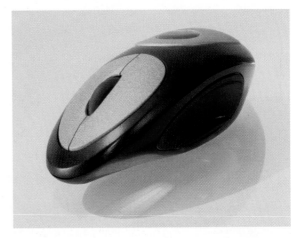

An optical mouse tracks movement with a light sensor.

- **Ctrl + drag:** A mouse technique that combines the mouse and the keyboard. Use the drag technique previously mentioned while holding down the Ctrl key on the keyboard to copy the items being selected and dragged.

Keyboard   As a transcriptionist, one of the most important computer skills to learn is keyboarding, that is, using the keyboard instead of the mouse to issue commands. The mouse is more intuitive and does not require as much memorization, but in the long run it is far more time-consuming to use compared to the keyboard. While transcribing, you will want to keep your hands on the keyboard as much as possible. Once you learn basic keyboarding conventions, you will be able to keyboard almost any Windows-based program.

Commands given to the computer using a keyboard are called keyboard shortcuts. Commands use the modifier keys Alt, Ctrl, Shift, and the Logo key to distinguish the keystroke as a command as opposed to typing the character itself. Several conventions are used to describe computer commands in written form. When the keys are written with a plus sign in between (e.g., Ctrl + C), you should press these keys at the same time (although you should aim for the modifier key slightly before the character key so that you don't accidentally type just the character). Commands written with a comma (e.g., Alt, F) should be typed in sequence, lifting off each key before pressing the next.

The following outlines basic conventions for using the keyboard:

- Commands on menus and dialog boxes have hot keys designated by the underscore character. Press the Alt key to activate (and/or display) the Menu bar and then press the underscored character in the menu's name. Once the menu drops down, press the next underscored character corresponding to the needed command. For example, File, Edit, and Insert use F, E and I, respectively.
- Within a dialog box, press Alt and the underscore character *at the same time* to select the needed command. You can also press the Tab

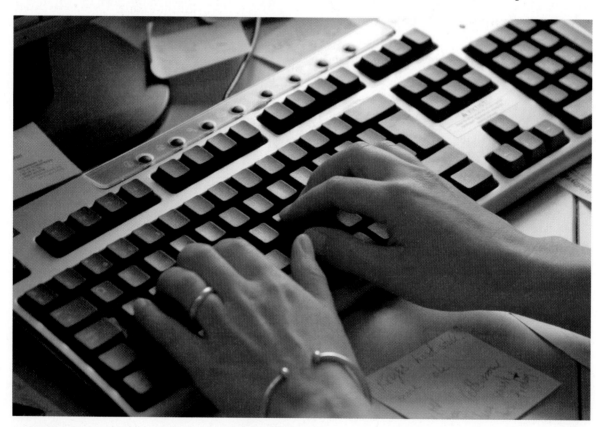

Accurate and quick keying is a skill that is essential to the medical transcriptionist, and shortcut keys can help improve a transcriptionist's efficiency.

key to move through a dialog box. The location of the cursor is indicated by a dotted line around the command name.

- Press the Spacebar to select or de-select a command in a dialog box when the command is surrounded by a dotted line. Press Esc to close a dialog box without making changes. Press the Enter key to close a dialog box and keep the changes.
- While commands on menu bars, drop-down menus, and dialog boxes always have designated hot keys, items created by the user (such as files and folders) do not have underscored characters, so the hot key is automatically the first letter of the item's name. In a folder window, press the first character of the file name to select that file. If more than one item in a window starts with the same character, press the character again until the item is selected. In Windows Vista, the cursor will automatically go to the Search box when you open a folder window, so begin typing the file name. Once the file is selected, press Enter to open the file and its corresponding application at the same time.
- To minimize a window, access the Control menu by pressing Alt, Spacebar. Press the letter N corresponding to the Minimize command.
- Use the navigation keys (right, left, up, and down arrows) to move around in a window in horizontal and vertical paths. Adding the Ctrl key to any of the arrow keys will move the cursor a level farther. For example, the right and left arrow keys move the cursor one *character* at a time, but adding the Ctrl key moves the cursor one *word* at a time. Hold down the Shift key while pressing any navigation key or Ctrl + navigation key in order to select text.
- The Home key always moves the cursor to the beginning of a line of text and End always moves to the end of a line of text. Ctrl + Home

will move to the top of the document or the top of the window. Ctrl + End moves to the end of the document or end of the window.

- The Logo key is used to open the Start menu using the keyboard. The Logo key is usually located to the right and/or left of the Spacebar and is marked with the Microsoft logo ⊞. Once the Start menu is open, press the first character of the item needed or use the arrow keys to move up and down the menu.
- To switch between open windows, hold down the Alt key and press Tab. Continue to hold the Alt key and tap the Tab key until the needed window's icon is selected and then release Alt and Tab. The selected item will become the active window. Versions of Windows Vista capable of running the high-tech Aero feature will switch between running windows using the key combination Logo + Tab. Instead of displaying icons as in Windows XP, each running window will be displayed as a holographic, 3-D image.

Table 2.3 lists some of the most useful shortcut keys for Windows and many Windows-based programs. As a helpful reminder, many shortcut keys are listed on drop-down menus to the right of the corresponding command. To maximize your keyboarding skills, you can print a complete list of shortcut keys for Windows and for the applications you use the most. Press Logo + F1 to access Windows Help. Search the Help files using the keywords "keyboard shortcuts." To see a list of shortcut keys for your favorite applications, open the application and press F1. Search the Help files using the same keyword. Incorporate shortcut keys into your daily routine a few at a time—you will be frustrated if you try to learn and use them all at once. After several days, you will notice a significant difference in your productivity as you decrease the use of your mouse.

Computer Maintenance

Your computer is the single most important tool as a transcriptionist. As such, it is imperative that you maintain your computer to assure reliability and performance. An important aspect of maintaining your computer is to limit the use of your computer

The cursor location is indicated in a dialog box with the use of a dotted line around a command name. When the option is selected, tap the spacebar to place a checkmark.

Table 2.3

Windows Shortcut Keys

To	Press	To	Press
Open the Start menu	⊞ (Logo key)	Accept the default	Press the Enter key while the button or command is surrounded by a dotted line
Open Windows Explorer	⊞ + E		
Return to the desktop (i.e., minimize all applications), toggle to return to initial program	⊞ + D		[Yes]
Start a search for files or folders in Windows	⊞ + F	Right-click an item using the keyboard (instead of the mouse)	Application key (located to the right of the Spacebar, marked with a small menu and arrow icon)
Open an item on the QuickLaunch bar (Windows Vista only)	Logo + 1 (for the first item) Logo + 2 (for the second item), etc.	Copy any item selected (text, shortcut icons, files, folders, graphics) and place the item on the Windows Clipboard	Ctrl + C
Search within a specific folder in Windows	Open the folder window and press F3. This will open the search pane and begin the search in the current folder	Paste the last item copied to the Windows Clipboard at the insertion point (see Copy Command)	Ctrl + V
Lock your computer	⊞ + L	Cut the selected item and place it on the Windows Clipboard (see Copy command)	Ctrl + X
Access Windows Help	⊞ + F1 (F1 is the universal key for Help in all Windows applications)	Undo the last command/action. For example, if you inadvertently deleted text, files or folders, you can immediately reverse the deletion using the Undo command	Ctrl + Z
Open System Properties to display information about your operating system and your computer	⊞ + Pause/Break (located in the upper right-hand corner of your keyboard)		
Close a file and/or an application	Alt + F4	Redo any action performed by the Undo command	Ctrl + Y
Select all (everything within the active window, including files, folders, graphics, text, or a combination of graphics and text)	Ctrl + A		
Return to previous window or previous Web page	Backspace		

to strictly transcription- and business-related tasks. For reasons of patient privacy as well as for the protection of your most important income-generating tool, family members should *never* be allowed to share or use a computer that is employed for medical transcription. Being without your computer while it is repaired or reloaded because of inappropriate use can cost you more in lost income and repair bills than the cost of a second computer. Repeated computer problems will decrease your employer's confidence in your ability to complete the work assigned to you.

Specific tasks should be performed routinely to assure the best computer performance. These tasks include setting up a backup of important files, deleting temporary files, and defragmenting files.

Backup Computer maintenance includes backing up important data. Files on a hard disk may be lost if the disk becomes defective or if the computer becomes disabled by a virus or other "malware" (software that hinders or prohibits optimum use of your PC). Backing up files means copying files to removable media (USB flash or CD) and storing the media in a safe place. Backing up a few files can be accomplished easily using a command called Send To. To do this, place a CD or other media in the appropriate drive slot in your computer, select the file(s) to be backed up, right-click and choose *Send To > [media]*, where [media] refers to the drive containing the media being used for a backup. Be sure to place the media in the appropriate drive *before* opening the Send To menu.

To perform a more extensive backup, use the backup utility that is included with Windows or purchase a third-party product specifically designed to back up large amounts of data. Be sure to place the backup media in a safe, fireproof container. For large amounts of critical data, offsite backup is also an option. Computer service companies sell space on data-storage servers located in highly secured buildings. Using an Internet connection, large amounts of data can be transferred for storage and retrieval as needed.

Disk Cleanup As you work, Windows creates temporary files that periodically need to be deleted.

Open Windows Explorer (Logo + E) and right-click the C drive. *Choose Properties > Disk Cleanup.* Select the file types to be deleted (read a description of each type in the bottom half of the dialog box) and then click OK. All of these files can be safely deleted without any loss of pertinent data.

Defrag As computer files are modified, the changes are added to the hard drive but not necessarily in the same area of the hard drive as the original file. This process "fragments" files so that pieces of an individual file may be scattered all across the disk. A heavily fragmented disk will run slower because Windows must scan the disk to reassemble the data before opening a file. Windows Vista performs the defragment process continuously, so theoretically the user should not need to perform this task unless the computer is running exceptionally slow. In Windows XP, periodically run the Defrag utility. To do this, open Windows Explorer and right-click the C drive. Choose *Properties > Tools > Defragment Now.*

Word Processing

The ability to use word processing software is a mandatory skill for medical transcriptionists. Mastery, not just a cursory understanding, of word processing software should be your goal, so you can work efficiently and without frustration. The two most common word processing software brands are Microsoft Word and Corel WordPerfect. Some transcription departments or services may use proprietary software (neither Word nor WordPerfect). Although it is difficult to predict exactly which word processing program you will be required to use on the job, there are fundamental skills that you can learn now which will apply to whatever software program you use.

To start a new document, open your word processing program. If a new, blank document does not appear, press Ctrl + N. To open an existing document, locate the document using Windows Explorer. Double-click the file icon to open the file and the corresponding application simultaneously. To open recently used documents, open the Start menu, choose Documents, and choose the file name from the submenu.

Format a Document Word processors are designed to allow text to flow from line to line automatically. Only use the Enter key to end a paragraph or to create a new, blank line between paragraphs. Word processing software includes specific commands for applying paragraph formats such as indents and hanging indents (see commands listed on page 47). It is not necessary (or good practice) to use the Tab character at the beginning of *every line of a paragraph* to create an indent (i.e., to move text away from the left margin). Figure 2.2 shows the Word 2007 document screen and Figure 2.3 demonstrates the most common formatting terms used in medical transcription. Each description actually demonstrates the format being described. Table 2.4 lists formatting shortcut keys used by Word and WordPerfect (and possibly other word processors) as well as common shortcut keys for moving around within a document.

Edit and Proof a Document Both Microsoft Word and Corel WordPerfect include tools to check the spelling and grammar of a document.

These software products install a reference list of English words to determine the correct spelling, but this reference list does not recognize medical and pharmaceutical terminology. Medical reference lists, called electronic medical spell checkers, can be purchased and installed on your PC so that you can easily spell check medical terms also. Words that are misspelled will be marked with a red line and grammar errors will be marked with a green or blue line. Right-click marked text (or use the Application key on the keyboard) to display a list of suggested corrections. Always use your medical and/or English dictionary to confirm the meaning of the words suggested by the spell checker to make sure you are choosing the word that fits the context. Grammar checking software is not reliable for medical reports because of the unique nature of the language and the structure of reports. Use the corrections offered by the word processor as suggestions, but always use your own judgment based on medical grammar and style when punctuating a medical report. Because the grammar checkers are typically unreliable, you may choose to turn off

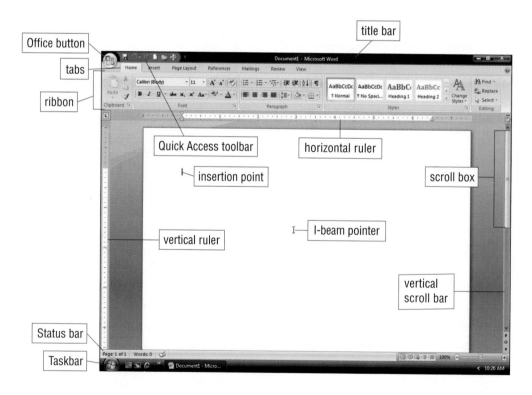

Figure 2.2 Microsoft Word 2007 Document Screen

this feature. Options for managing proofing tools can be found under the Tools menu of both Word and WordPerfect.

Figure 2.3   Formats Used in Medical Transcription

Table 2.4

Shortcut Keys Used in Microsoft Word and WordPerfect

Command	Shortcut Key
Bold	Ctrl + B
Italic	Ctrl + I
Underline	Ctrl + U
Toggle case	Shift + F3 (Word), Ctrl + K (WordPerfect)
Align text right	Ctrl + R
Align text left	Ctrl + L
Align text center	Ctrl + E
Justify	Ctrl + J
Indent	Ctrl + M (Word), F7 (WordPerfect)
Hanging indent	Ctrl + T (Word), Ctrl + F7 (WordPerfect)
Hard page break (forced page break)	Ctrl + Enter
Nonbreaking hyphen	Ctrl + Shift + -
Nonbreaking space	Ctrl + Shift + Space
Move to the beginning of a line	Home
Move to the end of a line	End
Move one word to the right	Ctrl + Right arrow (add Shift key to select text)
Move one word to the left	Ctrl + Left arrow (add Shift key to select text)
Move one line up	Up arrow
Move one line down	Down arrow
Save	Ctrl + S
Undo last action	Ctrl + Z
Redo last action	Ctrl + Y
Delete one word to the left	Ctrl + Backspace
Close current document	Ctrl + F4
Start new document	Ctrl + N
Print	Ctrl + P

Exercise 2.4   Name that Key

List the shortcut keys for the following commands.

1. Cut _____

2. Copy _____

3. Paste _____

4. Undo or reverse last action _____

5. Help feature access _____

6. Select one word to the left _____

7. Move to the top of the paragraph _____

8. Move to the beginning of a line _____

9. Move to the end of the document _____

10. Select all text and graphics on the web page or in the document _____

11. Save the current file _____

12. Select text to the end of the line _____

Exercise 2.5   What Do You Think?

How would a thorough knowledge of Windows and word processing software affect your income, employability, and accuracy of transcribed reports?

_____

_____

_____

The following sentences were taken from medical documents. One word in each sentence is spelled incorrectly. The words listed are those suggested by the word processor's spell check routine. Choose the correct word from the list of suggestions to correct the misspelled word. Use a medical or English dictionary to determine the correct word.

1. Her muscle spasms are sometimes relieed with chiropractic adjustment but seem to return pretty consistently.
   a. relied
   b. relieved
   c. relined
   d. relived

2. The patient has a remote history of tobacco abuse, but quiit about 25 years ago.
   a. quit
   b. quiet
   c. quite
   d. quits

3. The cholesterol-lowering medication effeced her liver, causing her doctor to change her prescription.
   a. effaced
   b. affected
   c. effected

4. He does not take any medications on a cronic basis.
   a. caronic
   b. cryonic
   c. chronic
   d. clonic

5. The patient had an extensive caiac workup including an echocardiogram at the hospital.
   a. carica
   b. cardiac
   c. celiac
   d. kaiak

6. I emphasized to the patient the critical importance of complianc with aspirin and Plavix.
   a. compline
   b. complices
   c. compliance
   d. complain

Productivity Tools

Transcriptionists must always strive for accuracy first, but the sheer volume of work and the shortage of qualified transcriptionists requires the working MT to perform as efficiently as possible. When you begin transcribing, it may seem slow and tedious, but with practice, you will increase your speed at a noticeable rate. On a typical day, a full-time transcriptionist may transcribe 30 to 50 documents. For any one dictator, the dictation is consistent and repetitive, so professional MTs take advantage of the repetition and create templates and text shortcuts to reduce the overall number of keystrokes required to complete a document. As described below, there are several software tools available to help you work more efficiently. Begin now to incorporate these tools into your routine.

Templates

A template is a document containing standard text that is used as a framework for future documents of the same type. The standard text is saved as a protected document or as a reusable block of text that can be used over and over without changing the original text. Using templates in medical transcription has several advantages.

Templates:
- ensure consistency from one document to the next
- promote standardization, making specific information easy to find within the document itself
- increase productivity
- improve accuracy

Instead of typing every element of a document each time you transcribe a report, create a template that contains the text that appears in all reports of that type, such as headings, subheadings, salutations, and signature lines. Using preformatted templates allows you to concentrate on keying the words being dictated rather than the mechanics of the document itself. Figure 2.4 is an example of a template. In the workplace, you may need to create your own templates or they may be supplied by your employer.

Templates can be a document file that you use repeatedly and rename each time you create a new file using that document. When using this approach, it is important that you immediately rename your template file (using the word processor's Save As command) *before* you begin transcribing the report; otherwise, you run the risk of changing your template by saving changes that do not belong in the template. Microsoft Word includes a built-in template feature that prevents the user from inadvertently changing templates. A template file in Word has the extension .dotx (or .dot) instead of the document file extension .docx (or .doc). The template file looks just like a document, but the different file extension protects the file from being inadvertently changed. To create a new document *based on a template file,* click the Office button and choose New (or File > New in versions prior to 2007). Select the template from the list of available templates and a new *document* will open which looks exactly like your template file. Even though you selected a template, a *document* (with the extension .docx) will open based on the information saved in the template file. The new document can be modified as needed without affecting the template file.

Some transcription companies integrate MS Word into their transcription software platform and disable the template feature. In this case, the templated text (i.e., headings, subheadings, standard text, and signature line) can be saved as a block of text using AutoCorrect, AutoText, or a text expander (described below).

As you work through this textbook, you will find that a specialized type of medical report is featured in each chapter. Also, there are other types of reports to transcribe at the end of each chapter. When transcribing the dictated reports, use the templates provided on the Dictations and Templates CD accompanying this text. These templates correspond to the model documents and standard formats of the various reports.

The templates provided on the Dictations and Templates CD were created in Word. They contain headings, signature lines, and other elements of a document that consistently appear in a document of that type. Navigate through these Word documents by pressing the F11 key, which will move the cursor to the next position within the document to begin typing. To display the "jump" points, press Alt + F9. Each jump point is represented by two brackets. Press Alt + F9 again to hide the jump points. Transcribe the reports with the jump points displayed.

In the transcribing reports activities, you will be prompted to key the dictated information after the headings. You may find that headings need to be added or changed to correspond with the dictation. Changing the headings and removing unused

PATIENT NAME: { }
DATE: { }

SUBJECTIVE
{ }

OBJECTIVE
{ }

ASSESSMENT
{ }

PLAN
{ }

_____

{ }

{ }/{ }
D: { }
T: { }

The braces ({ }) represent points where information will be keyed during the transcription process. These "jump" points can be viewed by clicking Alt + F9 in a document that contains this feature.

Figure 2.4   Office Note Template

headings are acceptable, but keep the headings in the recommended order. As a working transcriptionist, you will be required to use good judgment and critical thinking skills in order to place dictated information under the correct heading. Providers may dictate information out of order or in the wrong area of the document, but the MT should transcribe the information according to accepted standards. Using templates and standards allows other healthcare workers to easily locate information within the document. Individual institutions may use templates that vary from the formats provided with this text.

Macros

In computer terminology, the word "macro" refers to a computer technique of combining a series of keystrokes and/or commands into a single command. Both WordPerfect and Word include a tool for creating macros by "recording" a series of commands that can be "played back" using a single shortcut key combination. The software actually memorizes your exact keystrokes and repeats the

series of commands when the macro is executed. One of the most common macros used by transcriptionists is called a "jump." This macro uses the word processor's Find command to locate a specific character, such as an asterisk, and move the cursor to that point. The macro is assigned a shortcut key so that pressing the shortcut key moves the cursor to the next asterisk and then deletes the asterisk. This type of macro is used in conjunction with templates (as shown in Figure 2.4) to quickly navigate a document by "jumping" the insertion point to the next position in the template. Using "jumps" to navigate a document improves efficiency and increases productivity by reducing keystrokes (i.e., using the up, down, left, and right arrow keys) and eliminating mouse clicks. The templates included with this text use a slightly different method (although a similar concept) than the macro technique described here in order to navigate within the documents. Directions for navigating this book's templates were described previously (under Templates) and are also explained in more detail in Appendix B.

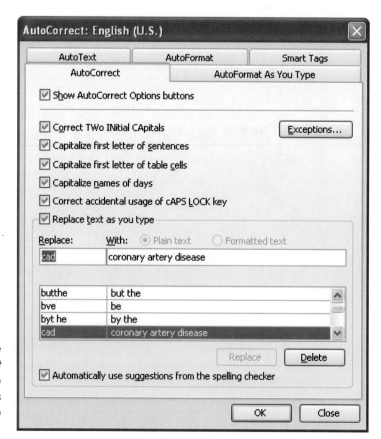

Create text expanions by using the AutoCorrect dialog box to direct Word to replace letters with common words or phrases. Here, Word is being directed to replace cad with coronary artery disease.

Text Expanders

As you continue to study medical transcription, you will notice that medical language makes extensive use of two- and three-word phrases such as "coronary artery disease," "congestive heart failure," and "liver function tests." Because phrases are used repeatedly in medical reports, efficiency-minded MTs use software tools that save common phrases as two- and three-letter short forms such as *cad*, *chf*, and *lft*. The short form is typed into the document where it "expands" into the complete phrase. Veteran transcriptionists often refer to these text shortcuts as "macros," even though they do not actually use the "macro" feature that is incorporated into word processing software (as described previously). AutoText, AutoCorrect, QuickWords, and QuickCorrect are tools within Word and WordPerfect (respectively) designed to expand short forms into complete phrases or blocks of text.

Text expanders are software programs (separate from the word processor software) designed specifically for inserting words and phrases into a document using a minimal number of keystrokes. They serve the same purpose as AutoText and QuickWords, but they offer several advantages. These programs work in concert with most word processing programs and many transcription platforms, so you can use your shortcuts regardless of the word processor or transcription platform your employer requires. It can be difficult, or even impossible, to transfer shortcuts from Word and WordPerfect to a different platform, and if you are unable to transfer your glossary of short forms, you will have to build a new one, which can be tedious and time-consuming. Text-expander programs are extremely stable, reliable, versatile, and capable of storing thousands of short forms. Text-expander software allows you to create multiple glossaries (lists of shortcuts) so you can separate short forms by specialty or by dictator. Using text expansion software requires some initial time and patience in order to develop the ability to hear a word or phrase and instantly translate and type the short form, but the time invested in developing this skill will pay you back many times over in the form of increased line counts and decreased hand fatigue. Two popular text expansion programs are Instant Text and SpeedType.

Exercise 2.7   Compare and Contrast

Describe a text expander. How is a text expander different from AutoCorrect and QuickCorrect?

_____

_____

_____

Exercise 2.8   What Is This?

Provide the correct terms for the following definitions.

1. a single command that represents a series of keystrokes or commands _____

2. a document containing text that appears on all reports of a particular type _____

3. a feature included in MS Word that converts typed text to a corrected or expanded form _____

4. a program that stores short forms and inserts expanded words and phrases into a document _____

Electronic Communications

Email, instant messaging, Internet forums, and electronic file transfers have become an integral part of most business processes. Knowing how to communicate electronically has become a required skill for most professionals, especially those who aspire to work from a home office. All electronic communications depend on computer networks to exchange information.

Networks

Networks consist of two or more computers that are connected by a network cable (called an Ethernet cable), an Internet connection, or through wireless technology called Wi-Fi. A local area network (LAN) typically involves several computers located in the same building. A wide area network (WAN) may involve hundreds of computers spread out across a wide geographic area and connected by both Ethernet cables and public utilities such as phone and cable lines. The Internet itself is a very large network of computers.

The Internet

To access the Internet, a computer must have a physical connection to the Internet in the form of a telephone line, cable, or satellite. These physical connections between your computer and the outside world are used to connect with an Internet service provider (ISP) who provides a gateway onto the Internet. AOL, MSN, and Yahoo! are popular ISPs. A modem (modulator-demodulator), which is physically positioned between your computer and the line connecting you to the ISP, is used to translate the electronic messages generated by your computer into a form that can traverse the Internet. The "speed" of a connection refers to how quickly information travels from point A to point B, and "fast" connections are often referred to as broadband connections. The different types of Internet connections include DSL, cable, satellite, and dial-up. A dial-up connection uses a standard phone line. The type of connection you use often depends on the availability in your community; not all service types are available in any given area. Cable connections are typically the fastest and most reliable. Satellite connections are usually fast but are vulnerable to extreme weather conditions. Dial-up connections, common in rural and sparsely populated areas, are extremely slow and may limit your use of some Internet features. Transcription employers prefer employees to have fast connections, such as DSL and cable, although some employers are able to work with transcriptionists who use dial-up Internet connections. The types of Internet connections available to you are an important point to discuss with a potential employer.

The computers in Figure 2.5 share an Internet connection through the wireless access point that connects to the Internet. Using Windows' networking tools will create a network between computers that will allow them to share files. When creating a home network, do not establish connections (shared folders) between your transcription computer and computers used by family members, as shared folders allow access to information as well as create pathways for malicious software to spread from one computer to another.

A browser is designed to locate and display information stored on the world-wide network of computers known as the World Wide Web (www). Internet Explorer is the most commonly used browser, and it installs with the Windows Operating System. Other browsers include Firefox and AOL. Information available as part of the World Wide Web is located using a Universal Resource Locator (URL), also referred to as the Web address.

Email

Email is the most common form of electronic communication. Most email accounts are provided by Internet Service Providers but may also be provided by an employer. Email basically takes two different forms: Web-based or client-based. Web-based email is accessed and managed through a Web site. This type of email account can be viewed from any computer connected to the Internet, not just your personal computer. Examples include G-mail, AOL, Hotmail, and Yahoo! mail. Client-based email is retrieved, displayed, and managed

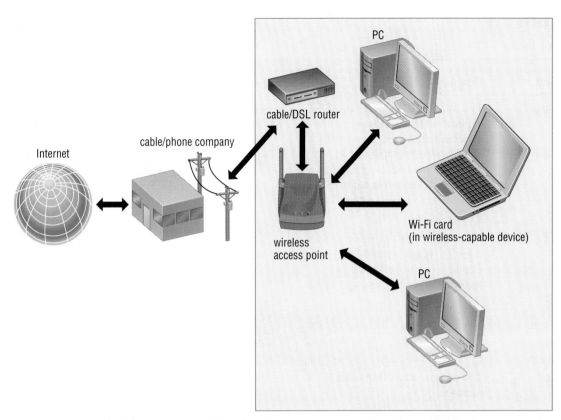

Wi-Fi–enabled devices can use a broadband Internet connection through a wireless access point.

Figure 2.5 A Wireless Network

using an email client, which is software designed specifically for email. Examples of email clients include Outlook, Eudora, and Windows Mail (previously called Outlook Express in Windows XP). Windows Mail and Outlook Express are free with the respective operating system. Client software is installed on your computer and, generally speaking, you must use your own computer to access your email.

The email type is determined by the email provider, not the user. If you use email provided by AOL, you must access it through the AOL Web site. If you have an email account that uses an email client, information for setting up the account will be provided by your Internet Service Provider or by your employer. Important email terms and commands are described in Table 2.5.

Email has its own form of "etiquette," which is a set of guidelines for promoting good communication and good will. Email exchanged between your employer and colleagues should always be handled in a business-like manner. Below is a list of basic email manners:

- Place the email address of the primary recipient(s) in the To: line. If you would like others to receive the email but do not expect them to reply, place their names in the Cc: line (courtesy copy). If you are sending an email to a large number of people, place your own email address in the To: line and place all the other names in the Bcc: line (blind courtesy copy).
- Do not use Reply All unless everyone is expecting or needing a reply.
- When forwarding email that was originally sent to a group of people, remove the email addresses from the message area of the forwarded copy.
- In order to keep up with the conversation, it is helpful to have previous messages (the message string) included in your reply. Including the relevant section from the original message helps the recipient place your reply in context. Set this option in your email program or copy and

Table 2.5

Email Terms

Term	Meaning	Term	Meaning
Inbox	The folder within an email application that receives incoming email messages. This term is a throwback to a traditional office setup where new papers to be reviewed were placed in a box labeled "In," completed work was placed in a box labeled "Out."	Forward	The command used to create a new email message using the text and attachments of another message. No addresses are automatically inserted in a forwarded message (as they are with Reply and Reply All). The abbreviation FWD: is typically inserted at the beginning of the Subject line.
To, Cc, Bcc	The address lines of an email message. To: is the primary recipient. The abbreviations cc: and bcc: stand for courtesy copy and blind courtesy copy.	Attachment	A file that accompanies an email message. The attachment is not part of the text of the message but is carried along for the ride. The icon representing an attachment is a paper clip.
Subject line	The text area in which to type the content or purpose of an email message.	String	A message and its replies—a way of describing a conversation by email.
Send	The command used to transmit a message.	Email server	A computer, operated by an Internet Service Provider, that handles email messages for all addresses on the same domain. Email addresses are always written in the format username@domain. (No spaces are ever allowed; capitalization does not matter.)
Receive	The command to retrieve messages from an email server.		
Reply	The command used to send a return message to the address that sent the original message. The original sender's email address is automatically inserted in the To: line of the reply message. The abbreviation Re: is usually filled in at the Subject line automatically to indicate the message is a reply.	Address book/ Contact list	A database associated with an email program for storing commonly used email addresses.
Reply All	The command used to send a return message to all email addresses that were included in the original message.		

paste pertinent parts of an email message into your reply.

- Use a meaningful and specific subject line that will allow the recipients to know the reason for your message and to prioritize his or her replies. Good subject lines allow recipients to easily sort and organize mail by topic.
- Do not use ALL CAPS when composing a message. This is considered yelling. Setting an occasional word in caps for emphasis is acceptable.

- For non-urgent messages, replies within 24 to 48 hours are considered reasonable. Also, replying immediately to confirm receipt of a message with a note stating you will write back as soon as possible is always appreciated. Your employer will expect prompt replies to messages concerning work assignments.
- Use common typefaces such as Callibri (Word 2007's default font), Arial, or Times New Roman. Avoid using stationery.

- Be sure to sign your email with your full name and contact information.
- Proof your email before you send it. Read the entire message for clarity and check for spelling errors. If you are answering an email, review the original message to make sure you are actually addressing the sender's question and that you have covered all necessary points. Poor spelling and grammar, even in an email message, will reflect negatively on your skills as an MT.
- Never escalate an argument or misunderstanding by firing off an angry email.

File Transfers

One of the most valuable aspects of the Internet is the ability to instantly move information from one place to another. Small files (individual files or aggregates of less than one megabyte) are often transferred by way of email attachments, but large audio dictation files and multiple transcribed documents are typically sent using other methods such as File Transfer Protocol (FTP). This method creates a direct connection between two computers and is the most secure and reliable method for transferring files, provided access to the site is password-protected. When moving files between two computers, the term download refers to the movement of files *toward* you and upload refers to the movement of files *away* from you.

Internet Explorer has minimal FTP capability built in, but does not offer sufficient controls necessary for routine use by medical transcriptionists. FTP software (also called an FTP client) provides better file management and more sophisticated control of file transfers. FTP clients are not expensive, and some can be downloaded from the Internet free of charge. To transfer files (e.g., sound files or documents), you will need an FTP "site" (also referred to as an FTP folder) located on an FTP server. Small businesses typically lease FTP sites from a computer services company. Larger companies with access to technical expertise establish their own FTP servers. To establish a connection and transfer files, open the FTP client software and fill in the FTP site name, username, and password. (This information will be supplied by the owner of the FTP server.) Once the connection is established, use the appropriate software commands to upload or download files. To transfer files between two individual workstations, the files are first uploaded to the FTP site and then downloaded or "retrieved" by the other user; the FTP site serves as a mutual access point between two workstations.

Some transcription software programs have FTP capability built-in, making it easy to retrieve sound files from an FTP site and then upload transcribed documents. Most large transcription companies use transcription management software that has FTP capability built in, making transfers "transparent" to the transcriptionist. Your employer will give you specific instructions on how to access files, but an understanding of FTP concepts is helpful.

Encryption

If you establish your own transcription service, you will need to use file encryption when sending personal health information (PHI) over the Internet, especially via email. PHI includes transcribed documents, audio files, and patient appointment sheets (provided to the MT by the clinic or hospital and used to verify patient names and date of service). Most small-business owners use an encryption service, since establishing an encryption protocol can be costly and requires technical expertise. Email encryption services are easy to use and cost-effective. Large transcription services and hospitals include encryption technology in their transcription management platforms, making the process transparent to the transcriptionist.

Facsimiles

Facsimiles (faxes) are still used extensively in the medical community. Healthcare facilities often send patient schedules (also called census sheets) to transcriptionists to aid with patient demographic information, such as the correct spelling of the patient's name, medical record number, date of birth, and other data needed to accurately transcribe medical reports. The transcriptionist may be required to routinely or occasionally fax a completed transcript to the dictator or to another physician caring for the patient. Always use a cover sheet when faxing reports and carefully confirm all fax numbers so information is not routed to the wrong recipient.

Exercise 2.9   The Ups and Downs

Define the terms *upload* and *download* in relation to moving files on an FTP site.

_____

_____

_____

Exercise 2.10   Making the Connection

What do these letters stand for?

1. LAN _____

2. WAN _____

3. ISP _____

4. WWW _____

5. URL _____

Exercise 2.11   You've Got Mail

Write a definition for the following email terms.

1. email client _____

2. forward _____

3. attachment _____

4. string _____

Computer Security

The ability to connect with anyone anywhere in the world is a major technological step forward that has changed the way every business practices, including medical transcription. But with this universal connectivity also come tremendous security issues. Medical transcriptionists have been guardians of patient confidentiality for years, and that role will no doubt continue as the percentage of Internet-based transcription continues to rise. It is imperative that MTs maintain adequate security measures on their PCs for optimum performance and to conduct business in ways that promote patient safety, privacy, and security. With each new type of security threat, software vendors respond by creating programs to counteract or defend against computer malfeasance. If you work from a home office using your own computer, you must be diligent in your efforts to secure your own computer. MTs who work in hospital transcription departments must follow the guidelines established by the information services department within the hospital. As a hospital employee, you may not be responsible for installing, updating, or otherwise managing security software, but you should be aware of the various types of security threats and understand basic security measures. No security software is 100% reliable or capable of detecting all possible threats, so every computer user should be cautious and skeptical, especially when receiving or responding to email messages or visiting Web sites. Regardless of your employment situation, security software will affect the way you use your computer and may sacrifice computer functionality in favor of safety.

In addition to using appropriate software for computer security, MTs working from a home office must restrict the use of their computer to transcription- and business-related tasks only. Computer hobbies such as shopping or exchanging music, playing Internet games, and other non-business activities should be conducted on a separate computer. Be extremely cautious about downloading free software, utilities, emoticons, coupons, and toolbars from the Internet. Do not share your transcription computer with anyone else in the household or allow anyone else to use it.

Viruses

Viruses consist of programing code intended to harm or disrupt the normal operation of a computer or a computer application. Viruses can be passed from one computer to another by embedding the malicious code in email messages, email attachments, and Web sites. Antivirus software is used to detect malicious programming and prevent it from harming the computer. Once installed, virus detection software must be updated weekly and subscriptions for updates renewed yearly in order to recognize any new threats.

Spam

Spam is unsolicited and unwanted email. A large number of spam messages can clog an email box, obscuring legitimate email. Spam is also a significant source of fraudulent schemes and phishing (baiting) ploys, which are attempts to get you to divulge confidential and/or financial information. Evaluate email with extreme skepticism and use spam-filtering software to decrease unwanted email.

Malware

Malware includes any software with malicious or undesirable intent such as adware or spyware. These types of software are capable of transmitting information on your PC without your permission as well as opening your system to hackers. Malware is typically a hidden payload with "free" software downloaded from the Internet. This type of unscrupulous software can present privacy and security issues for you and the patient reports stored on your computer. Malware can significantly reduce your computer's response time and performance. Windows Vista installs with Windows Defender, which will detect and remove malware. Windows XP users will need to purchase a software product designed specifically for this purpose. Free or low-cost detection software downloaded from the Internet is usually inadequate.

Windows Updates

Microsoft routinely issues software updates and service packs to seal security holes discovered since the software was first released. From the Control Panel, access Windows' Security Center to enable Automatic Updates. Be sure to maintain these updates at least weekly.

Firewall

Firewalls monitor information coming and going from your computer. A firewall is included with Windows and should remain enabled at all times. View the status of your firewall settings in the Security Center located in the Windows Control Panel.

Passwords

The use of passwords can also hinder security threats by network hackers or individuals who have direct access to your computer. Windows can be password-enabled, requiring a password to log on. When stepping away from the PC, "lock" your PC or set the PC to "sleep" after several minutes of inactivity, requiring a password to return to active work. Pass-

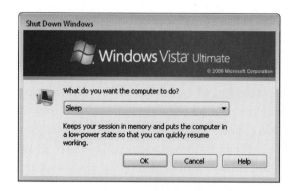

By selecting Sleep in the Shut Down Windows dialog box, the computer screen will go to black, and a password will need to be provided to gain access to the files again.

words should be changed routinely (every 60–90 days) and should be difficult to guess or decipher. "Strong" passwords consist of 6–8 characters, use a mixture of numbers and letters, alternate upper and lowercase letters, and are not related to commonly known information about the user such as name, date of birth, address, or telephone number. Passwords should be written down but stored out of sight and in a secure place.

Exercise 2.12   Anticipating Consequences

Explain the consequences of poor computer maintenance leading to computer failure.

1. How might this affect you? _____

    _____

2. How might this affect patient care? _____

    _____

3. How might this affect your employer? _____

    _____

Injury Prevention

Medical transcription is obviously a sedentary occupation. Working at a computer for long periods of time can produce sore muscles, headaches, eyestrain, tension, and fatigue. The good news is that you can arrange your workstation so that it is ergonomically designed and also develop specific habits that will help relieve physical and mental stress.

Posture and Body Mechanics

Maintaining the correct posture to prevent stress or strain on any particular muscle or joint is paramount to working comfortably. Figure 2.6 illustrates the correct monitor and keyboard positions. Provide support for your lower back with a lumbar cushion, a rolled up towel, or a small, thin, firm pillow. To encourage and maintain correct posture while transcribing, position your desk, monitor, keyboard, mouse, and chair with the following considerations in mind:

- Head and neck should be upright, in line with torso, and always facing forward.
- Monitor should be placed at eye level, approximately 20 inches from your eyes.
- Trunk should be straight (not twisted to the right or left) and perpendicular to the floor.

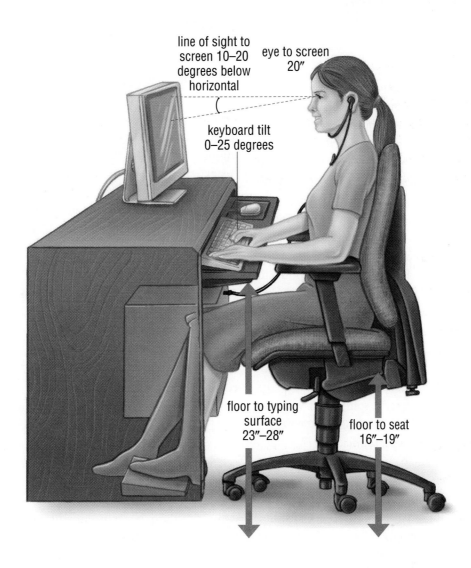

line of sight to screen 10–20 degrees below horizontal

eye to screen 20"

keyboard tilt 0–25 degrees

floor to typing surface 23"–28"

floor to seat 16"–19"

Figure 2.6   Correct Monitor and Keyboard Position

- Shoulders and upper arms should be close to the body and relaxed, not extended forward or raised upward. Elbows should be held close to the body.
- Forearms, wrists, and hands should be straight with forearms at about a 90-degree angle with the upper arm.
- Wrists should be level and should not angle outward toward the small fingers.
- Thighs should be parallel to the floor with lower legs perpendicular to the floor.
- Feet should rest flat on the floor or on a footrest.
- Bookshelves should be close by and positioned so as to prevent bending and twisting motions when reaching for books, especially large, heavy text books and dictionaries.

Computer Equipment

Choose computer equipment that promotes good posture and body mechanics as explained above. There are many keyboard and mouse designs to choose from. There is no particular style that is perfectly suited for transcription. Some MTs find the ergonomic, split-design keyboard very helpful; others do not. It may require some trial and error to find the keyboard that works best for you. Placement of the keyboard to meet the above posture requirements may be more important than the actual design of the keyboard. The mouse should fit comfortably under your hand and be placed so that you do not bend the wrist in any direction when using the mouse. As with the keyboard, placement may play a larger role than shape. Wrist rests for both the mouse and the keyboard may prove helpful for supporting the arms and keeping the wrists straight. Consider using wrist splints that will support the wrist and prevent "kinking" of the nerves that pass through the carpal tunnel.

The monitor should be large enough to comfortably see at a distance of about 20 inches. Larger flat-panel monitors take up much less space on the desktop than their CRT predecessors and are ideal for transcription. Items often overlooked are the level and direction of lighting. Lower lighting can be used for work limited to the computer. Lighting should be directed at the desktop and not the monitor. Move

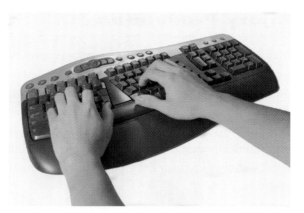

An ergonomically designed keyboard can reduce pain and injury.

your monitor away from the window or use drapes, blinds, or an antiglare screen. Adjust the intensity of the monitor to avoid a sharp contrast between the monitor lighting and the ambient light.

The Occupational Safety and Health Administration (OSHA) has helpful information on their Web site (www.osha.gov) for establishing a workstation that is designed to prevent occupational injuries. Search the OSHA site using keywords *computer workstation* to find a ergonomic workstation checklist to take with you to the store to evaluate equipment before you purchase. A link is also available at www.emcp.net/MedTrans3e.

Other Health Issues

Protect your eyes. The American Optometric Association recommends a 10-minute break for every hour or two spent staring at a computer screen. You may also take 30-second micro-breaks to focus on distant objects. Use eyeglasses with an antireflective coating to prevent glare. Consult with your eye-care professional about the most appropriate lenses for computer work. Computer workers blink at one fifth the normal rate while they are looking at the screen, causing dry, scratchy eyes. Make a conscious effort to blink more often, or moisten your eyes with a tear substitute (sold at drugstores).

Work in a quiet environment so you will not need to turn up the volume to overcome surrounding noise. Use high-quality earphones that do not create static, distort the sound, or require a high volume setting in order to hear clearly. Prevent ear infections by keeping your earphones clean and not allowing others to use them. If you are using digital audio files and a headset attached directly to your computer, turn off audible notifications in the programs you use, such as email or instant messaging. Turn off warning sounds in Windows to prevent sudden, startling noises directly in your ears. If working with cassette tapes, destroy and throw away old tapes that become worn or noisy.

Fatigue and discomfort are major contributors to decreased production and increased errors. Take short, frequent breaks to rest your eyes, squeeze your shoulders, stretch your back, and shake your arms. Develop a simple stretching routine that you can easily perform at your desk several times a day. Find an outside activity to relieve tension caused by stress. Eat a varied, nutritious diet, exercise regularly, and get enough sleep to improve your alertness, ability to think clearly, and comfort both on and off the job.

Exercise 2.13   Watch Your Back

Use the list of suggestions for creating an ergonomic workstation to evaluate the workstation that you will use while transcribing reports for this course. What pieces of equipment need to be modified or replaced? What personal habits do you need to change in order to prevent injury while transcribing?

_____

_____

_____

Three

Medical Terminology Review

The field of medicine has a specialized language with an enormous vocabulary of words identifying diseases, medical processes and procedures, body structures, and body systems. A solid knowledge of medical terms is essential for working in a healthcare environment.

Objectives

» Acquire basic knowledge of medical terms and their elements.

» Learn how the elements of terminology can be interchanged to meet specific needs.

» Become familiar with terms that map the human body.

» Learn the directional and positional terms used in diagnosis.

» Recognize the diagnostic importance of color and pain sensations and modern medical imaging procedures.

» Understand the basis of disease and the forms of treatment, including terminology related to pharmacology and surgical instruments.

Word Parts and How They Are Combined

A prerequisite for learning medical transcription is a course in medical terminology. In that course you learned many words and how they are used. Most importantly, you learned word parts and how they are combined to form a complete term. In this section you will find a brief review of some common root words, combining vowels and forms, prefixes, and suffixes. You will also find techniques for expanding your medical vocabulary throughout this course.

Root Words and Combining Forms

Root words provide the foundation of the medical term and are the source of its meaning. Each body system has a core of root words that will be provided in each of the sections of this book. Adding a combining vowel to a root word creates a word part called a combining form. These vowels make it easier to spell and pronounce medical terms and serve as links for root words when more than one root is needed to form the term. Additionally, a combining vowel may be used to join a root word and a suffix. Root words may be added to each other and function equally to serve as the foundation or contribute to the meaning of the original root. Table 3.1 provides a list of common root words and combining forms that you should know.

Prefixes

A prefix is a word part that comes before the root and begins the term. Prefixes further modify the root or roots; they often give an indication of direction, time, or orientation. Table 3.2 provides a list of common prefixes.

Suffixes

A suffix provides an ending that modifies and gives specific meaning to the root word. The suffixes presented in Tables 3.3, 3.4, and 3.5 are grouped by type: general; conditions, symptoms, or diagnoses; and procedures. Many of the anatomic and physiologic terms for each body system include one of the general suffixes, while names of conditions and diagnoses tend to use one of the condition-related suffixes that indicate disease actions. A special group of suffixes for procedures relate to some type of surgical cutting.

Suffixes are also used to create plural forms of words. In medical terminology, plural word forms can be confusing unless you understand one simple aspect: some plural terms are formed on the basis of Greek and Latin rules, while others are formed using English language rules. In English, plurals usually are constructed by simply adding *s* or *es* to the singular form (the plural of vein is veins). With Latin- and Greek-based words, plurals are formed by adding an ending based on the ending of the singular form (*stria,* meaning a discolored stripe on the skin, becomes *striae* as a plural). Singular words ending in *um* take an *a* in the plural form (*diverticulum,* a pouch or sac that has developed within the gut or bladder, becomes *diverticula* as a plural). Words ending in *nx* take an *nges* ending as plurals (*larynx,* part of the throat, becomes *larynges*).

The rules do not apply consistently, however, and for that reason the best strategy is to memorize the plural spelling for each new word you learn. Whenever you are uncertain of the correct plural form of a term, consult your medical dictionary. Table 3.6 lists some of the common plural forms.

Suggestions for Learning Medical Terms

In each specialty chapter in Part 2 of this text, a list of vocabulary terms that relate to the specialty is provided in a feature called the Terms Bank. Each term is listed with a definition and a pronunciation key. Note also that the word's part of speech is included in parentheses—for example, (n) for noun and (adj) for adjective; (pl) stands for plural. Words that are included in the transcription activities are highlighted in order to help you focus your study of these terms.

Every vocabulary word that may be difficult to pronounce is displayed with a phonetic pronunciation. As is common in dictionaries, the words are broken into syllables (indicated by hyphens), and **boldface** letters indicate which syllable(s) should receive the emphasis when you say the word out loud. The letters and letter combinations in Table 3.7 represent specific sounds in the phonetic pronunciations provided throughout this text.

As you study each specialty chapter's Terms Bank, follow these suggestions for learning and expanding your vocabulary.

1. Read and study each word for pronunciation and meaning.
2. Write each unfamiliar word from the list on a notecard, write the definition or a paraphrase of the definition on the back, and draw a simple picture to help you learn the word.

3. Study the pronunciation, spelling, and definition of each word on your notecard, then key each word twice for reinforcement. Check the spelling.
4. Add the terms to your word processor's spell checker.

Table 3.1

Common Root Words and Combining Forms

Root Word	Combining Form	Meaning	Root Word	Combining Form	Meaning
abdomin-	abdomin/o	abdomen	hepat-	hepat/o	liver
angi-	angi/o	vessel	irid-	irid/o	iris
bacteri-	bacteri/o	bacteria	kerat-	kerat/o	cornea; horny, hard
bi-	bi/o	life (Greek derivation)	lip-	lip/o	fat
			mast-	mast/o	breast
carcin-	carcin/o	cancer; cancerous	necr-	necr/o	death
cardi-	cardi/o	heart	nephr-	nephr/o	kidney
cephal-	cephal/o	head	onc-	onc/o	tumor
cyst-	cyst/o	sac or cyst containing fluid; urinary bladder	path-	path/o	disease
			pelv-	pelv/o	pelvic
cyt-	cyt/o	cell	radi-	radi/o	x-rays
electr-	electr/o	electricity	ren-	ren/o	renal, kidney
enter-	enter/o	intestines	sarc-	sarc/o	flesh
fibrin-	fibrin/o	fiber	sial-	sial/o	saliva, salivary glands
gnath-	gnath/o	jaw			
gynec-	gynec/o	woman, female	thromb-	thromb/o	clot
hem-	hem/o	blood	trache-	trache/o	trachea
hemat-	hemat/o	blood	uter-	uter/o	uterus

Table 3.2

Common Prefixes

Prefix	Meaning	Example	Prefix	Meaning	Example
a-	without, not, no	apnea—without breathing	con-	with; together	consanguineous—with blood (common ancestry)
an-		anhydrous—without water	sym-		symbiotic—with life
ab-	away from	abnormality—away from normal	syn-		synergy—with energy
ad-	toward, to, near	adduction—toward the center	de-	away from; down; removal of; cessation	decalcify—removal of calcium
ambi-	both	ambidextrous—use of both hands	dia-	across, through, completely	diathermy—through heat
ante-	before; forward; in front of	antepartum—before labor or childbirth	trans-		transurethral—across the urethra
pre-		prenatal—before birth	dis-	apart; separate	disease—separate from ease
pro-		procephalic—anterior part (before) of the head	dys-	faulty; painful; difficult; abnormal	dysuria—painful urination
anti-	against; opposed to	antibiotic—against bacteria	e-	out; away	efferent—conduction away from
contra-		contraindication—opposed to a certain treatment	ec-		ectomorphic—away from form
auto-	self	autoimmune—immunity to self	ex-		excrete— separate, cast out
bi-	two (Latin derivation); both	bilateral—both sides	ecto-	outside; away from	ectoderm—outer layer of skin
di-		didactylism—condition of two digits on a hand or foot	exo-		exothermic—release of heat
			extra-		extracellular—outside the cell
bio-	life	biology—study of life	en-	inside; within	enclosed—contained within
brady-	slow	bradycardia—slow heart rate	endo-		endocardium—innermost layer (lining) of the heart
circum-	around, surrounding; circular movement	circumorbital—around the orbit (eye)			
peri-		pericardium—around the heart	intra-	within; into	intra-abdominal—within the abdomen

continued

Table 3.2

Common Prefixes—continued

Prefix	Meaning	Example
epi-	upon; above; on	epigastric—upon (above) the stomach
eu-	normal or good	eupnea—normal breathing
hemi-	half	hemicardia—half of the heart (right or left)
semi-		semilunar—half moon
hyper-	above; excessive; extreme	hyperkalemia—excess potassium (in the blood)
hypo-	deficient; below	hypoglycemia—low blood sugar
infra-	under; below	inframammary—below the breast
sub-		subdural—below the dura mater
inter-	between	intercellular—between cells
mal-	bad	malaise—bad comfort; discomfort
meso-	middle	mesophlebitis—inflammation of the middle layer of the wall of a vein
meta-	beyond; after; change	metastasis—extension of disease from one part of the body to another
micro-	small	microcardia—small heart
mono-	one	mononuclear—one nucleus
uni-		unilateral—one side
neo-	new	neonatal—new birth
pachy-	thick; heavy	pachyderma—thick skin

Prefix	Meaning	Example
pan-	all	panimmunity—immune to all diseases
para-	abnormal; alongside; beside	paracystic—alongside the bladder
per-	through	percutaneous—through the skin
poly-	many	polycythemia—many red blood cells
multi-		multidisciplinary—many areas of study
post-	after	postmortem—after death
quadri-	four	quadriplegic—paralysis of all four limbs
tetra-		tetradactylism—condition of only four digits on a hand or foot
re-	again; back	resorb—absorb again
retro-	backward; behind	retroflexion—backward bending
sub-	under; below	subvaginal—below the vagina
super-	above; excessive	superficial—near the surface
supra-	outside; beyond	suprascleral—outside the sclera
tachy-	fast	tachycardia—rapid heart rate
tri-	three	trigeminy—three abnormal heartbeats
ultra-	beyond; excessive	ultrasonic—excessive sound

Table 3.3
Most Commonly Used General Suffixes

Suffix	Meaning	Example
-ac	pertaining to	hemophiliac—pertaining to an individual with hemophilia
-al		temporal—pertaining to the temporal lobe of the brain
-ar		clavicular—pertaining to the clavicle
-ry		sensory—pertaining to the senses
-eal		esophageal—pertaining to the esophagus
-ic		gastric—pertaining to the stomach
-ose		adipose—relating to fat
-ous		cutaneous—pertaining to the skin
-tic		spermatic—pertaining to sperm
-blast	immature	osteoblast—immature bone cell
-cyte	cell	osteocyte—bone cell
-e	noun marker (indicates this form of the word is a noun)	melanocyte—pigment-producing skin cell
-gram	record	electroencephalogram—record of brain activity
-graph	instrument for recording	electroencephalograph—instrument for recording brain activity
-graphy	process of recording	electrocardiography—process of recording the electrical activity of the heart
-meter	instrument for measuring	arthrometer—instrument for measuring motion in a joint

Suffix	Meaning	Example
-metry	process of measuring	arthrometry—process of measuring joint motion
-iatric	treatment	psychiatric—treatment of the psyche
-iatry	study of	psychiatry—study of the psyche
-logy	study of	urology—study of urine
-logist	one who specializes in the treatment or study of	cardiologist—one who specializes in the treatment or study of the heart
-icle	small	ventricle—small pouch or cavity, particularly within the heart or brain
-ole	small	arteriole—small artery
-ula		macula—small spot
-ule		pustule—small lesion (pimple) with pus
-ium / -eum	tissue or structure	periosteum—structure surrounding bone
-ize	make; use; subject to	anesthetize—subject to anesthesia
-ate		impregnate—make pregnant
-or	one who	mediator—one who mediates
-poiesis	formation	erythropoiesis—formation of red blood cells
-scope	instrument for examining	cystoscope—instrument for examining the bladder
-scopy	examination	cystoscopy—examination of the bladder
-stasis	stop; stand still; control	hemostasis—stop bleeding

Table 3.4

Suffixes Related to Conditions, Symptoms, or Diagnoses

Suffix	Meaning	Example
-algia	pain	myalgia—muscle pain
-cele	pouch; sac; hernia	cystocele—hernia of the bladder
-dynia	pain	arthrodynia—pain in a joint
-emesis	vomit	hyperemesis—excessive vomiting
-emia	condition of blood	anemia—condition of insufficient red blood cells
-form	like; resembling	vermiform—resembling worm-shaped vermin
-genesis	beginning; origin; production	pathogenesis—origin of disease
-genic	beginning; origin; production	pyogenic—production of pus
-ia	condition of	dysuria—condition of painful urination
-iasis	formation of; presence of	lithiasis—formation of stone
-ism	condition of	hirsutism—condition of excessive hair
-itis	inflammation	tendinitis—inflammation of a tendon
-lysis	breaking down	hemolysis—breaking down of blood
-malacia	softening	osteomalacia—softening of bone
-megaly	enlargement	cardiomegaly—enlargement of the heart
-oid	like; resembling	osteoid—resembling bone
-oma	tumor	osteoma—tumor of bone
-osis	condition	psychosis—condition of the psyche
-penia	abnormal reduction; lack of	leukocytopenia—abnormal reduction of white blood cells

Suffix	Meaning	Example
-phage	eat; devour	macrophage—large cell that devours
-phagia	eat; devour	geophagia—eating dirt
-phagy	eat; devour	aerophagy—swallowing air
-phile	attraction for; love for	pedophile—abnormal adult attraction to children
-philia		hemophilia—attraction for blood
-phobia	fear of	photophobia—fear of light
-plasia	formation; growth	dysplasia—faulty formation
-pnea	breathing	apnea—without breathing
-ptosis	drooping; falling or downward displacement	mastoptosis—drooping breast
-rrhage	to burst forth	hemorrhage—bursting forth of blood
-rrhagia		hemorrhagia—condition of bleeding
-rrhagic		hemorrhagic—relating to condition of bleeding
-rrhea	discharge; flow	amenorrhea—absence of menstrual flow
-rrhexis	rupture; breaking	trichorrhexis—breaking of hair
-spasm	involuntary contraction	laryngospasm—involuntary contraction of the larynx
-trophy	development; nourishment	hypertrophy—excess development (enlargement)
-y	condition; process of	ambulatory—process of ambulation (walking)

Table 3.5

Suffixes Related to Procedures

Suffix	Meaning	Example
-centesis	puncture to remove fluid	amniocentesis—puncture of the amniotic membrane to remove fluid
-desis	binding	arthrodesis—binding of a joint
-ectomy	excision; surgical removal	splenectomy—removal of the spleen
-pexy	surgical suspension or fixation	uteropexy—surgical fixation of the uterus
-plasty	surgical repair or reconstruction	hernioplasty—surgical repair of a hernia
-rrhaphy	suture	myorrhaphy—suture of muscle
-stomy	surgical creation of an artificial opening	colostomy—creation of an artificial opening in the colon
-tomy	incision	tracheotomy—incision into the trachea
-tripsy	crushing	lithotripsy—crushing of stones

Table 3.7

Phonetic Pronunciation Chart

Symbol	Pronunciation
a	the short a as in can
ay	the long a as in cane
ah	ah as in father
ai	ai as in fair
ar	ar as in far
aw	aw as in fall
e	the short e as in pen
ee	the long e as in me
i	the short i as in pin
I	the long i as in pine
o	the short o as in not
O	the long o as in note
oo	oo as in food
or	or as in for
ow	ow as in cow
oy	oy as in boy
u	the short u as in run
yoo	the long u as in cube
zh	zh as in casual

Table 3.6

Frequently Used Plural Forms

Singular	Ending	Plural
apex	-ex/-ices	apices
appendix	-ix/-ices	appendices
bacterium	-ium/-ia	bacteria
cardiopathy	-y/-ies	cardiopathies
condyloma	-a/-ata	condylomata
diagnosis	-is/-es	diagnoses
fungus	-us/-i	fungi
phenomenon	-on/a	phenomena
thorax	-ax/-aces	thoraces
vertebra	-a/-ae	vertebrae

Give the definition for each of the following word parts.

Suffixes

1. -iasis _____

2. -emesis _____

3. -phile _____

4. -malacia _____

5. -itis _____

6. -oid _____

7. -trophy _____

8. -rrhea _____

9. -ptosis _____

10. -phobia _____

Prefixes

11. tri- _____

12. pre- _____

13. brady- _____

14. auto- _____

15. dys- _____

16. syn- _____

17. bio- _____

18. ambi- _____

19. anti- _____

20. an- _____

Divide each of the following terms into prefixes, combining forms, and suffixes. Then define each term. You may need to look up some of the terms in a medical dictionary.

	Word Parts	**Meaning**
1. abdominocentesis	_____	_____
2. angiogram	_____	_____
3. melanocyte	_____	_____
4. carditis	_____	_____
5. cephalgia	_____	_____
6. cytorrhexis	_____	_____
7. dysuria	_____	_____
8. osteocyte	_____	_____
9. epigastric	_____	_____
10. esophageal	_____	_____
11. fibroid	_____	_____
12. gastric	_____	_____
13. hemigastrectomy	_____	_____
14. intracranial	_____	_____
15. urology	_____	_____

For this exercise, write a question using a medical term for each definition (What is ...?). Some of the word parts are provided. Reference the tables in this chapter and a medical dictionary as needed.

Diagnostic and Procedural Terms

-ectomy	mast-	oste-
-genic	-megaly	-otomy
hyper-	neo-	-phagy
-itis	-oma	-ptosis

1. excess development or enlargement _____

2. origin of or producing pus _____

3. inflammation of a tendon _____

4. bone tumor _____

5. enlargement of the heart _____

6. swallowing (eating) air _____

7. drooping breast _____

8. incision into the trachea _____

9. removal of the spleen _____

10. immediately after birth _____

Medical Specialties

cardi-	gastroenter-	neur-
dermat-	nephr-	

11. study of the heart _____

12. study of skin _____

13. study of the kidneys _____

14. study of the digestive system _____

15. study of nerves _____

Circle the proper noun in each sentence. Indicate whether the proper term is singular or plural.

1. When the physician examined the patient, he heard (rhonchi/rhonchus) in the lower lung fields.

2. The x-ray revealed obstruction in each of the (bronchus/bronchi).

3. After using the inhaler, the patient's (alveolus/alveoli) were cleared.

4. It was easy to see the single (hypha/hyphae) under the microscope.

5. The patient was infected with two types of (fungus/fungi).

6. The infant's left (naris/nares) was occluded.

7. The 3rd thoracic (vertebra/vertebrae) was injured in the accident.

8. The students reviewed the x-rays and became familiar with observing different sizes of (thorax/thoraces/thoraxes) of hundreds of patients.

9. There were lesions noted at both of the (apex/apices/apexes) of the lungs.

10. When looking at the eyes, the examiner notes whether the (conjunctiva/conjunctivae) in each eye is clear.

Anatomical Terms That Map the Human Body

The human body is a living organism made up of tiny microscopic cells to large systems that work together to make the body function. There are medical terms used to describe every part of the body—each cell, cavity, region, division—providing a map of the exact place and structure of that part. This section will describe the terms that are used to depict these elements and where they are located.

Levels of Organization

After the cell was defined as the unit of life in the human body, researchers could picture the way groups of cells make up a tissue, a group of tissues make up a body organ, and the organs make up functional systems such as the nervous system, the gastrointestinal system, the urinary system, and others. This concept is known as the *levels of organization* (see Figure 3.1). Note that each level becomes larger, or more complex, than the one below it.

As a foundation for your study of body systems, you will learn the general, whole-body terminology that you need to build your vocabulary of individual body system words. Transcription work for the specialty chapters in Part 2 will apply this terminology. Generally the terms related to cells and tissues and their structure are found in the transcribed pathology reports. Operative reports contain terms related to tissues and organs.

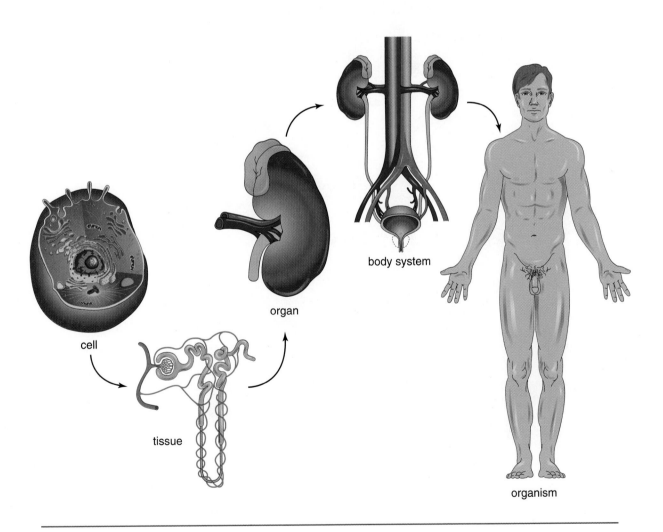

cell

tissue

organ

body system

organism

Figure 3.1   Levels of Organization

Cells   Cytology is the study of cells, including their origin, structure, functions, and pathology. (You may recall that the combining form *cyt/o* means "cell" and the suffix *-logy* means "study of.") The cell is the basic unit of all living things and is the smallest unit capable of independent life and reproduction (see Figure 3.2). All cells have certain similarities, but cells in the human body are highly specialized. Each has its own distinct outer membrane that maintains the cell and controls passage of materials into and out of the cell.

Inside the membrane is a substance that early scientists called protoplasm (*protos* = first or origi-nal; *plasma* = substance). Thanks to the discipline of microbiology (*micro-* = small; *bio-* = life; *-logy* = study of), we now know that this substance (cyto-plasm) is actually a collection of structures—called organelles—in a thick, fluidlike matrix. The organelles perform various activities that help maintain the cell and assist with cell reproduction.

The interior of the cell also contains the nucleus, a structure that controls activities of the cell and contains genetic material necessary for reproduction. DNA, or deoxyribonucleic acid, is a chemically complex substance that determines the heritable characteristics and the makeup and function of the cell.

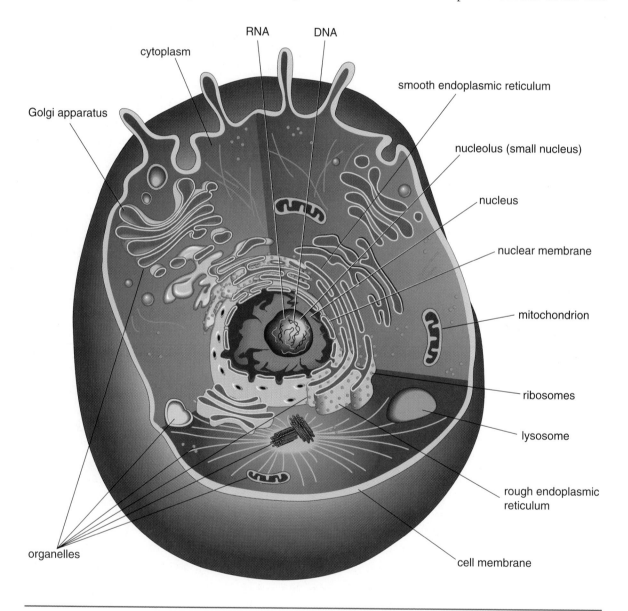

Figure 3.2   Cell Structure

The interior of a cell may also contain food particles (such as fat and starch), pigment granules, and special complexes of protein and vitamins. Humans consist of billions of cells that are grouped together and arranged to form tissues.

Tissues   A tissue is formed by a collection of specialized cells with similar structures and functions. A nonliving material called intercellular matrix joins the cells and fills the spaces between them. The matrix contains special substances, such as electrolytes, salts, and fibers, that give the tissue unique characteristics. Histology is a branch of science specializing in the microscopic study of tissues.

There are four basic types of tissue—epithelial, connective, muscle, and nerve—and the entire body is made up of combinations of these tissues.

- **Epithelial Tissue** Epithelial tissue (*epi-* = upon; above) is found throughout the body and makes up the covering of external and internal surfaces. The skin and the linings of the digestive system, urinary system, and respiratory system are all epithelial tissue. Histologists recognize several types of epithelial tissue and classify them according to the number of cell layers and the shape and other characteristics of the surface layer.
- **Connective Tissue** Connective tissue is the most widespread tissue type in the human body. It forms bones, cartilage, tendons, and ligaments. Connective tissue provides a framework for the body, holds organs in place, connects body parts, and allows for movement of joints. It also supports nerves and capillaries and plays an important role in the body's immune system. Fat, or adipose tissue, is a type of connective tissue that provides for storage of energy in the body and insulates against heat loss.
- **Muscle Tissue** There are three types of muscle tissue: smooth, skeletal or striated, and cardiac. The main function of muscle tissue is contraction, and the three muscle tissue types are categorized as voluntary (under the conscious control of the individual) or involuntary (individual has little or no control over the movement).

    Smooth muscle, which is involuntary, is found in the walls of hollow internal structures—such as the intestines, bladder, blood ves-

sels, and uterus. Skeletal muscle is voluntary and makes up the muscles that are attached to—and move—bones and joints. It is also called striated muscle because, viewed through a microscope, it appears to have stripes, or striae. When seen close up, cardiac muscle tissue also appears to have some striae, but the heart muscle is involuntary (not under conscious control). Found only in the heart, cardiac muscle is specialized to conduct the electrical impulses that cause the heart to contract rhythmically.

- **Nerve Tissue** Nerve tissue makes up the nerves and is specialized to conduct nerve impulses. Its cells are similar to those in cardiac or skeletal muscle tissue; it comprises the brain and spinal cord, in addition to nerves throughout the body.

Organs   These four tissue types—epithelial, connective, muscle, and nerve—combine in varying ways to produce organs, essential body structures that work in harmony within body systems and carry on the specialized functions of a living human. Examples of organs are the heart, liver, pancreas, lungs, stomach, and spleen. Internal organs of the body are called viscera and are located in the various body cavities. Not all organs are internal, and not all are as localized as the heart or liver. For example, sweat glands, hair, and skin are all considered body organs.

Body Systems   A body system is composed of several related organs that work together to perform a complex function. The concept of levels of organization provides scientists with a useful tool for thinking about how all parts of the body function and how the functions are interrelated. The chapters in Part 2 are organized by the medical specialty that refers to each body system.

Body Cavities and Regions

The medical language includes sets of terms commonly used to identify both general and specific areas of the body: body cavities, abdominopelvic regions and quadrants, and spinal column divisions. These terms are used in both verbal and written communication and may accompany diagrams. Table 3.8 lists the major body cavities and the organs or structures they contain and Figure 3.3 illustrates their locations. See Table 3.9 and Figure 3.4 for terminology related to body quadrants and Table 3.10 and Figure 3.5 for terminology related to abdominopelvic regions.

Divisions of the Spinal Column

The back is divided into five regions, corresponding with the divisions of the spinal column, or vertebral column (see Figure 3.6): cervical, thoracic, lumbar, sacral or sacrum, and coccygeal or coccyx. The vertebral column consists of a series of bony structures called vertebrae that encase and protect the spinal cord. There are a total of 24 separate vertebrae (vertebra is the singular form), with two sets of fused parts—five fused parts are in the sacrum and four are in the coccyx. Physicians use these divisional terms to identify problems with the spine and resulting impairments in function. For example, a major spinal cord lesion in the thoracic region (T1-T12) might tell a doctor that the patient is paraplegic (paralyzed in the lower half of the body). Table 3.11 lists the spinal divisions, their location, number of vertebrae, and the abbreviation.

Table 3.8

Body Cavities

Body Cavity	Organs and Structures
abdominal/ abdominopelvic cavity	stomach, liver, gallbladder, spleen, pancreas, small and large intestines
cranial cavity	brain
pelvic cavity	ureters, urinary bladder, urethra *female:* uterus, ovaries, fallopian tubes, vagina *male:* prostate gland, seminal vesicles, ejaculatory duct, vas deferens
spinal cavity	spinal cord
thoracic cavity	lungs, esophagus, trachea, bronchial tubes, thymus gland, aorta, heart

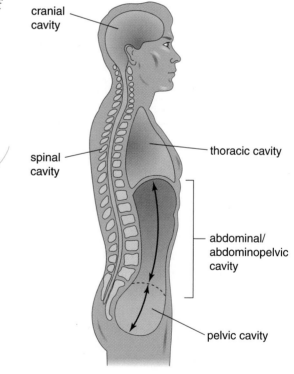

Figure 3.3 Body Cavities

Table 3.9

Body Quadrants

Quadrant	Organs and Structures
right upper quadrant (RUQ)	liver, gallbladder, duodenum, head of pancreas, right kidney and adrenal, hepatic flexure of colon, part of ascending and transverse colon
right lower quadrant (RLQ)	cecum, appendix *female*: right ovary and tube *male*: right ureter and right spermatic cord
left upper quadrant (LUQ)	stomach, spleen, left lobe of liver, body of pancreas, left kidney and adrenal, splenic flexure of colon, part of transverse and descending colon
left lower quadrant (LLQ)	part of descending colon, sigmoid colon *female*: left ovary and tube *male*: left ureter and left spermatic cord

Table 3.10

Abdominopelvic Regions

Region	Description of Location
right hypochondriac	upper right beneath the ribs
left hypochondriac	upper left beneath the ribs
epigastric	upper middle over the stomach
right lumbar	right middle near the waist (in back only)
left lumbar	left middle near the waist (in back only)
umbilical	around the navel
hypogastric	lower middle under the navel
right inguinal	right side near the groin
left inguinal	left side near the groin

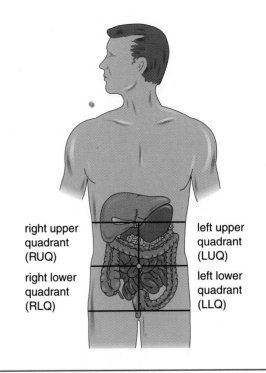

right upper quadrant (RUQ)

left upper quadrant (LUQ)

right lower quadrant (RLQ)

left lower quadrant (LLQ)

Figure 3.4 Body Quadrants

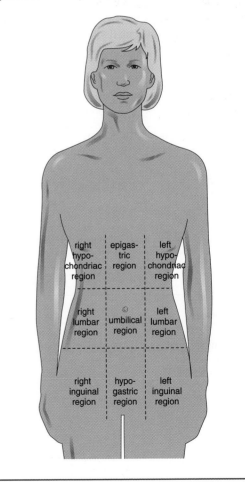

right hypochondriac region

epigastric region

left hypochondriac region

right lumbar region

umbilical region

left lumbar region

right inguinal region

hypogastric region

left inguinal region

Figure 3.5 Abdominopelvic Regions

Table 3.11

The Vertebrae

Spinal Division	Region of the Back	Number of Vertebrae	Abbreviation
cervical	neck	7	C (C1-C7)
thoracic	chest	12	T (T1-T12)
lumbar	loin	5	L (L1-L5)
sacral, sacrum	lower back	5 fused parts	S (S1-S5)
coc-cygeal, coccyx	tailbone	4 fused parts	

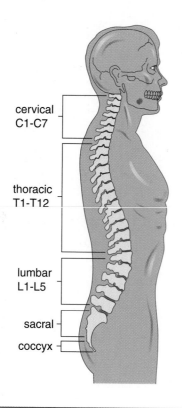

cervical
C1-C7

thoracic
T1-T12

lumbar
L1-L5

sacral

coccyx

Figure 3.6   Spinal Column Regions

Exercise 3.5   State Your Position

Provide definitions for the following positional and directional terms.

1. cephalic_____

2. ventral   _____

3. dorsal   _____

4. medial _____

5. distal _____

6. bilateral_____

7. plantar_____

8. superficial _____

9. parietal _____

10. visceral _____

Exercise 3.6   Use Your X-Ray Vision

Label the diagram with the appropriate cavity name and then list the major organ or organs contained within each body cavity.

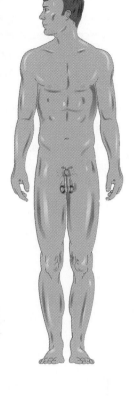

1. cranial cavity _____

2. spinal cavity _____

3. thoracic cavity _____

4. abdominal cavity _____

Exercise 3.7   Back Up What You Say

Identify the spinal division and region of the back that contain the following vertebrae.

1. C4 _____

2. C7 _____

3. T3 _____

4. T5 _____

5. T9 _____

Diagnostic Terms to Assess the Human Body

The language of medical communication includes words that describe the function of the human body as well as the physical parts. There are terms that describe the color of things seen in the body. It is also necessary to understand what the patient is feeling when there are problems that cause pain or discomfort. Further assessment is often needed through the science of medical imaging which provides an inside look at the cavities, tissues, bones, and internal organs.

Directional and Positional Terms

Medical personnel use positions and reference points to communicate about the human body. Anatomic position is used as a reference position in medical communication and assumes that the patient is standing, facing forward, with arms at the sides, palms out, legs straight, and feet flat on the floor with toes pointed forward. Figure 3.7 illustrates this orientation. Imagining a person in anatomic position gives uniform reference points for anyone describing areas of the body. The directional terms provided in Table 3.12 are part of the core medical vocabulary that is used to communicate about every body system.

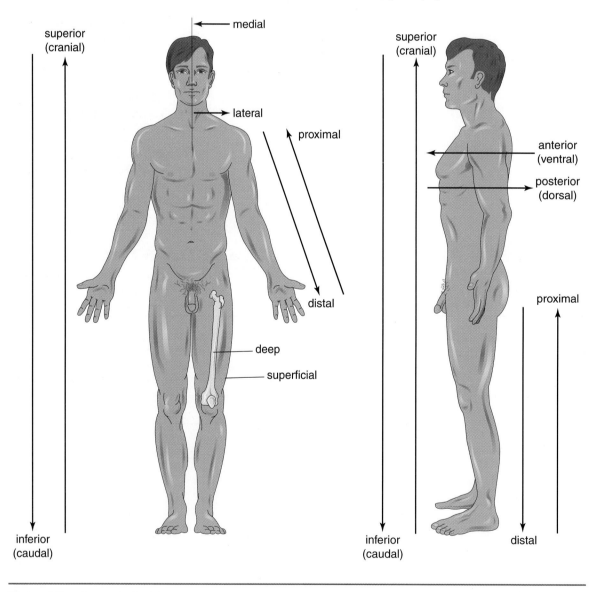

Figure 3.7 Anatomic Position

Table 3.12

Directional Terms

Term	Meaning and Usage	Term	Meaning and Usage
superior or cephalic	toward the head, the surface, or the upper portion of the body The heart is *superior* to the diaphragm.	bilateral	pertaining to both sides of the body or structure The kidneys are positioned *bilaterally* in the lower back.
inferior or caudal	toward the feet or lower portion of the body The kidneys are *inferior* to the adrenal glands.	unilateral	pertaining to only one side of the body or structure The heart is positioned *unilaterally*, on the left side of the chest.
anterior or ventral	toward the front of the body The sternum is *anterior* to the vertebral column.	palmar	pertaining to the palm of the hand The *palmar* surface of the hand may be heavily creased.
posterior or dorsal	toward the back The scapulae (shoulder blades) are *posterior* to the mammary glands.	plantar	pertaining to the sole of the foot The *plantar* surface of the foot is subject to thickening of the skin.
medial	toward the midline or center of the body or structure; The nose is *medial* to the cheekbone.	deep	toward the interior The heart is *deep* within the chest.
lateral	to the side of the body or structure The axilla (armpit) is on the *lateral* aspect of the chest, where the arm and chest join.	superficial	near the surface A scratch on the skin is *superficial*.
proximal	near the center of the body or structure The shoulder is *proximal* to the elbow.	parietal	the wall of a hollow organ or a body cavity The *parietal* peritoneum lines the abdominal cavity.
distal	away from the body The *distal* portion of the femur (thigh bone) is closer to the knee than to the hip.	visceral	the inner covering of the surface of an organ or body cavity The *visceral* peritoneum covers the stomach and other organs of the abdominal cavity.

Directional Planes Another set of terms that serve to describe the body and its parts are directional planes. The directional planes are imaginary cuts slicing through the body at various points and in various directions. Figure 3.8 illustrates the three planes.

- The sagittal plane divides the body into two parts lengthwise (right vs. left), though not necessarily into halves. The term *midsagittal plane* refers to the sagittal plane dividing the body into equal parts, or halves.
- The frontal (or coronal) plane divides the body into front and back sections from top to bottom.

The front side is referred to as anterior or ventral, and the back side is called posterior or dorsal.

- The transverse plane is also called the horizontal plane. It runs parallel to the floor, dividing the body into upper and lower portions. The upper portion is called superior or cephalic; the lower portion is referred to as inferior or caudal.

Movement Terms Figure 3.9 illustrates opposite actions or movements of body parts. Table 3.13 provides definitions and examples of usage.

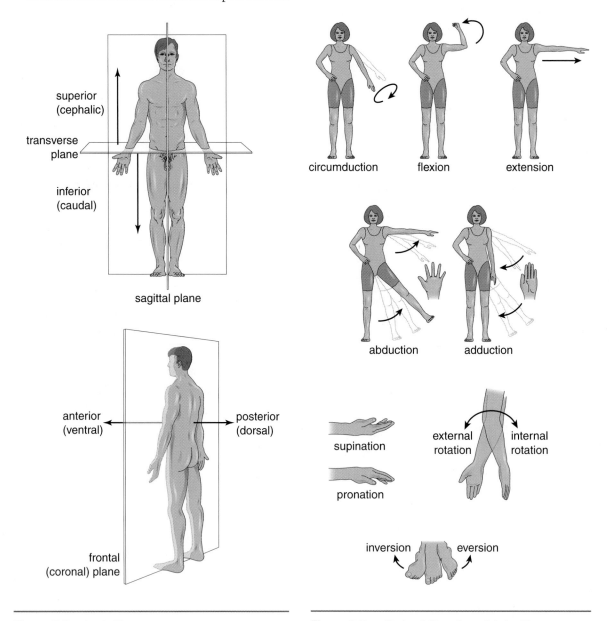

Figure 3.8 Body Planes

Figure 3.9 Skeletal Muscle and Joint Movements

Combining Forms Referring to Color

Combining forms referring to color are used in many areas of science and medicine. Dermatologists apply them to skin lesions, cytologists use them to discuss various cell types, and all physicians employ them to describe both normal and abnormal conditions. Table 3.14 shows the combining forms for color-related terms and gives examples of medical words based on those terms. Figure 3.10 provides examples of the colors.

Pain Assessment

Surveys show that over two-thirds of all American workers, or more than 80 million people, suffer from some sort of pain every year. Additionally, about 15 million Americans working full-time suffer from chronic pain—the ongoing or recurring pain that lasts six months or longer. These statistics have forced healthcare professionals to look closely at pain in their patients—asking questions about pain that they may be experiencing, assessing relief measures taken, and striving to provide adequate pain relief.

Today pain is considered the fifth vital sign, along with temperature, respirations, pulse or heart rate, and blood pressure. It is considered a subjective vital sign, and thus it is not as easily

Table 3.13
Movement Terms

Term	Meaning and Usage
flexion	bending of a joint When the hand is placed on the chest, the elbow is *flexed*.
extension	straightening of a joint When the hand is resting beside the thigh, the elbow is *extended*.
abduction	away from the midline of the body When the legs are spread apart, they are *abducted*.
adduction	toward the midline of the body When the legs are positioned together, they are *adducted*.
eversion	turned outward, frequently used to describe the movement of turning the eyelid outward to expose the inner side When the feet are *everted*, they point outward.
inversion	turned inward When a foot is turned inward, it is *inverted*.

Table 3.14
Color Combining Forms

Combining Form	Meaning	Example
cyan/o	blue	cyanosis: bluish discoloration of skin due to lack of oxygen
erythr/o	red	erythrocyte: red blood cell
leuk/o	white	leukocyte: type of white blood cell
melan/o	black	melanin: pigment portion of the skin
purpur/o	purple	purpura: a condition characterized by hemorrhaging into the skin, causing purple lesions
xanth/o	yellow	xanthopsia: an abnormal visual condition in which all objects appear yellow

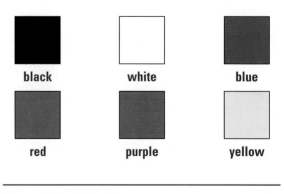

black	white	blue
red	purple	yellow

Figure 3.10 Color Names

measured as the other vital signs. However, when the patient is experiencing pain, there may be an increase in respirations, heart rate, and/or blood pressure. In order to assist the caregiver in assessing a patient's pain, several different scales can be used. Figure 3.11 provides examples of three different pain scales. By using one of these scales the patient can quantify the degree of his or her pain.

Some transcribed documents will include pain as an assessment as well as the pain intervention taken by the healthcare professional. There are many different terms to describe pain, and some of these are listed in Table 3.15. Descriptive terms can reflect the character (description) of the pain and the amount (frequency). The drug list included in each chapter in Part 2 will include pain-relieving medications.

Medical Imaging Terms

Medical imaging is a collective name for x-ray and computerized scanning techniques that permit visualization of the internal structures of the body. In the past, doctors often had to perform surgery just to accurately diagnose a problem inside the body. Advances in medical imaging have made it possible for physicians to view refined, detailed pictures of the body's interior without touching a scalpel. The new equipment and techniques have revolutionized medicine and have made diagnosis more accurate and safer for the patient.

Medical imaging results often appear in medical records as part of the diagnostic work. In hospital patient charts, there may be a separate section for medical imaging reports; in the problem-oriented medical record format, these reports appear in the database section. Although the report, or radiologist's interpretation of the pictures, is physically part of the medical record, the films themselves are usually stored separately from the chart. These films can be damaged or destroyed by exposure to certain substances and environmental conditions, so proper storage is essential. Generally, films are stored in the radiology or medical imaging department. Sometimes a physician requests that old films be retrieved for reinterpretation or comparison with more recent films.

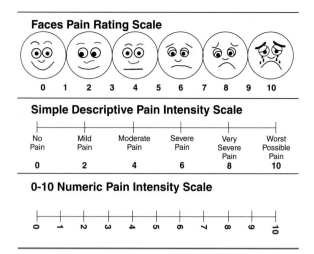

Figure 3.11 Pain Scale

Table 3.15

Terms to Describe Pain

Term	Meaning
ache (achy, aching)	a dull, steady pain
continuous	a pain that does not stop
discomfort (uncomfortable)	a feeling of being uncomfortable
dull	blunted; not sharp; not acute
intense	strong, sharp
intermittent	not continuous; stopping and starting
severe	strong, extreme
sharp	a pain that has a stabbing quality; usually described in one particular spot
stabbing	a pain that may be sharp in quality and stopping and starting
throbbing	a dull, steady pain with an intermittent exacerbation occurring periodically

Today, most medical institutions and practitioners use a PACS (picture archiving and communication system), replacing hard-copy film. A PACS is a computer or network dedicated to the storage, retrieval, distribution, and presentation of images, allowing off-site viewing and reporting of radiology tests, thereby providing quick reporting and turn-around by radiologist and requiring less storage space.

Radiologic imaging includes conventional x-rays and fluoroscopy, sonography (or ultrasound), computed tomography (CT), and magnetic resonance imaging (MRI). In some instances, the term *nuclear medicine* denotes the branch of medicine that uses radioactive emissions to produce images of the body for diagnosing and treating various illnesses.

Radiology   Radiology is the study of x-rays or other imaging modalities to screen for or diagnose abnormalities. X-ray films are produced by exposing sensitized film to the energy waves from an x-ray generator (a cathode ray tube). When part of the body is positioned between an x-ray source and sensitized film, the result is an image—actually a shadow—of that body part. Radiographs appear in various shades of black, white, and gray. The areas where x-rays strike the film directly appear black, whereas areas where the x-rays are blocked (by tissues of varying densities) appear in shades of white or gray. As a result, soft tissue—which is less dense—appears on the film as a shade of gray, and bone—which is relatively dense—appears as a shade of white. The films are usually taken by a technician and interpreted by a radiologist, a physician who specializes in radiology.

Fluoroscopy   Fluoroscopy is an imaging technique that uses a cathode ray tube to allow an observer to view a moving image. It is very similar to the traditional x-ray process, except that x-ray images are typically still, whereas fluoroscopy can provide images of moving body parts. Fluoroscopy is particularly useful in diagnosing problems of the gastrointestinal system and mobile areas or organs. Recording of fluoroscopy images can provide either still pictures or moving pictures (recorded on videotape or motion picture film).

Sonography   Sonography, or ultrasound imaging, uses sound waves above the frequency that can be heard by the human ear to produce images of body structures. A transducer (a device that produces the ultrasound waves) is placed over the body part to be imaged; the sound waves produced partially penetrate the structure to be examined and are reflected back to the transducer. The transducer senses these echoes and converts them into an image. As with fluoroscopy, ultrasound can produce a moving image, and that image can be recorded as a still or moving picture.

Ultrasound technology is used widely in gynecology and obstetrics to examine the uterus and adnexa as well as the developing fetus. Echocardiography is an ultrasound technique used to visualize the structures of the heart, especially the size of the chambers and the function of the valves.

Sound waves hitting a moving object create the Doppler effect, which allows the calculation of the speed and direction of the moving object. Doppler technology is often combined with ultrasonography to evaluate the flow and direction of fluids through vessels and cavities. Doppler color flow techniques display objects (e.g., red blood cells) on a monitor in different colors based on the direction of the object's movement. This technology is especially useful for diagnosing thromboses in the deep veins of the legs. Color flow Doppler combined with echocardiography is used to diagnose regurgitation (backward flow) of blood through the heart valves.

Computed Tomography   Computed tomography (CT) is a medical imaging technique that uses computer interpretations of x-rays to produce images of structures inside the body (see Figure 3.12). The body area is scanned in layers, using x-rays to penetrate the various structures. The computer calculates the densities of the structures from the x-rays and displays the results as an image. Comparing the scans of many layers of a body area produces a highly accurate representation of that area. Sometimes it is

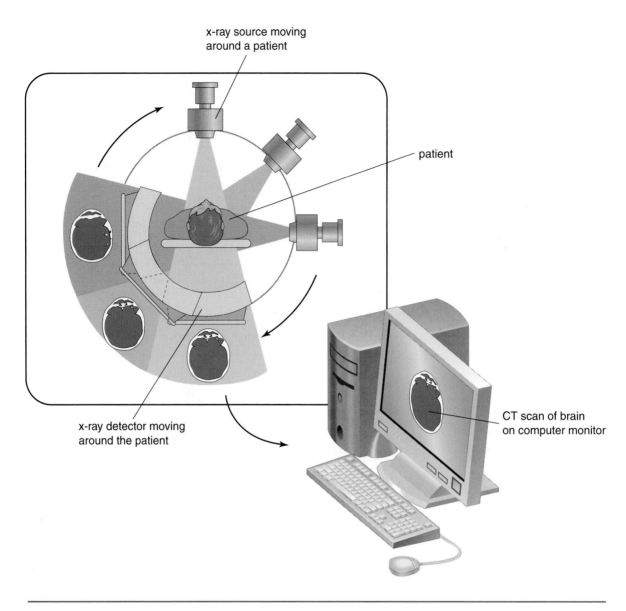

x-ray source moving
around a patient

patient

x-ray detector moving
around the patient

CT scan of brain
on computer monitor

Figure 3.12 Computed Tomography (CT) Scan

necessary to use a contrast medium, or dye, in conjunction with CT scanning to more accurately visualize the area. Positron emission tomography (PET) is a variation of computed tomography. CT scans are useful in delineating soft tissues and for identifying brain hemorrhages.

Magnetic Resonance Imaging   Magnetic resonance imaging (MRI), also called nuclear magnetic resonance (NMR), creates images from computer interpretations of the body's response to a strong magnetic field (see Figure 3.13). The patient is placed within the magnetic field, and the responses of the body's hydrogen atoms in the area being scanned are assessed by a computer to produce a highly accurate three-dimensional image. Since MRI is a noninvasive procedure, as are many of the imaging techniques, it is possible to gather a great deal of information with minimal risk to the patient.

MRI is useful for diagnosing tumors, especially in brain and liver tissue, as well as bone and joint disorders. Magnetic resonance arteriography (MRA) uses MRI technology combined with intravenous gadolinium (for contrast) to evaluate arteries, especially for aneurysms and stenosis.

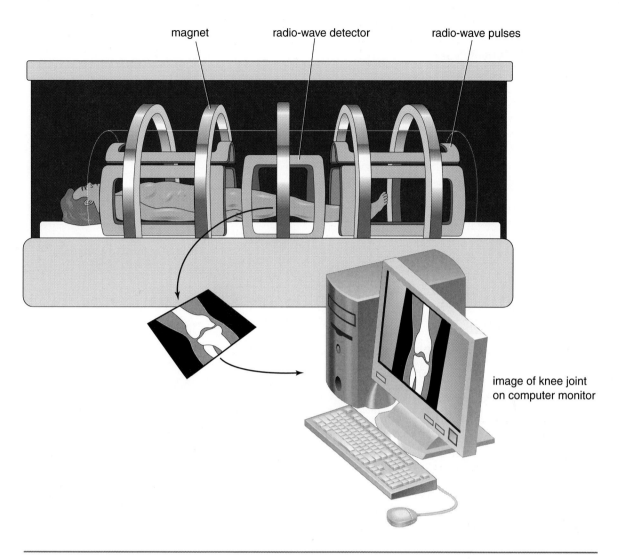

magnet   radio-wave detector   radio-wave pulses

image of knee joint
on computer monitor

Figure 3.13 Magnetic Resonance Imaging (MRI)

Nuclear Medicine Nuclear medicine is a medical specialty that uses radioisotopes for diagnostic and therapeutic purposes. The basic technique involves attaching a radioisotope, often technetium 99, to tracer molecules that are selectively used by different tissue types. After the tracer molecule is injected into the patient, the tracer is given time to be taken up by the tissue. The patient is then scanned using an instrument to detect the radioisotope, and the concentration and distribution of the radioisotope is measured. Areas of higher met-abolic activity take up higher concentrations of the tracer, showing areas of cancer, infection, or other abnormalities. Nuclear medicine techniques show functional changes in the tissues compared to x-ray and MRI techniques, which show structural changes (i.e., shape, size, fracture).

Tables 3.16–3.19 list common terms associated with radiology, nuclear medicine, and diagnostic imaging. Notice that most of the procedural and diagnostic test terms contain the suffixes *-graphy* (process of recording) or *-gram* (record).

Table 3.16

Equipment and Terminology

Terms	Meaning	Terms	Meaning
barium	contrast medium or dye, frequently used to provide enhanced images of body structures	radiogram	image on x-ray film
film	thin sheet of cellulose coated with light-sensitive chemicals used to take photos or x-rays	radioisotope	radioactive form of an element
		roentgen	unit of exposure to radiation (obsolete: replaced by the gray)
gray	international unit of measurement of ionizing radiation	shield	device used to protect against radiation
radioactive	emitting radiation energy	transducer	device for converting energy from one form to another

Table 3.17

Diagnostic Procedure Terminology

Terms	Meaning	Terms	Meaning
angiocardiography	process of viewing the heart and blood vessels by injecting radiopaque dye into circulating blood and exposing the chest to x-rays	myelograph	radiograph of the spinal cord
		pyelograph	radiograph of the kidney and ureter
angiography	process of recording a vessel (through the use of radiopaque dye and x-rays)	radiograph	image produced by ionizing radiation (x-rays) and radiation sensitive film
bronchography	process of viewing the bronchus (radiograph examination of the bronchus or bronchi)	radioimmuno-assay	measurement of antigen-antibody interaction using radioactive substances
cholangiogram	radiograph examination of the bile ducts	radiotherapy	treatment of disease using radiation; treatment for some cancers
cholecystogram	radiograph examination of the gallbladder	salpingograph	radiograph of fallopian tubes
echocardiogram	examination of the heart using ultrasound imaging	sonogram	image produced by sound waves reflected off of body structures (examination of a part of the body using sound waves)
echogram	examination of body structures using ultrasound imaging techniques		
fluoroscopy	examination of body tissues and deep structures by use of fluoroscope	tomograph	radiograph exam whereby the x-ray source is moved to view layers or slices of the body
lymphangiograph	radiograph of lymphatic vessels	ultrasonography	imaging technique that uses sound waves to study a portion of the body

Table 3.18

General Imaging Terminology

Terms	Meaning
radiologist	physician who specializes in use of x-rays; interprets radiographs
radiopaque	describing materials (such as lead) that are able to block x-rays
roentgenology	alternate term for x-ray technology
scan	repeated recording of emissions from radioactive substances onto a photographic plate in one specific area of the body
scintiscan	image created by gamma radiation, indicating concentration within the body
sonolucent	permitting the passage of ultrasound waves
tagging	attachment of radioactive material to a substance that can be traced as it moves through the body
therapeutic	treatment of disease
uptake	absorption of radioactive substance into tissue

Table 3.19

Directional Imaging Terminology

Terms	Meaning
anteroposterior	front to back (direction of x-rays passing through the chest when the patient is in a standard radiograph examination position)
axial	pertaining to around an axis
lateral decubitus	lying on the side
posteroanterior	from back to front (direction of x-rays)

Exercise 3.8   What's the Question?

Write a question using a medical term for each definition (What is…?).

1. bending of a joint _____

2. straightening of a joint _____

3. movement toward the midline of the body _____

4. movement away from the midline of the body _____

5. turned outward _____

Exercise 3.9   Color Me . . .

Give the correct color indicated by each of the following word parts.

1. xanth/o _____

2. leuk/o _____

3. cyan/o _____

4. erythr/o _____

5. melan/o _____

Exercise 3.10   This Is a Pain

Choose the descriptive term that best completes the following sentences.

ache	intense	stabbing
continuous	intermittent	throbbing
discomfort	severe	
dull	sharp	

1. Mr. Alverex went to the dentist because he had a tooth _____.

2. The migraine headache was described as intense pain with an intermittent, sharp, _____ pain occurring several times during each hour.

3. Surgical pain is usually _____ and without relief until pain medication is given.

4. There was a blunted, _____ quality to the pain of the sprained muscle.

5. A strong, sharp pain is also described as _____.

6. A pain that is not continuous is _____.

7. The difference between a _____ pain and a stabbing pain is that the former is pulsating and the latter is very sharp, intermittent, and usually felt in one spot.

8. If a person describes a feeling of being uncomfortable, it is described as _____.

9. A pain that has a stabbing quality, usually in one particular area is _____.

10. Very strong, extreme pain is described as _____.

Define each of the following medical imaging terms.

1. radioactive _____

2. transducer _____

3. echocardiogram _____

4. fluoroscopy _____

5. radiopaque _____

6. sonolucent _____

7. anteroposterior _____

8. sonogram _____

9. cholangiogram _____

10. pyelography _____

Basis of Disease and Forms of Treatment

The body strives to maintain homeostasis, a dynamic state of balance. A lack of homeostasis manifests as "disease." When faced with stress or imbalance, cells have many adaptive capabilities. Sustained stress typically leads to injury or cell destruction. Many diseases are named or described by the cellular response:

- atrophy—decrease in size of cell, structure, and/or organ caused by a lack of nutrients, decreased stimulation, or lack of use rendering it relatively nonfunctional
- dysplasia—abnormal size, shape, and appearance of cells
- hyperplasia—increase in the number of cells due to increased workload or increased stimulation
- hypertrophy—increase in cell size due to increased workload
- metaplasia—replacement of one adult cell type with another cell type more capable of dealing with the stressor; the replacement cell does not resume the function of the cell it replaced

Cells normally mature, function, and then die off, being replaced with new cells. This programmed cell death is called *apoptosis*. Malignant tumors are marked by a loss of this normal cellular control.

Treatment for illness or disease may be medical or surgical. Medical treatment may involve medications, lifestyle changes (diet, exercise), or physical therapy. Surgical treatment may involve excision, revision, repair, or replacement. Whenever possible, medical management is typically tried before surgical treatment. Physicians may also refer to "conservative" treatment measures, which is a treatment regimen with the lowest risk of adverse effects. Treatment may be preventive (e.g., vaccines, antihistamines), diagnostic (e.g., x-rays and contrast dyes), or therapeutic (e.g., antibiotics, pain relievers).

Pharmacology

Medical management most often involves the use of medications. Understanding pharmacology and recognizing medications, routes, forms, and dosages are an important part of producing an accurate medical document. Medications come in a variety of forms including tablet (sometimes abbreviated as tab), capsule (sometimes abbreviated as cap), cream, lotion, gel, ointment, powder, liquid, suspension (sometimes abbreviated as susp), and suppository. Routes for administering medications include oral, sublingual, nasogastric, rectal, vaginal, topical, transdermal, inhalation, parenteral (IV, IM, and subcutaneous), and intraarticular. Medication regimens are often described using Latin abbreviations. Table 3.20 lists the most common abbreviations used to describe medication regimens.

Drugs carry many different names: a chemical name, a generic name, and a trade or brand name. The chemical name describes their molecular structure. Because chemical names are often long and cumbersome, generic names are also assigned. Most laypersons are familiar with brand names of drugs because they are used for marketing purposes and associate the drug with a specific manufacturer. Example of drug names are given in Table 3.21. Many drug names are marketed with

initials along with the brand name to indicate their form of action. Examples include SR (slow release), LA (long acting), and ER (extended release). Generic names are written using lowercase type whereas the first letter of trade names are always capitalized, as they are considered to be proper nouns.

Pharmaceutical companies protect their investment in research and development of a new drug by patenting the drug. Patents are valid for 17 years, after which other companies may market the drug under the generic name or their own trade name.

Prescription medications that have a proven history of safety and efficacy and can easily be managed without physician oversight may be approved by the Food and Drug Administration (FDA) to be sold over-the-counter (OTC), meaning they can be purchased at lower doses without a prescription.

When describing a drug regimen, type the drug name, the dose and units, the route, the frequency, quantity, and refills (if dictated). Do not type commas between parts of a single drug regimen; use commas or semicolons to separate drug regimens in a list. For example, a prescription for 60 tablets of Dilantin 100 mg to be taken twice a day by mouth with 4 refills would be transcribed: Dilantin 100 mg p.o. b.i.d. (#60) with 4 refills.

As your knowledge and skills advance, you will learn to recognize drug classes (categories) and the

Table 3.20

Abbreviations and Latin Terminology Used in Pharmacology

Abbreviation	Latin Term	Meaning
a.c.	*ante cibum*	before meals
ad lib.	*ad libitum*	as needed
b.i.d.	*bis in die*	twice a day
h.s.	*hora somni*	hour of sleep, at bedtime
n.p.o.	*nil per os*	nothing by mouth
p.c.	*post cibum*	after meals
p.r.n.	*pro re nata*	as needed
q.h.	*quaque hora*	every hour
q.i.d.	*quarter in die*	four times a day
t.i.d.	*ter in die*	three times a day

Table 3.21

Examples of Drug Nomenclature

Trade or Brand Name	Generic Name	Chemical Name
FeverAll, Liquiprin, Tylenol	acetaminophen	N-(4-hydroxyphenyl) acetamide
PediaCare, Sudafed	pseudoephedrine	*DL*-threo-2-(methylamino)-1-phenylpropan-1-ol
Valium	diazepam	7-chloro-1, 3-dihydro-1-methyl-5-phenyl-2H-1,4-benzodiazepin-2-one

syllables within the drug names that give you clues as to their purpose or indication. Look for common syllables, especially in generic drug names, for clues as to their drug class. For example, several drugs used to reduce cholesterol are in the class called statins and their generic names include the class name (e.g., simvastatin, atorvastatin). See Table 3.22 for more examples. When searching for a drug name, it can be helpful to do a reverse search by looking under the class or the therapeutic category, such as analgesic, antiinfective, antihypertensive, antiinflammatory, steroid, narcotic, diuretic, or bronchodilator.

Surgery

Surgical intervention typically requires some type of anesthesia, which takes away the sensation of pain. General anesthesia causes a general loss of sensation by deep sedation of the central nervous system. General anesthesia may be induced by intravenous infusion or through intubation (inserting a tube through the throat into the lungs) and ventilation. A common approach to surgical procedures is monitored anesthesia care (MAC), which induces sedation and amnesia yet leaves the patient responsive when stimulated. Other forms of anesthesia include topical, local, regional, epidural, and spinal. These methods prevent the sensation of pain by blocking the flow of sodium ions across the nerve cell membranes, preventing conduction of nerve impulses.

Surgical procedures make use of myriad surgical instruments and devices. Although many instruments are specialized, there are several major categories of instruments that will be encountered

Table 3.22

Identifying Syllables for Drug Classes

Syllable	Drug Class	Example
-ase	enzymes	amylase, lipase
-azole	antifungal	clotrimazole
-caine	local/ regional anesthetic	cocaine
-cillin	penicillin or derivative	ampicillin
-iazide	thiazide diuretic	hydrochloro- thiazide
-olol	beta blocker	atenolol
-pramine	tricyclic antidepressant	imipramine
-profen	NSAID (nonsteroidal anti- inflammatory)	ibuprofen

routinely in surgical reports. Table 3.23 lists the most common surgical instruments. Suture materials include silk, catgut, nylon, and steel. Common brand names include Vicryl, Monocryl, PDS, and Prolene. Originally, suture sizes ranged from #1 (smallest diameter) to #6 (largest diameter). As manufacturing methods improved, suture diameters became smaller and smaller, so sizes below #1 are designated #0, #00 (2-0), #000 (3-0), etc., (listed largest to smallest). Surgeons will dictate these smaller sizes as "two oh," "three oh," etc.

Table 3.23

Common Surgical Instruments

Instrument	Use
rongeur	a strong, biting forceps for chipping away at bone
scissors	an instrument with two blades connected at a pivot, used for cutting and separating
needle	slender, solid, sharp-pointed instrument for pulling sutures; or a hollow, sharp-pointed instrument for administering fluids into tissues or vessels
trocar	an instrument used to withdraw fluid from a body cavity or for paracentesis, usually consisting of a cannula and an obturator with a sharp, three-cornered tip
drain	a flexible tube used to remove fluid from a cavity as the fluid forms, commonly placed after surgical procedures

Instrument	Use
Bovie	an instrument used for electrosurgical dissection and hemostasis; Bovie cautery separates tissues and coagulates (seals) vessels to minimize bleeding
forceps	an instrument used for grasping
blade	sharp-sided instrument used for cutting
elevator	an instrument used to raise or pry a body part away from another structure
retractor	an instrument used to pull apart edges of a wound or body parts to gain easier access to a surgical field
clamp	an instrument used to compress or hold
tenaculum	a clamp designed to grasp and hold a body part

Exercise 3.12   What Does This Mean?

Translate the following prescription orders using lay terms.

1. 2 cap q.a.m., 1 cap p.o. q.h.s. _____

2. 1 tab p.o. q.6 h. p.r.n. _____

3. 1 cap q.i.d. p.o. x7d _____

4. 1 tab p.o. a.c. _____

5. 1 tab ad lib. pain _____

6. apply h.s. _____

7. apply q.i.d. leg _____

8. 1 cap p.o. b.i.d. _____

9. 1 tab t.i.d. p.o. til gone _____

10. 1-2 tab p.o. q.3-4 h. p.r.n. pain _____

Four

Perfecting Your Editing Skills

Communication among medical personnel takes a number of forms—oral, dictated, written, and transcribed. For clarity of communication and continuity of care, the transmission of information must be accurate, concise yet detailed, and prompt. Accurate interpretation based on clinical knowledge and informed judgment is critical to partnering with the provider to produce a document that reflects the patient care encounter. In this chapter, you will develop your skills in applying rules of style, format, grammar, and punctuation. As you become familiar with these basics, you will have a deeper understanding of the way a medical transcriptionist contributes to the total process of care of the patient.

Objectives

» Define appropriate parameters for editing, correcting, and amending the patient record.

» Learn standards of style for medical transcription as developed by standard-setting industry organizations such as AHDI, The Joint Commission, and ASTM International.

» Apply standard rules for grammar and punctuation as they apply to the domain of clinical documentation.

» Develop proofreading and editing skills through transcription practice and evaluation.

Deciding When to Edit

There is the misperception among those who are not familiar with medical transcription that an MT is simply engaged in "typing what they hear." The reality is that the skill of applying clinical knowledge and developing an interpretive ear for what is being dictated is quite challenging. An MT must be engaged in the patient record, constantly applying informed judgment—judgment that has been shaped by extensive knowledge of medicine and the diagnostic process. A highly skilled MT will be expected to identify information that is incomplete, misplaced, or dictated in error. All of these scenarios represent judgments an MT will have to make to ensure these errors are not in the record itself.

When is it appropriate for an MT to change what has been dictated? There is some debate in the industry about the appropriate parameters for MT editing. Some facilities have adopted a verbatim policy, whereby the MT is not allowed to edit anything dictated, even if it is dictated in error. In those instances, the MT is simply required to leave a blank, flag the report, and refer that report back to the dictator for review and correction. However, most facilities recognize the editing skills of trained MTs and value their role in creating accurate medical records. In those settings, MTs are empowered to edit the record with defined parameters for what is appropriate and what is not.

In an environment where you will be expected to identify inconsistencies in the record, you will need to apply sound editing guidelines to promote clarity of meaning and preserve the healthcare provider's dictation style. Since an MT is not present at the time of the patient care encounter and is not qualified to make diagnostic decisions, the kind of information an MT is allowed to edit will be limited. An MT *is* empowered, however, to recognize and correct obvious errors in grammar, punctuation, style, terminology, and transposition of terms (Example: Blood pressure 98.6, temperature 128/72).

In cases where an MT has identified something is missing, information that is inconsistent within the context of the report, or words or terms clearly dictated in error, the MT is not expected to assume the role of the physician and add that information.

An MT should never guess or assume what is intended by the provider. In those instances, the MT is expected to (a) have the knowledge and skill to recognize the inconsistency, (b) flag the report for review, and (c) refer the report back to the dictator for review and correction.

Whether editing for clarity, recasting sentences to correct faulty grammar—including punctuation or formatting that is not provided by the dictator, or omitting erroneous punctuation or grammar instructions that *are* provided by the dictator—remember to always edit subtly. Make the least intrusive change necessary to correct the content and flow of the report. Make every attempt to preserve the dictation style of the physician or provider. The best editing is the kind that even the dictator does not recognize when signing off on the report.

This chapter will empower you to recognize errors in style, grammar, punctuation, and content and to correct those errors as you transcribe. Identifying those areas of dictation that will require editing will be important in understanding how to apply the rules for style and format.

Repairing Sentence Fragments and Run-On Sentences

One of the most common trouble spots in workplace documents such as letters and reports is faulty sentence construction. These problems take the form of either incomplete sentences (sentence fragments) or run-on sentences (two sentences that "run together" without the correct punctuation separating them). To be able to correct fragments and run-ons, you must know what makes a sentence complete. You also must know how to punctuate a sentence so the reader knows where it begins and ends.

It is important to keep in mind that while healthcare providers are experts in clinical care, they may not be expert writers. The MT can shape their often rambling, disjointed narrative into a clean, accurate record. In their defense, recounting a patient's entire care encounter and being able to dictate that encounter from start to finish in a sequential and organized way is very challenging! In addition, dictators whose primary language is not English and is built on an entirely different grammar and sentence structure will be challenged to dictate a narrative that reflects standard English. Some languages do not use personal pronouns, so you may encounter a provider who consistently uses "he" and "she" interchangeably in the same document. You will have to rely on clinical context to ensure that the appropriate pronoun is used.

You may make edits to the record that are subtle but promote clarity. Ignore dictator directions for punctuation unless you know they are correct. Following dictator instructions for periods, paragraph breaks, and commas can result in fragmented and run-on sentences you want to avoid. Always use the full context of the report to help you make informed editing decisions that aid in the flow of the report.

What Is a Sentence?

Every complete sentence contains a subject and a verb and expresses a thought. The subject is generally a noun or pronoun, and the verb always expresses some action or state of being *(am, was, will be, etc.)*.

In the following examples, the subject is in purple and the verb is in orange.

Bill worked.

Dr. Brown will see the patient.

You look tired.

My **physician** is unavailable on Fridays.

The **patient** and his **family** were informed of the diagnosis.
[compound subject]
A corporate healthcare **facility** seeks a full-time medical transcriptionist.

Sometimes the subject is implied but not stated. In the following sentences, for example, the subject *you* is understood.

Have a nice day.

Follow up with me next week.

Create a letterhead for all medical documents.

Fragments

A fragment is a group of words that expresses a partial thought and leaves the reader puzzled. It is not a complete sentence. If a sentence is incomplete in a dictation, a medical transcriptionist cannot complete the thought on behalf of the dictator. These examples are provided only as a comparison between fragments and complete sentences.

WRONG

The patient was instructed that if he develops a fever over 101 degrees or if he has increasing abdominal pain.
[This is a long dependent clause. What is missing is important information detailing what the patient should do in response to these symptoms.]

CORRECT

The patient was instructed to call the doctor's answering service if he develops a fever over 101 degrees or if he has increasing abdominal pain.

WRONG

After the examination, Mrs. Lawrence was told to see.
[This sentence is not complete. This fragment does not explain who Mrs. Lawrence was supposed to see.]

CORRECT

After the examination, Mrs. Lawrence was told to see the orthopedist for a followup if her hip pain continues.

Run-On Sentences

A run-on sentence consists of two sentences that are not separated by punctuation. If the second sentence is closely related, use a semicolon to connect them. Otherwise, key them as two individual sentences, each ending with a period (or a question mark or an exclamation mark).

WRONG

The patient's condition gradually improved on intravenous antibiotic therapy the speech therapist saw the patient in consultation.

CORRECT

The patient's condition gradually improved on intravenous antibiotic therapy. The speech therapist saw the patient in consultation.

WRONG

The nurses have alternative work schedules each shift is 7.5 hours.

CORRECT

The nurses have alternative work schedules. Each shift is 7.5 hours.

Exceptions to the Rules in Medical Reports

Certain sections of medical reports may contain incomplete sentences. For example, parts of the physical examination may or may not be in sentence form. Also, a doctor may dictate laboratory values that do not have to be written in sentence form.

CARDIOVASCULAR: Regular rate and rhythm. No murmurs, rubs, or gallops.

LABORATORY DATA
WBC 5500 with 45 segmented neutrophils, 15 basophils, 5 eosinophils, and 17 monocytes.

There are some sections of the report where fragments, or "clipped" sentences, are acceptable and some areas where they are not. Generally speaking, outpatient notes are less formal than other types of dictation and may be dictated in clipped sentences. A doctor may dictate without using subjects and articles. These notes should be transcribed as dictated, and would not require a heading. Such a note might look like this.

Seen for postoperative visit. Doing well. Wound healing, without signs of infection. Sutures removed. Will be seen again in 2 weeks. May return to work after that time.

Narrative sections of the report—those sections that "tell a story" like the History of Present Illness, Hospital Course, and Plan—need to be transcribed in complete sentences, particularly in the acute care setting. In private practice and clinic settings, you may encounter a physician who dictates the entire report, narrative sections included, in clipped sentences. In those informal settings, it is appropriate to yield to the physician's style and keep those sentences clipped as dictated.

Non-narrative sections, which are sections that typically lend themselves well to long lists of information (like the Past Medical History, Current Allergies, Medications, Review of Systems, Physical Examination, and Laboratory Data sections) are not expected to be transcribed in complete sentences.

PAST MEDICAL HISTORY
1. Status post coronary artery bypass grafting 5 years ago.
2. Bilateral hip pain.
3. History of hypertension, under good control on medical therapy.

No matter what, be consistent and always make sure the sentence or fragment reflects clarity of information and meaning.

Complete Exercise 4.1 to practice editing portions of transcribed medical records for correct sentence punctuation

Creating Subject-Verb Agreement

The subject and verb of a sentence must agree in number and person. Singular verbs require singular subjects, and plural verbs require plural subjects. Use first-person verbs with first-person subjects *(I, we)*, second-person verbs with second-person subjects *(you)*, and third-person verbs with third-person subjects. In the following examples, the subject is in purple and the verb is in orange.

I am confused.

[singular subject and verb]

The pronoun *you* can be either singular or plural in meaning, but it always takes a plural verb.

You are an excellent transcriptionist.

[singular subject and plural verb]

You are all excellent transcriptionists.

[plural subject and plural verb]

Read the following sentences and decide if any are run-on sentences or sentence fragments. Create complete sentences by combining groups of words or by changing the punctuation and then key the corrected sentences. Save the document as XXExercise04.01.doc, using your initials in place of the *XX* in the file name. Remember that as a transcriptionist, you must remain as true as possible to the original dictation while correcting obvious errors.

1. The patient's wife called 911, and the paramedics arrived some 10 minutes later to find the patient in a semiconscious state with an irregular heart rhythm the exact nature, of which is unknown.

2. Strict sterile precautions must be taken. Using only autoclaved instruments and adequate skin preparation.

3. CURRENT MEDICATIONS
   Lasix 20 mg per morning Micro-K 10 mEq twice per day Cardizem 30 mg per day Isordil 20 mg twice per day

4. The patient was extubated and noted to have purulent sputum and purulent urine and blood and urine cultures were positive for Klebsiella pneumoniae therefore the patient was started on gentamicin.

5. The patient was seen in routine followup. Six months since the last examination.

6. After informed consent was obtained the patient was brought to the operating room where general anesthesia was established and the lower abdomen was prepared and draped in the usual sterile fashion and an incision made just below the umbilicus.

7. The patient should apply the zinc oxide ointment directly to the lesions as often as needed to cool the burning sensation making sure she washes her hands before and after the application.

8. The patient is a 17-year-old female. A known IV drug abuser. She presents today to the emergency department she has an infected area on her left arm. The area is red and tender.

9. The head shows no deformities the nose and throat are clear the neck has no adenopathy the chest is clear with normal breath sounds the abdomen is soft and nontender extremities are normal skin shows no rash or redness.

10. This 35-year-old Hispanic male presented today with a 1cm laceration of the right hand at the web space between the middle and ring fingers.

Individuals who share a job must **have** similar work values and **be able** to cooperate with each other.

[plural subject and compound verb]

The two **physicians** who had similar practices **have** decided to merge.

[plural subject and plural verb]

Sometimes a subject "looks" plural but functions as one unit and is singular in meaning. This is a collective noun. Be sure you use a singular verb(s) in such cases.

I&D was performed.

[The procedure involves two steps, but together they make up *one* procedure; therefore, this subject is singular.]

Pediatrics is her specialty.

[Even though pediatrics has an *s*, it is the name of a single specialty and therefore requires a singular verb.]

A collective noun may also be singular in form but represents a group of individuals or things; therefore, it acts individually and takes a plural verb.

The **staff** are in disagreement on the best policy to imlement.

Complicating Factor: Inverted Order Sentences

Sentences are usually written with the subject before the verb. However, sometimes the sentence is inverted, meaning the verb comes first. This can cause some confusion in achieving subject-verb agreement. Many of these sentences begin with *Here* or *There*. Again, the subject is shown in purple and the verb in orange.

There is no **reason** to delay treatment.

Outside the clinic, there was a **crowd** waiting to be seen.

There was no **tenderness** to palpation.

Here are the patients' **files** that doctors need to keep.

Here are my **reasons** for declining the position.

Complicating Factor: Intervening Words and Phrases

In complicated sentences, first identify the verb and then the subject(s) of that verb. Then be sure you choose a singular verb for a singular subject or a plural verb for a plural subject. Disregard the parts of the sentence that come between the subject and the verb.

A verbal **report** of the biopsies was requested.

Resection of the malignant tumors was carried out.

The **patient**, along with his family, is pleased with the outcome of his surgery.

The **surgery** that occurred on Thursday caused a lot of pain.

The **celebration** that was planned for the couple was held in the hospital room following the birth of the baby.

Complete Exercise 4.2 to practice editing a medical report for proper subject-verb agreeement.

Creating Agreement between Pronouns and Antecedents

Remember that a pronoun takes the place of a noun in a sentence. Words such as *she, he, it, they, us, them, I,* and *you* are pronouns.

Pronouns must agree in person, number, and gender with the nouns they represent, which are called antecedents. In the sentences below, the pronoun is highlighted and the antecedents are underscored.

The patient reports that his headaches have been increasing.

The physician dictated the report and sent it to the transcriptionist.

Transcriptionists know they must keep their skills sharp.

Holly keeps her problems to herself.

Either Josephine or Maria will submit her findings of the survey.

Exercise 4.2   Editing for Subject-Verb Agreement

Read the following discharge summary section and circle the correct verbs from the choices in parentheses. Then key the report using correct subject-verb combinations. Save the document as XXExercise04.01. doc, using your initials in place of the *XX* in the file name.

SUBJECTIVE

The patient, a 56-year-old female with multiple medical problems, (presents/present) to the ophthalmology outpatient clinic with 24 hours of tearing and irritation of both eyes. Vision in both eyes (seems/seem) unimpaired. She has no history of allergies or URIs and (does/do) not wear contact lenses.

She has a thick mucous discharge in both eyes, which (causes/cause) the lashes to stick together. She denies any history of trauma to the eyes and no previous history of similar symptoms (is/are) noted.

OBJECTIVE

In each eye the conjunctiva (is/are) grossly inflamed and injected. There (is/are) moderate chemosis and some lid edema. Traces of mucopurulent discharge (is/are) noted on the eyelashes. Examination with tetracaine and fluorescein (reveals/reveal) no corneal abrasion. Funduscopy and slit-lamp exams (is/are) entirely normal.

ASSESSMENT

Acute bacterial conjunctivitis, both eyes.

PLAN

The patient, with her sister in attendance, (was/were) instructed to use sulfonamide ophthalmic solution 2 drops, both eyes, q.i.d. Techniques of careful handwashing and hygiene (was/were) explained to the patient. The patient will return if her symptoms (does/do) not improve.

Josephine and Maria agreed to discuss their findings with the group.

The pronouns *this*, *that*, *these*, and *those* must also agree with the nouns they modify.

this procedure	these procedures
that medication	those medications

The pronouns *them* and *their* are plural forms. Do not use these pronouns for singular meanings.

When gender is not known, try to create a sentence that does not require the awkward construction of *his/her*.

WRONG

The patient should be asked to remove their clothes prior to the exam.

CORRECT

The patient should be asked to undress prior to the exam.

WRONG

If the child completes the assignment, praise them for their efforts.

CORRECT

Praise children for their efforts in completing their assignments.

Pronouns as Subject or Object

A pronoun can represent a subject or an object. That is, the pronoun can be either the performer of an action or the recipient of the action. Subject pronouns are *I, you, he, she, it, we,* and *they.* Object pronouns are *me, you, him, her, it, us,* and *them.*

A predicate is either a verb or group of words that tells something about the action or state of being of the subject in the sentence. A predicate always has a verb and may also include helping verbs such as *has* or *have.*

Pronoun/Subject Agreement

Most people do not have difficulty achieving pronoun agreement in simple sentences that contain one pronoun in the predicate, e.g., Bill dislikes *me.* However, problems do come about when a sentence contains multiple nouns and pronouns, e.g., Bill dislikes *he/him* and *I/me.* To select the correct pronoun, simplify the sentence by looking only at the verb and the pronoun in question. Your ear should help you make the right choice.

dislikes *he* or *him*?	correct choice: dislikes him
dislikes *I* or *me*?	correct choice: dislikes me

Bill dislikes him and me.

The three supervisors usually meet monthly to review their productivity.

[This is a complete sentence. The words *usually* and *monthly* describe the verb *meet.* The complete predicate consists of the verb and all of the other words.]

Who versus Whom

Use the pronoun *who* for the subject of a verb; use *whom* for the object of a verb.

Who has the first appointment?
[Who is the subject.]

Whom did you assign to the emergency room?
[Whom is the object.]

In sentences or questions that contain a who/whom dilemma, check the sentence by substituting *he* for *who* and *him* for *whom* and then trust your ear.

Who will deliver these reports?

He will deliver these reports.

James will deliver these reports to whom?

James will deliver these reports to him.

Myself, Himself, and Other Reflexive Pronouns

Reflexive pronouns are formed by adding *-self* or *-selves* to a personal pronoun(s). *Myself, yourselves, herself,* etc., are reflexive pronouns, meaning that they must reflect back to a noun or pronoun within that same sentence. (*Mikey* wrapped the gift all by *himself.*) Many dictators mistakenly refer to themselves as myself instead of me. (He was seen by *myself* in the clinic.) Do not use a reflexive in a sentence when a simple personal pronoun is appropriate. (He was seen by *me* in the clinic.)

WRONG

The surgery was conducted by Dr. Jones, Dr. Roberts, and myself.

CORRECT

The surgery was conducted by Dr. Jones, Dr. Roberts, and me.

WRONG

The physician who had a middle ear infection treated her.

CORRECT

The physician who had a middle ear infection treated herself.

WRONG

The executive board discussed the issues among them.

Read each sentence and circle the word(s) in parentheses that correctly completes the sentence. Key the correct sentences. Save the document as XXExercise04.03.doc, using your initials in the place of the *XX* in the file name.

1. The patient and (I/me) have discussed the options for treatment.

2. (Who/whom) is my first patient today?

3. I will ask the nurse to arrange for my partner or (I/me) to see the child tomorrow.

4. A patient (who/whom) has a cholesteatoma may present with unilateral hearing loss.

5. The receptionist should always ask a new patient if (he or she/they) brought (his or her/their) records.

6. Do not assume that patients know how (his or her/their) medications are to be taken.

7. Both tympanic membranes were noted to be bulging, and (its/their) color was bright red.

8. This patient, (who/whom) I consider to be reliable, says that he was treated poorly by your department.

9. Please call if Dr. Adams or (I/me) can be of help.

10. A patient with chronic tonsillitis often has to have (his or her/their) throat cultured.

CORRECT

The executive board discussed the issues among themselves.

[The executive board acted as individuals, not as a single unit.]

Complete Exercise 4.3 to check your understanding of the proper use of pronouns and antecedents.

Punctuating with Commas, Semicolons, and Colons

In a spoken conversation, meaning is conveyed through tone of voice, gestures, and pauses. We pause and change the inflection in our voices to clarify meaning. In written language, punctuation marks serve as "road signs" for readers. Punctuation clarifies meaning and prevents confusion.

Commas: To Introduce

Use a comma to set off an introductory word or phrase.

Fortunately, the records were located.

Because his temperature spiked, the patient was not cleared for discharge.

Due to her rapid deterioration, the patient was transferred to the intensive care unit.

When Mr. Johnson arrived, we met with the doctors to discuss the case.

A sentence that is in the natural order (subject followed by verb and modifiers) does not contain an introductory clause and does not need an introductory comma.

I confirmed the patients' appointments for next week before leaving the office.

Your first-aid kit should be readily accessible in the event of a medical emergency.

We will replace the x-ray view box although the warranty is no longer in effect.

When a sentence is out of the natural order (inverted), a comma is needed to help the reader identify the important information of the sentence.

Before leaving the office, I confirmed the patients' appointments for next week.

In the event of a medical emergency, your first-aid kit should be readily accessible.

Be careful to place introductory phrases close to the word they modify; otherwise, your sentence may be grammatically incorrect and/or cause confusion to readers.

UNCLEAR
After pausing the audio file, the operative report was completed.

CLEAR
After pausing the audio file, he completed the operative report.

Commas: To Separate

Coordinate conjunctions (and, but, or, nor, for, so) join two main clauses into one sentence. Use a comma immediately before the coordinate conjunction. Remember that a main clause contains a subject, verb, and complement and can stand alone. (A complement completes the sense of the verb and explains or describes the subject.) The main clause is also called an independent clause.

The patient was prepared and draped in the usual sterile orthopedic fashion, and the tourniquet was inflated to 250 mmHg.

The patient has had intermittent confusion, so the home health nurse was assigned to dispense the patient's medications.

I do not know how long it will last, but the patient has stopped smoking.

We investigated several locations for the medical conference, but we selected the facility that would attract the largest number of physicians.

If the main clauses are very short, you may omit the comma.

The wound was cleaned and a dressing was applied.

In a series of three or more items, use a comma before the conjunction.

The patient's past medical history is significant for coronary artery disease, insulin-dependent diabetes mellitus, and peptic ulcer disease.

Dr. Johnson can see the patient on Monday, Wednesday, or Friday.

You will find paper, pens, and CDs in the storage room.

The supervisor explained the report formats to the new transcriptionists, assigned a dictation to each, and indicated when the reports should be completed.

Use a comma between consecutive adjectives that equally modify the same noun if *and* is omitted. Do not use a comma before the *and* in these examples.

She is a kind, dedicated nurse.

She is a kind and dedicated nurse.

Tomorrow the patient will have a long, painful procedure.

Tomorrow the patient will have a long and painful procedure.

Do not use a comma between two adjectives if you would not use *and*. Test this by saying the adjectives in a different order and insert *and* between them.

The patient is an elderly white female.
[We would not say she is an elderly *and* white female].

When placing commas, be sure you do not separate the subject from the verb. Even if the subject is several words long, it must not be separated from the verb by a comma.

WRONG

Patients who are afraid of hospitals and doctors because of past painful experiences, need to be given an extra dose of compassion.

CORRECT

Patients who are afraid of hospitals and doctors because of past painful experiences need to be given an extra dose of compassion.

Commas: To Enclose

Use commas to set off nonessential or interrupting words or phrases from the rest of the sentence. Think of commas that enclose as parentheses. By enclosing information in commas, you are telling the reader that the information is not vital to the meaning of the sentence.

I will graduate, unless I fail my chemistry class, next year.

The dose, at least according to my calculations, is 12.5 mg per hour.

The number of Internet users, according to the latest statistics, will continue to increase in the next decade.

Do not use commas to set off essential or restrictive words or phrases that give a clear meaning to the sentence.

The lady whose surgery I cancelled was understanding and willing to change the procedure date.
[The essential clause indicated which lady's surgery was cancelled.]

Semicolons

Semicolons are used in two situations: (1) to join two independent clauses and (2) to separate items in a series that have internal commas. Use one space after a semicolon in medical documents.

Use a semicolon to join two closely related independent clauses that are not joined by a coordinating conjunction (*and, or, but, nor*). Note that the clauses could also stand alone as sentences.

We have given the patient clear instructions; he will follow them explicitly.

When independent clauses are joined by *however*, *therefore*, etc., use a semicolon before the conjunctive adverb and a comma after it.

The patient has continued to take the medication; however, his condition has not improved.

Use a semicolon to separate items in a series when one or more of those items contains an internal comma.

He has written books about the use of blood during surgery, specifically the use of plasma expanders; tissue typing, his favorite topic; and hemophilia.

I have practiced medicine in Phoenix, Arizona; Portland, Oregon; and Seattle, Washington.

Colons

Colons are the neon signs of punctuation, alerting the reader to important information. Most commonly, they are used with report subheadings and in ratios. (Ratios will be covered later in this chapter.)

Use a colon after a report heading but only if the information follows on the same line. Key only one space after the colon. Capitalize the first letter after the heading. An example of a run-in subheading follows. It is excerpted from the Physical Examination section of a history and physical report.

HEENT: Pupils equal and reactive.

Use a colon after introductions to listed items such as *the following* and *as follows*. Again, only key one space after the colon.

The required skills for the job are the following: ability to communicate, knowledge of Microsoft Word, and ability to work on a team.

Complete Exercise 4.4 to practice your editing skills related to the correct use of commas, semicolons, and colons in medical documents.

Read the following sentences and add commas, semicolons, or colons where necessary for correct meaning. Key the corrected sentences. Save the document as XXExercise04.04.doc, using your initials in place of the XX in the file name.

1. Since the patient has improved with conservative management we will not consider operative intervention at this time.

2. Our latest project remodeling the waiting room is going to be more expensive than we had planned.

3. Past surgeries include hysterectomy cholecystectomy and appendectomy.

4. Surprisingly the patient's condition improved.

5. Laboratory tests to be ordered include a complete blood count chemistry panel and electrolytes.

6. The risks and benefits of the procedure were explained to the patient and his wife and the patient signed the consent forms.

7. The planned surgery has a very high success rate however I explained to the patient that any surgery has an element of risk.

8. Abdomen is soft no organomegaly is noted.

9. The patient is to return to the emergency department immediately if he develops nausea fever over 100 degrees or dramatically increased pain.

10. The patient has a history of coronary artery disease having undergone an angioplasty.

11. When testing the students should refrain from speaking.

12. After the induction of general anesthesia an endotracheal tube was placed.

13. The wound was then irrigated using normal saline and the deep muscles were closed using chromic sutures.

14. The experimental drug studies were carried out in San Diego California Denver Colorado Minneapolis Minnesota and Atlanta Georgia.

15. The patient is a young female college student.

16. Patients with AIDS who generally are underweight should receive nutritional counseling.

17. Thank you Dr. Smith for seeing this patient in pulmonary consultation.

18. Given the patient's overall debilitated condition and end-stage lung disease he wishes to be made a DNR.

Using Dashes, Quotation Marks, and Parentheses

Besides punctuation tools already covered, some transcribed reports will include dashes, quotation marks, and parentheses. Like commas, these symbols help the reader understand the intention of the author. It is important to use these special punctution tools correctly.

Dashes

Use dashes to set off interrupting phrases from the rest of the sentence. A dash indicates a change in thought or a side comment not essential to the meaning of the sentence. Use dashes sparingly, especially in any type of formal document.

> Thank you for seeing Mrs. Johnson—especially on such short notice—for evaluation of her chest pain.

> Many universities are focusing on online collaborative learning—it's exciting, informative, and a new approach to learning.

Key dashes with no spaces before or after them. Proportional fonts such as Times New Roman include a special dash character. If you are using a monospaced font such as Courier, create a dash by keying two hyphens.

Quotation Marks

Use quotation marks to surround the exact words someone has spoken. The marks should appear in pairs, with one set at the beginning of the quote and the other at the end.

The placement of other punctuation marks with quotes frequently causes confusion.

Always key a period and comma inside the quotation marks.

> The surgeon said, "We will first repair the heart valves and then deal with her coronary artery disease."

> "I want to go to observe the procedure next Friday," Stephanie said.

> "I cannot tolerate pain," the patient complained, "but I know I need this surgery."

> "The new medical journals," John said, "will be available for distribution next month."

Place a colon or semicolon outside quotation marks. Remember to set only a single space after a colon or semicolon.

> These are her "requirements": Arrive on time and attend all sessions.

> He said "thrombophlebitis"; I'm sure of it.

> The manager said, "A meeting will be held every Thursday on a monthly basis"; therefore, the supervisor needs to plan accordingly.

Place a question mark or exclamation mark outside the quotation marks if the entire sentence is a question or exclamation. Set the end punctuation inside the end quotation marks if only the quoted words are a question or exclamation.

> Was she the physician who said, "No two surgeries are alike"?

> "If the pain subsides in 2 days," she asked, "should I continue taking the medicine?"

> The director asked, "How long have you been employed?" [Omit final period.]

> Mr. Courtney was so surprised he said, "I can't believe you finished the project!" [Omit final period.]

History and physical reports may begin with a chief complaint. If the chief complaint is dictated in first person, key it in quotation marks.

> CHIEF COMPLAINT
> "I have been throwing up for 2 days."

If the quoted material is not a complete sentence, do not start the quote with a capital letter (unless the first word is a proper noun or an acronym).

> The patient says his left knee "doesn't feel right." [Contractions are acceptable in direct quotes but not in other dictation.]

> The patient said he had "some kind of x-ray test" on his back but did not know the name of the study.

Use quotation marks to draw attention to words and phrases or to designate slang, clichés, or nicknames.

The patient's condition was "touch-and-go" for the first 24 hours but then gradually stabilized.

I saw your patient Richard "Bud" Goodman for evaluation of his hypertension.

Use quotation marks to set off titles of magazine or newspaper articles and chapters of a book. The titles of magazines, newspapers, brochures, and books are placed in italics (in proportional spaced fonts such as Times New Roman) or underlined (in Courier).

All of our pregnant patients receive the *Eating for Two* brochure.

According to "Guide to a Healthy Heart," an article in the *Health Nuts* magazine, individuals who maintain a low-fat diet and who exercise regularly lower their risk of heart attack.

Parentheses

Use parentheses to enclose side thoughts or words not vital to the main idea of the sentence.

The sodium level was 131 (normal).

According to the surgery schedule (usually a reliable source), Michelle Brown will be admitted for excisional biopsy tomorrow.

Exercising on a daily basis (swimming, walking, aerobics) improves one's health.

Use parentheses to enclose acronyms or abbreviations.

Mr. Johnson underwent transurethral resection of the prostate (TURP) on the day of admission.

He will be referred for percutaneous transluminal coronary angioplasty (PTCA) of his right coronary artery lesion.

To become a certified medical transcriptionist (CMT), you have to pass the required examination.

Use parentheses to enclose numbers when a list is given in paragraph form.

The past history is remarkable for (1) coronary artery disease, treated with PTCA; (2) diabetes mellitus, controlled on insulin therapy; and (3) hypertension, not well controlled.

If parentheses enclose a complete sentence that does not interrupt another sentence, place the period inside the parentheses.

The risks and benefits of the procedure were explained to the patient, and he opted to proceed. (The signed consent form is on the chart.)

If parentheses enclose an interrupting statement within a sentence, do not place a period inside the parentheses.

The procedure and its risks (bleeding, infection, possible need for transfusion) were explained to the patient.

His risk factors for coronary artery disease include history of smoking (he quit 1 year ago), positive family history, and elevated cholesterol level.

Apply your understanding of the proper use of dashes, quotation marks, and parenthesis in the sentences from medical reports found in Exercise 4.5.

Using Modifiers to Achieve Correct Meaning

Modifiers are words, phrases, and clauses that describe or tell more about another word, phrase, or clause. Pay careful attention to the placement of modifiers to ensure clear meaning of sentences. However, be very careful when altering dictation. Reserve rewording for instances when the dictation is not clear because of the misplacement or misuse of a modifier. If you must edit, always use the dictator's original words for terms, procedures, instruments, and diseases. Too much editing can be considered tampering.

Read the following sentences from medical reports and add the appropriate special punctuation marks. Key the corrected sentences. Save the document as XXExercise04.05.doc, using your initials for *XX* in the file name.

1. CHIEF COMPLAINT

   I think I'm having a heart attack. [the patient's statement]

2. Gertrude Trudy Schmidt presented to my office today. [Indicate that Trudy is a nickname.]

3. Because her chest pain did not resolve with sublingual nitroglycerin, she was transported to the emergency department by a family member her son.

4. The patient states that his knee doesn't feel right when he walks. [a partial quote]

5. The patient's history has been well documented on previous admissions please see old records.

6. In accordance with his wishes, the patient was made a DNR do not resuscitate.

7. DISCHARGE DIAGNOSIS

   Acute bacterial endocarditis resolving.

8. Please set up an appointment with Dr. Edwards you can get his phone number from my secretary at your earliest convenience.

9. The patient has a history of one chronic obstructive pulmonary disease, two congestive heart failure, and three hypertension.

10. If the infection does not respond to amoxicillin, we may need to call in one of the big guns like cephalexin. [Mark the slang phrase.]

Related Words Should Be Placed Together

Place modifiers as close as possible to the words being modified.

UNCLEAR

Examination at that time of the esophagus was negative.
[What is "that time of the esophagus"?]

CLEAR

Examination of the esophagus at that time was negative.

UNCLEAR

The lady was a supervisor in the admitting department who wore a red suit.
[The clause *who wore a red suit* modifies the noun *lady.*]

CLEAR

The lady in the red suit was a supervisor in the admitting department.

Misplaced or Dangling Modifiers

Many transcription "bloopers" are caused by misplaced or dangling modifiers, particularly prepositional phrases or phrases beginning with *ing* words. These phrases are adjective phrases that modify a noun. Miscommunication occurs when the phrase is not placed next to the noun it modifies.

WRONG

The bleeder was clamped with a hemostat, hoping to achieve hemostasis.
[The phrase *hoping to achieve hemostasis* is an adjective phrase that refers to the surgeon—not to the bleeder, as is suggested in this sentence construction.]

CORRECT

The bleeder was clamped with a hemostat in the hope of achieving hemostasis.

WRONG

The driver was referred to a doctor with a severe head injury.
[The phrase *with a severe head injury* refers to the driver, not the doctor.]

CORRECT

The driver with a severe head injury was referred to a doctor.

Practice editing transcribed dictation for misplaced or dangling modifiers by editing the sentences in Exercise 4.6.

Forming Plurals

The first section of this chapter reviewed the guidelines for creating agreement between subjects and verbs. The guidelines are based on the principle that plural subjects require plural verbs and singular subjects require singular verbs. Since nouns and pronouns function as subjects of sentences, it is important to know the general rules for creating the plural forms of medical terms.

Generally, most nouns are made plural by adding *s* or *es* to the singular form. The same rules usually apply to nouns in medical reports. However, many medical words and terms are of Latin and Greek origin; therefore, they do not follow the English rules. For example, the plural form of *diagnosis* is not *diagnosises*; it is *diagnoses*. Consult a medical dictionary when necessary. If the dictionary lists more than one plural form, the first one listed is usually the preferred choice.

Rules for Plural Forms

As you become more familiar with the medical language, forming and/or recognizing plural forms will become easier. The following rules for making plural forms will be helpful.

- If the singular form ends in a, make the plural by adding e (vertebra/vertebrae, conjunctiva/conjunctivae).
- If the singular form ends in um, change the um to a (diverticulum/diverticula).
- If the singular form ends in us, change the us to i (fungus/fungi, embolus/emboli).
- If the singular form ends in is, change the is to es (diagnosis/diagnoses).
- If the singular form ends in ax or ix, change the x to ces (thorax/thoraces; cervix/cervices).

Revise and key the following dictated sentences to show the correct use and placement of modifiers.

1. The patient was referred to a gastroenterologist who, because of increasing complaints of esophageal reflux, ordered an upper GI.

2. In the left lateral Sims position, the doctor performed the rectal examination.

3. When 3 weeks post appendectomy, she called about her husband's inflamed incision.

4. X-ray this morning of the chest revealed moderate clearing of the infiltrate.

5. After improving on antibiotic therapy, surgery was deferred.

6. At 225 pounds, her doctor instructed her to eat smaller meals and to exercise more often.

7. A curved incision was made just above the umbilicus of 3 cm.

8. Feeling very nauseous, the nurse handed the patient an emesis basin.

9. With a family history of colon polyps, screening colonoscopy will be carried out every 2 years.

10. The doctor arranged for Mr. Smith's admission. Had he notified the insurance company, reimbursement would have been greater.

- If the singular form ends in ex, change the ex to ices (index/indices).
- If the singular form ends in nx, change the x to ges (phalanx/phalanges).
- If the singular form ends in en, change the en to ina (lumen/lumina).
- If the singular form ends in on, change the on to a (phenomenon/phenomena).
- If the singular form ends in ma, add ta (condyloma/condylomata). Note that it is sometimes acceptable to form plurals of words that end in ma by adding s (carcinoma/carcinomas).

Other Plural Forms

Very few plural forms contain an apostrophe, so do not be tempted to add one when keying a plural unless you are certain it is correct to do so.

Some words have only a singular or plural form. The word *adnexa* means appendages or auxiliary parts (plural), usually referring to the fallopian tubes and ovaries. So if you heard "right and left adnexa nontender" in a report of a pelvic examination, you would transcribe *adnexa*, not *adnexae* or *adnexi* because there are no such words. Also, the words *feces, genitalia, menses, scabies, tongs,* and *tweezers* are always plural in use. On the other hand, the words *circulation, vision, ascites,* and *herpes* are singular in meaning. *Biceps, forceps, scissors,* and *series* are spelled the same whether the meaning is singular or plural.

Forming Plural Abbreviations

Add *s* (no apostrophe) after all uppercase abbreviations.

Serial ECGs revealed no changes.

CBCs over the last 6 months have been abnormal.

Many radiologists select CDs to get a higher resolution and portability.

Add *s* to abbreviated forms such as *poly* or *seg* (polys, segs).

White count was 5500 with 67 segs, 7 monos, 2 eos.

Plural Numbers and Units of Measure

When pluralizing numbers, add *s* without an apostrophe unless the number is only one digit.

> She had her appendix removed in her 20s.
>
> Doctors have made many advances in the 1990s.
>
> Apgar scores of 8's and 9's are common.

Do not put an *s* on the end of an abbreviated unit of measure, no matter how large the value is, e.g., 1 mg or 1,000,000 mg.

> We removed 200 mL of fluid from the patient's peritoneal cavity.
>
> The incision measured 6 cm.

Correcting Dictation

Always consider the context of the dictation when choosing the singular or plural form of a noun. For instance, if you hear "conjunctiva clear," you would transcribe this in plural form (unless the patient only has one eye or the eye exams are being dictated individually).

Complete Exercise 4.7 to check your ability to use the correct plural form of various medical terms.

Using Capitals Correctly

Authors can use capitalization to signal to a reader that something is important or specialized. However, the overuse of capitals diminishes their effect and may confuse rather than help the reader. Transcriptionists need to know the basic rules of capitalization and how and when to apply them.

Proper Nouns

Capitalize formal names of persons, places, and organizations.

> John A. Smith, MD
>
> Mayo Clinic
>
> Coronado Hospital, San Diego
>
> the American Cancer Society

Capitalize languages and races. Do not capitalize skin color.

> French   black
>
> Caucasian   white
>
> Mexican American

Capitalize days of the week, months, and holidays. Do not capitalize names of seasons.

> Thursday, May 28
>
> spring 1997
>
> Independence Day

Capitalize trade or brand names, but do not capitalize generic drug names.

> Amoxil   amoxicillin
>
> Cardizem   diltiazem
>
> Xeroform dressing

Capitalize a job title only when it precedes a name and is used as that person's title. Do not capitalize the title when it replaces or renames the person.

> Director of Education Maria Jaeb will read the new nursing guidelines.
> [The job title precedes the name.]

> Maria Jaeb, education director, will read the new nursing guidelines.

> [*Maria Jaeb* identifies the person being discussed, and *education director* gives further information about (or renames) Maria.]

Capitalize a genus name when it appears with a species name, but do not capitalize the species name. Do not capitalize the genus name when it appears without a species name, such as when it is used as an adjective.

> Clostridium difficile
>
> Streptococcus aureus
>
> streptococcus infection

Write the appropriate plural form on the blank line after each word.

1. fossa _____

2. prognosis _____

3. appendix _____

4. labium _____

5. datum _____

6. salpinx _____

7. uterus _____

8. ovum _____

9. criterion _____

10. foramen _____

From the choices given, circle the correct plural or singular form for each word. Key the corrected sentences. Save the document as XXExercise04.07.doc, using your initials for the XX in the file name.

11. Colonoscopy revealed multiple (diverticulum/diverticula) in the ascending colon.

12. Hysterosalpingogram showed right (hydrosalpinx/hydrosalpinges).

13. Her history of intolerance to cold led to the diagnosis of Raynaud (phenomenon/phenomena).

14. She was treated with ampicillin 500 (mg/mgs) q.i.d. for 10 days.

15. Delivery of the infant was achieved using a (forcep/forceps).

16. James was told by his doctor that he had a (herpe/herpes) infection.

17. Examination of her cervix revealed the presence of different (fungus/fungi).

18. Babinskis/Babinski's were negative.

19. Serial (CBC/CBCs/CBC's) were obtained.

20. (Ascitis/Ascites) is a common condition in people with liver disease.

Do not capitalize hospital department names. When referred to as an entitiy, capitalize the name.

intensive care unit	operating room
emergency department	neurology service

The report from Pathology is due to arrive at noon.

Pharmaceutical Abbreviations

Because of The Joint Commission's National Patient Safety Goal, there have been many changes over the years to improve safety in drug delivery, packaging, labeling, and ordering of pharmaceuticals. These changes have come about through the study of abbreviations that are frequently misinterpreted or are otherwise involved in medication errors. The Institute of Safe Medication Practices (ISMP) is a nonprofit organization that has been instrumental in documenting these dangerous abbreviations in order to set policy to improve the safety in medication delivery to patients. A complete listing of the error-prone abbreviations, symbols, and dose designations identified by ISMP through the USP-ISMP Medication Error Reporting Program is available at www.ismp.org. While many of the errors occur in handwritten documents, it is appropriate to avoid these situations in both handwritten and typed records. In response to the recommendations made by ISMP and The Joint Commission, the dangerous abbreviations and notations listed in Table 4.1 should not be used by the transcriptionist.

Do not capitalize Latin abbreviations that deal with drug dosage (*b.i.d., a.c., p.o.*). According to *The Book of Style for Medical Transcription, Third Edition*, the correct form for Latin abbreviations is lowercase with a period after each letter.

h.s.	at bedtime
q.4 h.	every 4 hours
a.m.	morning
a.c.	before meals or food
q.12 h.	every 12 hours
t.i.d.	3 times a day
p.o.	by mouth
q.	every
p.m.	afternoon or evening
q.i.d.	4 times a day
b.i.d.	twice a day

These examples demonstrate the spacing to be used in transcribed reports. Notice the space before *h.* in *q.4 h.* and *q.12 h.*

Table 4.1

Dangerous Abbreviations and Notations

	Misinterpretation	Correct Form to Use
Dangerous Abbreviations		
μg	milligram	mcg or microgram
q.d.	q.i.d., 4 times a day	daily
q.o.d.	4 times a day or daily	every other day
U	0	unit
IU	IV, intravenous	International Unit
cc		mL or milliliter
MS	morphine sulfate or magnesium sulfate	magnesium sulfate or morphine sulfate
MgSO$_4$	morphine sulfate	magnesium sulfate
MSO$_4$	magnesium sulfate	morphine sulfate
Dangerous Notations		
>	7	greater than
<	L	less than
trailing zero (2.0 mg)	missed decimal point (20 mg)	2 mg
lack of leading zero (.X mg)	missed decimal point (2 mg)	0.2 mg
apothecary units		metric units
@	2	at

Source: Adapted from the official "Do Not Use List" created by The Joint Commission, www.jointcommission.org/PatientSafety/DoNotUseList. Additional dangerous abbreviations, symbols, and dose designations are listed at www.ismp.org.

Some hospitals direct their MTs to capitalize the abbreviation NPO, which stands for *nil per os* (nothing by mouth). The term is capitalized because it communicates very important information. If the term goes unnoticed in a patient's record, there could be life-threatening consequences. However, in this instance, as with other style issues, follow your employer's preference.

Abbreviate and capitalize courtesy titles when they appear with complete names or with last names only *(Mr., Mrs., Ms., Dr.)*. There is a trend toward dropping the periods with courtesy titles, but periods are still acceptable.

Mr. Jonathan Brendel is the incoming CFO of the entire hospital system.

Mrs. Mumford will prepare the address list.

Ms. Nancy Coletti is the new supervisor.

Dr. Sanders will be glad to accept your invitation to be keynote speaker at the convention.

Spell out all other titles used with personal names *(Senator, President, Governor, Captain)*.

Senator McCain

Governor George Byron

Always abbreviate *Jr* and *Sr* (without punctuation) when they follow personal names.

Dr. Frank Smith, Sr

Abbreviate *Esq.* and *MD* after a full personal name; however, never use a courtesy title before a full name.

INCORRECT
Dr. Courtney Lorenzo, MD
CORRECT
Courtney Lorenzo, MD
INCORRECT
Esq. Paul Mirando
CORRECT
Paul Mirando, Esq.

Abbreviated words used in routine correspondence and business forms are followed by a period and a space.

etc.	et cetera
vs.	versus
vol.	volume
fwd.	forward

When expressing time, use the abbreviations *a.m.* and *p.m.*

10 a.m.

4 p.m.

Acronyms

Acronyms are words formed by the first (or significant) letter of each term in a compound term. Examples include GERD (pronounced gurd), which stands for gastroesophageal reflux disease, and AIDS (pronounced aids), which stands for acquired immune deficiency syndrome. Capitalize all the letters of an acronym. No periods are required.

Abbreviations

Like acronyms, abbreviations are formed by the initial letters in a compound term. However, with an abbreviation, a word is not formed by the letters, and the individual letters are spoken. Capitalize all the letters of an abbreviation. No periods are required.

ASHD	atherosclerotic/arteriosclerotic heart disease
LVD	left ventricular dysfunction
CHF	congestive heart failure
LAO	left anterior oblique
MI	myocardial infarction

Some business terms are often abbreviated when used on business forms. Note that there are no periods used with these abbreviations.

ASAP	as soon as possible
CEO	chief executive officer
COD	cash on delivery
EOM	end of month
FDIC	Federal Deposit Insurance Company
FOB	free on board
FYI	for your information

However, when these terms are used within a sentence, use small letters with periods.

> This package arrived c.o.d.
>
> The invoice will be processed with other e.o.m. accounting procedures.

Eponyms

Eponyms are adjectives created from proper nouns. The terms usually derive from the name of the person who identified the disease, developed the protocol, or designed the instrument. The eponym can also be named after a patient. The eponym itself, but not the noun, is capitalized. The possessive form (Down's syndrome) has been replaced with the nonpossessive (Down syndrome) form. This transition is occurring with all eponyms. Do not use the possessive form.

Alzheimer disease	Foley catheter
Bruce protocol	Gram stain

While eponyms are capitalized when they precede and modify nouns, words that are derived from eponyms are no longer proper nouns and should not be capitalized.

> The patient exhibited symptoms of Parkinson disease.
>
> The patient's symptoms were parkinsonian.
>
> The specimen was sent for Gram stain and C&S, and it returned showing gram-negative rods.

Drug Allergies

The capitalization of the word *allergy* (or variations) and all letters of a drug name listed under an Allergies heading attracts the reader's attention.

> ALLERGIES
> The patient is ALLERGIC TO MORPHINE, which causes a rash.

Document Elements

Capitalize the first letter of a formal list.

> DISCHARGE INSTRUCTIONS
> 1. Activities ad lib.
> 2. Diet as tolerated.
> 3. Followup will be in 1 week in my office.
>
> DISCHARGE MEDICATIONS
> 1. Aspirin 325 mg 1 daily.
> 2. Hydrochlorothiazide 50 mg p.o. daily.

Keep headings and subheadings in all capital letters. Capitalize the first word after a heading.

> PHYSICAL EXAMINATION
> GENERAL: He is a slightly ill appearing white male who just turned 30 years old.
> VITAL SIGNS: Temperature 97.6 degrees Fahrenheit, pulse 80, respirations 20, blood pressure 140/80.
> HEENT: Pupils equal and reactive.

Correct a portion of a medical report containing multiple capitalization errors in Exercise 4.8.

Read the following partial discharge summary and circle all capitalization errors. Key the partial report with the errors corrected. Save the document as XXExercise04.08.doc, using your initials in place of XX in the file name.

history of present illness

the patient is a 55-year-old african american, who speaks french and chinese, presenting with a chief complaint of chest pain. he has been having mild chest pain since early autumn, but it has been increasing recently, especially over the holidays. he has been taking dyazide for blood pressure and also uses ibuprofen occasionally. on sunday, new year's day, he called his insurance company and was referred to south side hospital. the patient presented to the emergency department for evaluation and was noted to have t-wave inversions on his ecg. chest x-ray showed no pneumonia or pulmonary edema. he was given nitroglycerin sublingually x2, with resolution of his chest pain. cpk was shown to be elevated, and cardiology was called to evaluate this patient and assume his care. the patient was admitted to the intensive care unit at 0300.

past medical history

the patient has a diagnosis of early parkinson disease and is treated by a neurologist for this.

allergies

the patient is allergic to sulfa which causes hives.

physical examination

vital signs: blood pressure 110/95, pulse 75, respirations 18.

heent: normocephalic, atraumatic. pupils equal, round, reactive to light and accommodation. fundi clear, no av nicking. ears, nose, and throat clear.

neck: supple, no jvd, no lymphadenopathy.

thorax and lungs: clear to percussion and auscultation.

cardiovascular: s1 and s2 normal. there was a grade 2/6 systolic ejection murmur heard best at the left lower sternal border.

abdomen: supple. no organomegaly or rebound tenderness.

ano-rectal: deferred.

extremities: no clubbing, cyanosis, or edema.

(continued)

hospital course

the patient was taken to the cardiac catheterization laboratory on the morning of admission. this study revealed no areas of stenosis of the coronary arterial system. the patient was given nitroglycerin sublingually p.r.n. chest pain and was given procardia for his hypertension. his ecg normalized, and on tuesday he was subjected to a treadmill exercise test using the modified bruce protocol. this test was interpreted by the cardiologist as showing no signs of ischemia.

condition on discharge

the patient was discharged in excellent condition.

discharge medications

1. procardia 10 mg daily.

2. aspirin 325 mg 1 daily.

3. nitroglycerin sublingual p.r.n. chest pain.

plan

the patient is to follow up in 1 week with dr. smith at the south bay regional cardiac center.

Using Numbers in Word or Figure Form

In formal writing outside of the healthcare documentation domain, the general rule of spelling out numbers under 10 is appropriate. However, it is important to note that healthcare documentation does not fall within the parameters of most formal writing. Clarity of communication to eliminate ambiguity or potential misinterpretation is paramount, since the application of that information has a direct impact on coordination of care. Numbers that are spelled out are more apt to be overlooked or missed when a care provider is quickly scanning the chart for vital statistics and critical information. All clinically significant numeric values in the record should be expressed with Arabic numerals (with the exception of those few instances in the record where Roman numerals are

required). Since virtually all numbers in a medical record represent clinically important information (demographics, vital statistics, laboratory values, wound measures, drug dosages, classification descriptors, etc.), you will find that there are very few instances in a medical record where spelling out a number would be necessary or appropriate.

The patient will be seen again in 3 weeks.

She took 4 Advil this morning, which did little to resolve her headache.

Her staging PET scan revealed 3 nodular lesions in the right middle lobe.

There were 65 lymphocytes, 2 monocytes, and 5 eosinophils.

SOCIAL HISTORY
She has 2 cats and 3 dogs at home.

When consecutive numbers are dictated, spell out the first number to avoid confusion or misinterpretation.

> Exam revealed four 1 cm necrotic lesions on the right foot.
>
> We dressed the wound with three 4 x 4's.
>
> Three 1 L solutions were used.
>
> The surgeon made two 5 cm incisions.

When transcribing numeric values, avoid line breaks between the number and the unit of measure. If necessary, insert a nonbreaking space (Ctrl+Shift+Spacebar bar) between the number and the unit of measure. This is better than using a line break (Enter) or a manual line break (Shift+Enter) because it will not force a break if the text reflows in the document.

Dates

The date line of a business or consultation letter should be written in full (April 20, 20XX). At the top of reports, use the date format with slashes between the month, day, and year. For single digit months and days, insert a zero before the date.

> He has an appointment for 10/09/20XX.

Follow the dictated content for dates within the body of reports or letters. Only transcribe a date's year if the dictator states it. Use a cardinal figure when the day follows the month.

> Please arrange for surgery to be performed on October 3.
>
> Please keep July 1 open for graduation ceremonies.

A day that precedes a month should be expressed in ordinal numbers (numbers expressing place or position as in *first, second, third*) or in ordinal words.

> We have continued to follow this patient on the 5th of each month.
>
> The international oncology conference will be held in London from the fifth of October until the ninth.

It is preferred to use ordinal numbers in transcription, but using ordinal words is acceptable.

The military and international style for expressing dates reverses the day and month, with no commas in between. Follow this format if your client or employer prefers.

> The patient was admitted on 10 April 20XX.

Age

Express ages and other vital statistics in figures.

> She is a 21-year-old, well-developed, well-nourished white female. Height 5 feet 6 inches, weight 130 pounds, blood pressure 110/70, pulse 74, respirations 18.
> [Note that common nonmetric units of measurement (*feet, inches, pounds*) are spelled out.]

Time

Use figures to express times of day. No zeros are required when the time falls on the hour. Use a colon (with no spaces) to separate hours from minutes.

> The patient will be seen at 2 p.m.
>
> Surgery is scheduled for 7 a.m.
>
> The patient expired at 11:45 p.m.
>
> The meeting will be held from 9 a.m. to 12:30 p.m.

Many medical facilities follow the military style of expressing time. Military time uses no colons, and instead of starting over at noon, the clock continues to count to 2400 (stated as "twenty-four hundred hours"). If this confuses you, simply subtract 1200 to get "civilian" time, for example, 2350 − 1200 = 1150 a.m. Note the following dictated sentences and the times intended. Midnight is reported as 0000 (or "zero hundred").

DICTATED
The infant was delivered at fourteen forty-five.

TRANSCRIBED
The infant was delivered at 1445. [2:45 p.m.]

DICTATED

The last dose was given at zero three twenty hours.

TRANSCRIBED

The last dose was given at 0320. [3:20 a.m.]

Anatomic position may be dictated using a clock-face orientation (*o'clock*). Use figures in these expressions.

A suspicious mass was noted at the 3 o'clock position on the left breast.

The lesion appears at 12 o'clock on the right cheek.

Money

Use figures to express amounts of money. Do not include zeros in even dollar amounts.

The patient has a $5 copay.

He purchased $250 worth of equipment.

If similar functions are performed by numbers in a sentence, write them uniformly.

The pharmacy charged $75.50, $29.95, $55.00, and $60.00 for each of the medications.
[Note the consistent use of decimal points and places.]

When amounts of money include millions and billions of dollars, write out *million* or *billion*. Do not add *dollars*, but use the dollar symbol.

A $2.5 billion donation was given to the medical school.

Measurements, Mathematical Expressions, and Symbols

Use figures for measurements and ratios and in expressions involving symbols and abbreviations.

The mass on the head of the pancreas measured 2 x 3 cm.
[Note that the unit of measurement is expressed only once.]

It is an 8- by 14-foot room.

The patient's height is 5 feet 6 inches and her weight is 135 pounds.

The paper measures 8 inches by 11 inches.

The incision was closed with 3-0 Prolene.

The patient has 20/50 vision in the right eye and 20/70 in the left eye.

The solution was diluted 1:50.
[no space before or after the colon]

Pulses were 2+.
[Do not transcribe as ++.]

While it is acceptable and preferred to use the degree symbol (°) when transcribing angles and temperatures, there is a trend toward dropping the degree symbol and spelling out *degrees* in environments where technology interoperability protocols, which determine how data must be formatted in order to be exchanged between electronic systems, do not support use of some special characters and symbols. Where able and allowed to use the symbol, it is appropriate to do so. Keep in mind, though, that it is not acceptable to use the degree symbol with burn classifications.

She had a second-degree burn on the palmar aspect of her right hand.

Temperatures should be expressed with Arabic numbers (except for zero). Use the word *minus*, not the symbol, to express temperatures below zero. Include the temperature scale (Celsius, Kelvin, Fahrenheit, or Centigrade) only if dictated. Transcribe the word degrees (or the symbol) only if the word is dictated. If the temperature scale is dictated, spell it out if spelling out *degrees* and abbreviate if using the degree symbol. Do not put a space between the degree symbol and the scale abbreviation.

zero degrees

37° or 37 degrees

98 degrees Fahrenheit

minus 10 °F

Vertebrae

Express vertebral levels using a capital C, T (or D), L, or S followed by an arabic numeral, as in T2. Do not use a hyphen. Do not superscript or subscript the numeral. It is preferable to repeat the letter before each numbered vertebra in a list. It is not necessary to repeat the letter before the second vertebra if the letters are the same, but it may be transcribed if dictated.

C4, C5, and C6   C1-2 or C1-C2

Use a hyphen to express the intervertebral space (space between two vertebrae), as in L5-S1 or L2-L3. This could be dictated with or without the word "to" representing the hyphens.

Decimals and Fractions

Use figures to express decimals. If a decimal less than 1 is dictated, transcribe a zero before the decimal point, even if it is not dictated. When whole numbers are dictated, do not add a decimal point and zero.

DICTATED

The patient takes digoxin point 125 milligrams daily.

TRANSCRIBED

The patient takes digoxin 0.125 mg daily.

DICTATED

She was given five point zero milligrams of Valium.

TRANSCRIBED

She was given 5 mg of Valium.

When a metric measurement is dictated as a fraction, convert the fraction to a decimal. Common fractions and decimal equivalents include the following: ¼ = 0.25, ½ = 0.5, and ¾ = 0.75.

INCORRECT

Local anesthesia was achieved using ½ percent Xylocaine.

CORRECT

Local anesthesia was achieved using 0.5% Xylocaine.

Write fractions standing alone as words.

At least two-thirds of the patients were scheduled to have blood work done at their next visit.

When a dictation refers to a fraction that is an estimate or a general amount, not a specific measurement, use words to express the fraction.

INCORRECT

The upper ½ of the esophagus appeared normal.

CORRECT

The upper one-half of the esophagus appeared normal.

INCORRECT

The distal ⅔ of the esophagus revealed no abnormalities.

CORRECT

The distal two-thirds of the esophagus revealed no abnormalities.

Use a colon to express a ratio. Do not key a space before or after the colon.

DICTATED

The ECG revealed a two-to-one block.

TRANSCRIBED

The ECG revealed a 2:1 block.

DICTATED

Xylocaine with one-to-one hundred thousand epinephrine was instilled for local anesthesia.

TRANSCRIBED

Xylocaine with 1:100,000 epinephrine was instilled for local anesthesia.

Numeric Ranges

Ranges are dictated frequently in patient records to express values that fall within certain parameters. Use a hyphen between the values of a range only when all of the following conditions have been met:

- The phrases "from...to," "from...through," "between...and" are **not** used.
- Decimals and/or commas do not appear in the numeric values.
- Neither value contains four or more digits.
- Neither value is negative.
- Neither value is accompanied by a symbol.

The word "to" may be used instead, even when all these conditions are met.

Applying the rules for correctly transcribing numbers in medical reports can be challenging. Test your editing skill by completing Exercise 4.9.

Edit the discharge summary shown in Figure 4.1 on pages 127 and 128 for the correct use of numbers. Circle the correct number expressions from the choices in parentheses, then key the report with the errors corrected. Save the document as XXExercise04.09, using your initials in place of the *XX* in the file name.

Using Abbreviations Correctly

An abbreviation is a quicker or shorter way to say or write a word or phrase. Abbreviations save space and may speed up communication, but they can also cause confusion and misinterpretation.

In the rush of documenting care for a provider to dictate shortened forms of common clinical words. Typically, these newly coined abbreviated forms start out as slang and evolve over time through trend and usage to become acceptable brief forms. Slang terms should be expanded and spelled out in full. Short forms, however, have evolved in many cases to such widespread usage and adoption as to become acceptable in the medical record. Be careful to consult appropriate references to determine if a word is either a slang or brief form and transcribe according to that reference.

Your medical transcription library should include an abbreviations reference. Keep context in mind as you search for abbreviations to ensure that the extended form you choose is the appropriate term.

Generally, transcribe abbreviations in full capital letters without punctuation and without spaces between the letters. Short forms, such as *segs* for *segmented neutrophils* or *lymphs* for *lymphocytes*, are transcribed as dictated.

SLANG

cath'd (catheterized)
foley'd (had a Foley placed)
appy (appendectomy)
epi (epinephrine)
D/C'd or D/C (discontinued)

BRIEF FORMS

lab
exam
segs
monos
eos
prep

Keep in mind that many abbreviations in clinical medicine are dictated as acronyms. An acronym is an abbreviation that is pronounced as a word rather than by its individual letters. As an MT, you will need to be familiar with common abbreviations and acronyms and be careful to correlate what is dictated to the clinical context of the report.

DICTATED

The patient has a past medical history that is significant for cabbage times 4 at the age of 59.

TRANSCRIBED

The patient has a past medical history that is significant for CABG x4 at the age of 59.

DICTATED

She had an extended hospital stay, complicated by nosocomial mersa infection.

TRANSCRIBED

She had an extended hospital stay, complicated by nosocomial MRSA infection.

To Abbreviate or Not to Abbreviate

In medical reports, there are some areas in which abbreviations are not used even if they are dictated. Do not use abbreviations in any impression, assessment, admitting or discharge diagnosis, or preoperative or postoperative diagnosis. Do not use abbreviations in the title of the procedure for an operative report.

DICTATED

ADMITTING DIAGNOSIS
S/P CVA.

PATIENT NAME: Juan Juarez
MR #:   12-34-56
ADMISSION DATE: (April 4 20XX; 04/04/20XX)
DISCHARGE DATE: (April 6 20XX; 04/06/20XX)

DISCHARGE DIAGNOSIS
Herniated nucleus pulposus, (L-5-S-1; L5-S1).

HISTORY OF PRESENT ILLNESS
This is a (fifty; 50)-year-old Hispanic male who presented with a (four; 4)-month history of progressive low back pain. Over the past (one; 1) month, he has had worsening symptoms and now has numbness, tingling, and pain radiating down his right leg.

PAST MEDICAL HISTORY
His history is significant for (two; 2) episodes of pneumonia (five; 5) years ago, and he has chronic asthma.

SOCIAL HISTORY
The patient smokes (one; 1) pack of cigarettes per day and has done so for the past (twenty; 20) years. He drinks (2 6-packs; two six-packs; two 6-packs; 2 six-packs) of beer per week.

ALLERGIES
CODEINE, which causes a rash.

CURRENT MEDICATIONS
1. Theo-Dur (three hundred milligrams; 300 milligrams; 300 mg) (tid; t.i.d.; TID).
2. Proventil inhaler (two; 2) puffs (q12h; q. 12 h.; q.12 h.)

PHYSICAL EXAMINATION
GENERAL: This is a slightly obese Hispanic male appearing slightly older than his stated age of (fifty-years; 50-years; 50 years).
VITAL SIGNS: Blood pressure (one hundred twenty over sixty; 120 over 60; 120/60), pulse (eighty; 80) and regular, respirations (twelve; 12), temperature (ninety eight; ninety-eight; 98) degrees.
HEENT: Pupils equal and reactive to light. The left tympanic membrane was (one plus/1+) injected. Nares were patent bilaterally.
NECK: Right shotty supraclavicular lymph node approximately (two, 2) cm wide. Trachea midline.
THORAX AND LUNGS: Clear to percussion and auscultation.
CARDIOVASCULAR: Auscultation revealed a grade (two over six; 2 over 6; 2/6) systolic ejection murmur. PMI is at the (fifth; 5th) intercostal space.
ABDOMEN: Slightly obese, (one plus; 1 plus; 1+) tenderness in the epigastrium. Bowel sounds were present, no hepatosplenomegaly.
MUSCULOSKELETAL: Negative CVA tenderness. There was (two plus; 2+) tenderness in the (L-4-L-5; L4-L5) area. Straight leg raising was negative on the left, positive on the right at (forty five; forty-five; 45) degrees.
EXTREMITIES: No clubbing, cyanosis, or edema. Distal pulses were good.
NEUROLOGIC: Cranial nerves (two through twelve; II-XII; 2-12) were intact. The patient was alert and oriented (times three; x3).

(continued)

Figure 4.1   Discharge Summary

DISCHARGE SUMMARY
PATIENT NAME: Juan Juarez
MR #: 12-34-56
DISCHARGE DATE: (April 6 20XX; 04/06/20XX)
Page 2

LABORATORY DATA
Admission CBC revealed WBC of (fifty-eight hundred; 5800) with (seventy-one; 71) polys,
(two; 2) bands, (one; 1) eosinophil, and (twenty-six; 26) lymphs. Hemoglobin was (thirteen; 13),
hematocrit (thirty-nine percent; 39 percent; 39%). BUN was (eight; 8), creatinine (point nine; .9; 0.9).

HOSPITAL COURSE
Lumbar myelogram on day of admission revealed significant disk herniation at the (L-4-L-5;
L4-L5; L4-5) level. The patient was taken to the operating room where right partial (L-4; L4)
hemilaminectomy with excision of herniated disk was performed.

Postoperatively the patient had a temperature spike to (101 degrees; one-hundred one degrees) and
was started on Ancef. He had no further temperature elevations and his chest x-ray remained clear. He
had good resolution of his symptoms.

DISCHARGE INSTRUCTIONS
The patient was discharged to home to be followed in clinic in (five; 5) days. Instructions were given for
no heavy lifting. It was suggested that a (thirty; 30)-minute walk be taken daily.

DISCHARGE MEDICATIONS
1. Vicodin (one; 1) p.o. (q. three to four hours; q.3-4 h.) p.r.n. pain.
2. Theo-Dur and Proventil as previously.

_____
Nancy Sprans, MD

NS/XX
D: 04/08/20XX
T: 04/09/20XX

Figure 4.1   Discharge Summary (Continued)

TRANSCRIBED

ADMITTING DIAGNOSIS
Status post cerebrovascular accident.

DICTATED

NAME OF OPERATION
ORIF, right hip fracture.

TRANSCRIBED

NAME OF OPERATION
Open reduction and internal fixation, right hip fracture.

Do not abbreviate any medical term that is dictated in full except for metric units of measure (*milligrams, milliliters*) preceded by a number (for example, transcribe 5 mg, not 5 milligrams). Metric units of measure most often appear in laboratory results and drug dosages.

Units of Measure

Use abbreviations when a numeric quantity precedes metric units of measure. Metric units of measure are abbreviated in technical and scientific work, in tables, and on business forms (L, mL, g). Do not add *s* or *'s*. When a metric unit of measure is preceded by a numeric value, abbreviate the unit of measure, and do not use punctuation (such as apostrophes or hyphens).

DICTATED

ampicillin five hundred milligrams capsule

TRANSCRIBED

ampicillin 500 mg capsule

DO NOT USE

500 mg. capsule
500-mg capsule
500 mgs capsule
500 mg's capsule

Spell out metric units of measure when they are not preceded by numerals.

The patient's weight was reported in kilograms.

The volume was measured in milliliters.

Spell out common nonmetric units of measure, like foot, inch, ounce, and so on, except in tables.

Do not abbreviate or use an apostrophe or quotation marks to indicate feet or inches except in tables. Follow the rules for using a hyphen with a compound modifier when using written-out units of measure.

The child's height was 4 feet 2 inches.

The infant weighed 8 pounds 8½ (or 8-1/2) ounces.

A 5-inch incision was made.

Punctuation with Abbreviations

Usually, no punctuation is used with abbreviations. The exception is the group of Latin abbreviations that deal with medication administration. These are always keyed in lowercase with periods in between.

b.i.d.   p.r.n.   q.12 h.

If more than one Latin abbreviation is dictated together, put a space between the two abbreviations.

Zantac 150 mg p.o. b.i.d.

DICTATED

She takes Valium five milligrams p-o-b-i-d-p-r-n anxiety.

TRANSCRIBED

She takes Valium 5 mg p.o. b.i.d. p.r.n. anxiety.

Plural Abbreviations

Abbreviations in capital letters do not require an apostrophe before the *s* (*WBCs, ECGs, VCRs, CDs, CPAs*). Add an apostrophe to words that could be misread (for example, *CPS's*). Add an *s* to short forms for laboratory terms (*lymphs, monos, segs*).

Abbreviations That Have Multiple Meanings

Do not guess. If an abbreviation with multiple meanings is dictated—for example, PT—you may or may not be able to determine the intended meaning based on the context of the report. To figure out the meaning, read the rest of the report to see if the full term has been dictated elsewhere, or look at the patient's record if you have easy access to it. If you are unsuccessful, leave the term in the abbreviated form, even in a diagnosis. It is better to leave an abbreviated form that knowledgeable people will be able to interpret than to transcribe a full term that is incorrect.

If the abbreviation itself is not clear (CVP? CPT? CCP?), try the same methods as above. Again, do not guess. It is better to leave a blank than to guess incorrectly.

Shorthand Dictation

Physicians sometimes use a verbal "shorthand" for certain words or expressions that appear regularly in medical reports. For example, the terms *discharged*, *discontinued*, and *identified* may be dictated as "dee seed" [DC'd] and "i deed" [ID'd]. The terms should be transcribed in full:

DICTATED
Streptococcus was ID'd on blood culture.

TRANSCRIBED
Streptococcus was identified on blood culture.

DICTATED
The patient was DC'd from the hospital today.

TRANSCRIBED
The patient was discharged from the hospital today.

DICTATED
Physical therapy was DC'd because the patient complained of severe pain.

TRANSCRIBED
Physical therapy was discontinued because the patient complained of severe pain.

Complete Exercise 4.10 to practice editing abbreviations in transcribed medical records.

Using Apostrophes Correctly

Apostrophes are used to denote omitted letters in contractions, to express an abbreviated year, to show possession, and to form some plurals.

Contractions

Use contracted forms in medical reports only in a direct quote; otherwise, write out the words.

DICTATED
I don't feel the patient is improving.

TRANSCRIBED
I do not feel the patient is improving.

DICTATED
The patient said, "I don't feel I'm improving."

TRANSCRIBED
The patient said, "I don't feel I'm improving."

Remember that *it's* means *it is*, while the word *its* is a singular possessive pronoun. Because *it's* is a contraction, do not use it in a medical report.

The central venous line was placed and its ports were flushed with saline.

It is important that the bandages be changed every 2 hours.

Whose is a relative pronoun that can function in various ways, including as a connector between a subordinate clause and a main clause. *Who's* is a contraction for the two words *who is*. Note the differences in use:

She is a physician whose research is widely regarded as the best in the field.
[*Whose* connects the subordinate clause with the main clause.]

He is a new employee whose surgical acumen was highly rated.
[possessive pronoun]

It is not important who's speaking at the conference, as long as the field of candidates is carefully selected.
[*Who's* stands for *who is*.]

Who's responsible for taking the minutes for the meeting?
[*Who is* responsible?]

Who said they're booking a room for the meeting?
[*They are* booking.]

Use your abbreviations references, if available, to find the appropriate extended forms. Otherwise, use the abbreviations appendix at the end of the book. Then key the report extracts with the abbreviations spelled out, even if it would be acceptable to use the abbreviation in the transcribed report. Save the document as XXExercise04.10.doc, using your initials in place of the *XX* in the file name.

1. The patient was diagnosed with ALS, a degenerative neurologic disease commonly known as Lou Gehrig disease.

2. Because of her symptoms of left hemiparesis and confusion, Mrs. Smith was believed to have suffered a CVA.

3. An EEG, a test showing the electrical activity of the brain, was performed to rule out seizure disorder.

4. HEENT: PERRLA. Extraocular movements intact.

5. The patient suffers from weakness, paresthesias, and speech disturbances secondary to MS, a degenerative neurologic disorder.

6. The patient is alert and oriented, in NAD, resting comfortably.

7. The patient is n.p.o. in preparation for surgery; do not serve him breakfast.

8. The infant's PKU test was positive, so he will require a diet very low in phenylalanine to prevent mental retardation.

9. The patient has had several episodes of TIAs with neurologic deficits.

10. The myelogram revealed HNP at the L3-L4 level, with a significant disk protrusion.

Years

When a single year is expressed without the century, precede it with an apostrophe ('97). Use an apostrophe preceding expressions of decades of the century (in the '90s), but not when referring to decades of a patient's life (in his 50s).

Possessive Forms

Apostrophes indicate ownership, either literally or figuratively. When the noun is singular, add an *'s* to create the possessive.

> The patient's laboratory tests were normal.
> [possessive singular noun: 1 patient, his tests]

> He will be seen in 1 day's time.
> [the time belonging to 1 day]

Add only an apostrophe to form the possessive of singular nouns that end in *s*.

> Meredith Dobbs' cart crashed down the ramp.

Some singular nouns *(Mr. Harris)* become difficult to pronounce when you add *'s* because the addition makes an extra syllable. In this case, add only an apostrophe to show possession.

> Mrs. Billings' condition is stable.

When a possessive is an abbreviation, use *'s* just as you would with a singular word.

> The HMO's policies are clear.

As with singular nouns that end in *s*, add only an apostrophe to express the possessive of plural nouns that end in *s*.

> The physicians' opinions were varied.
> [more than one physician]

> All of the AIDS patients' study results were compiled.
> [possessive plural noun: more than one patient, their results]

However, add *'s* to plural nouns that do not end in *s* to make them possessive.

> The conference dealt with children's issues.

> More and more, women's rights are being protected and continuing to increase.

Use *'s* after the last word in a hyphenated, compound, and possessive term.

> Her mother-in-law's health was failing.

> Her daughters-in-laws' schedules were conflicting.
> [the schedules of both daughters-in-law]

The Book of Style for Medical Transcription, Third Edition, states not to use *'s* with eponymic terms (Alzheimer disease, not Alzheimer's disease). This has been widely accepted by all medical writing authorities, and this style will be followed for the transcription work in this text. However, defer to the wishes of your client or employer. It should be noted, though, that eponymic surgical terms generally do not require *'s*.

Plurals

In some instances, *'s* forms plurals that are not possessives. For example, use *'s* to form plurals of single letters or numbers. Without the apostrophe, *As* could be read as the word *as*.

> Three A's, two B's, and two C's.

> Mind your p's and q's.

> He rates his pain as mostly 1's and 2's on a scale of 1-10.

However, do not use an apostrophe to form the plural of capital letter abbreviations or numbers of two characters or more.

> Serial ECGs showed no change.

> Her hematocrits have been in the high 30s.

Plural nouns that act as descriptive terms in the name of a company or organization may or may not require an apostrophe. Determine the organization's preference and follow their usage.

Physicians Lounge

Physician's Lounge.

Complete Exercise 4.11 to check your ability to select the correct use of the apostraphe in Medical reports.

Using Hyphens Correctly

Hyphens are commonly used to form compound adjectives, nouns, and verbs. In these cases, hyphens help readers understand that a combination of words has a single meaning and function in the sentence, as in the phrase *24-year-old patient*. Hyphens are also occasionally used to connect prefixes to root words, especially when an unhyphenated spelling may confuse the reader. Finally, hyphens are used in fractions and in certain medical technical terms to communicate a continuation such as L1-L2.

Using hyphens to create compounds can be complicated because so many variables are involved and because the construction of a compound may change as it becomes widely used. For these reasons, you should always consult a current dictionary when you question the spelling of a compound word. The rules below provide general guidelines.

Compound Adjectives

The joining of two or more words to form a single adjective modifier that describes a noun is called a *compound adjective*. Compound adjectives are distinct from other adjectives because they represent the joining of two or more words that, individually, do not modify or describe the noun. It is only when they are joined together that they form a

Exercise 4.11   Editing for Correct Apostrophe Use

Circle the letter beside each correctly written sentence below. Some items may have more than one correct answer.

1. (a) Its important to rule out malignancy in this case.
   (b) It's important to rule out malignancy in this case.
   (c) It is important to rule out malignancy in this case.

2. (a) CBC's have continued to show decreased hemoglobin and hematocrit.
   (b) CBCs have continued to show decreased hemoglobin and hematocrit.
   (c) CBCS have continued to show decreased hemoglobin and hematocrit.

3. (a) The CMT's knowledge was evident in her reports.
   (b) The CMTs knowledge was evident in her reports.
   (c) The CMTs' knowledge was evident in her reports.

4. (a) The physician who's patients' records were transferred is Dr. Che.
   (b) The physician whose patients records were transferred is Dr. Che.
   (c) The physician whose patients' records were transferred is Dr. Che.

5. (a) The patients CD4s have been decreasing.
   (b) The patient's CD4's have been decreasing.
   (c) The patient's CD4s have been decreasing.

6. (a) "I don't think the rash has gotten worse."
   (b) "I do not think the rash has gotten worse."
   (c) "I dont think the rash has gotten worse."

7. (a) The patient whose family just arrived was discharged from the hospital today.
   (b) The patient who's family just arrived was discharged from the hospital today.

8. (a) He had an appendectomy in his '40s.
   (b) He had an appendectomy in his 40s.
   (c) He had an appendectomy in his 40's.

9. (a) She was first diagnosed with lupus in the late 80s.
   (b) She was first diagnosed with lupus in the late '80s.
   (c) She was first diagnosed with lupus in the late '80's.

10. (a) She will be followed up in 2 days time.
    (b) She will be followed up in 2 day's time.
    (c) She will be followed up in 2 days' time.

11. (a) Her son-in-laws all came to visit her.
    (b) Her sons-in-law's all came to visit her.
    (c) Her sons-in-law all came to visit her.

12. (a) Mr. Jones's condition is stable.
    (b) Mr. Jone's condition is stable.
    (c) Mr. Jones' condition is stable.

unique adjective expression.

> The x-ray emitted a high-power field.

> The injury occurred when she fell from her second-story window.

In the above example, the hyphen is needed because neither the word *second* nor the word *story* have a modifying relationship with the noun *window*. Only when they are joined with a hyphen do they form a single adjective that describes the window.

Compound adjectives are used frequently, and you will encounter them often in dictation. Most compound adjectives are hyphenated when preceding the nouns they modify. The only exception is when a compound modifier is preceded by an adverb, in which case the hyphen is dropped.

> He had a well-developed sense of humor.

> He had a very well developed sense of humor.

Some compound modifiers retain their hyphenation when they follow their nouns or are placed somewhere else in the sentence. Regardless of where they are placed, if they retain their modifying relationship with the noun, they retain their hyphens.

> The surgeon used bone-biting forceps.

> The forceps the surgeon used were bone-biting.

Some compound modifiers contain participles (verb forms functioning as adjectives). These modifiers retain their hyphens only when they precede, but not when they follow, the nouns they modify. In those instances, the verb forms cease to be participles and revert to their function as verbs.

> Examination revealed a well-healed scar.

> On examination, her scar was well healed. [The verb "was healed" is modified by the adverb "well."]

The Book of Style for Medical Transcription, Third Edition has outlined recommendations for hyphenating compound modifiers that are based on the parts of speech of each word in the modifying phrase. Recognizing and understanding basic

parts of speech will be critical to applying the rules for hyphenation of compound modifiers.

Do not hyphenate adverb-adjective combinations. You can identify these combinations by checking if the first word ends in *ly*, which usually means it is an adverb. In the phrase, *a slowly enlarging lesion*, for example, *slowly* is not an adjective but an adverb, so the modifying phrase is not hyphenated.

> She bought a poorly constructed house on Main Street.

Compound adjectives using the prefixes *self-* or *all-*, or the suffix *-free* should always be hyphenated, whether or not they precede a noun.

self-esteem	all-encompassing
self-limiting	all-inclusive
symptom-free	pain-free

You may decide to rewrite a sentence to omit some of the hyphenated words. Do this cautiously and only when absolutely necessary.

DICTATED

The patient has a 2-pack-per-day-times-30-year cigarette-smoking history.

TRANSCRIBED

The patient has a history of smoking 2 packs of cigarettes per day for 30 years.

Prefixes and Suffixes

As explained in Chapter 3, prefixes are syllables that are added to the beginning of a word. Suffixes are syllables that are attached to the end of a word.

Do not hyphenate words with the prefix *non* unless the following element is capitalized or starts with a number. An exception is *non-insulin-dependent diabetes*.

nontender	non-Hodgkin lymphoma
nonnarcotic	non-A hepatitis
nonsteroidal	non-MD members
nonprofessional	non-2002 graduates

Do not hyphenate words with the prefix *extra* unless the word can be easily misread.

extradural	extra-large
extrapapillary	extra-apical
extraordinary	extra-base hit

Do not use a hyphen with the prefixes *ante-, anti-, bi-, dis-, co-, infra-, inter-, intra-, mid-, mini-, multi-, non-, out-, over-, post-, pre-, pro-, pseudo-, re-, semi-, sub-, super-, supra-, trans-, tri-, ultra-, un-,* and *uni-* unless the word that follows begins with the same vowel that ends the prefix; it may cause confusion and be misread. Generally, no hyphens are added when a prefix is the first element of a compound or a suffix is the last element.

PREFIX

interoffice	nonessential
antiemetic	
anti-inflammatory drug	
antibiotic	

SUFFIX

leadership	excitement

Do not hyphenate words with the suffix *-like* unless the word is capitalized, ends in *l* or a vowel, or has three or more syllables.

AIDS-like	slitlike
flu-like	Parkinson-like
plate-like	

Hyphenate words with the prefix *ex-* when *ex-* means former. Otherwise do not hyphenate.

ex-husband	excision
ex-president	expression
ex-patient	exogenous

Hyphenate words that would be misread without a hyphen. If the lack of a hyphen makes a word difficult to interpret, hyphenate the word.

re-cover (to cover again, not to return to normal)

re-create (to make again, not to play)

It was time to re-cover the chair.

Try to re-create the Titanic and enter it into the contest.

non-neoplastic

pre-clotting

Some words are so commonly used together that they are read as a unit without hyphenation. A few examples are listed below. Check your dictionary when in doubt, since there are no firm guidelines.

arterial blood gas	blood pressure readings
deep tendon reflex	exercise tolerance test
jugular venous distention	left upper lobe
low back pain	normal sinus rhythm
status post cellulitis	red cell count

Suspended Hyphens

Suspended hyphens connect two or more prefixes or adjectives to the same term. Use a suspended hyphen after each prefix or word in the series.

full- and split-thickness skin grafts

2- and 3-inch lengths

Boxes of 5-, 10-, and 15-pound books will be sent to you by FedEx.

Specific Words

The verb, adjective, and noun variations of the words *follow up* can cause confusion if not transcribed correctly.

VERB
The patient will follow up with me next week.

ADJECTIVE
He will have a followup chest film to document resolution of his pneumonia.

NOUN
Followup will be with her primary physician.

Other Uses of the Hyphen

Hyphenate fractions expressed in words.

The lower one-third of the right lung was removed.

Three-fourths of my patients are nonsmokers.

Use a hyphen to express the space between two vertebrae.

C4-C5

L5-S1

Use hyphens with most suture sizes. Include the number symbol (#) if the physician dictates the word *number*.

DICTATED

The fascia was reapproximated with three oh Vicryl.

TRANSCRIBED

The fascia was reapproximated with 3-0 Vicryl.

DICTATED

The skin was closed with number seven Ethibond.

TRANSCRIBED

The skin was closed with #7 Ethibond.

In numeric and alphabetic ranges, use a hyphen in place of the word *to* if it separates two consecutive units. Refer back to page *XX* for the rules of using hyphens for numeric ranges.

The child brought to the emergency room appeared to be 2-3 years old.

The construction will take from 10-12 hours.

Complete Exercise 4.12 to practice editing a medical report for proper use of compound modifiers, compound words, and other uses of hyphens.

Exercise 4.12   Editing for Correct Use of Hyphens

Edit the following text placing hyphens where needed. Also correct those words written as two words that should be written as one word. Key the body of this corrected history and physical report with the correct hyphenation and word format. Save the document as XXExercise 04.12.doc, using your initials in place of the *XX* in the file name.

HISTORY OF PRESENT ILLLNESS

This 30 year old white male reported to clinic today for a routine follow up appointment, with diagnosis of HIV disease.

He was initially diagnosed in mid August 20XX. Additional diagnoses include major depression, chronic serous otitis media, chronic active hepatitis, low back pain, and headaches.

Since his previous examination, the patient has continued to have active medical problems. With regard to his HIV infection, the patient continues to have a decreasing CD4 count. He is followed by a physician in Los Angeles, and his most recent CD4 count was an absolute value of 250. The patient notes a 10 to 12 week history of increasing night sweats. The patient, at present, is on no anti retro viral therapy, having discontinued AZT therapy 2 months ago.

(continued)

The patient also had a long recovery complicated by infection following a scar revision of his lower lip earlier this year. He also continues to be followed for his diagnosis of chronic active hepatitis. He also is followed for chronic depression, for which he is treated with Zoloft therapy. The patient continues to be affected by right sided migraine like headaches; a recent CT scan was negative for any intra cranial pathology.

SOCIAL HISTORY

The patient continues to work but on a part time basis. He works at home using his computer. He is a non drinker. He was a one pack per day smoker until two years ago, when he stopped.

FAMILY HISTORY

Non contributory.

PHYSICAL EXAMINATION

GENERAL: He is a slightly ill appearing white male who just turned 30 years old.

VITAL SIGNS: Temperature 97.6 degrees, pulse 80, respirations 20, blood pressure 140/80.

HEENT: Pupils equal and reactive. Extra ocular movements are intact.

NECK: Mild supraclavicular adenopathy. No jugular venous distention.

THORAX AND LUNGS: Mild end expiratory wheezes, worse on the left.

CARDIOCVASCULAR: Regular rate and rhythm. PMI is in the 5th left inter costal space at mid clavicular line.

ABDOMEN: Soft, non tender on the left with some mild right sided pain. Liver span is 2 finger breadths below the costal margin. Back reveals mild tenderness at the L4 L5 level. No costo vertebral angle tenderness.

PELVIS: Normal male phallus with descended testes bilaterally.

ANO-RECTAL: Rectal exam reveals normal anal sphincter tone with a few mild external and internal hemorrhoids.

PERIPHERAL VASCULAR: Pulses, including brachio radialis, femoral, popliteal, and dorsalis pedis, normal.

LABORATORY DATA

White blood cell count is 4.1, hematocrit 45.5, hemoglobin 15.6, platelet count 181,000. Differential shows 52% segs, 34% lymphocytes, 12% monocytes, and 2% eosinophils. The urinalysis revealed 1 to 2 white cells per high power field, otherwise normal.

(continued)

The liver function tests are normal. The CD4 count is 210 with a CD4 percentage of 15%. Intradermal skin testing reveals the patient to be anergic. VDRL is nonreactive.

IMPRESSION

1. Human immuno deficiency virus infection.
2. Chronic hepatitis B.
3. History of major depression.
4. Migraine like headaches.
5. History of chronic middle ear infections.

PLAN

The patient will follow up in 6 months for clinic visit and repeat labs. We have discussed appropriate short and long term goals for this patient. He will continue to work part time, as he enjoys this and is having no difficulty performing his job related activities.

Part Two

Transcribing for the Specialties

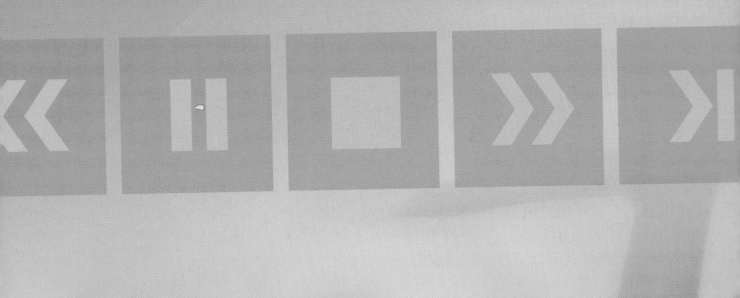

8.6 —
<u>Office Note</u>

drug —
Albuteral inhaler.
   w/ inspeiec

asthma exacerbt

Five

Dermatology

Dermatology encompasses the entire integumentary system, which includes the skin, hair, and nails. Because the skin can reflect the general health of the patient, it is the first part of the assessment by the healthcare professional.

Objectives

» Identify and understand the anatomy and function of the skin.

» Identify lesions and rashes that affect the skin.

» Recognize microbial pathogens that infect the skin.

» Differentiate the three types of skin biopsies.

» Pronounce and correctly spell terminology related to dermatology.

» Transcribe dictation related to the medical specialty of dermatology.

» Describe an Office Note, including typical content, format, and turnaround time.

The skin is the largest organ of the body and is considered the body's first line of defense against organisms. It is an important area of medical attention since approximately 5–10 percent of all ambulatory patient visits in the United States are for skin-related complaints.

Structure and Function

The skin forms a barrier between the internal organs and the outside environment. It is rich with sensory nerve endings that constitute the four cutaneous senses: touch pressure (sustained touch), cold, warmth, and pain. It communicates with the external openings of the digestive, respiratory, and urogenital systems through the mucous membranes.

The skin is composed of three layers, or strata: the epidermis, the dermis, and the subcutaneous tissue, as shown in Figure 5.1. The epidermis is the external layer of the skin composed of squamous epithelial cells. These cells divide continuously, pushing the older, dead cells closer to the surface and completely replacing them every three to four weeks. Skin cells contain keratin, an insoluble, fibrous protein that makes up the horny layer of the epidermis and helps protect the body. There are different amounts of keratin in different areas of the body. The palms of the hands and soles of the feet contain more keratin than other parts of the body. This extra thickness increases with use and results in callus formation.

Cells within the epidermis called melanocytes produce melanin, which gives skin its color. The more melanin present, the darker the skin color. Melanin can absorb ultraviolet light, protecting the person from the harmful effects of sun exposure. People with lighter skin have an increased risk of sunburn after sun exposure. On the positive side, the ultraviolet rays of sunlight react with vitamin-D precursors within the skin to convert them into the active form of vitamin D. Vitamin D aids in the absorption of calcium, helping to form and maintain strong bones.

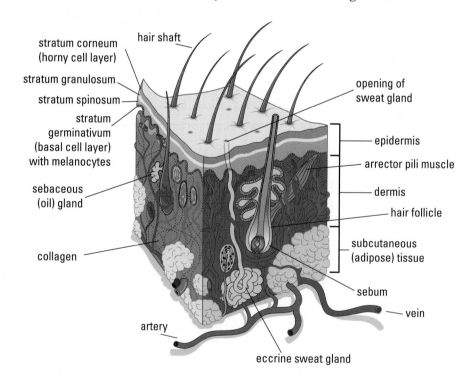

Figure 5.1 Anatomic Structures of the Skin

The dermis lies immediately under the epidermis and is composed of collagen and elastic fibers, blood and lymph vessels, nerves, sweat and sebaceous glands, and hair roots. The subcutaneous layer is composed of adipose, or fat, tissue. This layer is important in the regulation of body temperature and connects the skin to the muscles and bones.

The glands of the skin are within its layers. The sebaceous glands drain oily secretions into an area between each hair follicle and its hair shaft to make the hair soft and pliable. Sweat glands are found within the skin and are classified into two categories: eccrine and apocrine. Eccrine sweat glands are found all over the body and have ducts that open directly onto the surface of the skin. They secrete a watery fluid in response to warm temperatures and are controlled by the sympathetic nervous system (see Chapter 14). Apocrine sweat glands, which become active at puberty, secrete a milky sweat that is broken down by bacteria, producing a characteristic body odor. Specialized apocrine sweat glands produce cerumen, the wax found in the ear.

Hair is composed of keratin. It appears all over the body except on the palms and soles. Hair grows from a root within a cavity known as a hair follicle. The follicle is located in the dermis; the hair shaft extends beyond the skin. Hair grows in two phases: a growing phase (anagen) and a resting phase (telogen). About 80 percent of the body's hair follicles on the scalp are in the anagen phase at any given time.

The nails are composed of hardened keratin. The nail grows from a root within the cuticle, a thin fold of skin at the base of the nail. Nails protect the very sensitive areas of the fingers and toes. Nail growth is relatively slow. Fingernails take about 180 days to completely regenerate; toenails take up to 18 months.

Physical Assessment

Assessment of the skin involves the entire body. The physician inspects and palpates the patient's skin, mucous membranes, hair, and nails to observe appearance, color or pigmentation, temperature, and turgor. Turgor includes motility, elasticity, and moisture or dryness. The practitioner or examiner notes vascularity and inspects the skin thoroughly for abnormalities or lesions (Figure 5.2).

Diseases and Conditions

Since the skin is the first line of defense to protect the inner organs of the body from outside pathogens, early diagnosis and treatment of skin disorders are essential. The most common skin problem is pruritus, or itching, which can indicate either local or systemic problems. Scratching and irritation due to pruritus can cause skin breakdown. Local disorders causing pruritus include allergies to food; medications; and soaps, creams, and other topical chemicals. Contact dermatitis, miliaria (prickly heat), dry skin, and poison ivy are examples of conditions that cause pruritus. It is not always easy to find the cause of pruritus, but it is beneficial to determine the allergen in order to avoid further irritations.

Pruritus may be associated with urticarial and erythematous lesions. Commonly, varicella (chickenpox) and herpes zoster (shingles) viruses are accompanied by itching, redness, burning, and pain. Many "childhood" viral illnesses such as measles, rubella, and "fifth disease" display a red rash, usually without pruritus.

Several bacterial, fungal, and yeast infections cause skin eruptions. *Staphylococcus aureus* and *streptococcus* species are common bacteria found on the skin. These organisms can cause skin lesions such as folliculitis, furuncles, carbuncles, bullae, and impetigo. Tinea corporis (ringworm), tinea pedis, tinea manus, tinea cruris, tinea capitis, and tinea unguium are all dermatophyte infections, caused by *Microsporum*, *Trichophyton*, and *Epidermophyton* species. Intertrigo is a fungal infection commonly caused by *Candida* species, which occurs in areas where skin touches skin such as the axillae and under pendulous breasts. Symptoms include erythema, papules, pustules, and eventually erosion of skin.

Psoriasis is a chronic, noninfectious inflammatory skin disease characterized by an increase in the rate of growth of epidermal cells. Although it

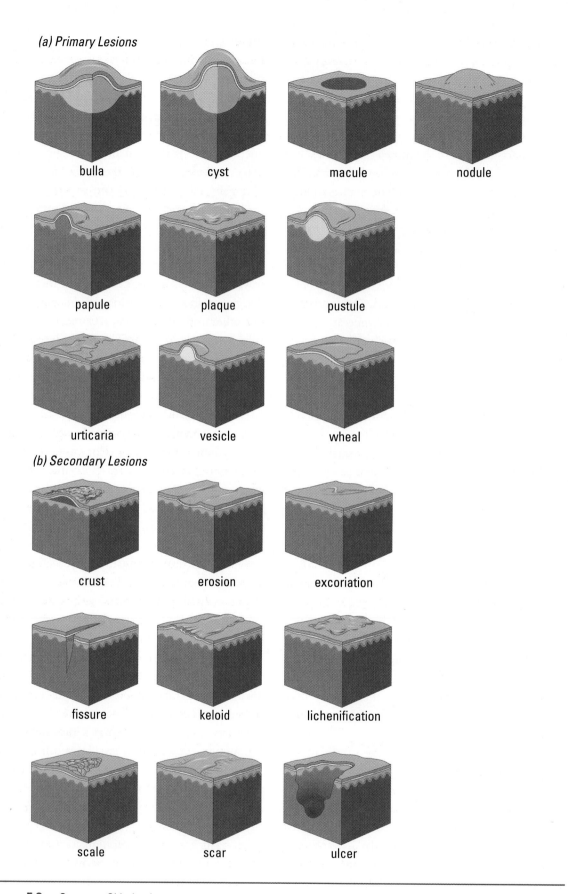

(a) Primary Lesions

bulla   cyst   macule   nodule

papule   plaque   pustule

urticaria   vesicle   wheal

(b) Secondary Lesions

crust   erosion   excoriation

fissure   keloid   lichenification

scale   scar   ulcer

Figure 5.2   Common Skin Lesions

is one of the most common skin diseases, the exact cause is unknown. There may be a combination of genetic and environmental stimuli to precipitate the onset. The immune system, emotional stress, and seasonal and hormonal changes have been implicated in the exacerbation of psoriasis.

Atopic dermatitis, also known as eczema, is a chronic, intermittent skin condition characterized by rough, red, itchy, dry skin. Untreated, eczema may cause skin to become leathery, or lichenified. Eczema may be the result of food allergy. Treatment is typically topical corticosteroids, antihistamines when needed for pruritus, and avoidance of the offending allergen.

Seborrheic keratosis produces benign, beige to brown or black plaques that appear to be "stuck" or "pasted" on top of the skin. These plaques are common in sun-exposed areas of the body. Other benign, pigmented lesions include nevi (singular, nevus), freckles, and lentigines (singular, lentigo).

There are several forms of precancerous and cancerous lesions that affect the skin. Actinic keratosis produces a small, scaly patch that feels like sandpaper and is tender when rubbed. Actinic keratosis is considered a precancerous lesion and is treated with liquid nitrogen. Melanoma is the deadliest of the skin cancers. Melanomas may be recognized using the "ABCD" mnemonic. Malignant lesions are typically **a**symmetric, have irregular **b**orders, have variation in **c**olor, and increase in **d**iameter. Tumor thickness at the time of diagnosis is prognostic. Excision is the treatment of choice. Basal cell carcinoma and squamous cell carcinoma are the other two common forms of skin cancer, but they have a much better prognosis. Basal cell carcinoma (BCC) rarely metastasizes. Squamous cell carcinoma (SCC) is invasive, destructive, and is known to metastasize.

There are some systemic diseases and/or conditions that are manifested by rashes or lesions of the skin. Patients with lupus erythematosus may display a butterfly-shaped rash on both cheeks and over the bridge of the nose. A bull's-eye rash may appear on the back of a patient who is in the early phase of Lyme disease. Tattoos and body piercings are extremely common today, especially among adolescents. Some of the complications seen as a result are rejection, local skin irritation, allergic reactions, keloid formation, granulomas, local or systemic infection, and viral infection including human papillomavirus, herpes simplex virus, and even HIV.

Common Tests and Surgical Procedures

Physicians routinely order allergy skin testing such as scratch tests, patch tests, and intradermal tests to determine which allergens are responsible for causing allergic reactions. KOH (potassium hydroxide) preparation is used to diagnose fungal infections, and Tzanck smear is used to diagnose viral skin vesicles. In addition, the dermatologist performs three types of biopsies: excisional (complete removal of a skin lesion), incisional (partial removal of a lesion by cutting out part of the lesion), and punch (removal of a portion of skin containing a lesion by means of a special surgical instrument). Many skin cancers can be treated with Mohs chemosurgery. This procedure removes and immediately examines thin layers of skin one by one until the frozen-sections no longer show malignant cells.

Cosmetic surgery is commonly performed nowadays. Laser treatment to remove unwanted hair, varicose veins, and other lesions is also common. Dermabrasion and chemical peels are methods used to remove the upper skin layers in order to eradicate scars, tattoos, and fine lines.

Procedures such as Botox, collagen, and Restylane (hyaluronic acid) injections are commonplace, "quick-fix" methods to smooth fine lines and wrinkles. Botox is made from the *Clostridium botulinum* toxin and actually causes local paralysis of the underlying muscle, decreasing the appearance of lines around the eyes, across the forehead, and around the mouth. Collagen and hyaluronic acid injections under the skin fill in the lines on the face to achieve a younger-looking appearance. These procedures are especially enticing because they can be performed in the physician's office without general anesthesia.

Terms Bank

These terms and abbreviations provide a foundation for the language and transcription skills you will develop in the following sections of this chapter. Terms marked with » will be included in the reports transcribed in the Building Transcription Skills section.

abrasion
(a-**bray**-zhun) (n) scraping away of skin or mucous membrane by friction

abscess
(**ab**-ses) (n) a pus-filled cavity, usually because of a localized infection

acne
(**ak**-nee) (n) an eruption of papules or pustules on the skin, involving the oil glands

adipose
(**ad**-i-pOz) (adj) containing fat

albinism
(**al**-bi-nizm / al-**bin**-izm) (n) a congenital lack of melanin in the skin, hair, and eyes

allergen
(**al**-er-jen) (n) a substance that produces an allergic reaction

alopecia »
(al-O-**pee**-shee-a) (n) partial or total loss of hair

alopecic
(al-O-**pee**-sik) (adj) relating to alopecia

anagen
(**an**-a-jen) (n) the actively growing phase of the hair growth cycle

angioedema
(an-jee-O-e-**dee**-ma) (n) periodically recurring episodes of noninflammatory swelling

angioma »
(an-jee-**O**-ma) (n) a swelling or tumor composed primarily of blood vessels; spider, strawberry, cherry angiomas

anhidrosis
(an-hI-**drO**-sis) (n) the suppression or absence of perspiration

antecubital
(an-te-**kyoo**-bi-tal) (adj) front of the elbow; often the site for drawing blood

apocrine
(**ap**-O-krin) (adj) relating to sweat glands

assessment
(as-**ses**-ment) (n) a complete evaluation of the patient; diagnosis

bedsore
(**bed**-sor) (n) an infected wound on the skin that occurs at pressure points in patients confined to bed

biopsy
(**bI**-op-see) (n) the removal of tissue and/or fluid from the body for microscopic study; the specimen obtained

Botox
(**bO**-tawks) (n) Clostridium botulinum toxin A, injected into the skin around the eyes, forehead, and lips to remove facial lines

bullae
(**bul**-ee) (n, pl) blisters of the skin containing clear fluid

café-au-lait spots »
(kaf-ay-O-**lay** spots) (n) light brown spots of patchy pigmentation of the skin

callous
(**kal**-us) (adj) being hardened and thickened, having calluses; also feeling no emotion or sympathy.

callus
(**kal**-us) (n) thickened skin which develops at points of pressure or friction; the bony substance which develops around the broken ends of bone during healing

candidal rash
(**kan**-di-dal rash) (n) a rash which usually includes itching, a white discharge, peeling, and easy bleeding; caused by the yeastlike fungus *Candida;* common examples are diaper rash, thrush, and vaginitis

carbuncle
(**kar**-bung-kl) (n) subcutaneous, pus-filled interconnecting pockets, caused by staphylococcal infection; eventually discharges through an opening in the skin

carcinoma »
(kar-si-**nO**-mah) (n) a cancerous growth or malignant tumor that occurs in epithelium (cell layers covering outside body surfaces)

caruncle
(**kar**-ung-kl) (n) small, fleshy outgrowth

cellulitis
(sel-yoo-**lI**-tis) (n) inflammation of the connective tissue caused by infection

cephalocaudal
(**sef**-a-lO-**caw**-dal) (adj) relating to the axis of the body from the head to the base of the spine

cerumen
(se-**roo**-men) (n) earwax

chancre
(**shang**-ker) (n) hard sore; the sore that develops at the site of entry of a pathogen

chloasma
(klO-**as**-ma) (n) light brown patches on the face and elsewhere; commonly associated with pregnancy

cicatrix
(**sik**-a-triks) (n) scar

circumscribed »
(**ser**-kum-skrIbd) (adj) having a boundary; confined

cirrhosis
(sir-**rO**-sis) (n) a degenerative liver disease characterized by damaged cell function and impaired blood flow

collagen
(**kol**-a-jen) (n) the protein which forms the tough white fibers of connective tissue, cartilage, and bone

comedo »
(**kom**-i-dO) (n) in a hair follicle or oil gland, a plug of dead cells and oily secretions; blackhead; comedones (com-i-**dO**-neez) (pl)

concussion
(kon-**kush**-un) (n) an injury resulting from violent striking or shaking, especially an injury to the brain

confluent
(**kon**-floo-ent) (adj) merging together; connecting

congenital »
(kon-**jen**-I-tal) (adj) present at birth

contusion
(kon-**too**-zhun) (n) a bruise

cryosurgery
(**krI**-O-ser-jer-ee) (n) the use of extreme cold to destroy tissue

cutaneous »
(koo-**tay**-nee-us) (adj) pertaining to the skin

cuticle
(**kyoo**-ti-kl) (n) the edge of thickened skin around the bed of a nail; the sheath surrounding the base of a hair follicle

cyanosis
(cI-a-**nO**-sis) (n) bluish cast to the skin and/or mucous membranes due to decreased amount of oxygen in the blood cells

dermabrasion
(**der**-ma-bray-zhun) (n) peeling of skin done by a mechanical device with sandpaper or wire brushes

dermatitis »
(der-ma-**tI**-tis) (n) inflammation of skin often evidenced by itching, redness, and lesions

dermatitis medicamentosum
(der-ma-**tI**-tis med-i-ka-men-**tO**-sa) (n) a skin eruption caused by ingestion, injection, or inhalation of a drug

dermatology
(der-ma-**tol**-o-jee) (n) the study of the skin, hair, and nails

dermatophyte
(**der**-ma-tO-fIt) (n) a parasitic fungus that causes skin disease

desiccate
(**des**-i-kayt) (v) to dry out

diagnosis
(dI-ag-**nO**-sis) (n) deciding the nature of a medical condition by examination of the symptoms; diagnoses (pl)

diaphoresis
(**dI**-a-fO-ree-sis) (n) profuse perspiration or sweating

discrete
(dis-**kreet**) (adj) separate; distinct

ecchymosis
(ek-im-**O**-sis) (n) reddish or purplish flat spot on the skin; a bruise; ecchymoses (pl)

eccrine
(**ek**-rin) (adj) relating to sweat glands

eczema
(**ek**-si-ma/**eg**-ze-ma) (n) inflammatory condition of the skin characterized by blisters, redness, and itching

electrodesiccation
(el-ek-trO-de-si-**kay**-shun) (n) destruction of tissue by the use of electrical current; fulguration

electrolysis
(el-ek-**trol**-i-sis) (n) destruction of a hair follicle by passing an electrical current through it

ellipse »
(el-**lipz**) (n) a conic section taken either parallel to an element or parallel to the axis of the intersected cone; an oval

ephelides
(ef-**ee**-lI-deez) (n, pl) freckles

epidermis
(ep-i-**der**-mis) (n) the top or outer layer of the skin

epinephrine »
(ep-I-**nef**-rin) (n) a hormone of the adrenal medulla that acts as a strong stimulant and blood vessel constrictor

epithelial
(ep-i-**thee**-lee-al) (adj) relating to or composed of epithelium

epithelium
(ep-i-**thee**-lee-um) (n) cell layers covering the outside body surfaces as well as forming the lining of hollow organs (e.g., the bladder) and the passages of the respiratory, digestive, and urinary tracts

erythema
(er-i-**thee**-ma) (n) redness of the skin; inflammation

erythema infectiosum
(er-i-**thee**-ma in-fek-shee-**O**-sum) (n) a mild, infectious disease characterized by an erythematous rash; also called fifth disease

erythematous »
(er-i-**them**-a-tus/er-i-**thee**-ma-tus) (adj) relating to or having erythema; reddened; inflamed

erythrocyte
(e-**rith**-rO-sIt) (n) mature red blood cell

erythroderma
(e-rith-rO-**der**-ma) (n) any skin condition associated with unusual redness of the skin

exanthema
(eg-zan-**thee**-ma) (n) a disease, such as measles or chickenpox, accompanied by a general rash on the skin, which may have particular characteristics specific to the disease

excisional biopsy »
(ek-**sizh**-un-al **bI**-op-see) (n) surgical removal of a tissue for microscopic examination

excoriation
(eks-kO-ree-**ay**-shun) (n) a scratching or scraping injury to the skin

familial »

(fa-**mi**-lee-al) (adj) pertaining to a disease or characteristic that is present in some families

fifth disease

(n) erythema infectiosum; a mild, infectious disease characterized by an erythematous rash

fistula

(**fis**-tyoo-la) (n) abnormal opening or channel connecting hollow organs or leading from an internal organ to the outside or a cavity; such as a urinary fistula

follicle

(**fol**-i-kl) (n) pouch-like cavity, such as a hair follicle in the skin enclosing a hair

folliculitis

(fol-i-kyoo-**lI**-tis) (n) inflammation of the hair follicles

fossa »

(**fos**-a) (n) channel or shallow depression; fossae (pl)

fulguration

(ful-gyoo-**ra**-shun) (n) destruction of tissue by the use of electrical current; electrodessication

furuncle

(**fyoo**-rung-kl) (n) a localized, pus-forming infection in a hair follicle or gland

gangrene

(**gang**-green) (n) death of cells or tissue due to obstruction of blood supply

gland

(n) organ that secretes one or more substances not needed by the organ itself

glans

(n) the head of the penis; "glans penis"

hemangioma

(he-man-jee-**O**-ma) (n) a congenital benign tumor consisting of a mass of blood vessels

hematology

(hee-ma-**tol**-o-jee) (n) the study of blood

hemosiderin »

(hee-mO-**sid**-er-in) (n) an iron-containing pigment derived from hemoglobin when red blood cells disintegrate

herpes zoster

(**her**-peez **zos**-ter) (n) a viral infection causing inflammation along the path of nerve with associated painful vesicles (blisters) on the skin above; shingles

hirsutism

(**hur**-soot-izm) (n) excessive body hair

hyperpigmentation »

(hI-per-pig-men-**tay**-shun) (n) darkening of the skin due to excessive pigment in the skin

hypertrophy

(hI-**per**-trO-fee) (n) increase in size

impetigo

(im-pe-**tI**-gO) (n) a streptococcal or staphylococcal infection of the skin characterized by lesions, usually on the face, which rupture and become covered with a thick yellow crust; highly contagious

incised »

(in-**sIzd**) (adj) cut with a knife

incisional biopsy

(in-**si**-zhun-al **bI**-op-see) (n) removal of part of a lesion for microscopic examination

incision and drainage

(n) commonly dictated "I and D"; procedure of cutting through an infected lesion and allowing it to drain

intertriginous

(in-ter-**trij**-i-nus) (adj) characterized by intertrigo

intertrigo

(in-ter-**trI**-gO) (n) irritation (dermatitis) of juxtaposed surfaces of skin such as between the thighs, folds of skin, or under pendulous breasts caused by retained sweat, moisture, friction, and concomitant overgrowth of microorganisms such as *Candida* species

integumentary

(in-teg-yoo-**men**-ta-ree) (adj) relating to the skin

jaundice

(**jawn**-dis) (n) yellowish skin and whites of the eyes

keloid

(**kee**-loyd) (n) a mass of scar tissue

keratin

(**ker**-a-tin) (n) a tough, fibrous protein in skin, hair, and nails

keratosis

(ker-a-**tO**-sis) (n) a condition in which the skin thickens and builds up with excessive keratin

keratotic »

(ker-a-**tot**-ik) (adj) relating to keratosis

lesion »

(**lee**-zhun) (n) general term for any visible, circumscribed injury to the skin; such as a wound, sore, rash, or mass

macrophage »

(**mak**-ro-fayj) (n) a large scavenger cell (phagocyte) that digests microorganisms and cell debris

macule

(**mak**-yool) (n) a small discolored spot on the skin

maculopapular »

(mak-yoo-lO-**pap**-yoo-lar) (adj) describing skin lesions that are raised in the center

malformation

(mal-for-**may**-shun) (n) abnormal development or structure of the body or a part

melanin

(**mel**-a-nin) (n) naturally-occurring dark brown or black pigment found in the hair, skin, and eyes

melanocyte »

(**mel**-an-O-sIt) (n) a cell that produces melanin

melanocytic »

(mel-a-nO-**sit**-ik) (adj) pertaining to or composed of melanocytes

melitis

(mee-**lI**-tis) (n) inflammation of the cheek

milia

(**mil**-ee-a) (n, pl) whiteheads, due to obstruction of the outlet of hair follicles or sweat glands

miliaria
(mil-ee-**ay**-ree-a) (n) a skin eruption of small vesicles and papules; heat rash

motility
(mO-**til**-i-tee) (n) ability to move spontaneously

mycosis
(mI-**kO**-sis) (n) disease caused by a fungus

neuromuscular »
(noor-O-**mus**-kyoo-lar) (adj) pertains to the muscles and nerves

nevus »
(**nee**-vus) (n) congenital discoloration of the skin; birthmark or mole; nevi (pl)

obese »
(o-**bees**) (adj) very fat

onycholysis
(on-ee-**kol**-i-sis) (n) loosening of the nails from their beds

papule »
(**pap**-yool) (n) a small, solid, raised skin lesion, as in chickenpox

paraplegia »
(par-a-**plee**-jee-a) (n) paralysis of the lower portion of the body and of both legs

paronychia
(par-O-**nik**-ee-a) (n) infected skin around the nail

pathogen
(**path**-O-jen) (n) any microorganism or substance capable of producing a disease

pemphigus
(**pem**-fi-gus) (n) a distinctive group of diseases marked by successive crops of bullae

perineum »
(**per**-i-**nee**-um) (n) the external region between the urethral opening and the anus, including the skin and underlying tissues

peritoneum
(per-i-tO-**nee**-um) (n) lining of the abdominal cavity

petechia »
(pe-**tee**-kee-a / pee-**tek**-ee-a) (n, sing.) tiny reddish or purplish flat spot on the skin as a result of a tiny hemorrhage within the skin (usually used in the plural form, petechiae)

petechial
(pee-**tee**-kee-al / pee-**tek**-ee-al) (adj) relating to or having petechiae

pigment »
(**pig**-ment) (n) any organic coloring substance in the body

pigmented »
(**pig**-men-ted) (v) colored by a pigment

presents »
(pre-**sents**) (v) appears; shows; displays; the symptoms displayed are the presenting symptoms

pruritic
(pru-**ri**-tic) (adj) itching

pruritus
(proo-**rI**-tus) (n) itching skin condition

psoriasis
(sO-**rI**-a-sis) (n) chronic skin disease in which reddish scaly patches develop

punch biopsy
(punch **bI**-op-see) (n) a special instrument is used to take a small cylindrical piece of tissue for microscopic examination

pustular »
(**pus**-choo-lar) (adj) relating to or having pustules

pustule
(**pus**-chool) (n) small pus-containing elevation on the skin

Restylane
(**res**-sti-layn) (n) an injection of hyaluronic acid used to decrease the appearance of facial lines

rhinophyma
(rI-nO-**fI**-ma) (n) enlargement of the nose from severe rosacea

rubella
(roo-**bel**-a) (n) a contagious viral disease with fever and a red rash; German measles

scabies
(**skay**-beez) (n) contagious rash with intense itching; caused by mites

scrotal
(**skrO**-tal) (adj) relating to the scrotum

scrotum »
(**skrO**-tum) (n) the pouch of skin containing the testes

sebaceous
(see-**bay**-shus) (adj) relating to sebum

seborrhea »
(seb-O-**ree**-a) (n) overactivity of the oil glands of the skin

sebum
(**see**-bum) (n) an oily secretion of the oil glands of the skin

sequela »
(see-**kwel**-a) (n) a condition following and resulting from a disease; sequelae (pl)

serosanguineous »
(**see** row sang win ess) (adj) characterized by blood and serum

Staphylococcus aureus
(staf-il-O-**kok**-us **awr**-ee-us) (n) a common species of Staphylococcus (a bacteria), present on nasal mucous membranes and skin that causes pus-producing infections

streptococcus
(strep-tO-**kok**-us) (n) a genus of bacteria; many species cause disease in humans

subcutaneous »
(sub-kyoo-**tay**-nee-us) (adj) under the skin

subjective data
(sub-**jek**-tiv **day**-tah) (n) information revealed by the patient to the health care provider

suture »
(**soo**-chur) (n and v) natural seam, border in the skull formed by the close joining of bony surfaces; closing a wound with a sterile needle and thread

syndrome »
(**sin**-drOm) (n) the signs and symptoms that constitute a specific disease

telogen

(**tel**-O-jen) (n) the resting phase of the hair growth cycle

texture

(**teks**-chur) (n) character, structure, and feel of parts of the body

tinea

(**tin**-ee-a) (n) fungal infection; such as tinea pedis or athlete's foot

torso

(**tor**-sO) (n) trunk of the body

turgor

(**ter**-gOr) (n) fullness; the normal resiliency of the skin

Tzanck smear

(tsangk smeer) (n) a method to help diagnose skin lesions by the miscroscopic examination of material from them

urticaria »

(er-ti-**kar**-ee-a) (n) hives; an eruption of itching red, raised lesions

urticarial

(er-ti-**kar**-ee-al) (adj) relating to or having urticaria

varicella

(var-i-**sel**-a) (n) chickenpox; a highly contagious viral disease

varicose veins »

(var-I-kOs vaynz) (n) veins that become distended, swollen, knotted, tortuous, and painful because of poor valvular function

vascularity

(vas-kyoo-**lar**-i-tee) (n) the blood vessels in a part of the body

vesicle

(**ves**-i-kl) (n) blister; small, raised skin lesion containing clear fluid

vesiculopustular »

(ves-**ick**-you-low-**pus**-to-ler) (adj) characterized by vesicles and pustules

vitiligo

(vi-ti-**lee**-gO) (n) white patches, due to loss of pigment, appearing on the skin

wheal »

(hweel) (n) a raised, red circumscribed lesion usually due to an allergic reaction; usually accompanied by intense itching; welt

xanthoma

(zan-**thO**-mah) (n) yellowish nodules in or under the skin, especially in the eyelids

xerosis

(zer-**O**-sis / zee-r**O**-sis) (n) dry skin

Xylocaine »

(**zI**-lO-kayn) (n) trade name for lidocaine hydroxhloride

Abbreviations

BCC	basal cell carcinoma	HSV-2	herpes simplex virus type 2
Bx	biopsy	I&D	incision and drainage
C&S	culture and sensitivity	KOH	potassium hydroxide
CA	cancer; carcinoma	S aureus	*Staphylococcus aureus*
derm.	dermatology	SCC	squamous cell carcinoma
FS	frozen section	strep	streptococcus
HIV	human immunodeficiency virus	ung.	ointment
HPV	human papillomavirus	UV	ultraviolet
HSV-1	herpes simplex virus type 1		

Building Language Skills

Complete the following exercises, drawing on the information learned in the Exploring Dermatology section of this chapter and referencing the Terms Bank.

Exercise 5.1   Matching Sound and Spelling

The numbered list that follows shows the phonetic spelling of hard-to-spell words. Sound out the word, then write the correct spelling in the blank space provided. Check your answers in the Terms Bank or other appropriate reference.

1. er-i-**thee**-ma _____

2. see-**bay**-shus _____

3. er-ti-**kar**-ee-a _____

4. **des**-i-kayt _____

5. al-O-**pee**-shee-a _____

6. **kon**-floo-ent _____

7. pe-**tee**-kee-a/pe-**tek**-ee-a _____

8. **kom**-i-dO _____

9. **per**-i-**nee**-um _____

10. eks-kO-ree-**ay**-shun _____

11. an-te-**kyoo**-bi-tal _____

12. sel-yoo-**ll**-tis _____

13. **ap**-O-krin _____

14. sO-**rl**-a-sis _____

15. ek-im-**O**-sis _____

Below is a list of frequently used words that look alike and/or sound alike. Study the meaning and pronunciation of each set of words, then read the following sentences carefully and circle the word in parentheses that correctly completes the meaning.

cirrhosis	disease of the liver	**patient**	(n) an individual who is receiving medical treatment
psoriasis	skin condition	**patient**	(adj) behaving calmly
cirrhosis	liver disease		
xerosis	dry skin	**perianal**	around the anus
		perinatal	relating to the time shortly before and after birth
discreet	cautious, careful with speech or behavior		
discrete	separate, distinct; "discrete mass"	**perineum**	pelvic floor and associated structures
glands	organs or groups of cells that produce or secrete substances	**peritoneum**	serous membrane lining the walls of the abdominal and pelvic cavities
glans	head of the penis; "glans penis"		
		vesical	(adj) relating to a bladder
malaria	acute blood disease caused from bite of tropical mosquito	**vesicle**	(n) blister
milia	white raised "pimple" found on skin of infants	**wheal**	raised, red lesion on the skin
miliaria	eruption of vesicles and papules at the sweat glands	**wheel**	circular frame of hard material that can turn on an axle (as on a car)
patience	ability to suppress restlessness; to be patient		
patients	individuals who are receiving medical treatment		
patient's	possessive form of noun patient		

1.   We will refer the patient to the dermatologist regarding his (cirrhosis/xerosis).

2.   Due to the patient's (cirrhosis/psoriasis), we need to repeat her liver function tests.

3.   It is important to be (discreet/discrete) when transcribing patient care documentation.

4.   I noted a few (discreet/discrete) papular lesions on the patient's left arm.

5.   The examination of the (perineum/peritoneum) shows that the patient's episiotomy is well healed.

6.   A family physician sometimes sees up to 40 (patients/patient's) a day.

7.   When transcribing difficult dictation, (patience/patients) is important.

8.   He is having some irritations of the foreskin and (glands/glans).

9.   A (vesical/vesicle) is beginning to form at the burn site.

10.   Apparently she is allergic to amoxicillin because she developed pruritic (wheals/wheels) on her trunk a few hours after taking the first dose.

When transcribing dictation, the medical transcriptionist frequently needs to consider the situation when determining the word that correctly completes the sentence. From the list of words below, select the term that meaningfully completes each statement.

acne	follicle	pruritic
adipose	integumentary	sebaceous
comedo	nevus	subcutaneous
erythematous	perineum	torso
excoriations	pigment	vesicle

1. He has a rash with many _____, due to constantly scratching the area.

2. The patient is complaining of a (an) _____ rash and would like a medication to relieve itching.

3. He had a (an) _____ that opened and drained a clear fluid.

4. The _____ system is the first system noticed when the patient appears in the physician's office.

5. This _____ on my nose has caused me much embarrassment.

6. The patient has a (an) _____ rash sprinkled across the nose.

7. The patient has a (an) _____ that she would like removed from her chin. She states it has been there since birth.

8. The _____ shows scarring from the episiotomy performed during the birth of her first child.

9. The _____ glands clog and cause acne.

10. The 16-year-old girl consulted the dermatologist because the over-the-counter medications she used to treat her _____ were not effective.

From this list, locate the term that best matches each of the following definitions. Write the term in the space provided beside the definition.

alopecia	erythema	pruritus
cephalocaudal	hyperpigmentation	rhinophyma
confluent	I&D	torso
dermatitis	onycholysis	urticaria
ephelides	petechiae	wheal

1. patchy light brown spots in pigmentation of skin   _____

2. from head to tail   _____

3. loss of hair   _____

4. redness   _____

5. tiny reddish or purplish spots appearing on the skin resulting from tiny hemorrhages   _____

6. a raised, red, circumscribed lesion   _____

7. pertaining to merging of tissues, pustules, or lesions   _____

8. unusual darkening of the skin   _____

9. inflammation of the skin   _____

10. trunk of a body   _____

Exercise 5.5   Creating Terms from Word Forms

Combine prefixes, root words, and suffixes from this list to create medical words that fit the following definitions. Fill in the blanks with the words that you construct. The first word is done for you.

adip/o	fat	**-cyte**	cell
bi/o	life	**-ema**	condition of
caudal	referring to tail	**-ia**	condition
cephal/o	head	**-itis**	inflammation
derm/a	skin	**-logy**	study of
dermat/o	skin	**-opsy**	view of
erythr/o	red	**-ose**	related to
hyper-	above or excessive	**-osis**	condition
kerat/o	horny tissue	**-ous**	pertaining to
melen/o	black	**-rrhea**	discharge
seb/o	oil	**-trophy**	development
pigmentation	coloring	**-y**	condition or process of
tension	pressure		

1. study of skin, hair, and nails _____ *dermatology* _____

2. excessive growth _____

3. condition in which skin thickens and builds up with excessive keratin _____

4. peeling of skin with sandpaper _____

5. containing fat _____

6. skin condition associated with abnormal redness of skin _____

7. inflammation of skin _____

8. condition caused by over-activity of the sebaceous glands _____

9. red blood cell _____

10. removal of tissue and/or fluid from the body for microscopic study _____

11. a darkened skin cell _____

12. excessive pigment in the skin _____

As a medical transcriptionist, you are responsible for producing quality work. One of the most important skills you need to develop is proofreading, which involves checking for all types of mistakes in the document and correcting them. You must carefully read for accuracy of content, omission of words, consistency of format, English usage, spelling, punctuation, capitalization, word choice, and typographical errors.

Read the following report excerpts and look for and correct incomplete sentences and errors in spelling and punctuation. Mark the corrections on this page and key the excerpts with all errors corrected. Save the documents as XXExercise05.06-1 and XXExercise05.06-2 using your initials in place of the *XX* in the file names.

1. Thank you for referring Kyle Sanderson to me. This baby is truely in pain with scrotal inflammation and excoriation of the perineum. I have instituted Burow soaks to the area q.i.d., with Mycostatin ointment after each soak. If this does not clear the rash I would be concerned about an secondary infection. I would expect to see improvement within 1 week otherwise I feel the baby should be admitted to the hospital and more aggressive antifungal agents be used to clear this rash.

2. Robert is a very cooperative, gregaris youngster. Examination reveals normal vitle signs and the cuteanus lesions noted above. Aside from his nuromuculer deficit his exam was otherwise un-remarcable.

Read this scenario carefully and then select the most appropriate response. Write an explanation for why you think your choice is the best answer.

You work from home as an independent contractor using your own computer and reference materials to transcribe reports for a multispecialty clinic in your community. The clinic sends sound files to you through an FTP site and you transcribe reports using a pedal and headset connected to your PC. Your son is working on an audiovisual project for school and wants to use your PC to download music off the Internet. After downloading, he will also need to edit the music and adapt it to his presentation. He has found the song he needs on a site that offers free music as well as software for downloading and sharing music. What should you do?

---

a. Download the software, retrieve the music, and then remove the music and the software from your PC.

b. Create a new profile on your computer for your son and allow him to finish his school project under his own user name and password.

c. Drive to the store, purchase the CD, and copy the song from the CD to the PC and allow your son to complete his project.

d. None of the above.

Best response: _____

Explanation: _____

_____

_____

_____

_____

You will apply the medical specialty and language information you learned in this chapter to transcription work in this section. After you learn the formatting recommendations of an office note, you will transcribe eight reports related to eight different patient studies.

Introducing the Office Note

An office note typically describes an office visit and becomes part of the patient's chart. Figure 5.3 is an example of an office note. Sometimes the office note may describe a minor procedure performed in the physician's office.

These notes are not always written using complete sentences, especially in the section describing the physical exam. Often, sentences are "clipped" at the beginning, leaving off "The patient." For example, the practitioner may say, "States she has not had these symptoms before." If the subject of the sentence is not dictated, it is acceptable to transcribe an incomplete sentence, but complete sentences should always be punctuated using standard rules of grammar. If a practitioner dictates a patient's name within the body of an office note, it is important to transcribe the name as "the patient" to protect the patient's rights to privacy.

Refer to page 469 of Appendix A for a complete list of headings found in the office note template along with descriptions of the type of information found under each heading. Not every heading will be included in every transcribed report.

The format displayed in Figure 5.3 uses the SOAP (Subjective, Objective, Assessment, Plan) format. Note that if the report is short, it is sometimes acceptable to add a colon after each SOAP heading and key the text on the same line.

Preparing to Transcribe

To prepare for transcribing dictation, review the common dermatology terms, drugs, and abbreviations presented in this chapter's Terms Bank. Then, study the format and organization of the model document shown in Figure 5.3, and key the model document, using the office note template on the Dictations and Templates CD as a starting point. Save the document as XXFigure05.03, using your initials in place of the XX in the file name. Proofread the document by comparing it with the printed version. Categorize the types of errors you made and document them on a copy of the Performance Comparison Chart. A template of this chart is available on the Dictations and Templates CD.

Transcribing Reports

Transcribe, edit, and correct each report in the following patient studies. Consult reference books for words or formatting rules that are unfamiliar.

As you work on the transcription assignment for this chapter, fill in the Performance Comparison Chart that you started when you keyed the model document. For at least three of the reports, categorize and document the types of errors you made. Answer the document analysis questions on the bottom of the chart. With continuous practice and assessment, the quality of your work will improve.

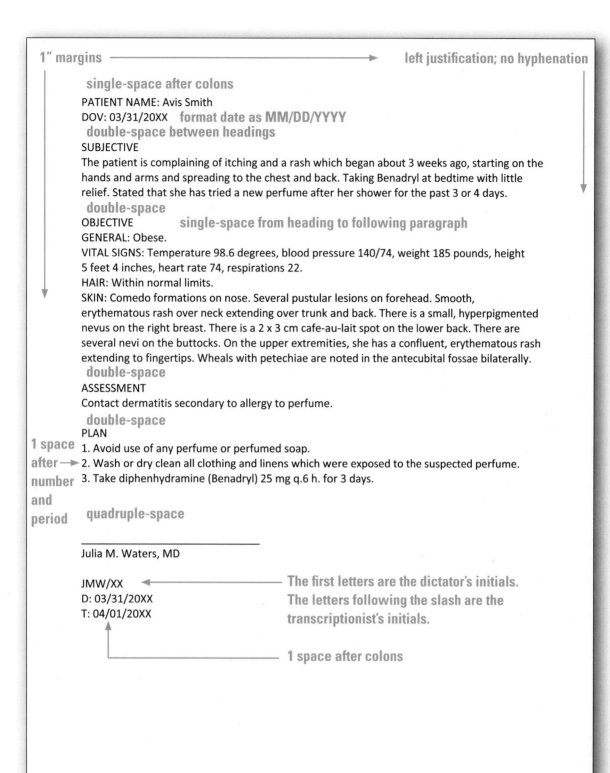

PATIENT NAME: Avis Smith
DOV: 03/31/20XX   format date as MM/DD/YYYY
double-space between headings

1" margins ———————————————→ left justification; no hyphenation

single-space after colons

SUBJECTIVE
The patient is complaining of itching and a rash which began about 3 weeks ago, starting on the hands and arms and spreading to the chest and back. Taking Benadryl at bedtime with little relief. Stated that she has tried a new perfume after her shower for the past 3 or 4 days.
double-space
OBJECTIVE   single-space from heading to following paragraph
GENERAL: Obese.
VITAL SIGNS: Temperature 98.6 degrees, blood pressure 140/74, weight 185 pounds, height 5 feet 4 inches, heart rate 74, respirations 22.
HAIR: Within normal limits.
SKIN: Comedo formations on nose. Several pustular lesions on forehead. Smooth, erythematous rash over neck extending over trunk and back. There is a small, hyperpigmented nevus on the right breast. There is a 2 x 3 cm cafe-au-lait spot on the lower back. There are several nevi on the buttocks. On the upper extremities, she has a confluent, erythematous rash extending to fingertips. Wheals with petechiae are noted in the antecubital fossae bilaterally.
double-space
ASSESSMENT
Contact dermatitis secondary to allergy to perfume.
double-space
PLAN
1 space after → 1. Avoid use of any perfume or perfumed soap.
number 2. Wash or dry clean all clothing and linens which were exposed to the suspected perfume.
and 3. Take diphenhydramine (Benadryl) 25 mg q.6 h. for 3 days.
period
quadruple-space

_____
Julia M. Waters, MD

JMW/XX ←———————————————— The first letters are the dictator's initials.
D: 03/31/20XX   The letters following the slash are the
T: 04/01/20XX   transcriptionist's initials.

——————————————————— 1 space after colons

Figure 5.3   Office Note

Ms. Avis Smith is a 45-year-old woman who presents with a 3-week history of generalized itching and a maculopapular, erythematous rash, most prominent on the torso.

REPORT 5.1   Office Note

Use the Report0501.mp3 audio file and the office note template (Office_Note) when transcribing this report. Save the document as XXReport05.01, using your initials in place of *XX* in the file name.

This dictation includes a measurement of body temperature. It is acceptable to use either the degrees symbol or the word *degrees* if dictated, but do not use the degrees symbol unless directed by your instructor. Do not transcribe Fahrenheit or Celsius unless the provider says the word as part of the dictation. If the degree symbol is used, abbreviate *Fahrenheit* as *F* and *Celsius* as *C*; otherwise, do not abbreviate the temperature scale name. If using the degrees symbol with the temperature scale name abbreviation, do not insert a space between the symbol and the abbreviation (101°F).

For clarity, do not allow lines to break between numbers and units of measure. Avoid such problematic breaks by inserting a nonbreaking space (Ctrl + Shift + Space) instead of a standard space. Adding a nonbreaking space is better than inserting a hard return to force a line break. This is because line breaks may change depending on the font size, line length, or viewing format of the transcribed document.

When the word "times" is dictated and can be replaced with *for*, it should be transcribed as such. However, when the word "times" means the number of times something was done, use the letter *x*.

In this dictation, the practitioner says "times 3 days." *Times 3* can be replaced with the word *for*; therefore, it should be transcribed as "for 3 days." If the practitioner ordered Phenergan 12.5 mg "times 2," you would transcribe "Phenergan 12.5 mg x2." (The patient was given 2 doses of Phenergan 12.5 mg, for a total of 25 mg.) In order to make the expression easier to read, no space is set between the *x* and the number. However, when *x* is used in a dimensional measurement, set a space before and after it (2 x 3 inches).

Mr. Albert Alvarez, a 45-year-old male, was referred to dermatologist Anthony Palmer, MD, by his internist for assessment of several lesions. Although Dr. Palmer found none of the lesions suspicious, he removed them, as they were inflamed.

REPORT 5.2   Office Note

Use the Report0502.mp3 audio file and the office note template (Office_Note) when transcribing this report. Delete or change the template's headings within the report to match the content of the dictation. Delete headings without corresponding dictated text. Save the document as XXReport05.02, using your initials in place of *XX* in the file name.

Listen for these terms:
   excision
   keratotic papules

Remember to avoid using the patient's name within the body of a report, even if the name is dictated.

Ms. Sanderson's 3-month-old infant, Kyle, was referred to Dr. Palmer by the pediatrician for evaluation of a persistent rash on his scalp, behind his ears, and in the diaper area.

REPORT 5.3 Office Note

Use the Report0503.mp3 audio file and the office note template (Office_Note) when transcribing this report. For this report, the dictated headings and the template's headings will not align perfectly. When a template's heading is synonymous to the dictated heading, use the template's heading. If a synonymous heading is not available, transcribe the dictated heading. Save the document as XXReport05.03, using your initials in place of *XX* in the file name.

Listen for these terms:
    alopecic (adjective) and alopecia (noun)
    perineum
    seborrheic (adjective) and seborrhea (noun)

PMD means "primary medical doctor." This common medical abbreviation should be transcribed only when it is dictated. Do not change "primary medical doctor" to PMD and do not change "PMD" to primary medical doctor. The same rule applies to other abbreviations such as BP (blood pressure).

In general, abbreviations should be avoided unless the abbreviation is a widely used and accepted abbreviation. Do not abbreviate phrases that have been dictated in full. Expand dictated abbreviations only when absolutely certain of the intended meaning. If in doubt, transcribe exactly as dictated. The diagnosis and impression sections of a document should not contain abbreviations. The Joint Commission requires facilities to establish a list of acceptable abbreviations, and this list should be followed.

Drug dosages are expressed in Latin abbreviations, for example, q.i.d., which means four times a day, or b.i.d., which means twice a day. The dictator will pronounce the letters rather than say "four times a day." Transcribe the abbreviation in lowercase letters with periods and no internal spaces. See Chapter 4 for more information on transcribing medications and capitalization rules.

Ramon Yates, a 45-year-old construction worker, sought medical help after he noticed a small, raised bump in his groin area.

REPORT 5.4   Office Note

Use the Report0504.mp3 audio file and the office note template (Office_Note) when transcribing this report. Save the document as XXReport05.04, using your initials in place of *XX* in the file name. Note that lidocaine, epinephrine, and silver nitrate are generic drug names and should not be capitalized.

See Chapter 4 for more information on numbers.

In this report, you will hear "point five cee cees" dictated. The abbreviation for cubic centimeters is on the Joint Commission's list of dangerous abbreviations. Change this abbreviation to the acceptable abbreviation as explained on page 118 of Chapter 4. Also, follow appropriate style guidelines for transcribing decimals.

Recently, Ms. Mahoney visited her local clinic to have a mole removed from her forearm.

REPORT 5.5   Office Note

Use the Report0505.mp3 audio file and the office note template (Office_Note) when transcribing this report. Save the document as XXReport05.05, using your initials in place of *XX* in the file name.

Steri-Strips is a brand name and thus should be capitalized. Benzoin is a generic drug name and should be capitalized only if it starts a sentence.

John Smith is a teenager who was brought to the neighborhood health clinic after his mother noticed a small lump on his scalp while cutting his hair. He had not bumped his head or sustained any other injuries that could have caused the lump to occur.

REPORT 5.6   Office Note

Use the Report0506.mp3 audio file and the office note template (Office_Note) when transcribing this report. Save the document as XXReport05.06, using your initials in place of *XX* in the file name.

Listen for these terms:
  angioma
  parietal

The physician dictates the patient name as "Smith comma John," but transcribe the patient's name as John Smith for consistency with other reports. This style will be used for all transcribed documents.

Compound modifiers are made up of an adverb or an adjective and a participle. For example, well-defined and oval-shaped, require a hyphen. See Chapter 4 for a discussion of compound modifiers.

Robert Charles is an 8-year-old male brought to the dermatology clinic for evaluation of skin lesions. His past medical history includes a familial spastic paraplegia syndrome.

REPORT 5.7   Office Note

Use the Report0507.mp3 audio file and the office note template (Office_Note) when transcribing this report. Delete or change headings to match what is dictated. If a synonymous template heading is available, use the template's heading. Save the document as XXReport05.07, using your initials in place of *XX* in the file name.

Listen for these terms:
    antihistamines
    cutaneous
    cyproheptadine
    gregarious
    hydroxyzine
    neuromuscular
    urticaria pigmentosa

In the first paragraph of the dictation, a wrong word form is dictated. In the transcribed report, change the word "erythemas" to the adjective form.

Remember to use a hyphen to indicate a numerical range when the following rules are met (*The Book of Style for Medical Transcription*):

- Comparative phrases *from & to*; *from & through*; *between & and* are not used.
- None of the numbers contain decimals or commas.
- Numbers contain 3 or fewer digits.
- None of the numbers are negative.
- No other symbols are used in the expression.

If the above criteria are not met, use the word *to* to separate numbers in a range (e.g., the temperature dropped from 25 to –5 degrees; normal potassium values are 3.5 to 4.5).

Alberta Mariano is a young woman who had been diagnosed with childhood leukemia as a young child. She presented to the dermatologist with a pigmented lesion on her left breast.

REPORT 5.8 Operative Report

Use the Report0508.mp3 audio file and the operative report template (Operative_Report) when transcribing this report. The operative report will be introduced in Chapter 7. Look ahead to Figure 7.6 on page 207. Use the template's headings if the dictated headings are synonymous. Delete any unneeded headings. Save the document as XXReport05.08, using your initials in place of XX in the file name.

Listen for these terms:
Bacitracin
epinephrine
expeditiously
Monocryl suture
sequelae
Xylocaine

Metric measurements are abbreviated when used with an actual number. If no specific number is dictated, write out the complete word (e.g., I excised a few millimeters of tissue; I excised 1 cm of tissue).

Review the use of the noun and adjective form *followup* and the compound verb *follow up*. The noun or adjective form was once hyphenated, but is now accepted as one word.

Ophthalmology

The professionals within this specialty include the ophthalmologist, the medical doctor (MD) who diagnoses and treats eye disorders; the optometrist, the doctor of optometry (OD) who specializes in refraction of the eyes to determine the extent of vision and prescribes glasses; and the optician who takes the prescription from the MD or OD, grinds the lenses, and fits the glasses.

Objectives

» Identify and understand the anatomy and function of the eye.

» Recognize instruments and pharmacological agents used to examine the eye.

» Identify diseases and conditions affecting the eye.

» Describe treatments for vision problems and eye diseases.

» Pronounce and correctly spell terminology related to ophthalmology.

» Transcribe dictation related to the medical specialty of ophthalmology.

» Describe a consult letter, including typical content, format, and turnaround time.

Exploring Ophthalmology

The word *ophthalmology* is derived from a Greek root, *oculus*, for eyeball. This specialty encompasses the study of the eyeball, along with vision, the eyelids, the eye sockets (orbits), and the related parts of the face, brain, sinuses, nose, and throat.

Structure and Function

Working in partnership with the brain, the eye is the organ of sight. Vision is possible when the retina converts light into nerve impulses.

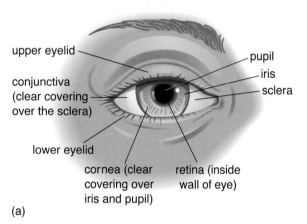

upper eyelid
conjunctiva (clear covering over the sclera)
lower eyelid
cornea (clear covering over iris and pupil)
retina (inside wall of eye)
pupil
iris
sclera

(a)

The main parts of the eye include the sclera, cornea, lens, retina, pupil, and iris (see Figure 6.1). The sclera is the "white" of the eye, the outer protective layer of the eyeball. The cornea is the transparent center, allowing light to enter the eye and directing it through the lens to the retina at the back of the eye. The cornea is the protective membrane at the center of the exterior eye and is important in the refractive system. The lens focuses the light; the pupil and iris control the amount of light that enters the eye.

Vision occurs when the retinas of both eyes send pictures to the brain, which merges the information into one image. Diplopia, or double vision, occurs when there is failure to merge the images.

Physical Assessment

The physician assesses the eye by examining the eyeballs and surrounding structures, including the eyebrows, upper and lower eyelids, and eyelashes. The patient's eyes may reflect feelings such as pain or fear as well as the individual's general health.

After the initial observation, the physician makes a closer inspection by asking the patient to

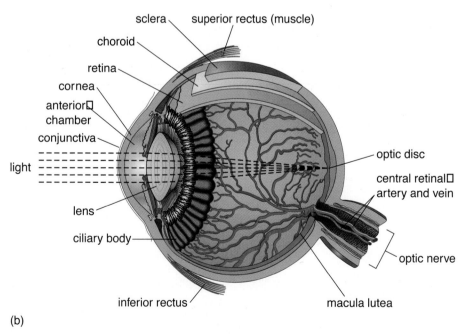

sclera
superior rectus (muscle)
choroid
retina
cornea
anterior chamber
conjunctiva
light
lens
ciliary body
inferior rectus
optic disc
central retinal artery and vein
optic nerve
macula lutea

(b)

Figure 6.1   The Eyeball   (a) Anterior view (b) Sagittal view

perform certain tasks to reveal facial neuromuscular coordination. The patient's squinting, blinking, raising and lowering of eyebrows, and making faces, such as a grimace, can reveal if there are any neuromuscular problems related to the eyes. These movements test the cranial nerves and are also performed by the neurologist (see Chapter 13).

There should be no pain or tenderness on palpation over the forehead, around the eye sockets, or across the lids and eyeballs. The eyeballs should feel firm, round, and bouncy to the touch.

The examination includes the observation of the sclerae, which should be white. Icteric (yellow-colored) sclerae can indicate jaundice. Very thin, blue-appearing sclerae can occur in some connective tissue disorders. The physician inspects the cornea with a light to determine if there are any irregularities, foreign bodies, or scars. The pupils are inspected for size, equal appearance, and reaction to light, an assessment that appears in the medical record as PERRLA (pupils equal, round, reactive to light and accommodation). The patient will be asked to look at the examiner's finger about 15 cm from the eyes and then look at a distant object. The pupils should narrow when looking close and widen when looking at a distance.

A Snellen, or "E," chart tests visual acuity. The chart has lines of letters with numbers on the side to represent how far a person can be from the chart to

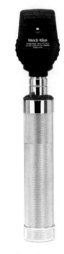

An ophthalmoscope is used to examine the retina.

read that line. Therefore, if the patient is seated 20 feet away from the chart and can read the line marked 20 feet, the person is said to have 20/20 vision. That is the distance that a normal eye can read at 20 feet. Central and peripheral visual fields are also tested. An Amsler grid is used to evaluate the central visual field.

The ophthalmoscope is the instrument used to look at the retina. By observing the veins and arteries directly, the examiner can check for

The Snellen eye chart is used to test visual acuity.

damage associated with hypertension, diabetes, and other diseases. The pupils may be dilated using mydriatic drops in order to perform a thorough examination.

The nerve fibers in the cornea make it extremely sensitive to pain. Examining the cornea requires a slit lamp that magnifies and illuminates the lens, cornea, and iris. A local anesthetic is used to relieve pain during the examination. It may be necessary to use fluorescein staining to outline any epithelial defects.

Diseases and Conditions

Examination of the eye is difficult from infancy to young school age. Frequently, the physician must sedate the young patient in order to complete the examination. The diagnosis of strabismus (crossed eyes) is usually made in childhood. This condition is typically the result of a weakness in one of the muscles controlling eye movement. Diplopia (double vision) is most common and can lead to reversible amblyopia (decreased vision) if diagnosed before the age of about seven years. Other deviations of eye control include esotropia (inward

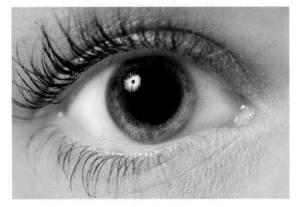

The dilated pupil remains open during the retinal examination.

turning of the eyes), exotropia (outward turning of the eyes), and hypertropia (upward squinting).

The eyelids protect the eyeball; therefore, it is important to seek medical attention when there are abnormalities of the eyelid. There can be irritation, inflammation, or infection of the eyelid, including blepharitis, an inflammation of the margins of the lid, and chalazion, a sterile granulomatous inflammation of the meibomian gland. A sty (or stye), called a hordeolum, is an infection of the lid usually caused by *Staphylococcus aureus*.

Conjunctivitis is an inflammation of the conjunctiva and can be caused by bacterial, viral, fungal, or parasitic organisms. There is usually hyperemia (redness), discharge, tearing, itching and/or burning, and a feeling of having a foreign body present in the eye.

Trachoma, caused by the organism *Chlamydia*, is a type of conjunctivitis that affects millions of people. It is rare in the United States, but is endemic to Africa, the Middle East, and Asia. Trachoma is the world's leading cause of blindness. It is very contagious through direct contact with infected individuals or materials they have touched and possibly through insect carriers, but it can be prevented by good hygiene and education. The symptoms of this disease include inflammation, blurred vision, and increasing pain and discomfort. Treatment consists of tetracycline or sulfonamides.

Uveitis is the inflammation of the structures of the uveal tract caused by allergens, bacteria, fungi, viruses, chemicals, or eye trauma. It is characterized by pain, photophobia, blurred vision, and erythema. A physician will prescribe corticosteroid drops to reduce inflammation and proper systemic treatment to treat the underlying cause.

Corneal abrasions occur from trauma, foreign bodies, including contact lenses, or any defect to the flow of protective tears. Keratitis is an infection of the cornea and can be caused by any organism that has entered the cornea through an abrasion. Because there is easy entry of infectious agents through the eye into the body, patients with severe infectious keratitis are hospitalized and placed on antibiotic therapy.

Keratoconus is a progressive thinning of the cornea that first shows up in puberty and affects

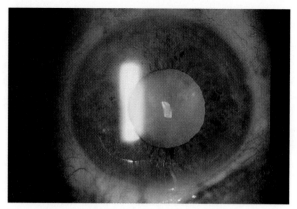

This eye's lens is clouded with a cataract. Surgical removal of the cataract is usually done as an outpatient procedure.

women more than men. Vision is distorted, leading to astigmatism and myopia that are difficult to correct even with eyeglasses. Surgery may be necessary to correct this problem.

Corneal transplants are performed using corneas from deceased (cadaveric) donors. A circular blade called a trephine is used to incise the cornea. The new cornea is sutured into place. Healing may be slow because of the decreased blood supply of the cornea. A transplant eye bank has been established to make donated corneas available.

Glaucoma, characterized as an increase in intraocular pressure, is a leading cause of blindness. The increased intraocular pressure damages the optic nerve, but proper management of glaucoma can prevent blindness. There are two forms of glaucoma: open angle and angle closure. Acute, angle-closure glaucoma prevents adequate drainage of aqueous humor into the trabecular meshwork resulting in increased fluid within the posterior chamber, thereby raising the intraocular pressure (IOP). Acute, closed-angle glaucoma must be treated emergently to prevent blindness. Open-angle glaucoma is typically a chronic and progressive disorder that is thought to be hereditary and usually affects both eyes. In this form of glaucoma, the angle is open, so there is no obstruction to the flow of aqueous humor through the uveoscleral outflow tract into the trabecular meshwork. Chronic glaucoma may be treated with prostaglandin analogs or with beta-adrenergic receptor antagonists. Laser trabeculectomy may be used to create an additional opening through the trabecular meshwork in order to drain aqueous humor.

A cataract is a clouding of the crystalline lens. The opaque lens scatters light rather than producing a fine, sharp image. Vision becomes blurred and distorted. While a cataract is usually associated with aging, it can be caused by systemic disease, such as diabetes mellitus, hypoparathyroidism, radiation exposure, or sickle C syndrome.

Retinal detachment is a separation of the neurosensory retina, or rods and cones, from the epithelial, or nourishment layer of the retina; it results in partial or total loss of vision in the affected eye. The most common type of detachment is rhegmatogenous, or a tear-induced detachment, which occurs in 1 out of 10,000 persons between 40 and 70 years old.

Diabetic retinopathy is a common complication of diabetes mellitus. The risk for this complication increases with the duration of the diabetes.

Macular degeneration is caused by damage to the photoreceptor cells in the area of the macula. It may be hereditary and is the leading cause of severe visual impairment for people over 65 years of age.

Common Tests and Surgical Procedures

Gonioscopy is used to visualize the uveoscleral angle to assess glaucoma. Tonometry measures intraocular pressure. Ophthalmoscopy is used to visualize the posterior chamber and a slit lamp is used to evaluate the anterior eye. Snellen charts are used to assess visual acuity and Amsler grids are used to assess visual fields, especially when macular degeneration is suspected. Fluorescein dye is used to diagnose disorders of the cornea or may be used in angiography to assess the vasculature.

Many eye disorders can be treated with conservative measures including antibiotic drops, antifungal and antiviral drops, antihistamine drops for allergic conjunctivitis, wetting drops for dry eyes, and steroids for inflammatory reactions. Nonsteroidal antiinflammatory drops are used to treat postoperative inflammation following cataract extraction and laser corneal surgery. As described above, glaucoma is commonly treated with eyedrops to reduce intraocular pressure. Patching of one eye may be used to encourage visual activity and increase visual acuity in the unpatched eye.

Surgical procedures to treat glaucoma include trabeculoplasty or trabeculectomy. Other surgical procedures include laser iridotomy, peripheral iridectomy, and gonioplasty. Other procedures that are commonly performed as outpatient surgical procedures include laser vision correction using laser-assisted in-situ keratomileusis (LASIK), photorefractive keratectomy (PRK), and radial keratotomy (RK). Lens implants are used to address cataracts.

Terms Bank

These terms and abbreviations provide a foundation for the language and transcription skills you will develop in the following sections of the chapter. Terms marked with » will be included in the reports transcribed in the Building Transcription Skills section.

accommodation
(ah-kom-o-**day**-shun) (n) the eye's ability to focus or see

afferent »
(**af**-er-ent) (adj) inward or toward a center, as a nerve; carrying a sensory impulse

amblyopia »
(am-blee-**O**-pee-a) (n) decreased vision in one or both eyes; not correctable

Amsler test
(**ahm**-zler) (n) used to evaluate visual field defects

anterior »
(an-**teer**-ee-or) (adj) front of a part, organ, or structure

aqueous humor
(**ak**-wee-us **hu**-mer) (n) the watery fluid that fills the anterior and posterior chambers of the eye

astigmatism
(a-**stig**-ma-tizm) (n) visual condition in which light rays entering the eye are bent unequally, preventing a sharp focus point on the retina

blepharectomy
(blef-ar-**ek**-tO-mee) (n) excision of a lesion of the eyelid

blepharitis
(blef-a-**rI**-tis) (n) inflammation of the eyelid

calcification »
(kal-si-fi-**kay**-shun) (n) a hardening of tissue resulting from the formation of calcium salts within it

cataract
(**kat**-a-rakt) (n) clouding of the lens of the eye, resulting in loss of transparency

chalazion
(ka-**lay**-zee-on) (n) a chronic inflammatory granuloma of the meibomian gland

chemosis
(kee-**mO**-sis) (n) an accumulation of fluid in the eye, causing swelling around the cornea

chemotherapy »
(kem-O-**thayr**-a-pee / **keem**-O-thayr-a-pee) (n) treatment of disease with drugs

choroid
(**kO**-royd) (n) a vascular membrane surrounding the eyeball, between the retina and sclera

conjunctiva »
(kon-junk-**ti**-va) (n) the mucous membrane covering the front of the eyeball and inside the eyelids; conjunctivae (pl)

conjunctival »
(kon-**junk**-ti-val (adj) pertaining to the conjunctiva

conjunctivitis »
(kon-junk-ti-**vI**-tis) (n) inflammation of the conjunctiva

cornea
(**kor**-nee-a) (n) the outer, transparent portion of the eye through which light passes to the retina

cupping
(**cup**-ping) (n) formation of a hollow or cup-shaped excavation

diabetes insipidus »
(dI-a-**bee**-tez in-**sip**-i-doos) (n and adj) disease caused by insufficient secretion of antidiuretic hormone (AHD) from the posterior pituitary gland

diplopia
(di-**plO**-pee-a) (n) double vision; may be monocular

enucleation
(ee-noo-klee-**ay**-shun) (n) removal of a tumor or structure as a whole, as in removal of the eyeball

epiphora
(ee-**pif**-O-ra) (n) overflow of tears

esotropia »
(es-O-**trO**-pee-a) (n) a condition in which one or both eyes appear to turn inward; cross eye(s)

exophthalmos
(ek-sof-**thal**-mos) (n) protrusion of the eyeball(s)

exotropia
(ek-sO-**trO**-pee-a) (n) outward turning of one eye relative to the other

extraocular »
(**ek**-stra-**ok**-yoo-lar) (adj) outside the eye

floater »
(**flO**-ter) (n) spot in the visual screen when one stares at a blank wall; caused by bits of protein and other debris moving in front of the retina

fluorescein »
(**floor**-ess-scene) (n) a yellow dye which glows in visible light

fundus
(**fun**-dus) (n) that part of the interior of the eyeball exposed to view through an ophthalmoscope; lowest part; fundi (pl)

funduscopic »
(fun-dus-**skop**-ik) (adj) relating to funduscopy

funduscopy
(fun-dus-**kop**-ee) (n) examination of the fundus of the eye using a funduscope; ophthalmoscopy

glaucoma »
(glaw-**kO**-ma) (n) disease of the eye in which intraocular pressure increases, damaging the optic nerve; can lead to blindness

Goldmann perimeter screen test
(n) assesses patient response when a light comes into view

gonioplasty
(gO-ni-O-**plas**-tee) (n) procedure that contracts the peripheral iris to eliminate contact with the trabecular meshwork

gonioscopy
(gO-ni-**O**-skOp-ee) (n) procedure that allows viewing of the anterior chamber angle

histiocyte ≫
(**hiss**-tee-O-cyte) (n) a cell that participates in the body's reaction to infection or injury; found in connective tissue

hordeolum
(hor-**dee**-O-lum) (n) a stye; a suppurative inflammation of a gland of the eyelid

hydrocephalic
(hI-drO-se-**fal**-ik) (adj) relating to or having hydrocephalus

hydrocephalus
(hI-drO-**sef**-a-lus) (n) increased accumulation of cerebrospinal fluid within the ventricles of the brain

hydrocephaly
(hI-drO-**sef**-a-lee) (n) the condition of having hydrocephalus

hyperopia
(hI-per-**O**-pee-a) (n) farsightedness

hypertropia
(hI-per-**trO**-pee-a) (n) a type of squint in which the eye looks upward

hypotropia ≫
(hI-pO-**trO**-pee-a) (n) a type of squint in which the eye looks downward

icteric
(ik-**ter**-ik) (adj) related to or affected with jaundice

infundibulum ≫
(in-fun-**dib**-yoo-lum) (n) a funnel-shaped opening

intraocular pressure ≫
(in-tra-**ok**-yoo-lar **presh**-er) (n) the pressure of the fluid within the eye

iris ≫
(**I**-ris) (n) colored portion of the eye that regulates the amount of light entering through the pupil; irides (**ir**-i-deez) (pl)

keratoplasty
(**ker**-a-tO-**plas**-tee) (n) surgery on the cornea, especially transplant of a cornea

laser iridotomy
(ir-i-**dot**-O-mee) (n) cutting some of the fibers of the iris with a laser

LASIK
(**lay**-sik) (n) acronym for laser-assisted in-situ keratomileusis

macula ≫
(**mak**-yoo-la) (n) small discolored spot on the retina

metastasis
(me-**tas**-ta-sis) (n) spread of a tumor from its site of origin to distant sites

metastatic ≫
(met-a-**stat**-ik) (adj) relating to metastasis

motility ≫
(mO-**til**-i-tee) (n) ability to move spontaneously

mydriatic
(mi dree-**at**-ik) (n) pharmaceutical agent which dilates pupil

myopia
(mI-**O**-pee-a) (n) nearsightedness; visual defect in which parallel rays come to a focus

myelocyte ≫
(**my**-e-lo-cyte) (n) immature granulocytic leukocyte normally found in bone marrow and present in the circulatory blood in certain diseases, e.g., myelocytic leukemia

nystagmus
(nis-**tag**-mus) (n) involuntary, rhythmic oscillation of the eyeballs

oblique
(ob-**leek**) (adj) slanting

ophthalmologist ≫
(of-thal-**mol**-o-jist) (n) a physician specializing in diseases of the eye

ocular ≫
(**ok**-yoo-lar) (adj) concerning the eye or vision

ophthalmoscopy
(of-thal-**mos**-ko-pee) (n) procedure used to examine the optic nerve head for color, shape, and vascularization

ophthalmus
(of-**thal**-mus) (n) the eye

optic ≫
(**op**-tik) (adj) pertaining to the eye or sight

optic chiasm
(**op**-tik **kI**-azm) (n) the point of crossing of the optic nerves

optometrist
(op-**tom**-e-trist) (n) a professional who tests visual acuity and prescribes corrective lenses

osteosarcoma ≫
(os-tee-O-sar-**ko**-ma) (n) a tumor of the bone, usually highly malignant

palsy ≫
(**pawl**-zee) (n) an abnormal condition characterized by partial paralysis

papilledema ≫
(**pap**-ill-e-dee-ma) (n) edema and inflammation of the optic nerve at its point of entrance into the eyeball

papillopathy ≫
(pap-i-**lop**-a-thee) (n) the blood supply to the optic disk and retina is obstructed; often producing low-tension glaucoma

peripheral iridectomy
(per-**if**-er-al ir-i-**dek**-tO-mee) (n) procedure that creates a hole in the iris; used to relieve high intraocular pressure

phacoemulsification
(fak-O-ee-mul-si-fi-**kay**-shun) (n) process that disintegrates a cataract using ultrasonic waves

photophobia
(fO-tO-**fO**-bee-a) (n) marked intolerance to light

pilocarpine

(pI-lO-**kar**-peen) (n) a parasympathomimetic agent used to treat glaucoma

platelet »

(**playt**-let) (n) disc-shaped, small cellular element in the blood that is essential for blood clotting

presbyopia

(prez-bee-**O**-pee-a) (n) farsightedness associated with aging

prognosis

(prog-**nO**-sis) (n) the expected outcome of a disease

pterygium

(ter-**ij**-ee-um) (n) web eye; an outward growth of tissue of the eye

ptosis »

(**tO**-sis) (n) sagging of the upper eyelid

pupil

(**pyoo**-pil) (n) the round opening in the center of the iris which opens or closes to adjust to light

pupillary »

(**pyoo**-pi-layr-ee) (adj) relating to the pupil of the eye

radial keratotomy

(**ray**-dee-al ker-ah-**tot**-O-mee) (n) incision(s) in the cornea radiating out from the center

radiotherapy »

(ray-dee-O-**thayr**-a-pee) (n) the treatment of disease by application of radium, ultraviolet, and other types of radiation

recession

(ree-**sesh**-un) (n) the withdrawal of a part from its normal position

rectus »

(**rec**-tus) (adj) relating to the rectus muscle of the eye

referral

(ree-**fer**-al) (n) a physician's sending of a patient to another physician

reflex »

(**ree**-fleks) (n) an involuntary response to a stimulus

regression »

(ree-**gresh**-un) (n) returning to an earlier condition

retina

(**ret**-i-na) (n) innermost layer of the eyeball that receives images formed by the lens and transmits visual impulses through the optic nerve to the brain; composed of light-sensitive nerves

retinal hemorrhage »

(**ret**-i-nal **hem**-or-age) hemorrhage of the retina

retinitis pigmentosa

(ret-in-**I**-tis pig-men-**toe**-saw) (n) an inflammation of the retina with pigment changes, eventually leading to blindness

retinoblastoma »

(**ret**-i-nO-blas-**tO**-ma) (n) malignant sarcoma or neoplasm of the retina; hereditary and generally occurring in young children

retinopathy »

(ret-i-**nop**-a-thee) (n) any disorder of the retina without inflammation

retinoscopy

(ret-i-**nos**-ko-pee) (n) light beam test used to detect refractive errors

sclera »

(**skle**-rah) (n) white of the eye; the tough, outer covering of the eye

sclerostomy

(skle-**ros**-tO-mee) (n) surgical formation of an opening in the sclera

scotoma »

(skO-**tO**-ma) (n) a blind spot; a small area of defective vision

seed

(n) as related to oncology, it is the beginning of a tumor

seeding

(n) the local spreading of immature tumor cells

Seton procedure

(n) placing of a tube in the anterior chamber to drain fluid and decrease the intraocular pressure

slit lamp »

(n) instrument consisting of a microscope and a thin, bright beam of light; used to examine the eye

sphincterotomy

(sfink-tur-**ot**-O-mee) (n) procedure that produces cuts in the iris sphincter muscle to allow pupillary enlargement

sporadic »

(spO-**rad**-ik) (adj) occurring occasionally or in isolated situations

strabismus »

(stra-**biz**-mus) (n) improper alignment of eyes; crossed eye(s)

sty

(stI) (n) an infection of a marginal gland of the eyelid; stye

tangent screen test

(n) maps the field of vision using a marker

thrombocytopenia »

(**throm**-bO-cy-to-**pee**-nee-a) (n) abnormal decrease in the number of blood platelets

tonometry

(tO-**nom**-et-ree) (n) a test that measures intraocular pressure

trabeculectomy

(tra-bek-yoo-**lek**-tO-mee) (n) surgical removal of a section of the cornea to decrease intraocular pressure in patients with severe glaucoma

trabeculoplasty

(tra-**bek**-yoo-lO-**plas**-tee) (n) surgical procedure that decreases intraocular pressure in open-angle glaucoma

unilateral »

(yoo-ni-**lat**-e-ral) (adj) affecting or occurring on only one side

uveitis

(yoo-vee-**I**-tis) (n) inflammation of the uvea, including the choroid and the iris

viable »

(**vI**-a-bl) (adj) capable of surviving; living

visual acuity

(**vizh**-yoo-al a-**kyoo**-i-tee) (n) clearness of vision, e.g., 20/20 visual acuity

vitreous

(**vi**-tree-us) (adj) resembling glass

vitreous humor »
(**vit**-ree-us **hyoo**-mer) (adj) glassy; gelatin-like substance within the eyeball

Xalatan
(**zal**-a-tan) (n) eyedrops used to treat glaucoma by increasing drainage of aqueous humor.

xanthopsia
(zan-**thop**-see-a) (n) yellow vision; a condition in which everything seen appears yellowish

Abbreviations

ACC	accommodation		OS	left eye *(oculus sinister)*
D	diopter		OU	both eyes *(oculus uterque)*
DCR	dacryocystorhinostomy		PAN	periodic alternating nystagmus
ECCE	extracapsular cataract extraction		PERLA	pupils equal, reactive to light and accommodation
Em	emmetropia			
EOM	extraocular muscles; extraocular movements		PERRLA	pupils equal, round, reactive to light and accommodation
ERG	electroretinography			
ICCE	intracapsular cataract extraction		PRK	photorefractive keratectomy
IOL	intraocular lens		REM	rapid eye movement
IOP	intraocular pressure		ROP	retinopathy of prematurity
L&A	light and accommodation		ST	esotropia
LASIK	laser assisted *in-situ* keratomileusis		VA	visual acuity
my	myopia		VF	visual field
OD	right eye *(oculus dexter);* doctor of optometry		XT	exotropia

Building Language Skills

Complete the following exercises, drawing on the information learned in the Exploring Ophthalmology section of this chapter and referencing the Terms Bank.

Exercise 6.1   Matching Sound and Spelling

The numbered list that follows shows the phonetic spelling of hard-to-spell words. Sound out the word and then write the correct spelling in the blank space provided. Check your answers in the Terms Bank or other appropriate reference.

1. kal-si-fi-**kay**-shun _____

2. **ret**-i-nO-blas-**tO**-ma _____

3. yoo-ni-**lat**-e-ral _____

4. **pyoo**-pi-layr-ee _____

5. ob-**leek** _____

6. hI-drO-**sef**-a-lus _____

7. blef-a-**rI**-tis _____

8. **vit**-ree-us _____

9. fO-tO-**fO**-bee-a _____

10. me-**tas**-ta-sis _____

11. nis-**tag**-mus _____

12. ek-sof-**thal**-mos _____

13. **os**-tee-O-sar-**kO**-ma _____

14. pap-i-**lop**-a-thee _____

15. mO-**til**-i-tee _____

Below is a list of frequently used words that look alike and/or sound alike. Study the meaning and pronunciation of each set of words, read the following sentences carefully, and then circle the word in parentheses that correctly completes the meaning.

afferent	conducting (as a nerve) or progressing toward the center	**hyper -**	(prefix) more, greater
efferent	conducting (as a nerve) or progressing away from the center	**hypo-**	(prefix) less, smaller
		LASIK	surgical procedure
affluent	having wealth	**Lasix**	diuretic
effluent	something that flows out	**loop**	a shape
anterior	front	**loupe**	a magnifying lens
inferior	below; lower	**macula**	a small, yellowish spot on the retina at the back of the eye
posterior	back; behind	**macule**	a spot discoloration or thickening of the skin
superior	above		
appraise	to set a value on; to give an expert judgment of the value or merit of	**metastases**	plural form of metastasis
		metastasis	spread of a tumor to different parts of the body
apprise	to notify; to tell	**metastasize**	to invade by metastasis
ectropion	rolling outward	**metastatic**	relating to metastasis
entropion	turning inward	**papillary**	relating to papillae
esotropia	inward turning of the eye	**pupillary**	relating to the pupil
exotropia	outward turning of the eye	**recession**	withdrawal of part from its normal position
fundus	part farthest from the opening	**resection**	cutting out part of an organ
fungus	organism		

1. The head is (inferior/superior) to the chest.

2. Your face is located on the (anterior/posterior) part of your body.

3. The legs are (inferior/superior) to the head.

4. The spine is (anterior/posterior) to the chest.

5. Examination of the face revealed a 1 cm (macula/macule) on the cheek.

6. Due to her (hyperthyroidism/hypothyroidism), she requires thyroid supplementation.

7. The patient's (hypertension/hypotension) is under good control on the Calan SR.

8. On ophthalmic exam, the (fundus/fungus) appeared normal.

9. This patient has metastatic colorectal carcinoma with (metastases/metastasis) diagnosed in the liver, lung, and brain.

10. The patient is status post craniotomy for removal of tumor (metastasis/metastatic).

Choosing Words from Context

When transcribing dictation, the medical transcriptionist frequently needs to consider the situation when determining the word that correctly completes the sentence. From the list below, select the term that meaningfully completes each of the following statements.

conjunctivitis	nystagmus	retinopathy
diplopia	optic	scotoma
enucleation	optic chiasm	strabismus
epiphora	osteosarcoma	
esotropia	radiotherapy	

1. The patient is status post _____ of the left eye, with a poorly fitted prosthesis in place.

2. The right fundus showed a flame hemorrhage superior to the _____ nerve.

3. She had an amputation of the right leg below the knee because she was diagnosed with a malignancy called _____.

4. She describes a blind spot in the right eye; this is most likely a _____.

5. When you have _____, your eyes may deviate either toward the nose or to the outside of midline.

6. The patient's allergic _____ seems to be controlled on the antibiotic eyedrops.

7. It was recommended that Joseph have _____ treatments to the eye, rather than have an enucleation.

8. A mild form of _____, where the eye turns inward, can often be corrected with exercises for the eye.

9. The funduscopic exam showed no signs of _____.

10. The MRI revealed an enhancing lesion surrounding the _____.

Exercise 6.4   Pairing Words and Meanings

From this list, locate the term that best matches each of the following definitions. Write the term in the space provided by each definition.

amblyopia	hydrocephalus	pupillary
calcification	macula	rectus
cornea	nystagmus	retina
diplopia	ophthalmus	retinopathy
extraocular	optic	seed
funduscopy	papilledema	

1. outer, transparent portion of the eye   _____

2. pertaining to vision   _____

3. pertaining to pupil of eye   _____

4. accumulation of cerebrospinal fluid
   within ventricles of brain   _____

5. examination of the base of the eye   _____

6. small, yellowish spot on retina   _____

7. hardening of tissue resulting from calcium salts   _____

8. beginning of a tumor   _____

9. any disorder of the retina without edema   _____

10. a muscle of the eye   _____

11. swelling of the optic nerve in the eye   _____

12. double vision   _____

Exercise 6.5   Creating Terms from Word Forms

Combine prefixes, root words, and suffixes from this list to create medical words that fit the following definitions. Fill in the blanks with the words you construct.

angi/o	vessel	**retina**	nerve tissue layer of eye
blephar/o	eyelid	**thromb/o**	platelet
conjunctiv/o	mucous membrane lining inner eyeball and eyelids	**-a**	word ending
		-ectomy	removal
cyt/o	cell	**-itis**	inflammation
extra	outside	**-pathy**	disease
hyper	above or excessive	**-penia**	deficiency
hypo	below or deficient	**-phobia**	excessive fear
kerat/o	hard or cornea	**-plasty**	surgical repair
ocul/o	pertaining to the eye	**-scopy**	examination
ophthalm/o	eye	**-tropia**	condition of turning
phot/o	light		

1. disease of the retina_____

2. type of squint when the eye looks downward _____

3. inflammation of the membrane lining the inner
   eyelid and the eyeball_____

4. excision of a lesion on the eyelid_____

5. light beam test that detects refractive errors _____

6. operation to correct defect in eyelids_____

7. visualizes the optic nerve for color and shape _____

8. mucous membrane lining the inner surface of the eye _____

9. inflammation of the eyelid _____

10. corneal transplant _____

11. outside the eye _____

12. deficiency of platelet cells (decreased platelets) _____

Read the following report excerpts and look for errors in punctuation, spelling, plural vs. singular word forms, run-on sentences, and subject-verb agreement. Mark the corrections on this page and key the excerpts with all errors corrected. Save the documents as XXExercise06.06-1 and XXExercise06.06-2, using your initials in place of XX in the file names.

1.   **OBJECTIVE:**

On examination visual aquity at distance was 20/20 in both eyes. The interocular pressure was 20 in both eyes. Motility was strait with full versions and the pupils was normal. External exam revealed fat pertrusion on the lateral aspect of the upper and lower lids on both eye. There was a firmness on the right eye. The contacts were centered will with good movement, slit lamp exam revealed white conjunctiva, with clear cornia. The lenses had some cortical changes. Dilated funduscopic exam revealed normal cup-to-disc ratio with normal macule, blood vessels, and peripheral retina.

2.   I found him to have papilodema as well as retinale hemorrhages. He occasionally notes some transient visual bluring when he suddenly goes from sitting to standing and occasional vertical deplopia.

Read this scenario carefully and then select the most appropriate response. Write an explanation for why you think your choice is the best answer.

You have successfully completed a one-year internship and have been given the opportunity to work from home. After your first week of working from home, your neighbor notices your car in the driveway and recognizes that you are home during the day. Since you are home all day, she asks if you would babysit her toddler three days a week while she works. Should you accept the opportunity to make more money and help your neighbor?

---

a. No, do not agree to care for the child. Explain that you are working also, just not working in an office away from the house.

b. Yes, but only for a limited time. Agree to help your neighbor for a week or two until she makes other arrangements.

c. Agree to care for the child and set up a play area and TV in the same room where you are transcribing so you can keep an eye on the child while you work.

Best response: _____

Explanation: _____

_____

_____

_____

_____

You will apply the medical specialty and language information you learned in this chapter to transcription work in this section. After you learn the formatting recommendations of a consultation letter/report, you will transcribe nine reports related to six different patient studies.

Introducing the Consultation Letter

The consultation letter (Figure 6.2) is a report that a patient's primary or attending physician requests of a specialist. Dictated in either letter or report form, this document provides an opinion on a particular problem or diagnosis. The specialist dictates the letter/report and addresses it to the primary physician.

Required Headings/Content

The Joint Commission guidelines require no special headings in consultation letters; the format varies among institutions. The content includes sections similar to a history and physical, including date of consultation, reason for consultation, present history, past history, physical and laboratory evaluation, and the consultant's impression and recommendations. At the end of the dictation, physicians often add a phrase such as *Thank you for referring this patient to me.*

Turnaround Time

For emergency department situations, specialists' consultations are available within approximately 30 minutes; initial consultation through two-way voice communication is acceptable. Consulta-

tions should be dictated within 24 hours from the time the request is received by the physician, and the report should be transcribed and on the chart within the next 24 hours. This guideline varies among institutions.

Preparing to Transcribe

To prepare for transcribing dictation, review the common ophthalmology terms, drugs, and abbreviations presented in this chapter's Terms Bank. Then, study the format and organization of the model document shown in Figure 6.2, and key the model document, using the consultation letter template on the Dictations and Templates CD as a starting point. Save the document as XXFigure06.02, using your initials in place of *XX* in the file name. Proofread the document by comparing it with the printed version. Categorize the types of errors you made, and document them on a copy of the Performance Comparison Chart. A template of this chart is available on the Dictations and Templates CD.

Transcribing Reports

Transcribe, edit, and correct each report in the following patient studies. Consult reference books for words or formatting rules that are unfamiliar.

As you work on the transcription assignment for this chapter, fill in the Performance Comparison Chart that you started when you keyed the model document. For at least three of the reports, categorize and document the types of errors you made. Answer the document analysis questions on the bottom of the chart. With continuous practice and assessment, the quality of your work will improve.

November 29, 20XX

2 or more line spaces, depending on length of letter

Albert J. Eisner, MD
Brookfield University Medical School
One University Place
Fort Worth, TX 76104-3223
ds
RE: Lawrence Johnson, Jr.
ds
Dear Al:
ds
We rechecked the above-named patient under anesthesia on November 21. It has been
9 months since he completed his course of external beam radiation therapy as management of
unilateral sporadic retinoblastoma in the left eye.
ds
On our exam today, our findings remain the same as on our prior exam in August. The tumor is
completely regressed, and there is no evidence of viability. There are no new tumors in the left
eye. The optic disk is healthy, and there are no signs of radiation retinopathy or papillopathy.
ds
The right eye is perfectly normal with no evidence of retinoblastoma. Regarding the visual
prognosis, because of the macular location of the regressed retinoblastoma, his visual
prognosis is very guarded. We will try patching of the right eye in an attempt to stimulate any
possible vision in the left eye.
ds
Thank you for allowing us to assist in his care.
ds
Very sincerely yours,

quadruple-space

Richard Sowers, MD
ds
RS/XX

Figure 6.2   Consultation Letter

Lawrence Johnson is an infant who was diagnosed with retinoblastoma by Dr. Richard Sowers at Wills Eye Hospital. He was referred to Dr. Albert J. Eisner at Brookfield University Medical School for followup care. After his examination, Dr. Eisner sent Lawrence to Dr. Jorge Frieze, a specialist in radiation oncology, for radiotherapy.

REPORT 6.1   Consultation Letter

Use the Report0601.mp3 audio file and the consultation letter template (Consultation_Letter) when transcribing this report. Save the document as XXReport06.01, using your initials in place of *XX* in the file name.

Listen for these terms:
    enucleation
    unilateral sporadic retinoblastoma

Measurements of tumors are done with metric terms, as in 15 by 15 by 5.9 mm. Transcribe "by" as x with one space before and after. The abbreviation for millimeters requires no period, and the abbreviation should be keyed only once—at the end of the measurement.

REPORT 6.2   Letter of Referral

Use the Report0602.mp3 audio file and the consultation letter template (Consultation_Letter) when transcribing this report. Save the document as XXReport06.02, using your initials in place of *XX* in the file name.

The word *followup* functions as a noun or an adjective, and *follow up* functions as a verb. Key the term as one word when used as a noun or adjective and as two words when used as a verb. A hyphenated construction (*follow-up*) is also acceptable for adjective uses, but one word is preferred. In this report, *followup* is used three times as a noun. See Chapter 4 for a more complete discussion of compound words.

REPORT 6.3   Consultation Letter

Use the Report0603.mp3 audio file and the consultation letter template (Consultation_Letter) when transcribing this report. Save the document as XXReport06.03, using your initials in place of *XX* in the file name.

Ronald Jones is a 21-year-old male diagnosed with osteosarcoma. While hospitalized for administration of chemotherapy, he developed difficulty with his vision. A specialist in ophthalmology, Dr. Regina Smyth, was called as a consultant to assist with this complication.

REPORT 6.4   Chart Summary

Use the Report0604.mp3 audio file and the chart summary template (Chart_Summary) when transcribing this report. The chart summary will be introduced in Chapter 15. The function of this type of report is similar to the office note. However, in this template, there are no internal headings. Key the headings as dictated, but keep the date as the last identifying heading at the top of the report. Save the document as XXReport06.04, using your initials in place of *XX* in the file name.

This report will include subheadings within an Examination section. Key these subheadings in all capital letters followed by a colon and one space to the dictated information. Do not set an extra line space below the Examination heading and before the first subheading or between subheadings. Refer to the format shown in Figure 4.1 on pages 127 and 128.

Listen for these difficult terms:
    metastatic osteosarcoma
    scotoma

Visual acuity results are dictated as two numbers ("twenty twenty") and transcribed as two numerals separated by a virgule (diagonal slash), as in 20/20.

If a dictation includes a sentence that begins with a number, the transcriptionist may recast the sentence to improve the word order.

The word *re-examine* requires a hyphen since the prefix ends with the first letter of the following word, *examine*.

REPORT 6.5   Consultation Letter

Use the Report0605.mp3 audio file and the consultation letter template (Consultation_Letter) when transcribing this report. Save the document as XXReport06.05, using your initials in place of *XX* in the file name.

This consultation letter is taken from the consultation report and is turned into a letter to be sent back to the referring physician. As with all letters, this is written in a formal style with complete sentences.

Reling Quang is a 47-year-old secretary who reports that she has been finding it more difficult to see her computer screen and that her eyes tire easily. She has never worn glasses but thinks that it may be necessary now.

REPORT 6.6 Office Note

Use the Report0606.mp3 audio file and the consultation letter template (Office_Note) when transcribing this report. Save the document as XXReport06.06, using your initials in place of *XX* in the file name.

When transcribing visual acuity test results, separate the abbreviation (for example, OD) and the numbers with a space but no comma. However, include a comma between the results for the right and left eyes, as in OD 20/20, OS 20/20.

When speaking, we often do not pronounce the correct form of the noun (singular or plural), but the correct form should always be transcribed. When transcribing this report, be sure to transcribe the singular or plural form of nouns and their corresponding verbs as required by the context. Note when the dictator is reporting results on both eyes or just one eye and transcribe nouns and verbs accordingly.

Elizabeth Hammers has been referred to an ophthalmologist for an opinion about her dimness of vision in the right eye. Although the problem has been present since birth, Elizabeth's primary physician wanted to ensure that no disease process was occurring in the eye.

REPORT 6.7 Consultation Letter

Use the Report0607.mp3 audio file and the consultation letter template (Consultation_Letter) when transcribing this report. Save the document as XXReport06.07, using your initials in place of *XX* in the file name.

Listen for these terms:
    afferent
    amblyopic
    cup-to-disk ratio
    disk edema
    dot-and-blot hemorrhage
    fluorescein angiogram
    ischemia
    pupillary
    rubeosis

When using a plus sign (+) to grade a reflex or other observation, always use a numeral either before or after the plus sign: 2+, +2; not ++ or two plus.

As in Report 6.6, listen for places in the dictation where a singular form is used instead of the intended plural form. Be sure to correct these errors in the transcribed document.

Glen Brian is a child who has a disorder of the eye because of increased pressure within the brain. His pediatrician, Dr. Richard Golden, has referred him to Sanford Guterman, MD, an ophthalmologist, for treatment.

REPORT 6.8   Consultation Letter

Use the Report0608.mp3 audio file and the consultation letter template (Consultation_Letter) when transcribing this report. Save the document as XXReport06.08, using your initials in place of *XX* in the file name.

Listen for these terms:
>   bimedial rectus recession
>   esotropia
>   hydrocephalus
>   oblique over-action
>   strabismus

Ordinals may be written out (e.g., sixth) or written with a numeral and plain or superscript suffix (e.g., 6th or 6th). *The Book of Style for Medical Transcription* recommends using numbers. Use of superscript is acceptable if available within the word processor and compatible with the receiving electronic record. For this text do not use superscript.

Christopher Barney is a young man who is diagnosed with acute myeloblastic leukemia. He is being evaluated by the ophthalmologist for followup for visual problems resulting from retinal hemorrhages.

REPORT 6.9   Consultation Letter

Use the Report0609.mp3 audio file and the consultation letter template (Consultation_Letter) when transcribing this report. This dictator will include headings in the body of the letter. Set headings in all capital letters followed by a single hard return, but set a blank line space above each heading. Save the document as XXReport06.09, using your initials in place of *XX* in the file name.

This letter will go onto a second page. Use the template's second page's running head jump fields to set the patient's name and the date of the letter at the top of the second page. A continued line is not necessary in consultation letters.

Listen for these terms:
>   afferent pupillary defect
>   dot-to-blot
>   irides (plural of iris)
>   papilledema
>   vitreous heme

Seven

Otorhinolaryngology

The ears, nose, and throat are important passageways into the body that can be affected by a variety of medical conditions. Otorhinolaryngology, from the Greek for ear *(oto)*, nose *(rhis)*, and larynx *(larynx)*, is the medical specialty that deals with these passageways. Physicians who practice in this area are called otorhinolaryngologists or ENT (ear, nose, and throat) specialists.

Objectives

» Identify and understand the anatomy and function of the ears, nose, and throat.

» Distinguish the two types of hearing loss.

» Recognize diseases that affect the ears, nose, and throat.

» Recognize common microbial pathogens that infect the ear, nose, sinuses, and throat.

» Pronounce and correctly spell terminology related to otorhinolaryngology.

» Transcribe dictation related to the medical specialty of otorhinolaryngology.

» Describe an operative report, including typical content, format, and turnaround time.

The specialty of otorhinolaryngology is concerned with diseases of the ears, nose, and throat. Because many common illnesses affect the ears, nose, and throat, people frequently visit the doctor with complaints of symptoms affecting these areas. In addition, because the ears and nose are so visible and prominent, people often seek corrective treatment for deformities or malformations of these structures.

Structure and Function

The ear is the organ of hearing and equilibrium. It has three parts: the external, middle, and inner ear. Figure 7.1 shows the sections of the ear, consisting of the external auricle, or pinna, and the external ear canal. The auricle is designed to collect sound waves from the air and conduct them through the external auditory canal (EAC) into the middle ear. Figure 7.2 shows the structures of the inner ear.

When sound waves enter the ear canal, they strike against the tympanic membrane, or eardrum, which is located at the outer end of the middle ear (also called the tympanic cavity). From the tympanic membrane, the sound waves vibrate three bones called the ossicles. The ossicles include the malleus (hammer), the incus (anvil), and the stapes (stirrup). These three bones are referred to as the *ossicular chain*. All of the parts of the ossicular chain (group of three ear bones) must be working properly for the sound-pressure ratio to be in balance and for hearing to be in the normal range.

The structures of the inner ear, or labyrinth, include the cochlea, the vestibule, and the semicircular canals, as well as the auditory and vestibular receptors of the 8th cranial nerve (CN VIII), also called the vestibulocochlear nerve. The inner ear receives sound waves when the stapes gently pushes on the membrane of the oval window, or fenestra ovalis, forcing fluid to move within the cochlea. The cochlea contains tiny hairs (cilia) that move forward and back as the sound waves move through the cochlea. Movement of the cilia excites the hair cells within the organ of Corti, thereby generating

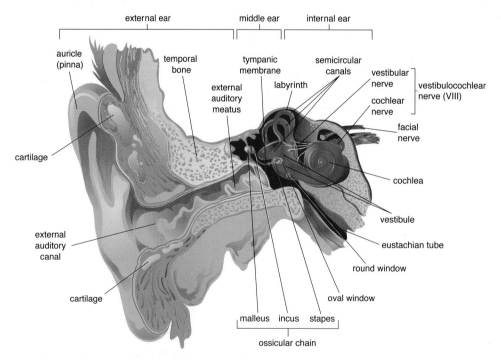

Figure 7.1   Divisions of the Ear: External, Middle, and Inner Ear

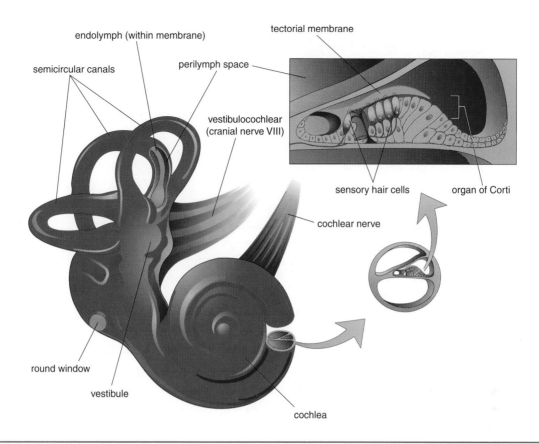

endolymph (within membrane)

semicircular canals

tectorial membrane

perilymph space

vestibulocochlear
(cranial nerve VIII)

sensory hair cells

organ of Corti

cochlear nerve

round window

vestibule

cochlea

Figure 7.2 Structures of the Inner Ear

neural impulses detectable by the cochlear nerve. Impulses move from the cochlear nerve to the vestibulocochlear nerve and are routed to the brain where they are interpreted as sound.

Cerumen, or ear wax, is a normal byproduct of a healthy ear. It prevents foreign particles from entering the passageway. Cerumen is produced by glands in the middle ear.

The eustachian tube connects the middle ear with the nasopharynx. The tube opens and closes as needed to equalize the pressure on either side of the eardrum and allows for drainage of fluid from the middle ear. The "popping" sound heard when ascending and descending in airplanes is actually the eustachian tube opening and closing.

The nose is an important structure with multiple functions. Besides being the organ of smell, the nose is the passageway for air into the respiratory tract and is the disposal system for tears. The nasal passages contain olfactory nerves, which send messages to the brain to help identify odors. The nose also assists with the production of sound

during speech. Mucous membranes lining the nasal passages contain goblet cells, which secrete mucus. To protect the lungs from particulates in the air, the mucus and cilia trap dust and particles and "sweep" them toward the nasopharynx and down the esophagus. Sneezing also helps to rid the upper respiratory tract of contaminants.

A cartilaginous structure called the septum divides the nose into right and left nasal cavities. The lateral wall of the septum contains three bony structures: the inferior, middle, and superior turbinates, or conchae. The nasal cavities open into the paranasal sinuses—frontal, maxillary, ethmoidal, and sphenoidal sinuses (see Figure 7.3). The open, airy spaces created by the sinuses lessen the weight of the skull, provide a space for air to become warm and moist before entering the lungs, and also contribute to the resonance and tone of a person's voice.

The nasal cavities are separated from the mouth by the hard and soft palates which make up the "roof" of the mouth. The hard palate is located just

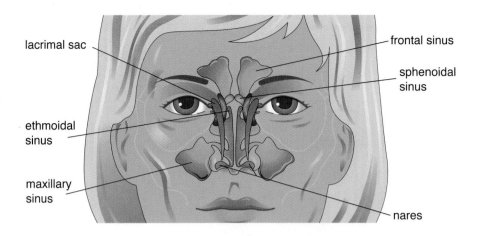

lacrimal sac

frontal sinus

sphenoidal sinus

ethmoidal sinus

maxillary sinus

nares

Figure 7.3 The Paranasal Sinuses

behind the upper front teeth and the soft palate is located toward the back of the mouth. Above and behind the tongue is the fauces, an arch-shaped area bounded by the anterior and posterior tonsillar pillars, tongue, and soft palate. The area posterior to the nose and mouth is divided into two areas: the nasopharynx and the oropharynx (visible when the mouth is open). The tonsils, made of lymphoid tissue, form a protective ring in the mouth and back of the throat where they form the first line of defense against infection. Figure 7.4 shows the three sets of tonsils: the palatine tonsils, located on each side of the throat; the pharyngeal tonsils, or adenoids, located on the posterior wall of the nasopharynx; and the lingual tonsils, located on both sides of the base of the tongue.

The larynx, or voice box, is located between the pharynx and the trachea. The epiglottis closes over the aperture of the larynx during swallowing to prevent food from entering the glottis. The glottis consists of folds of membranous tissue that make up the vocal cords. The larynx is supported by cricoid cartilage, as shown in Figure 7.5. The principal function of the larynx is vocalization.

The upper jaw bone is called the maxilla and the lower jaw bone is the mandible. The temporomandibular joint (TMJ), located just anterior to the ear, is the articular surface formed by the mandible and the temporal bone. This may be a source of pain and headache if this joint becomes malaligned.

Physical Assessment

The practitioner assesses the ears, nose, and throat using an otoscope. The otoscope is equipped with a bright light which illuminates and magnifies internal areas. The practitioner also observes the external areas of the ears, nose, and throat for abnormalities such as low-set ears (which may indicate genetic syndromes), malformations, or discharge. The face is palpated to assess for tenderness and swelling of the sinuses.

During physical examination of the ear, the speculum is inserted into the external auditory meatus. The practitioner can see a portion of the tympanic membrane and important landmarks: the malleus, the annulus, and Wilde triangle, which is a triangular area that under normal conditions reflects the otoscope's light. A normal tympanic membrane should be flat or concave and pearly gray in color. It should reflect a good cone of light.

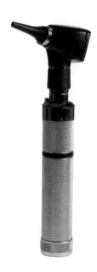

The otoscope's bright light allows the physician to examine the patient's ears, nose, or throat.

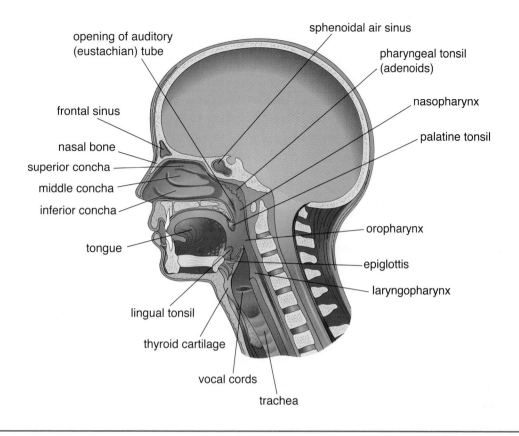

Figure 7.4   Sagittal View of the Head and Neck

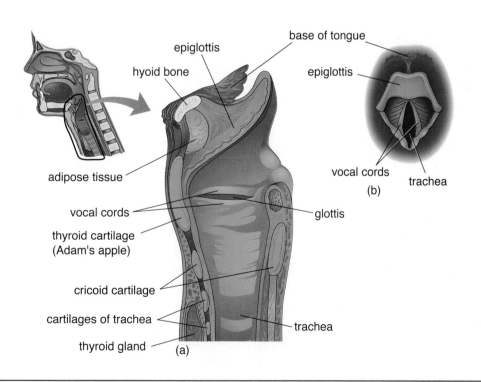

Figure 7.5   Structures within the Neck   *(a) Sagittal view (b) Superior view*

The nasal cavity is also examined using the otoscope. The turbinates are examined for erythema, congestion, exudates, and polyps. The mouth is examined for ulcers, leukoplakia (white patches), and abnormalities of the tongue, including position (in or away from the midline) and movement. The oropharynx is assessed for erythema, swelling, exudates, and drainage from the nasal cavities and sinuses.

Diseases and Conditions

One of the most common complaints of the ear is otitis media, an inflammation of the middle ear. In adults, the eustachian tube slants downward from the middle ear, allowing fluid to drain. Infants and toddlers are especially prone to otitis media because the eustachian tube tends to be more horizontal, making it more difficult to adequately drain, especially in the presence of an upper respiratory infection (URI). The increase in fluid within the middle ear and eustachian tube causes pressure and pain. Also, the shorter tube in children allows easy migration of pathogens from the mouth and nose to the middle ear, leading to infection. Occasionally, the eardrum will rupture and release fluid into the external auditory canal. To prevent rupture of the tympanic membrane and promote drainage, children suffering from recurrent bilateral otitis media (BOM) are often treated surgically with myringotomy tubes, also called PE tubes. Left untreated, otitis media may lead to mastoiditis, an infection of the mastoid bone. Otitis media can also result in hearing loss. Serous otitis media (SOM) may result from mechanical or functional obstruction of the eustachian tube. In these cases, a decongestant helps to relieve congestion of the tissues, and surgical placement of ventilation tubes helps equilibrate pressure on the eardrum.

Hearing loss is categorized as conductive or sensory. Conductive hearing loss may be due to an obstruction in the ear canal or the result of damage to the tympanic membrane or ossicular chain. Common causes of conductive hearing loss include otosclerosis, the hardening of the spongy bone surrounding the oval window; cholesteatoma, a mass in the middle ear consisting of epithelial cells and cholesterol; and cerumen impaction in the external auditory canal. Sensory hearing loss is caused by damage to the cochlear or auditory nerve (CN VIII). Causes for sensory loss include ototoxic drugs, advanced age (presbyacusis), and noise trauma.

Labyrinthitis is an inflammation of the inner ear resulting in vertigo. Ménière disease (endolymphatic hydrops) is a disturbance of the labyrinth that is characterized by vertigo with or without tinnitus, hearing loss, and nausea and/or vomiting. Balance may also be affected.

Because the nose is often exposed to the sun's dangerous ultraviolet light, it is one of the most common sites of basal cell or squamous cell carcinomas, both malignant skin tumors.

The common cold is a viral infection of the upper respiratory system. URIs account for about half of all work absences. Winter is the most common time for colds to appear. There are many different cold viruses and they are constantly mutating, which makes it difficult for a person to become completely immune to "the common cold." The usual signs and symptoms of a URI are rhinitis, pharyngitis, and laryngitis lasting from 5–14 days. Coryza (acute rhinitis) is the term for an acute head cold.

Congenital malformations of the nose or the septum (nasoseptal deformity, septal deviation) may result in difficulty breathing through the nose or improper drainage of the nasal cavities. Congestion, exudates, and turbinate hypertrophy caused by an upper respiratory infection or allergic rhinitis can block sinus openings, leading to sinusitis. Polyps may also impede normal drainage. The symptoms of sinusitis include pressure and pain over the affected sinus areas, with or without purulent nasal secretions. Left untreated, sinusitis may spread to the meninges causing meningitis.

Although pharyngitis is caused by a viral pathogen at least 70 percent of the time, group A beta-hemolytic *streptococcus* (GABHS) is the most common cause of bacterial pharyngitis. Symptoms include pain, fever, swollen tonsils with exudate, and enlarged and often tender lymph nodes. Early and complete treatment of "strep throat" is important in order to prevent rheumatic fever and glomerulonephritis, two autoimmune diseases caused by cross-reacting antibodies to GABHS.

Obstruction of the pharynx can occur from severe allergic reactions, foreign bodies, or epiglottitis, usually caused by *Haemophilus influenzae*. Epiglottitis can create a partial or complete airway obstruction, leading to a medical emergency. Other common conditions of the upper airway include sleep apnea syndrome, tonsillitis, and chronic cryptic tonsillitis.

Common Tests and Surgical Procedures

Hearing may be tested using a tuning fork placed on the midline of the head (Weber test) or next to the ear (Rinne test). A patient's hearing at various sound frequencies can be assessed through audiometry, which measures nerve conduction. Electronystagmography (ENG) and caloric stimulation (placing hot and cold air or water into the external auditory canal) are used to evaluate vertigo. The Romberg test is used to screen for balance disorders.

Airway obstructions are cleared in an emergency by means of the Heimlich maneuver, designed to force food or other obstructions from the airway; severe obstructions may require an emergency tracheotomy to create an artificial airway.

Epistaxis (nosebleed) is usually self-limiting and easily managed with compression to the bridge of the nose (nasal ala). Severe or protracted epistaxis may require emergent treatment with silver nitrate or nasal packing.

Common surgical procedures include tonsillectomies and adenoidectomies, which may be performed in patients who have had recurrent bouts of tonsillitis resulting in enlarged tonsils and adenoids or in those who have hearing loss from frequent infections. In cancers of the larynx, an ENT specialist may perform a laryngectomy, which can involve partial or complete removal of the larynx. ENT physicians also perform numerous constructive or reconstructive surgeries: otoplasty to correct an ear deformity, myringoplasty and tympanoplasty to reconstruct the eardrum, and myringotomy, most common in small children, to place a small tube into the eardrum in order to provide proper drainage of fluid from the middle ear. Dacryocystorhinostomy is a surgical procedure for creating an opening into the nose for the drainage of tears. Rhinoplasty is the surgical restructuring of the nose, which can be performed for cosmetic reasons or for medical necessity—to improve breathing, for example.

Terms Bank

These terms and abbreviations provide a foundation for the language and transcription skills you will develop in the following sections of this chapter. Terms marked with » will be included in the reports transcribed in the Building Transcription Skills section.

adenitis
(ad-e-**nI**-tis) (n) inflammation of a lymph node or gland

adenoidectomy
(ad-e-noy-**dek**-tO-mee) (n) surgical removal of the adenoids from the nasopharynx

ala nasi
(a-la **nay**-sI) (adj) the outer flare of each nostril; alae nasi (**a**-lee) (pl)

allergen »
(**al**-er-jen) (n) a substance that produces an allergic reaction

amphotericin »
(**am**-fO-tear-a-sin) (n) a toxic antibiotic reserved for use in serious, potentially fatal infections of fungi and protozoa; amphotericin B

amplitude
(**am**-pli-tood) (n) the extent of a vibrating or alternating movement or wave from the average to the extreme; a louder sound has a greater amplitude

annulus
(**an**-yoo-lus) (n) a circular structure or opening

anosmia
(an-**ahz**-mee-a) (n) inability to smell

Antivert
(**an**-ti-vert) brand name for meclizine; used to treat vertigo

arytenoid
(ar-i-**tee**-noyd) (n) cartilage and muscles of the larynx

audiologic »
(aw-dee-O-**loj**-ik) (adj) pertaining to hearing disorders or loss

audiometry
(aw-dee-**om**-e-tree) (n) test used to measure hearing (using an audiometer)

aural
(**aw**-ral) (adj) relating to the ear

auricle
(**aw**-ri-kl) (n) external ear; pinna

barotrauma
(bair-O-**trah**-ma) (n) injury caused by increased pressure

Bovie »
(**bO**-vee) (n) an instrument used for electrocautery

buccal »
(**buk**-al) (adj) relating to the area inside the cheek

cavernous sinus thrombosis
(**kav**-er-nus **sI**-nus throm-**bO**-sis) (n) a group of symptoms caused by an obstruction in the cavernous intracranial sinus

cerumen
(se-**roo**-men) (n) earwax

cholesteatoma
(kO-les-tee-a-**tO**-ma) (n) a tumor-like mass of scaly epithelium and cholesterol in the middle ear

ciliary action
(**sil**-ee-ar-ee) (n) the lashing movement of a group of cilia, which can produce a current of movement in a fluid

cochlea
(**kok**-lee-a) (n) a spiral-shaped cavity in the internal ear

concha
(**kon**-ka) (n) a shell-shaped anatomical structure, such as the auricle of the ear; conchae (pl)

conductive deafness
(n) hearing impairment due to obstruction of sound waves; the sound waves are not passed on to the inner ear

coryza
(ko-**rI**-za) (n) acute rhinitis; acute head cold; inflammation of the mucous membrane of the nose with sneezing, tearing, and watery nasal discharge

cricoid cartilage
(**krI**-koyd) (n) a ring-shaped cartilage in the lower part of the larynx

culture
(**kul**-chur) (n) propagation of microorganisms in a solid or liquid medium

dacryocystorhinostomy
(**dak**-ree-O-**sis**-tO-rI-**nos**-tO-mee) (n) a surgical opening to provide drainage between the tear duct and the nasal mucosa

debride »
(da-**breed**/dee-**brId**) (v) to remove unhealthy tissue and foreign material to prevent infection and permit healing

distress
(n) trouble; mental or physical suffering

dysgeusia
(dis-**goo**-see-a) (n) dysfunctional sense of taste

dysphagia
(dis-**fay**-jee-a) (n) difficulty swallowing

en bloc »
(ahn blok) (adj) as a whole, in one piece

epiglottis
(**ep**-I-**glot**-is) (n) flap of elastic cartilage at the back of the mouth that covers the opening to the windpipe during swallowing, thereby preventing choking.

epiglottitis
(ep-i-glot-**tI**-tis) (n) inflammation of the epiglottis, causing potentially fatal airway obstruction, especially in small children

epistaxis
(**ep**-i-**stak**-sis) (n) nosebleed

ethmoidal »
(eth-**moy**-dal) (adj) relating to the ethmoid bone or ethmoid sinus

eustachian tube
(yoo-**stay**-shun / yoo-**stay**-kee-an) (n) a tube leading from the middle ear to the nasopharynx; thus air pressure is equalized on both sides of the tympanic membrane

excision »
(ek-**si**-zhun) (n) cutting out; surgical removal of all or part of a lesion, structure, or organ

exudate »
(**eks**-oo-dayt) (n) any fluid that has oozed out of a tissue, usually due to inflammation or injury

exudative »
(**eks**-oo-dayt-iv) (adj) relating to exudate

fenestra ovalis
(fe-**nes**-tra O-**val**-is) (n) an oval opening between the middle ear and the vestibule; closed by the base of the stapes

fixation
(fik-**say**-shun) (n) process of securing a part, as by suturing

foramen »
(fO-**ray**-men) (n) hole or opening, especially in a bone or membrane

gingival »
(**jin**-ji-val) (adj) relating to the gums

glossopharyngeal neuralgia
(**glos**-O-fa-**rin**-jee-al noo-**ral**-jee-a) (n) a condition of sharp spasmic pain in the throat or palate

helix
(**hee**-liks) (n) the folded edge of the external ear

incus
(**ing**-kus) (n) the anvil-shaped bone in the middle ear

jugular »
(**jug**-yoo-lar) (adj) relating to the throat or neck

labial »
(**lay**-bee-al) (adj) relating to the lips

labyrinth »
(**lab**-i-rinth) (n) an anatomical structure made up of a complex of cavities, such as the inner ear

labyrinthitis
(**lab**-i-rin-**thI**-tis) (n) inflammation of the inner ear (labyrinth) or ethmoidal labyrinth (nose)

lacrimation
(**lak**-ri-**may**-shun) (n) secretion of tears

laryngectomy
(**lar**-in-**jek**-tO-mee) (n) surgical removal of the larynx

laryngostomy
(**lar**-ing-**gos**-tO-mee) (n) surgically creating an opening into the larynx

larynx
(**lar**-ingks) (n) the voice box, located between the pharynx and the trachea

leukotrienes
(loo-kO-**trI**-eens) (n) mediators of inflammation

lucency »
(**loo**-sen-see) (n) the quality or state of being lucent

lucent
(**loo**-sent) (adj) bright, clear, allowing light to pass

lymph »
(limf) (n) fluid that bathes the tissues of the body and circulates through lymphatic vessels

malleus
(**mal**-ee-us) (n) the largest of the three inner ear bones; club-shaped; attached to the tympanic membrane

mandibular
(man-**dib**-yoo-lar) (adj) relating to the lower jaw

mastoiditis
(mas-toy-**dI**-tis) (n) inflammation of the mastoid process (part of the temporal bone behind the ear)

maxilla
(mak-**sil**-a) (n) the upper jaw

maxillary sinus
(**mak**-si-layr-ee **sI**-nus) (n) an air cavity in the body of the upper jaw bone; connects with the middle passage (meatus) of the nose

meatus
(mee-**ay**-tus) (n) a passage or channel, especially with an external opening

Ménière disease
(mayn-**yairz**) (n) a disease of the inner ear with attacks of dizziness, nausea, ringing in the ear, and increasing deafness

meninges
(me-**nin**-jeez) (n) membranes covering the brain and spinal cord

meningitis
(men-in-**jI**-tis) (n) inflammation of the meninges

mucoperiosteum
(**myoo**-kO-per-ee-**os**-tee-um) (n) the mucous membrane covering the hard palate at the front of the roof of the mouth

mucosa »
(myoo-**kO**-sa) (n) mucous membrane

myringitis
(mir-in-**jI**-tis) (n) inflammation of the tympanic membrane; tympanitis

myringoplasty
(mi-**ring**-gO-**plas**-tee) (n) surgical repair of the eardrum

myringotomy »
(mir-ing-**got**-o-mee) (n) surgical incision into the tympanic membrane

nafcillin »
(naf-**sill**-in) (n) an antibiotic; one of the varieties of penicillin

naris »
(**nay**-ris) (n) nostril; nares (**nay**-rees) (pl)

neoadjuvant »
(nee-O-**ad**-joo-vant) (adj) used in conjunction with other types of therapy

neuroblastoma »
(**noor**-O-blas-**tO**-ma) (n) malignant (cancerous) tumor containing embryonic nerve cells

neuroectodermal »
(**noo**-rO-ek-tO-**der**-mal) (adj) embryonic tissue that gives rise to nerve tissue

node »
(nOd) (n) a small knot of tissue, distinct from surrounding tissue; a lymph node

orbital cellulitis
(**or**-bit-al sel-yoo-**lI**-tis) (n) inflammation of tissue around or behind the eye

organism
(**or**-ga-nizm) (n) a living plant, animal, or microorganism

orifice
(**or**-i-fis) (n) an opening

ossicles
(os-i-kls) (n) small bones, such as the auditory ossicles (the three bones of the inner ear)

ostectomy »
(os-**tek**-tO-mee) (n) surgical removal of all or part of a bone

otalgia
(O-**tal**-jee-a) (n) earache

otitis externa
(O-**tI**-tis eks-**ter**-na) (n) inflammation of the external ear

otitis media »
(O-**tI**-tis **mee**-dee-a) (n) inflammation of the middle ear

otorhinolaryngology
(O-tO-**rI**-nO-lar-in-**gol**-o-jee) (n) study of the ears, nose, and throat

otosclerosis
(**O**-tO-sklee-**rO**-sis) (n) a growth of sponge-like bone in the inner ear, eventually leading to deafness

otoscope
(**O**-tO-skOp) (n) an instrument for examining the eardrum

otoscopy »
(O-**tos**-kO-pee) (n) visual examination of the ear with an otoscope

ototoxic »
(O-to-**tok**-sic) (adj) harmful to the organs of hearing or auditory nerve

palpable »
(**pal**-pa-bl) (adj) able to be identified by touch

palate
(**pal**-at) (n) the roof of one's mouth, composed of the hard palate (front) and the soft palate (back)

pathogen »
(**path**-O-jen) (n) any microorganism or substance that can cause a disease

periauricular »
(**per**-ee-aw-**rik**-yoo-lar) (adj) around the ear

pharyngitis
(far-in-jI-tis) (n) inflammation of the pharynx

pharynx
(**far**-ingks) (n) throat; passageway for air from nasal cavity to larynx, and food from mouth to esophagus

pinna
(**pin**-a) (n) the external ear; auricle; pinnae (**pin**-ee) (pl)

polyp
(**pol**-ip) (n) an outgrowth of tissue from a mucous membrane

presbycusis
(**prez**-bee-**koo**-sis) (n) the loss of hearing acuity due to aging

pseudoephedrine
(soo-dO-i-**fed**-rin) (n) a generic drug; decongestant

pterygoid plate
(**ter**-i-goyd) (n) wing-shaped bones at the back of the nasal cavity

purulent
(**pyoor**-u-lent) (adj) relating to, containing, or forming pus

resection »
(ree-**sek**-shun) (n) surgical removal of a portion of a structure or organ

rhinitis
(rI-**nI**-tis) (n) inflammation of the mucous membrane of the nose

rhinoplasty
(**rI**-nO-plas-tee) (n) surgery to correct a defect in the nose or to change its shape

Rinne test
(**rin**-ne) (n) also Rinne's (**rin**-ez); a hearing test comparing perception of air and bone conduction in one ear with a tuning fork; normally air conduction is more acute

Romberg
(**rahm**-berg) (n) a simple test requiring the patient to stand with feet close together while opening and closing their eyes

semicircular canals
(**sem**-ee-**sir**-kyoo-lar ka-**nals**) (n) three fluid-filled loops in the labyrinth of the inner ear, associated with the body's sense of balance

sensorineural deafness
(**sen**-sOr-i-**noor**-al) (n) hearing impairment due to nerve disturbance

septum
(**sep**-tum) (n) division between two cavities or two masses of tissue, such as the nasal septum; septa (pl)

serous
(**seer**-us) (adj) relating to or having a watery consistency

serous otitis media
(**seer**-us O-**tI**-tis **mee**-dee-a) (n) inflammation of the middle ear accompanied by production of a watery fluid (serum)

shotty
(**shot**-ee) (adj) resembling shot (hard pellets) to the touch; as shotty nodes

sinus
(**sI**-nus) (n) a passageway or hollow in a bone or other tissue

sinusitis
(sI-nu-**sI**-tis) (n) inflammation of the nasal sinuses, occurring as a result of an upper respiratory infection, an allergic response, or a defect of the nose

sleep apnea syndrome
(**ap**-nee-a) (n) breathing stops, briefly and periodically, due to partial upper airway obstruction during sleep

speculum
(**spek**-yoo-lum) (n) an instrument used for examining the interior of a cavity

sphenoidal sinus
(sfee-**noy**-dal) (n) one of two sinuses in the sphenoid bone opening to the nasal cavity

stapes
(**stay**-peez) (n) the smallest and innermost of the three auditory bones in the inner ear; stirrup

strep
(n) short form of Streptococcus, a genus of bacteria; many species cause disease in humans

submandibular
(sub-man-**dib**-yoo-lar) (adj) under the lower jaw

supratentorial »
(**soo**-pra-ten-**tO**-ree-al) (adj) located above the tentorium, a tentlike structure

symphysis
(**sim**-fi-sis) (n) joint in which fibrocartilage firmly unites the bones

thyroid
(**thI**-royd) (n) a gland in the neck that secretes thyroid hormone

tinnitus
(ti-**nI**-tus) (n) noise, such as ringing, in the ears

tonsils »
(**ton**-silz) (n) lymphoid tissue structures in the oropharynx

trachea
(**tray**-kee-a) (n) the windpipe

tracheostomy
(**tray**-kee-**os**-tO-mee) (n) a surgical opening into the trachea

tracheotomy
(**tray**-kee-**ot**-O-mee) (n) the surgical procedure in which a tracheostomy is created

tragus
(**tray**-gus) (n) the small projection of cartilage in front of the external opening to the ear canal

turbinate
(**ter**-bi-nayt) (n) one of several thin, spongy, bony plates within the walls of the nasal cavity

tympanic membrane
(tim-**pan**-ik) (n) eardrum

tympanometric »
(**tim**-pa-nO-**met**-rik) (adj) pertaining to tympanometry, a procedure for evaluation of motility of eardrum and middle ear disorders

tympanoplasty
(**tim**-pa-nO-plas-tee) (n) surgical repair of the middle ear

umbo
(**um**-bO) (n) the inner surface of the tympanic membrane where it connects with the malleus in the middle ear

unremarkable
(adj) nothing unusual is noted

upper respiratory infection (URI)
(n) an infection of the upper respiratory tract such as the common cold, laryngitis, sinusitis, and tonsillitis

uvula
(**yoo**-vyoo-la) (n) small, fleshy mass hanging from the soft palate in the mouth

uvulitis
(yoo-vyoo-**lI**-tis) (n) inflammation of the uvula

uvulopalatopharyngoplasty
(**yoo**-vyoo-lO-**pal**-a-tO-fa-**rin**-gO-plas-tee) (n) UPPP for short; a surgical treatment for sleep apnea for patients who cannot tolerate or respond to medical therapies

vertigo
(**ver**-tigO) (n) dizziness

vestibulum
(ves-**tib**-yoo-lum) (n) the central cavity of the labyrinth in the inner ear, between the cochlea and the semicircular canals

vibrissae
(vI-**bris**-a) (n) nose hairs

Weber test
(**web**-er) (n) a hearing test performed with a tuning fork placed at points in the middle of the skull to determine where the vibration is heard (not where it is felt)

xerostomia
(zeer-O-**stO**-mee-a) (n) dryness of the mouth

Abbreviations

AC	air conduction		ENG	electronystagmography
AD	right ear (auris dextra)		ENT	ear, nose, and throat
AOM	acute otitis media		GABHS	group A beta-hemolytic *streptococcus*
AS	left ear (auris sinistra)		PE tubes	pressure-equalizing tubes
BOM	bilateral otitis media		SAR	seasonal allergic rhinitis
C&S	culture and sensitivity		SOM	serous otitis media
CN	cranial nerves		T&A	tonsillectomy and adenoidectomy
dB	decibel		TM	tympanic membrane
dbHL	decibel hearing level		TMJ	temporomandibular joint
EAC	external auditory canal		UPPP	uvulopalatopharyngoplasty
EENT	eye, ear, nose, and throat		URI	upper respiratory infection

Building Language Skills

Complete the following exercises, drawing on the information learned in the Exploring Otorhinolaryngology section of this chapter and referencing the Terms Bank.

Exercise 7.1 — Matching Sound and Spelling

The numbered list that follows shows the phonetic spelling of hard-to-spell words. Sound out each word, then write the correct spelling in the blank space provided. Check your answers in the Terms Bank or other appropriate reference.

1. nee-O-**ad**-joo-vant _____

2. **pyoor**-u-lent _____

3. yoo-**stay**-shun _____

4. **aw**-ri-kl _____

5. fO-**ray**-men _____

6. **per**-ee-aw-**rik**-yoo-lar _____

7. **nay**-ris _____

8. **ver**-ti-gO _____

9. tim-**pan**-ik **mem**-brayn _____

10. **sim**-fi-sis _____

11. O-**tal**-jee-a _____

12. **mal**-ee-us _____

13. ti-**nI**-tus _____

14. **loo**-sen-see _____

15. ep-i-**stak**-sis _____

Below is a list of frequently used words that look alike and/or sound alike. Study the meaning and pronunciation of each set of words, then read the following sentences carefully, and then circle the word in parentheses that correctly completes the meaning.

assistance	aiding, helping	**osteal**	bony or bonelike
assistants	individuals who give aid and support	**ostial**	relating to an ostium (a small opening, e.g., eustachian tube)
aural	pertaining to the ear	**palate**	roof of mouth
oral	pertaining to the mouth	**pallet**	a portable platform or a temporary bed
auricle	external ear		
oracle	a wise person; a god-like person	**passed**	past tense of verb pass; to move, to accomplish
C&S	abbreviation for culture and sensitivity	**past**	time that has gone by
CNS	abbreviation for central nervous system	**serious**	not joking
		serous	resembling serum
dysphagia	difficulty swallowing	**shoddy**	inferior or imitation goods
dysphasia	difficulty using language due to injury or disease	**shotty**	resembling shot to the touch
		subtle	hard to detect
dysphonia	difficulty in speaking	**supple**	limber
dysphoria	depression		
		tendinitis	
laryngitis	inflammation of the larynx	**or tendonitis**	inflammation of a tendon
pharyngitis	inflammation of the pharynx	**tinnitus**	ringing in the ears
malleolus	a rounded bone on either side of the ankle		
malleus	a structure in the inner ear		

1. (Aural/Oral) examination revealed cerumen in the canal.

2. Examination of the mouth reveals no (aural/oral) lesions.

3. The patient complains of tenderness around the (auricle/oracle).

4. Examination of the neck revealed a few (shoddy/shotty) nodes.

5. I feel great. I (passed/past) my exam!

6. The patient thinks his (tendinitis/tinnitus) and headache symptoms may be associated with his high blood pressure.

7. Examination of the face revealed only (subtle/supple) changes in the pigmentation of the skin.

8. NECK: (Subtle, Supple) without masses.

9. We will be adding three new medical (assistance/assistants) to the staff this month.

10. Could you please give me some (assistance/assistants) in lifting this patient?

11. While the patient was making a (serious/serous) effort to get out of bed, we noticed the (serious/serous) drainage from his ear.

12. The eustachian tube is blocked, the eardrum is retracted, and the (malleolus/malleus) looks shorter and more horizontal.

13. The injury resulted from a rolling bowling ball, which caused a fractured (malleolus/malleus).

14. A sore throat with (dysphagia/dysphasia) made the child uncomfortable when eating solid foods.

15. The patient's (osteal/ostial) opening was about 1.2 cm.

Exercise 7.3   Choosing Words from Context

When transcribing dictation, the medical transcriptionist frequently needs to consider the situation when determining the word that correctly completes the sentence. From the list below, select the term that meaningfully completes each of the following statements.

buccal	jugular	otitis
culture	laryngostomy	palpable
erythematous	mandibular	purulent
excision	mastoiditis	shotty
exudate	node	

1. Examination of the external ear showed a periauricular lymph _____ .

2. DIAGNOSIS

   Upper respiratory infection with acute bilateral _____ media.

3. The central line was changed from her right subclavian to her right internal _____.

4. Her throat is slightly red; however, no drainage or _____ is noted.

5. The patient's throat _____ came back positive for strep.

6. The examining physician found a (an) _____ mass in the abdomen.

7. The tympanic membrane on the right is _____ and bulging.

8. The en bloc _____ to remove the tumor left a large scar.

9. I instructed the patient to call us promptly if she develops any _____ drainage from the wound site.

10. The patient had large open sores on his gingiva and _____ cavity on the right side of his mouth.

From this list, locate the term that best matches each of the following definitions. Write the term in the space provided by each definition.

aural	mandibular	pathogen
cerumen	mastoiditis	periauricular
coryza	myringotomy	tracheostomy
gingival	neuroblastoma	
labial	otitis	

1. waxy secretion of the external auditory canal _____

2. acute rhinitis _____

3. opening created surgically in the trachea _____

4. relating to the gums _____

5. relating to the lower jaw _____

6. substance capable of producing a disease _____

7. pertaining to the lips _____

8. infection of the mastoid bones _____

9. surgical incision into tympanic membrane _____

10. malignant tumor of nerve cells _____

Exercise 7.5　　　　Creating Terms from Word Forms

Combine prefixes, root words, and suffixes from this list to create medical words that fit the following definitions. Fill in the blanks with the words you construct.

a-	without, absence	-pharyng/o	throat
dys-	difficult	-auricular	pertaining to the ear
ex-	out	-blastoma	malignant cell/tumor
oto-	ear	-cision	to cut
peri-	around	-ectomy	removal of body structure
rhin-	nose	-gen	to produce
sub-	beneath, under	-itis	inflammation or infection
laryng/o-	larynx	-mandibular	lower jaw
neur/o-	nerve	-phonia	voice; sound
or/o-	mouth	-stomy	artificial or surgical opening
oste/o-	bone		

1. loss of voice _____

2. difficulty in speaking _____

3. cut out _____

4. surgical opening into the larynx _____

5. portion of the pharynx posterior to the mouth _____

6. surgical excision of a bone _____

7. inflammation of the ear _____

8. middle of the throat, between roof of mouth and upper edge of epiglottis _____

9. surrounding the ear _____

10. inflammation of the nasal mucosa _____

Exercise 7.6   Proofreading Review

Read the following report excerpts and look for errors in format, usage, and spelling. Mark the corrections on this page and key the excerpt with all errors corrected. Save the document as XXExercise07.06, using your initials in place of *XX* in the file name.

CHIEF COMPLAINT

The patient Had been well until about four wks ago when he devlloped a runy nose, sore throat, and pain in both ears. He was seen by peditritian, who gave him an antibiotic for seven days. Two week later the ear pain has not resolved.

PAST MEDICAL HX

Noncontributory.

PHYSICAL EXAMINATION

L TM is injected with whitish exadate. Palpable shoddy L submandibalar lymph nodes and a 2 centimeter firm periaurcular lymph node. Physical exam is otherwise within normal limits.

Exercise 7.7   Thinking Like a Professional

Read this scenario carefully and then select the most appropriate response. Write an explanation for why you think your choice is the best answer.

You have just started transcribing for a new physician. You have been given a template that includes standard text for the Review of Systems and the Physical Examination sections of the report. The former transcriptionist tells you that she uses the paragraph of text already typed under these headings on all reports by that physician. As you begin to transcribe the reports, you realize that the standard text in the template is similar but not exactly what is being dictated. What should you do?

---

a. Use the standard text as is since these are the instructions given to you by the previous transcriptionist.

b. Use the standard text as is and only modify what seems to be significantly different.

c. Contact the physician to determine expectations.

d. Do not use the standard text and transcribe exactly what is being dictated.

Best response: _____

Explanation: _____

_____

_____

_____

Building Transcription Skills

You will apply the medical specialty and language information you learned in this chapter to transcription work in this section. After you learn the formatting recommendations of an operative report, you will transcribe nine reports related to eight different patient studies.

Introducing the Operative Report

The operative report (Figure 7.6) is a narrative description of an operation or other invasive procedure. The surgeon or an assistant to the surgeon dictates the report. This type of document is often quite long and detailed. It is likely to be the most technically demanding report a medical transcriptionist will encounter.

Required Headings/Content

Operative reports are variously structured but usually include the surgeon's name, preoperative and postoperative diagnoses, the name of the procedure, the anesthesia, the indications for surgery, the specimen removed, and the actual description of the surgery, called the procedure. The report usually documents a sponge count and an estimate of blood loss.

The operative report may include the assistant surgeon's name, the name of the anesthesiologist, type of incision, drains used, and complications. The operative report may also include information on when an informed consent document was presented by the surgeon and signed by the patient.

Many hospitals break down the operative description into three sections: (1) positioning, prepping and draping, and opening the incision; (2) the internal operation; and (3) the closing. Refer to page 469 of Appendix A for a complete list of headings found in the operative report template along with descriptions of the type of information found under each heading. Not every template heading will be included in every transcribed report.

Turnaround Time

An operative report is dictated or written in the medical record immediately after surgery and ideally transcribed within six hours. This guideline applies to all surgical procedures done in hospitals, outpatient surgical centers, and clinics.

Preparing to Transcribe

To prepare for transcribing dictation, review the common otorhinolaryngology terms, drugs, and abbreviations presented in this chapter's Terms Bank. Study the format and organization of the model document shown in Figure 7.6, and key the model document, using the operative report template on the Dictations and Templates CD as a starting point. Save the document as XXFigure07.06 using your initials in place of XX in the file name. Proofread the document by comparing it with the printed version. Categorize the types of errors you made, and document them on a copy of the Performance Comparison Chart. A template of this chart is available on the Dictations and Templates CD.

Transcribing Reports

Transcribe, edit, and correct each report in the following patient studies. Consult reference books for formatting rules or words that are unfamiliar.

As you work on the transcription assignment for this chapter, fill in the Performance Comparison Chart that you started when you keyed the model document. For at least three of the reports, categorize and document the types of errors you made. Answer the document analysis questions on the bottom of the chart. With continuous practice and assessment, the quality of your work will improve.

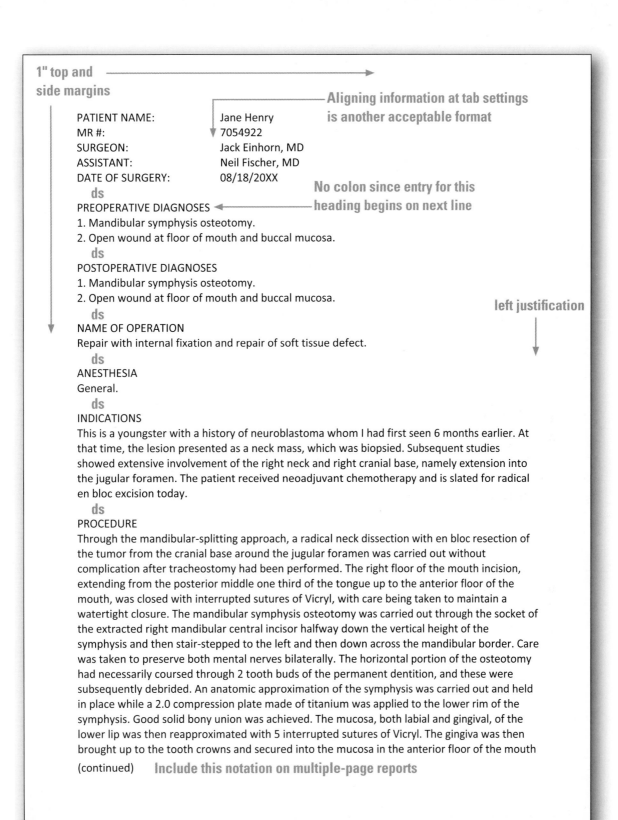

1" top and side margins ────────────────────────────►

Aligning information at tab settings is another acceptable format

PATIENT NAME: Jane Henry
MR #:   7054922
SURGEON: Jack Einhorn, MD
ASSISTANT: Neil Fischer, MD
DATE OF SURGERY: 08/18/20XX
        ds
PREOPERATIVE DIAGNOSES ◄───── **No colon since entry for this heading begins on next line**
1. Mandibular symphysis osteotomy.
2. Open wound at floor of mouth and buccal mucosa.
        ds
POSTOPERATIVE DIAGNOSES
1. Mandibular symphysis osteotomy.
2. Open wound at floor of mouth and buccal mucosa.   **left justification**
        ds
NAME OF OPERATION
Repair with internal fixation and repair of soft tissue defect.
        ds
ANESTHESIA
General.
        ds
INDICATIONS
This is a youngster with a history of neuroblastoma whom I had first seen 6 months earlier. At that time, the lesion presented as a neck mass, which was biopsied. Subsequent studies showed extensive involvement of the right neck and right cranial base, namely extension into the jugular foramen. The patient received neoadjuvant chemotherapy and is slated for radical en bloc excision today.
        ds
PROCEDURE
Through the mandibular-splitting approach, a radical neck dissection with en bloc resection of the tumor from the cranial base around the jugular foramen was carried out without complication after tracheostomy had been performed. The right floor of the mouth incision, extending from the posterior middle one third of the tongue up to the anterior floor of the mouth, was closed with interrupted sutures of Vicryl, with care being taken to maintain a watertight closure. The mandibular symphysis osteotomy was carried out through the socket of the extracted right mandibular central incisor halfway down the vertical height of the symphysis and then stair-stepped to the left and then down across the mandibular border. Care was taken to preserve both mental nerves bilaterally. The horizontal portion of the osteotomy had necessarily coursed through 2 tooth buds of the permanent dentition, and these were subsequently debrided. An anatomic approximation of the symphysis was carried out and held in place while a 2.0 compression plate made of titanium was applied to the lower rim of the symphysis. Good solid bony union was achieved. The mucosa, both labial and gingival, of the lower lip was then reapproximated with 5 interrupted sutures of Vicryl. The gingiva was then brought up to the tooth crowns and secured into the mucosa in the anterior floor of the mouth

(continued)   **Include this notation on multiple-page reports**

Figure 7.6   Operative Report

OPERATIVE REPORT

PATIENT NAME: Jane Henry   **Include a header on second and succeeding pages**

MR #: 7054922

DATE OF SURGERY: 08/18/20XX

Page 2

ds

with sutures. These sutures encircled the teeth and created a nice watertight seal with no exposure of the underlying mandible. The lip was then prepared, and the remainder of the neck closure was carried out by Dr. Fischer.

ds

ESTIMATED BLOOD LOSS

Negligible.

ds

COMPLICATIONS

None.

ds

SPECIMENS

None.

qs

_____

Jack C. Einhorn, MD

ds

JCE/XX

D: 08/18/20XX

T: 08/18/20XX

Figure 7.6   Operative Report (Continued)

Pediatrician Marcus Green, MD, treats 5-year-old Mark Rankin for ear pain. Dr. Green refers Mark to Dr. Joseph Strong, otorhinolaryngologist, for consultation.

REPORT 7.1   Office Note

Use the Report0701.mp3 audio file and the office note template (Office_Note) when transcribing this report. Save the document as XXReport07.01, using your initials in place of *XX* in the file name.

CBC stands for complete blood count, a common laboratory test that measures levels of red blood cells (RBCs or rbc's), white blood cells (WBCs or wbc's), and platelets.

The measurement unit, cubic millimeters, should be transcribed as mm with a superscript 3. Because not all equipment allows superscripts, the form *cu mm* is the preferred alternative.

The shortened forms *polys, lymphs,* and *monos* can be transcribed as dictated.

Listen for this word:
    exudate

When a template's heading is synonymous to the dictated heading, the transcriptionist should use the template's heading. For example, if the dictator uses the headings *History of Present Illness*, *Physical Examination*, and *Impression*, it is appropriate to use the office note template's Subjective, Objective, and Assessment headings. If a synonymous heading is not available in the template, transcribe the dictated heading.

In this report, the dictated heading "HPI" stands for History of Present Illness and "PE" stands for Physical Examination. The heading "Labs" can be typed in the short or long form, but use Laboratory Data for this report's internal heading.

If a dictator says the short form of laboratory from within the body of the report, it is acceptable to transcribe "lab." However, the term *laboratory* should be transcribed in its place in headings or subheadings.

REPORT 7.2   Office Note

Use the Report0702.mp3 audio file and the office note template (Office_Note) when transcribing this report. Save the document as XXReport07.02, using your initials in place of *XX* in the file name.

Listen for these words:
    exudate (noun) and exudative (adjective)
    mastoiditis
    myringotomy
    periauricular
    submandibular

Yarvella Harves is an 11-week-old girl who had been well until a few days ago. She had a neck mass that did not appear to be painful, but it had been growing steadily for several days. The baby was referred to the specialist from the pediatrician's office.

REPORT 7.3   Consultation Letter

Use the Report0703.mp3 audio file and the consultation letter template (Consultation_Letter) when transcribing this report. Save the document as XXReport07.03, using your initials in place of *XX* in the file name.

BUMC stands for Brookfield University Medical Center. Do not use the abbreviation in the transcribed report.

Nafcillin is the generic name of a penicillin antibiotic.

CT scan refers to computerized tomography scan and CAT scan refers to computerized axial tomography scan. These scans are dictated by pronouncing the letters "CT," or the word "cat." Both CT scan and CAT scan are acceptable in transcribed reports.

The letters "OR" refer to the operating room. OR is acceptable in transcribed reports.

The letters *IV* stand for intravenous. When typed, IV can look like the Roman numeral IV (4), but if the meaning is clear in context, then using IV for intravenous in a transcribed report is acceptable.

Jane Henry is a 2-year-old girl who was diagnosed with a neuroblastoma arising from the floor of the mouth and extending to the neck and lower base of the skull. She has been treated with chemotherapy and is now undergoing surgery to remove any residual tumor. Dr. Einhorn is an otorhinolaryngologist who is performing the surgery with the assistance of a plastic surgeon, Dr. Fischer.

REPORT 7.4   Operative Report

Use the Report0704.mp3 audio file and the operative report template (Operative_Report) when transcribing this report. Save the document as XXReport07.04, using your initials in place of *XX* in the file name.

Run-on sentences are common in this type of dictation. Extra care must be taken when transcribing and editing these reports. The language used actually allows the reader to visualize the surgical procedure.

The surgeon dictates a "two point zero compression plate," and this should be transcribed as "2.0 compression plate." The exactness of measurement is relevant in this instance, so the zero should be transcribed.

Fifty-three-year-old Julia Wang is seeing the physician regarding a snoring problem that disrupts her sleep, leaving her feeling chronically tired. She also thinks she may have allergies or a sinus infection because of an annoying drainage into her throat.

REPORT 7.5   Office Note

Use the Report0705.mp3 audio file and the office note template (Office_Note) when transcribing this report. Remember that office notes are sometimes referred to as SOAP notes. Use the template's headings, not the dictated letters. Save the document as XXReport07.05, using your initials in place of *XX* in the file name.

Listen for these terms:
    apnea
    somnolence

Vancenase Nasal Spray and Allegra are brand-name drugs.

Cynthia Mancini is a 35-year-old woman who was in an automobile accident 5 years ago. At that time she had a fracture of the septum, causing a deviation. She presents to the surgeon for correction of the nasal obstruction.

REPORT 7.6   Operative Report

Use the Report0706.mp3 audio file and the operative report template (Operative_Report) when transcribing this report. Save the document as XXReport07.06, using your initials in place of *XX* in the file name.

Listen for these words:
    Bovie cautery
    hemitransfixion
    in-fractured
    mucoperichondrial
    mucoperiosteal
    out-fractured
    rongeurs
    Takahashi
    vomerine

Every operative report must contain a preoperative and postoperative diagnosis, the name of the procedure, the name of the surgeon, and a description of the procedure.

In many operative reports, the preoperative and postoperative diagnoses are the same. Most hospitals require that the diagnosis be repeated, even if the dictator says "same." Do this efficiently by blocking and copying the item.

Suture size is dictated as "four Oh" and should be transcribed as 4-0.

This procedure uses epinephrine, which is dictated as one to one-hundred-thousand. Type this dilution (ratio) with a colon (1:100,000).

Rosa Valdez is seeking relief for recurring headaches and dizziness, for which she has been treated in the past. This 30-year-old ad agency account manager leads a hectic work life and wants to resolve her medical problem before it worsens and requires her to miss work for an extended period of time.

REPORT 7.7   Office Note

Use the Report0707.mp3 audio file and the office note template (Office_Note) when transcribing this report. Save the document as XXReport07.07 sing your initials in place of *XX* in the file name.

Listen for this term:
    vestibulitis

Listen for these drug names:
    Antivert
    Bactrim DS
    Beconase

The abbreviation PO stands for *postoperative*. In other instances, this abbreviation can stand for *by mouth* (p.o.) from the Latin phrase *per os*.

Case Study 7.G   **Sara Vagts**

Sara Vagts is a 44-year-old woman who has been seen by her primary physician for recurrent sinusitis. A consultation with the ENT specialist results in a recommendation for an ethmoidectomy and a different antibiotic.

REPORT 7.8   Phone Call Note

Use the Report0708.mp3 audio file and the office note template (Office_Note) when transcribing this report. Since it is a brief documentation of a phone call, none of the headings within the report will be needed. Save the document as XXReport07.08, using your initials in place of *XX* in the file name.

Aspergillus is the genus name of a fungus. According to *The Book of Style for Medical Transcription*, species and genus names are not italicized in transcribed reports. Aspergillosis is an infection caused by that fungus.

Listen for these drug names:
    amphotericin
    vancomycin

Irene Callahan is a 16-year-old with a diagnosis of a brain tumor. She was sent to the audiology clinic for evaluation of her hearing status prior to beginning chemotherapy, which may potentially cause some hearing loss.

REPORT 7.9   Chart Summary

Use the Report0709.mp3 audio file and the chart summary template (Chart_Summary) when transcribing this report. The function of this type of report is similar to the office note. However, in this template there are no internal headings. Save the document as XXReport07.09, using your initials in place of *XX* in the file name.

Decibels is abbreviated dB and hertz is abbreviated Hz. Use abbreviations (without periods) when the terms are dictated immediately following a number. Spell out these terms when not preceded by a number.

The abbreviation dBHL means decibel hearing level.

"Minus 5 to 10" is transcribed as -5 to 10. The use of a hyphen to indicate a negative is acceptable in this instance.

chapter

Eight

Pulmonology

Pulmonology derives from the Latin word for lung, *pulmo* Pulmonology is the medical specialty that deals with the respiratory system. The respiratory system functions with the circulatory system to transport oxygen and carbon dioxide between the lungs and tissues of the body. The organs of the respiratory system include the nose, mouth, pharynx, larynx, epiglottis, trachea, lungs, bronchi, bronchioles, and alveoli. The physician who specializes in the respiratory tract is called a pulmonologist.

Objectives

» Identify the anatomy of the respiratory system.

» Understand the mechanics of respiration.

» Describe diseases and conditions affecting the bronchial tree and the lungs as well as their common causes.

» Recognize classes of pharmaceuticals used to treat obstructive airway diseases.

» Pronounce and correctly spell terminology related to pulmonology.

» Transcribe dictation related to the medical specialty of pulmonology.

» Describe a discharge summary, including typical content, format, and turnaround time.

Our bodies need oxygen to function properly. The air we breathe, inhaled through the nose and mouth, contains oxygen. Cells throughout the body use oxygen to create energy and produce carbon dioxide as a byproduct of metabolism. The respiratory system exchanges oxygen and carbon dioxide between the alveoli in the lungs and the blood, thereby supplying the tissues with oxygen and removing carbon dioxide waste. Each step of the respiratory process is essential for good health.

Structure and Function

The respiratory system is made up of two main tracts (Figure 8.1). The central part of the respiratory system the lower respiratory tract, is located in the chest, or thorax, which contains the sternum, ribs, thoracic vertebrae, and lungs. The muscles of the respiratory system are important as they These muscles expand the thoracic cavity during inspiration.

Air enters the body through the nose or mouth, at the top of the respiratory tract. Air then passes through the pharynx and into the trachea, or windpipe. The air is warmed, humidified, and filtered of particulates. It then passes into the tracheobronchial tree. This tree, so named because of its branching into the left and right bronchi, is further divided into bronchioles, which terminate as air sacs, called alveoli. Adjacent to the alveoli lie tiny capillary beds (Figure 8.2). These circulatory beds enable exchange of oxygen from the alveoli to the blood and carbon dioxide from the blood to the alveoli.

During the normal respiratory cycle, there is an inspiratory phase that requires active muscle movement followed by a passive expiratory phase. During inspiration, the diaphragm contracts, pressing the abdominal contents downward and expanding the rib cage, thereby increasing the volume of the thoracic cavity. The increased thoracic volume decreases the intrathoracic pressure, causing air to be drawn into the lungs. The work of the diaphragm is supported by the external intercostal muscles (between the ribs). When more vigorous breathing is required,

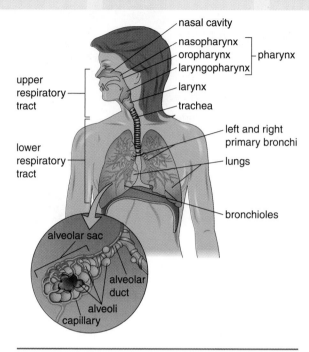

Figure 8.1   Respiratory System

accessory muscles of respiration are also used. These include the intercostal muscles, sternocleidomastoid muscle, platysma, and neck muscles. The recoiling of the thoracic cavity expels the air (expiration). In the normal adult, there is a 6 to 8 cm expansion during each of the 16–20 cycles per minute.

Respiration is divided into the external and internal processes. External respiration is the exchange of oxygen and carbon dioxide between the person and the environment. Internal respiration takes place on a cellular level, exchanging the oxygen carried within the red blood cells with the carbon dioxide in the tissues. After this dual exchange takes place, the lungs eliminate the carbon dioxide.

Physical Assessment

Assessment begins with visualization of the nose, observing for deviated septum or other abnormalities that would decrease the amount of air entering the passages. Inspection of the chest includes counting the respirations, observing the movement of the chest during inspiration and expiration, and

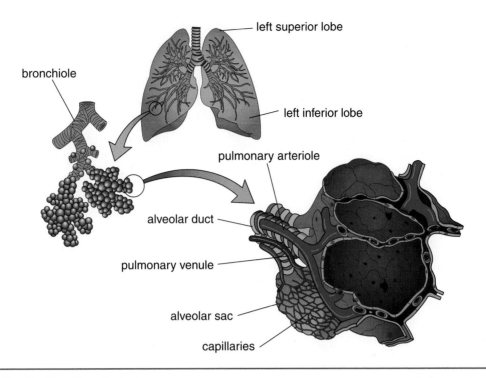

left superior lobe

bronchiole

left inferior lobe

pulmonary arteriole

alveolar duct

pulmonary venule

alveolar sac

capillaries

Figure 8.2 Capillary Beds in the Lungs

noting the general shape of the thorax and symmetry of expansion. Posture, contour, and movement are important elements in proper air exchange.

Examination includes palpation, percussion, and auscultation of the chest and back. The rate, rhythm, and depth of respiration are noted. Palpation of the back should include feeling for fremitus, the vibrations caused by breathing. A resonant sound should be produced when tapping on the chest over the area of the lungs. Tapping, or percussing, on the ribs and sternum produces a dull sound. On auscultation, the physician listens with a stethoscope for breath sounds. Normal lung sounds are called vesicular, while abnormal lung sounds are called adventitious. Abnormal sounds include wheeze (high-pitched, musical), rhonchi (low-pitched, sonorous), and crackles.

The extremities are also examined for clubbing and cyanosis. Cyanosis (blue coloring) results from decreased oxygen attached to the hemoglobin molecule.

Diseases and Conditions

Chronic obstructive pulmonary disease (COPD), or chronic obstructive lung disease (COLD), is characterized by the obstruction of proper airflow due to chronic bronchitis and/or emphysema. Symptoms include dyspnea, cough, and sputum production. The disease is progressive. In late stages of this disease, the patient may become very debilitated and require oxygen to be delivered continuously via a nasal cannula or mask. Smoking is the most common cause of COPD.

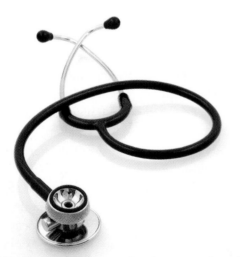

Physicians use a stethoscope when listening to breath sounds.

Inflammation of the bronchi is known as bronchitis. Acute bronchitis is usually caused by a viral or bacterial pathogen. Symptoms include cough, usually productive, and chest pain. Chronic bronchitis is characterized by excess mucus production and productive cough for three or more months. Bronchiolitis is inflammation of the bronchioles and is usually found in children.

Emphysema is defined as the permanent and abnormal enlargement of the air sacs (alveoli) and destruction of the alveolar walls. Air becomes trapped in the interstitial spaces of the lung and expands the lung tissue. This constant expansion leads to the characteristic "barrel chest." During periods of difficult breathing, the patient must remain erect, either sitting up continuously or in an orthopneic position, leaning over a table with arms resting on the surface and extended over the head. This position allows for better air exchange.

Asthma, also referred to as reactive airway disease (RAD), is a common obstructive airway disease producing intermittent attacks that usually are reversible. It is characterized by a narrowing of the airways, resulting in dyspnea, cough, chest tightness, and wheezing in response to various stimuli. An asthma attack may be triggered by a variety of stimuli such as allergens, exercise, upper respiratory infection (URI), or emotions. Asthma treatment includes long-term control and "rescue" treatments in the case of an acute attack. The goal of ongoing, long-term treatment is to prevent or lessen airway inflammation. Agents include inhaled and systemic corticosteroids (Azmacort), cromolyn sodium and nedocromil, Serevent, Proventil, theophylline, and leukotriene modifiers (Singulair, Accolate). Acute attacks are treated with bronchodilators including albuterol (Proventil and Ventolin), terbutaline, and Atrovent. Metered-dose inhalers are used to deliver inhaled medications.

Pneumonia is an inflammatory process affecting the tissue of the lung. Community-acquired pneumonia is caused by infectious organisms. The types of pneumonia are described by the causative agent: bacterial, viral, fungal, or parasitic. Most common agents include *Streptococcus pneumoniae, Haemophilus influenzae, Staphylococcus aureus, Klebsiella pneumoniae,* pseudomonas species. Patients with AIDS (acquired immunodeficiency syndrome) or other immune deficiencies often suffer from TB (*Mycobacterium tuberculosis*) or PCP.

PCP was originally the abbreviation for *Pneumocystis carinii* pneumonia, but this organism has been renamed *Pneumocystis jiroveci.* The abbreviation "PCP" has remained in common use and now means "pneumocystis pneumonia." The abbreviation still refers to the same disease. It is dictated as letters "P C P." Scientific literature will use italic type when writing out the full genus and species of an organism, but *The Book of Style for Medical Transcription* recommends avoiding italic typeface because it is more difficult to read. On the job, MTs should follow the specifications of their employers.

Other causes of pneumonia include chemical inhalations or aspirated foreign material. Manifestations may include cough, with or without sputum production; lethargy; fever; pain in the chest; changes in the respiratory rate; grunting; and nasal flaring. Assessment includes adventitious (abnormal) breath sounds, increased tactile fremitus, dullness on percussion, bronchovesicular breath sounds, egophony, and pectoriloquy. A diagnostic evaluation includes physical examination, chest x-ray, sputum culture if productive cough exists, and blood culture if bacteremia is a concern.

Respiratory distress syndrome (RDS) is seen in premature infants. It is characterized by very rapid breathing, cyanosis, nasal flaring, grunting, and retractions of the intercostal muscles. Premature infants are at risk because their immature lung tissue has not yet developed surfactant, the substance that prevents alveoli from completely collapsing between inspiration and expiration. Without surfactant, respiration is physically demanding and exhaustion and respiratory failure ensues. The prognosis of premature infants has improved with the administration of surfactant.

Cystic fibrosis is a hereditary disorder affecting the lungs and digestive system. Within the lungs, thick, viscous mucus is produced, blocking the airway and trapping air in the lungs. Within the digestive system, pancreatic enzymes are not produced, causing problems with digestion including fatty, frequent, foul-smelling stools. Presently, lifelong treatment with pancreatic enzyme replacement, respiratory or pulmonary toilet including postural drainage, and antibiotic therapy for frequent, associated pneumonia is necessary. The genetic abnormality causing this disease has been discovered and progress is being made to replace the aberrant gene in order to develop a cure for persons affected with cystic fibrosis. Some cystic fibrosis patients may receive lung transplants.

Pulmonary embolism is a common, life-threatening complication resulting from thrombus formation in the venous circulation. Thrombi (blood clots) pass through the venous circulation and become lodged in the venous circulation of the lungs. Treatment involves administration of anticoagulants and thrombolytic therapy.

Lung cancer is the leading cause of deaths due to cancer. By far, cigarette smoking causes the majority of cases. Over 90% of lung cancer cases fall into two major classifications: small cell carcinoma and non-small cell carcinoma (squamous cell carcinoma, adenocarcinoma, and large cell carcinoma).

Sarcoidosis is a disorder of unknown etiology that can affect any organ in the body. Ninety percent of patients with sarcoidosis (also called sarcoid) have pulmonary involvement characterized by shortness of breath, chronic cough, hoarseness, wheezing, tightness, and chest pain.

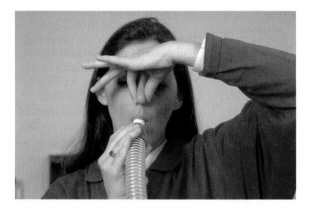

Patient pinches nose and mouth-breathes, allowing spirometer to measure and record airflow.

Common Tests and Surgical Procedures

X-ray imaging of the chest is one of the most commonly used procedures to diagnose conditions such as pneumonia, tuberculosis, and abnormalities of the lungs and surrounding structures. The physician may request both AP (anterior to posterior) and PA (posterior to anterior) views, indicating the body plane which faces the source of the x-ray. CT scans are also important for diagnosing lung disease. V/Q scans have been used to diagnose pulmonary embolism in the past, but this procedure is being supplanted by helical CT scans.

Pulmonary function tests are essential to diagnosing chronic obstructive pulmonary disease and other lung ailments. These tests measure airflow rates, lung volumes, and the ability of the lung to transfer gas across the alveolar-capillary membrane. Spirometry measures the flow and volume of air during inspiration and expiration. Asthma patients are diagnosed using a bronchial provocation test which provokes an asthmatic attack in susceptible patients.

Another common procedure is bronchoscopy. The examination is usually performed with a flexible bronchoscope that allows the physician to see even the small airways and to remove pieces of tissue for biopsy or culture. A brush biopsy, which uses a brush to pick up cells, may be performed at the same time as a bronchoscopy. The same type of instrument is used to view the trachea and esophagus for signs of disease and abnormalities.

Thoracentesis is a surgical procedure to remove fluid from the pleural cavity. Pneumonectomy, or pulmonectomy, is an excision of all lobes of a lung in a single operation while a lobectomy is the removal of a part (lobe) of a lung.

Pulse oximetry uses a small, portable, non-invasive monitoring device that measures the percent of oxygen saturation of hemoglobin. Capnography is the measurement of exhaled carbon dioxide and the capnogram is the visual display of the exhaled carbon dioxide.

idiopathic
(i-dee-O-**path**-ik) (adj) describes a disease in which the cause is unknown

infiltrate »
(in-**fil**-trayt) (v) to pass into or through a substance or a space

inspiratory »
(in-**spI**-ra-tO-ree) (adj) relating to inhalation, drawing air into the lungs

latissimus »
(la-**tis**-i-mus) (n) denoting a broad anatomical structure, such as a muscle

linear »
(**lin**-ee-ar) (adj) pertaining to or resembling a line

lobectomy
(lOb-**ek**-tO-mee) (n) the removal of a lobe from an organ or gland

lytic »
(**lit**-ik) (adj) pertaining to lysis, a gradual subsidence of the symptoms of an acute disease

mediastinal »
(mee-dee-as-**tI**-nal (adj) related to the mediastinum, a septum or cavity between two principal portions of an organ

metaphyseal »
(met-a-**fiz**-ee-al) (adj) relating to a metaphysis

metaphysis »
(me-**taf**-i-sis) (n) a conical section of bone between the epiphysis and diaphysis of long bones

metaplasia »
(me-ta-**play**-zee-a) (n) conversion of a tissue into a form that is not normal for that tissue

metastasis »
(me-**tas**-ta-sis) (n) the shifting of a disease from one part of the body to another, especially in cancer; metastases (pl)

multinucleated »
(mul-ti-**noo**-klee-ay-ted) (adj) possessing several nuclei

nasopharynx »
(**nay**-zO-**far**-ingks) (n) open chamber behind the nose and above the palate

nebulization »
(**neb**-yoo-li-**zay**-shun) (n) production of fine particles, such as a spray or mist, from liquid

opacity »
(O-**pas**-i-tee) (n) state of being opaque, impenetrable by visible light rays or by forms of radiant energy, such as x-rays

organomegaly »
(**Or**-ga-nO-**meg**-a-lee) (n) abnormal enlargement of an organ, particularly an organ of the abdominal cavity, such as the liver or spleen

orthopnea »
(Or-thop-**nee**-a) (n) difficulty in breathing when lying down

oximetry »
(ok-**sim**-i-tree) (n) a method of measuring the amount of oxygen combined with the hemoglobin in a blood sample

pancrelipase »
(pan-kree-**lip**-ase) (n) standardized preparation of enzymes with amylase and protease, obtained from the pancreas of hogs

parenchymal »
(pa-**reng**-ki-mal) (adj) pertaining to the distinguishing or specific cells of a gland or organ contained in and supported by the connective tissue framework

parietal »
(pa-**ree**-e-tal) (adj) pertaining to the inner walls of a body cavity

pathogen »
(**path**-O-jen) (n) any microorganism or substance that can cause a disease

pathologic »
(path-O-**loj**-ik) (adj) pertaining to pathology, the medical science concerned with all aspects of disease, especially with the structural and functional changes caused by disease

pectoriloquy
(pek-tO-**ril**-O-kwee) (n) voice sounds transmitted through the pulmonary structures, clearly audible on auscultation

pectus carinatum
(**pek**-tus kar-i-**nay**-tum) (n) forward protusion of the sternum; pigeon breast

pectus excavatum
(**pek**-tus eks-ka-**vay**-tum) (n) markedly sunken sternum; funnel breast

percussion
(per-**kush**-un) (n) a technique of physical examination in which the sound of fingers or a small tool tapping parts of the body is used to determine position and size of internal organs and to detect the presence of fluid

perihilar »
(per-i-**hI**-lar) (adj) occurring near the hilum, the part of an organ where the nerves and vessels enter and leave

pharynx
(**far**-ingks) (n) throat; passageway for air from nasal cavity to larynx, and food from mouth to esophagus

pleura
(**ploor**-a) (n) membrane lining the chest cavity and covering the lungs

pleural »
(**ploor**-al) (adj) relating to the pleura

pleurisy »
(**ploor**-i-see) (n) inflammation of the pleura; pleuritis

pneumonia
(noo-**mO**-nee-a) (n) inflammation and congestion of the lung, usually due to infection by bacteria or viruses

pneumonitis »
(noo-mO-**nI**-tis) (n) inflammation of the lungs

pneumothorax »
(noo-mO-**thor**-aks) (n) abnormal presence of air or gas in the chest cavity

protuberant »
(prO-**too**-ber-ant) (adj) pertaining to a part that is prominent beyond a surface, like a knob

Pseudomonas »
(soo-dO-**mO**-nas) (n) a genus of gram-negative rods, which is a significant human pathogen

lifelong treatment with pancreatic enzyme replacement, respiratory or pulmonary toilet including postural drainage, and antibiotic therapy for frequent, associated pneumonia is necessary. The genetic abnormality causing this disease has been discovered and progress is being made to replace the aberrant gene in order to develop a cure for persons affected with cystic fibrosis. Some cystic fibrosis patients may receive lung transplants.

Pulmonary embolism is a common, life-threatening complication resulting from thrombus formation in the venous circulation. Thrombi (blood clots) pass through the venous circulation and become lodged in the venous circulation of the lungs. Treatment involves administration of anticoagulants and thrombolytic therapy.

Lung cancer is the leading cause of deaths due to cancer. By far, cigarette smoking causes the majority of cases. Over 90% of lung cancer cases fall into two major classifications: small cell carcinoma and non-small cell carcinoma (squamous cell carcinoma, adenocarcinoma, and large cell carcinoma).

Sarcoidosis is a disorder of unknown etiology that can affect any organ in the body. Ninety percent of patients with sarcoidosis (also called sarcoid) have pulmonary involvement characterized by shortness of breath, chronic cough, hoarseness, wheezing, tightness, and chest pain.

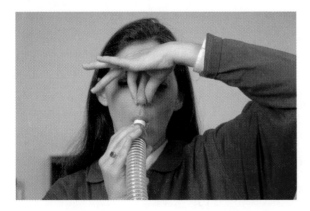

Patient pinches nose and mouth-breathes, allowing spirometer to measure and record airflow.

Common Tests and Surgical Procedures

X-ray imaging of the chest is one of the most commonly used procedures to diagnose conditions such as pneumonia, tuberculosis, and abnormalities of the lungs and surrounding structures. The physician may request both AP (anterior to posterior) and PA (posterior to anterior) views, indicating the body plane which faces the source of the x-ray. CT scans are also important for diagnosing lung disease. V/Q scans have been used to diagnose pulmonary embolism in the past, but this procedure is being supplanted by helical CT scans.

Pulmonary function tests are essential to diagnosing chronic obstructive pulmonary disease and other lung ailments. These tests measure airflow rates, lung volumes, and the ability of the lung to transfer gas across the alveolar-capillary membrane. Spirometry measures the flow and volume of air during inspiration and expiration. Asthma patients are diagnosed using a bronchial provocation test which provokes an asthmatic attack in susceptible patients.

Another common procedure is bronchoscopy. The examination is usually performed with a flexible bronchoscope that allows the physician to see even the small airways and to remove pieces of tissue for biopsy or culture. A brush biopsy, which uses a brush to pick up cells, may be performed at the same time as a bronchoscopy. The same type of instrument is used to view the trachea and esophagus for signs of disease and abnormalities.

Thoracentesis is a surgical procedure to remove fluid from the pleural cavity. Pneumonectomy, or pulmonectomy, is an excision of all lobes of a lung in a single operation while a lobectomy is the removal of a part (lobe) of a lung.

Pulse oximetry uses a small, portable, non-invasive monitoring device that measures the percent of oxygen saturation of hemoglobin. Capnography is the measurement of exhaled carbon dioxide and the capnogram is the visual display of the exhaled carbon dioxide.

Terms Bank

These terms and abbreviations provide a foundation for the language and transcription skills you will develop in the following sections of this chapter. Terms marked with » will be included in the reports transcribed in the Building Transcription Skills section.

abscess
(**ab**-ses) (n) a pus-filled cavity, usually because of a localized infection

aerosol
(**ayr**-O-sol) (n) a liquid or solution dispensed as a fine mist or a product dispensed from a pressurized container as a fine mist

afebrile »
(ay-**feb**-rIl) (adj) without fever

albuterol »
(al-**byoo**-ter-ol) (n) bronchodilator available in oral and inhalent forms to be used in asthma, emphysema, and other lung conditions

alveolus
(al-**vee**-O-lus) (n) tiny chambers of the lungs where the exchange of oxygen and carbon dioxide takes place; alveoli (al-**vee**-O-lI) (pl)

anicteric »
(an-ik-**ter**-ik) (adj) without jaundice or icterus (a yellowing of the skin and whites of the eyes)

anorexia »
(an-O-**rek**-see-a) (n) loss of appetite

arytenoid »
(ar-i-**tee**-noid) (adj) resembling a ladle or pitcher mouth; the muscle and cartilage of the larynx

asthma
(**az**-ma) (n) respiratory disorder with temporary narrowing of the airways, resulting in difficulty in breathing, coughing, gasping, wheezing

atelectasis »
(at-e-**lek**-ta-sis) (n) condition in which lungs are unexpanded

atraumatic
(ay-traw-**mat**-ik) (adj) without injury or trauma

auscultation »
(aws-kul-**tay**-shun) (n) act of listening through a stethoscope to sounds from within the body, including lungs, heart, and abdomen

bacteremia
(bak-ter-**ee**-mee-a) (n) the presence of bacteria in the blood

bibasilar »
(bI-**bays**-i-lar) (adj) occurring in both bases

bifurcation
(bI-fer-**kay**-shun) (n) forking into two branches

bleomycin »
(blee-O-**mI**-sin) (n) antitumor agents

bolus »
(**bO**-lus) (n) a mass of something such as masticated (chewed) food or substance that is ready to be swallowed; an amount of medication

brachial »
(**bray**-kee-al) (adj) pertaining to the arm

bronchial
(**brong**-kee-al) (adj) relating to the bronchi

bronchiectasis
(brong-kee-**ek**-ta-sis) (n) persistent, abnormal widening of the bronchi, with an associated cough and spitting up of mucus

bronchiole
(**brong**-kee-Ol) (n) one of the smaller subdivisions of the bronchi

bronchitis
(brong-**kI**-tis) (n) inflammation of the bronchi

bronchovesicular
(**brong**-kO-ve-**sik**-yoo-lar) (adj) relating to the bronchioles and alveoli in the lungs

bronchus
(**brong**-kus) (n) the divisions of the trachea leading to the lungs; bronchi (**brong**-kI) (pl)

bulla »
(**bul**-a) (n) large bleb in the skin that contains fluid; bullae (pl)

cannula »
(**kan**-yoo-la) (n) a tube for insertion into a duct or cavity to allow the escape of fluid

cannulate »
(**kan**-yoo-layt) (v) to introduce a cannula through a passageway

capillary »
(kap-i-**layr**-ee) (n) tiny blood vessel connecting arterioles and venules

capnography
(cap-**nog**-ra-phy) (n) measurement of exhaled carbon dioxide via a capnogram which produces a visual display of the exhaled carbon dioxide

ceftazidime »
(sef-**taz**-i-deem) (n) antibiotic used in the treatment of moderate to severe infections

cilium
(**sil**-ee-um) (n) a short hairlike extension of a cell surface, capable of lashlike movement, which aids in the movement of unicellular organisms and in the movement of fluids in higher organisms; eyelash; cilia (pl)

clavicular »
(kla-**vik**-yoo-lar) (adj) pertains to the clavicle, or collarbone

clubbing »
(**klub**-ing) (n) condition of the fingers and toes in which their ends become wide and thickened; often a sign of disease, especially heart or lung disease

radiograph »
(**ray**-dee-O-graf) (n) a negative image in photographic film made by exposure to x-rays or gamma rays that have passed through matter or tissue

rales
(rahls) (n) abnormal sounds, such as rattling or bubbling, heard on auscultation of the lungs

rectal
(**rek**-tal) (adj) relating to the rectum, the lower part of the large intestine

regimen
(**rej**-i-men) (n) plan of therapy, including drugs

respiration
(res-pi-**ray**-shun) (n) inhalation and exhalation; the exchange of gases—oxygen and carbon dioxide—between an organism and the environment

respiratory »
(**res**-per-a-tOr-ee) (adj) relating to respiration

respiratory distress syndrome
(**res**-pi-ra-tOr-ee dis-**tres sin**-drOm) (n) acute lung disease, especially in premature newborn babies, caused by a lack of surfactant in the lung tissue

rhinorrhea »
(rI-nO-**ree**-a) (n) a watery discharge from the nose

rhonchus »
(**rong**-kus) (n) abnormal sound heard on auscultation of the chest, usually during expiration; rhonchi (pl)

sarcoidosis
(**sar**-koid-O-sis) (n) a systemic disease of unknown cause resulting in interstitial fibrosis involving the lungs, lymph nodes, skin, liver, spleen, eyes, phalangeal bones, and parotid glands

sclera »
(**skleer**-a) (n) a fibrous coat that covers approximately five-sixths of the outer tunic of the eye; sclerae (pl)

sclerotic »
(skle-**rot**-ik) (adj) relating to sclerosis, or induration; in neuropathy, induration of nervous and other structures by a hyperplasia of the interstitial fibrous structures

squamous »
(**skway**-mus) (adj) scale-like

septum
(**sep**-tum) (n) division between two cavities or two masses of tissue, e.g., nasal septum; septa (pl)

sputum
(**spyoo**-tum) (n) spit; expectorated material

sternum
(**ster**-num) (n) the breast bone

supraglottic »
(soo-pra-**glot**-ik) (adj) located above the glottis, the sound-producing apparatus of the larynx

tachycardia »
(**tak**-i-**kar**-dee-a) (n) rapid heart rate

tachycardiac »
(**tak**-e-**kar**-dee-ak) (adj) relating to or suffering from an abnormally rapid heart rate

tachypnea
(tak-ip-**nee**-a) (n) rapid rate of breathing

theophylline »
(thee-**off**-i-lin) (n) a drug used in chronic obstructive lung disease

thoracotomy »
(thor-a-**kot**-O-mee) (n) surgical incision of the chest wall

thoracoscopy »
(thor-a-**kos**-kO-pee) (n) diagnostic examination of the pleural cavity with an endoscope

thorax »
(**thor**-aks) (n) the chest

thyromegaly »
(thI-rO-**meg**-a-lee) (n) enlargement of the thyroid gland

tibia »
(**tib**-ee-a) (n) larger bone of the lower leg; shin bone

tibial »
(**tib**-ee-al) (adj) relating to the tibia

tobramycin »
(tO-bra-**mI**-sin) (n) an antibiotic drug

trachea »
(**tray**-kee-a) (n) the windpipe

turbinates »
(**ter**-bi-naytz) (n) three scroll-shaped bones that form the sidewall of the nasal cavity

turgor »
(**ter**-gOr) (n) normal tension in a cell; swelling

tympanic membrane »
(tim-**pan**-ik) (n) eardrum

vincristine »
(vin-**kris**-teen) (n) an antineoplastic drug that disrupts cell division and is used to treat many cancers, especially those of the lymphatic system.

wheezing »
(**hweez**-ing) (n) breathing with difficulty and with a whistling sound; can be heard aloud and/or on auscultation

Wright peak flow »
(n) maximum flow of expired air as measured by the Wright flowmeter

Abbreviations

A&P	auscultation and percussion		FIO_2	fractional inspired oxygen concentration
ABG	arterial blood gas (gases)		FVC	forced vital capacity
AFB	acid-fast bacilli		FVL	flow volume loop
AIDS	acquired immunodeficiency syndrome		IPPB	intermittent positive pressure breathing
AP	anterior posterior		IS	incentive spirometry
ARDS	acute respiratory distress syndrome		MDI	metered dose inhaler
BiPAP	bilevel positive airway pressure		O_2	oxygen
BOOP	bronchiolitis obliterans with organizing pneumonia		PA	posterior anterior
			PAP	positive airway pressure
CO_2	carbon dioxide		PCP	pneumocystis pneumonia
COLD	chronic obstructive lung disease		PEEP	positive end expiratory pressure
COPD	chronic obstructive pulmonary disease		PEF	peak expiratory flow
CPAP	continuous positive airway pressure		PND	paroxysmal nocturnal dyspnea
CPR	cardiopulmonary resuscitation		RAD	reactive airway disease
CT	computed tomography		RDS	respiratory distress syndrome
CXR	chest x-ray		SIDS	sudden infant death syndrome
DNR	do not resuscitate		SMR	submucosal resection
FEF	forced expiratory flow		SOB	shortness of breath
FEF_{25-75}	forced midexpiratory flow during the middle half of the FVC		TB	tuberculosis
			URI	upper respiratory infection
FEV	forced expiratory volume		VC	vital capacity
FEV_1	forced expiratory volume in one second		V/Q	ventilation/perfusion
FEV_3	forced expiratory volume in three seconds			

Building Language Skills

Complete the following exercises, drawing on the information learned in the Exploring Pulmonology section of this chapter and referencing the Terms Bank.

Exercise 8.1   Matching Sound and Spelling

The numbered list that follows shows the phonetic spelling of hard-to-spell words. Sound out the word and then write the correct spelling in the blank space provided. Check your answers in the Terms Bank or other appropriate reference

1. tak-i-**kar**-dee-a _____
2. **ploor**-al _____
3. an-ik-**ter**-ik _____
4. thee-**off**-i-lin _____
5. brong-kee-**ek**-ta-sis _____
6. noo-mO-**nl**-tis _____
7. **rong**-kus _____
8. aws-kul-**tay**-shun _____
9. tak-ip-**nee**-a _____
10. thl-rO-**meg**-a-lee _____
11. **nay**-zO-**far**-ingks _____
12. hee-**mop**-ti-sis _____
13. di-**fyoos** _____
14. **tray**-kee-a _____
15. **Or**-ga-nO-**meg**-a-lee _____

Below is a list of frequently used words that look alike and/or sound alike. Study the meaning and pronunciation of each set of words, read the following sentences carefully, and then circle the word in parentheses that correctly completes the meaning.

afebrile	(adj) without fever	**loss**	(n) something that is missing
a febrile	(adj) with fever	**lost**	(v) past tense of lose
		lost	(adj) missing as in "a lost watch"
breath	(n) air taken into the lungs		
breathe	(v) to take air into the lungs	**perfuse**	to force blood or other fluid to flow; "toes are well perfused"
coarse	rough; "coarse breath sounds"	**profuse**	abundant; "the patient had profuse bleeding"
course	progress or duration of time		
dose	(n) a measure	**presence**	(n) attendance; close proximity
doze	(v) to nap	**presents**	(n) gifts
		presents	(v) manner in which the patient appears to the caregiver
expiratory	breathing out from the lungs		
inspiratory	breathing into the lungs	**vicious**	(adj) mean
		viscous	(adj) sticky
loose	(adj) free from anything that restrains	**viscus**	(n) a hollow, multilayered, walled organ such as an organ of the digestive system or the heart
lose	(v) to miss something		

1. The patient is to take 3 (doses/dozes) of the medication daily.
2. It was unfortunate that she (dosed/dozed) through the lecture.
3. The patient (presence/presents) for followup of his colitis.
4. On cardiac examination, I detected the (presence/presents) of a systolic murmur.
5. As the patient inhaled, I noted (expiratory/inspiratory) wheezing.
6. She is complaining of shortness of (breath/breathe) on exertion.
7. When she exercises, she feels like she cannot (breath/breathe) as easily.
8. We will have her complete her full (coarse/course) of antibiotics.
9. When she cut her finger, she noted (perfuse/profuse) bleeding.
10. The patient was directed to (loose/lose) 10 pounds by her next visit.

Exercise 8.3   Choosing Words from Context

When transcribing dictation, the medical transcriptionist frequently needs to consider the situation when determining the word that correctly completes the sentence. From the list below, select the term that meaningfully completes each of the following statements.

afebrile	diffuse	nebulizer
alveoli	effusion	radiograph
auscultation	erythema	respiratory distress
bolus	hemoptysis	rhonchi
cyanosis	infiltrate	tachycardic
cyanotic	mediastinal	tachypneic

1. Upon presentation to the emergency room, the patient was in severe _____, making breathing painful.

2. On _____ of the lungs, I heard rhonchi and rales.

3. Her fingernails were _____, indicating that she needed oxygen.

4. Mrs. Smith is _____ today, with a temperature of 98.6 degrees on exam.

5. The chest x-ray showed improvement in her pleural _____.

6. The patient has had two episodes of _____, when he noticed flecks of blood in his sputum.

7. Although she complains of rapid breathing, she is not _____ on exam.

8. On auscultation, there were _____ heard in the lower lung fields.

9. Jackie has developed a lot of chest congestion over the past 24 hours, with an increase in her wheezing. She has been using her _____ at home but no other medications.

10. The patient is _____, with a heart rate of 160.

11. The _____ revealed a pleural effusion.

12. The CT scan showed a large _____ mass in the center of the chest.

13. The color of the lips revealed _____, an indication that there was an airway obstruction.

14. The chest x-ray revealed a left hilar _____.

15. The medication was given very quickly by _____ injection.

From this list, locate the term that best matches each of the following definitions. Write the term in the space provided by each definition.

bronchiole	esophagus	theophylline
cystic fibrosis	hemothorax	trachea
edema	hyperemia	tympanic membrane
effusion	pathogen	Ventolin
epiglottis	*Pseudomonas*	

1. a drug resembling caffeine that dilates blood vessels _____

2. a genus of small, motile bacilli _____

3. a muscular canal that carries food from the mouth to the stomach _____

4. one of the smaller divisions of the bronchial tubes _____

5. a transparent membrane that separates the outer ear from the middle ear _____

6. abnormal collection of fluid in spaces between cells _____

7. a disease in which the passageways (including pancreatic and bile ducts, intestine, and bronchi) become clogged with thick mucus _____

8. cartilage at the back of the mouth cavity that covers the windpipe during swallowing _____

9. increased blood supply in part of the body _____

10. a substance or organism capable of producing disease _____

Exercise 8.5   Creating Terms from Word Forms

Combine prefixes, root words, and suffixes from this list to create medical words that fit the following definitions. Fill in the blanks with the words you construct.

bronch/o	airway	**thyroid**	gland
cyt/o-	cell	**-capnia**	carbon dioxide
hyper-	above or excessive	**-cyte**	cell
hypo-	below or deficient	**-ectomy**	removal of anatomical structure
oxa- or **oxy-**		**-emia**	blood condition
or **oxo-**	oxygen	**-ia**	condition of
pneum/o or		**-itis**	inflammation or infection
pneumon/o	air or lung	**-plasia**	formation; growth
pulmon/o	lung		

1. excision of the thyroid _____

2. reduction of oxygen supply to tissue _____

3. excision of entire lung _____

4. increase in number of cells, enlarging the organ _____

5. excess of carbon dioxide_____

6. underdevelopment of organ growth _____

7. excess of red blood cells _____

8. inflammation of thyroid gland _____

9. deficiency of carbon dioxide_____

10. inflammation of the mucosa of the bronchi _____

Read the following medical report extracts and look for and correct errors in word use, spelling, the use of commas, pronoun and reference agreement, and subject and verb agreement. Also check for incomplete sentences. Mark the corrections on this page and key the excerpts with all errors corrected. Save the documents as XXExercise08.06-1 and XXExercise08.06-2, using your initials in the place of *XX* in the file names.

1.   **PHYSICAL EXAMINATION:** Plus of 120, respertory rate of 30, temperature of 99 degrees and weight 40.6 kg. She is a thin, pale, adolescence female in mild respiratory distress. Head is normocephalic and a traumatic. Pupil are equal, round and reaction to light. Extraocular movements are full. Sclera are anicteric. Conjunctavae is not injected. Nose is without discharge. No flareing. Her mouth has pale pink and moist mucosa. No legions. Her lips were cyanotic. His face had a flush over the cheek bones. Her neck was supply, without palpable limph nodes.

2.   Within the proxmal right humoral metaphysys ther is a mixed litic and sclerotic lesion. Since the previous exam this has worsened significantly, and is consistent width pathologic fracture.

Read this scenario carefully and then select the most appropriate response. Write an explanation for why you think your choice is the best answer.

As part of a dictated report, a physician states, "The patient spent three days in ICU, probably because the nurse gave him the wrong dose." What should you do?

---

a.   Finish transcribing the report exactly as dictated.

b.   Finish the report but leave the comment out of the final transcript.

c.   Contact your supervisor (or the risk management officer) about the dictation.

d.   Delete the report and ask the doctor to re-dictate the file because the first audio file was lost.

Best response: _____

Explanation: _____

_____

_____

_____

_____

You will apply the medical specialty and language information you learned in this chapter to transcription work in this section. After you learn the formatting recommendations of a discharge summary, you will transcribe ten reports related to nine different patient studies.

Introducing the Discharge Summary

Sometimes called a dismissal summary or summary of hospitalization, the discharge summary (Figure 8.3) provides a review of the patient's hospitalization, including the reason for entering the hospital, the patient's medical history, and a description of the procedures and treatment performed during the stay.

Required Headings/Content

The discharge summary report includes documentation about the patient's discharge diagnosis, the history of the present illness, the care given in the hospital (called the hospital course), and discharge instructions. Instructions for continuing care can include information on therapy, diet, activity, the plan for future visits or medical care. If medications are prescribed on discharge, this listing is included in the report. The report usually also includes details of a physical examination, which is either presented in paragraph or list format. (Figure 8.3 shows the report's Physical Examination section in paragraph format.) The report might also include information about the patient's past medical history, diagnostic or laboratory tests performed during the hospital stay, and the patient's condition on discharge.

Refer to page 470 of Appendix A for a complete list of headings found in the discharge summary template along with descriptions of the type of information found under each heading. Not every heading will be included in every transcribed report.

Turnaround Time

Medical records for discharged patients are to be completed within a time period specified by the hospital, but the time period is not to exceed 30 days. Because subsequent medical care can proceed without the discharge summary, the turnaround time on this report is typically three to seven days, which is longer than for other, more critical hospital reports.

Preparing to Transcribe

To prepare for transcribing dictation, review the common pulmonology terms, drugs, and abbreviations presented in this chapter Terms Bank. Then, study the format and organization of the model document shown in Figure 8.3 and key the model document, using the discharge summary template on the Dictations and Templates CD as a starting point. Save the document as XXFigure08.03, using your initials in the place of XX in the file name. Proofread the document by comparing it with the printed version. Categorize the types of errors you made, and document them on a copy of the Performance Comparison Chart. A template of this chart available is on the Dictations and Templates CD.

Transcribing Reports

Transcribe, edit, and correct each report in the following patient studies. Consult reference books for words or formatting rules that are unfamiliar.

As you work on the transcription assignment for this chapter, fill in the Performance Comparison Chart that you started when you keyed the model document. For at least three of the reports, categorize and document the types of errors you made. Answer the document analysis questions on the bottom of the chart. With continuous practice and assessment, the quality of your work will improve.

PATIENT NAME: tab   Jaheem Arnold
MR #:   tab   7013920
ADMISSION DATE: tab   02/13/20XX
DISCHARGE DATE: tab   02/20/20XX
    ds

Aligning name,
dates, and
record numbers
is another
acceptable
format

left justification

ADMITTING DIAGNOSIS
Reactive airway disease.
    ds
DISCHARGE DIAGNOSIS
Reactive airway disease.
    ds
HISTORY OF PRESENT ILLNESS
The patient is a 19-month-old African American male who had been well until 2 days prior to admission, when he developed a loose cough. Mother gave him an over-the-counter children's cough remedy several times each day. He was afebrile during this time. During the day, the child had increased difficulty breathing, and wheezing was noted in the late p.m. when the child was brought to the emergency room. In the ER, the child was found to have a fever of 102 degrees Fahrenheit rectally. He was found to be in respiratory distress and was given Ventolin nebulization and admitted.
    ds
PHYSICAL EXAMINATION
Physical examination showed a patient sitting in bed with mild respiratory distress. He was alert. Respiratory rate was 40, heart rate was 115, temperature was 102.3 degrees. Right tympanic membrane was slightly erythematous. There was slight nasal flaring. Throat was slightly injected. On auscultation, the lungs were found to have diffuse inspiratory and expiratory wheezes. The heart showed the presence of normal heart sounds with mild tachycardia.
    ds
HOSPITAL COURSE
Reactive airway disease. The patient was admitted, started on theophylline, given a bolus of theophylline 1 mg/kg, and subsequently put on a maintenance dose of theophylline. High-flow nebulization was also given p.o. every 2 hours. With this management, the patient showed rapid improvement and his respiratory treatments were gradually spaced out so that, subsequently, the patient was changed to oral medication of theophylline. Theophylline levels were monitored during the hospital course.
    ds
CONDITION ON DISCHARGE
The child was discharged after a 1-week hospitalization on theophylline. Condition at time of discharge was improved.
    ds
DISCHARGE INSTRUCTIONS
Mother was instructed to bring him to our office in 1 week.

    qs

_____

Mencer Alcott, MD
    ds
MA/XX
D: 02/22/20XX
T: 02/29/20XX

Figure 8.3   Discharge Summary

Jaheem Arnold is a 19-month-old African American male who came to the emergency room (ER) of the hospital with a history of cough for 2 days. He had begun wheezing and having increased difficulty breathing for 1 hour prior to coming to the ER.

REPORT 8.1   Discharge Summary

Use the Report0801.mp3 audio file and the discharge summary template (Discharge_Summary) when transcribing this report. Transcribe the Physical Examination section of the report in paragraph format, as dictated. (Do not include the template's subheadings for this section of the report.) Save the document as XXReport08.01, using your initials in place of *XX* in the file name.

Listen for these drug names:
theophylline
Ventolin

When the dictator refers to nebulization given "pee oh," transcribe this abbreviation for *by mouth* as p.o.

This physician dictates the word "bolused," which is a "back formation" of the word "bolus." Changing a noun into a verb is common among dictators. Sometimes, the back formation becomes so prevalent, a new term is added to the medical dictionary. "Bovied" is a good example of an accepted back formation of the noun Bovie. Although bolused may be commonly used, in this report transcribe the phrase using the word bolus, making slight changes to the syntax as necessary.

It is important to use the template's headings to accurately identify the dictated content. In this report, the provider will dictate the heading "Disposition." Use a heading from the template that more closely aligns with the dictated content. Similarly, use the template's heading for the discharge instructions given to the patient's mother.

Charles Ingrid is a 4½-year-old male who was diagnosed with cystic fibrosis several months ago. He had a history of frequent colds with large amounts of thick nasal discharge and thick respiratory sputum. His growth was slow, and his mother noticed that he had very sticky bowel movements. The diagnosis of cystic fibrosis was made after the pediatrician sent him for a sweat test that was positive for the disease. Charles is being admitted to the hospital because of a respiratory tract infection, which is common for persons with cystic fibrosis.

REPORT 8.2   Physical Examination Section of Discharge Summary

Use the Report0802.mp3 audio file and the discharge summary template (Discharge_Summary) when transcribing this report. This is a partial report, so delete the unneeded heads within the report according to the dictated content. Save the document as XXReport08.02, using your initials in place of *XX* in the file name.

The HEENT examination is a review of the patient's head, eyes, ears, nose, and throat. Many providers will dictate the content of the HEENT portion of the physical examination collectively, with the information run-in without internal headings separating the separate parts of the exam. If the provider itemizes the parts of the examination with headings, it is appropriate to list out the sections with each heading set in all capital letters, followed by a colon. If there is no collective HEENT content, delete that heading.

PERRL and PERRLA are common abbreviations in the HEENT examination. They stand for *pupils equal, round, and reactive to light* or *pupils equal, round, and reactive to light and accommodation.* This means that the pupils are equal in size and round in shape and that they constrict when a light is shined into the eyes. Accommodation refers to the changing shape of the lens in response to the patient focusing on an object across the room and then on an object a foot or two away.

Pulse is dictated as "92 per minute" but may be transcribed as "92 beats per minute." Temperature may be transcribed with a degree symbol (if available in your word processor) or written out as "97 degrees."

Note the spelling of funduscope, funduscopy, funduscopic.

For some of the headings within the Physical Examination section, you will replace the dictated heading with the template's heading. Follow the template as closely as possible. For example, use the template's heading *Thorax and Lungs* instead of the dictated "Chest." Also, use the template's *Pelvis* heading for the dictated "Genitalia."

Refer to Chapter 14 for notes on the transcription of cranial nerves and reflexes.

REPORT 8.3   Consultation Letter

Use the Report0803.mp3 audio file and the consultation letter template (Consultation_Letter) when transcribing this report. This report format was introduced in Chapter 6. Save the document as XXReport08.03, using your initials in place of *XX* in the file name.

continued on next page

REPORT 8.3 Consultation Letter *continued*

Physicians sometimes use the words *regime* and *regimen* interchangeably in dictation. However, *regimen* is the word that is usually intended. A regime is a system of government or a social system. A regimen is a daily routine, as in a *medication regimen.*

Drug names tobramycin and ceftazidime should be transcribed with lowercase letters because they are generic names, and the drug name Bactrim is transcribed with a capital B because it is a brand name.

Listen for dictated dangerous abbreviations, and be sure to use the acceptable replacement.

Patient Study 8.C

Denise Sultan

Denise Sultan is a 17-year-old girl diagnosed 1 year ago with lymphoma (also called Hodgkin disease). She has been receiving chemotherapy for the past year. She was admitted to the hospital for difficulty breathing. She was diagnosed with pneumonia and had a complicated hospital course.

REPORT 8.4 Discharge Summary

Use the Report0804.mp3 audio file and the discharge summary template (Discharge_Summary) when transcribing this report. Save the document as XXReport08.04, using your initials in place of *XX* in the file name.

Use the order and content of the template's headings as you transcribe this report. For example, when the dictator says "History," use the template's History of Present Illness heading. Within the Physical Examination section, use the subheadings from the template even though they are not dictated. Insert dictated content after the appropriate subheading. Note that this dictator does not dictate the details of the physical examination in the order of the template, which is common problem faced by transcriptionists.

Dictators will often bounce back and forth from heading to heading, or forget something and have to go back. Medical transcriptionists need to learn to recognize what type of information is being dictated and insert it under the appropriate heading, using the appropriate template.

Replace the dictated Impression on Admission heading with the template's Hospital Course heading. Because of the narrative style of this report, do not separate out the diagnostic studies or laboratory data. As dictated, these lab results are central to the decision-making process and the report would lose continuity if they were split out. However, do use the template's Discharge Medications heading and Plan heading where appropriate. (These headings are not dictated.)

REPORT 8.4   Discharge Summary *continued*

Listen for these shortened terms for blood cells in the CBC results:

basos

eos

lymphs

monos

segs

Blood gases are transcribed using the chemical abbreviations and numbers. The dictator may use the full term (for example, carbon dioxide) for some gases and may pronounce the letters of the abbreviation for others. In this report, the blood gases should be transcribed as pH of 7.5, pCO_2 of 31, pO_2 of 35, CO_2 of 24, and an O_2 saturation of 84.2.

The abbreviations for oxygen and carbon dioxide include the number 2, which may be transcribed as a subscript or directly on the line. The preferred method is subscript (CO_2, O_2) if your word processor has that capability; otherwise, transcribe as O2, CO2.

The dictator uses the acronym "MOPP" for the chemotherapy regimen of mechlorethamine (also called nitrogen mustard), Oncovin, prednisone, and procarbazine.

Patient Study 8.D   Janis Miller

Janis Miller is a tour guide and part-time college student who has been feeling ill for about a week. She has had a runny nose and shortness of breath.

REPORT 8.5   Office Note

Use the Report0805.mp3 audio file and the office note template (Office_Note) when transcribing this report. This report format was introduced in Chapter 5. Add headings or subheadings that are dictated but are not included in this report. Save the document as XXReport08.05, using your initials in place of *XX* in the file name.

Listen for these terms:

rhinorrhea

Wright peak flow

Listen for the word "guttur," which means "throat." It could easily be confused with the similar-sounding "gutter," meaning "a trench."

The reports containing numbered lists are transcribed with one space after the number (and period). Do not use the Microsoft Word AutoFormat feature when keying numbered lists. Also, do not set the item that runs over onto a second line with a hanging indent. The second line should be flush left.

A third-grader with chronic asthma, Rhonda Bentz is returning for a checkup following treatment for pneumonia.

REPORT 8.6   Office Note

Use the Report0806.mp3 audio file and the office note template (Office_Note) when transcribing this report. Use the template's headings in place of the dictated SOAP letters. Save the document as XXReport08.06, using your initials in place of *XX* in the file name.

Listen for these pharmaceutical terms:
    albuterol inhaler with InspirEase
    Azmacort

Jordan White is an 11-year-old boy with Hurler syndrome. Over the past months, he has been hospitalized several times with recurrent bronchitis. On this admission, he will undergo laryngoscopy and bronchoscopy to rule out tracheal granulomas.

REPORT 8.7   Operative Report

Use the Report0807.mp3 audio file and the operative report template (Operative_Report) when transcribing this report. This report format was introduced in Chapter 7. Save the document as XXReport08.07, using your initials in place of *XX* in the file name.

Listen for these terms:
    arytenoids
    cannulate
    KTP laser

Because the surgeon and assistant are both listed as doctors in the Physician Directory on the Dictations and Templates CD, add the credentials after the physicians' names.

The provider doesn't use the Informed Consent heading in the dictation, but since the heading is available in the template, it should be included in the report.

Also, use the template's Complications heading even though the heading is not dictated. Transcribe the dictated comment about complications under the heading.

Thomas Kalamara is a 17-year-old young man who complained of severe pain on the right side and immediately collapsed. He was rushed to the emergency room. Chest x-ray revealed a collapse of his right lung. He is being taken to the OR for immediate surgery.

REPORT 8.8   Operative Report

Use the Report0808.mp3 audio file and the operative report template (Operative_Report) when transcribing this report. Save the document as XXReport08.08, using your initials in place of *XX* in the file name.

Listen for these terms:
   2-0 Vicryl
   4-0 Monocryl
   apical
   blebs
   bullous
   emphysematous bullae
   latissimus
   pneumothoraces
   pneumothorax
   Scarpa layer
   Surgiport

Listen for at least one dictated dangerous abbreviation, and be sure to use the acceptable replacement.

Numbers may be written as arabic numerals or written out depending on their usage and/or placement in the sentence. Apply the correct rule for transcribing the number "two" in this report.

Rychena Karina is referred for a repeat chest x-ray by Dr. Ellinger. She has had recent surgery and has a pulse oximeter reading of 87% on room air.

REPORT 8.9   Radiology Report

Use the Report0809.mp3 audio file and the radiology report template (Radiology_Report) when transcribing this report. Save the document as XXReport08.09, using your initials in place of *XX* in the file name.

Listen for these terms:
    lytic
    metaphysis
    metastasis
    perihilar
    sclerotic

This report format will be introduced in Chapter 9. Review information about the radiology report on page 471 of Appendix A.

The name of the test is to be keyed within the first field in the template's body, following the identifying information at the top of the report. Since this is a chest x-ray, set that test name in all capital letters on a line by itself. The technique (details about the test) and findings (what the radiographer observed) will be dictated without headings, but include the headings in the transcribed report. The Impression heading is dictated. The template's Indication heading will not be used in this report.

Remember that an impression is a type of diagnosis. When a report contains more than one diagnosis, the diagnoses should be listed in a numbered list in the transcribed report.

Jeffrey has been diagnosed with a kidney tumor and is sent for CT scan to determine if there are metastases in his lungs. Dr. Barney notes that there are some small pleural effusions.

REPORT 8.10   Radiology Report

Use the Report0810.mp3 audio file and the radiology report template (Radiology_Report) when transcribing this report. Save the document as XXReport08.10, using your initials in place of *XX* in the file name.

Listen for these terms:
    atelectasis
    parenchymal
    postop (postoperative)

As with Report 8.9, the test name (CT chest) should be set in all capital letters on the first line of the body of the report. Include the template's Technique and Findings headings, even though they are not dictated.

Nine

Cardiology

Cardiology is the study of the heart and the blood vessels that carry blood throughout the body. Cardiovascular diseases are the major cause of death in the United States and many other Western societies. Over the last few decades, however, advances in surgical techniques and knowledge about lifestyle and diet effects on the cardiovascular system have resulted in a significant decline in the death rate from heart disease. Medical transcriptionists working in cardiology are constantly challenged by the changing terminology for procedures, new drugs, and technology.

Objectives

» Identify and understand the anatomy and function of the heart.

» Distinguish the different forms of heart disease and their treatment.

» Recognize drug classes used in the prevention and treatment of heart disease.

» Recognize laboratory tests used to evaluate and monitor heart disease.

» Identify invasive and noninvasive procedures used in the diagnosis and treatment of heart disease.

» Pronounce and correctly spell terminology related to cardiology.

» Transcribe dictation related to the medical specialty of cardiology.

» Describe a radiology report, including typical content, format, and turnaround time.

Cardiology is the study of the heart and the vessels surrounding the heart. The heart is a muscular pump that circulates blood through the body via the pulmonary and systemic circulation. The physician who specializes in this field is the cardiologist. Subspecialists include interventional cardiologists, who assess the function of the heart through invasive and noninvasive procedures, and cardiovascular surgeons, who operate on the heart and its vessels.

Structure and Function

The function of the heart is to pump blood throughout the body. The blood vessels are arranged so that each contraction of the heart pumps blood through the pulmonary circulation and the systemic circulation simultaneously, although each has a distinct purpose.

The heart and great vessels are located between the lungs in the middle of the thoracic rib cage, which is called the mediastinum (Figure 9.1). The normal heart extends from the second to the fifth intercostal space and from the right sternal border to the left midclavicular line. The heart is shaped like a triangle with the wider portion, called the base, located on the top, and the point, or apex, pointing downward and to the left.

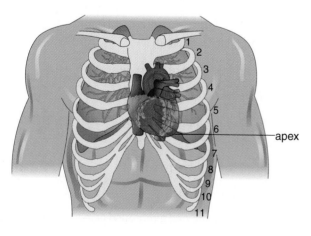

Figure 9.1 Position of the Heart in the Thoracic Cavity

The heart is surrounded by several layers of tissue. The pericardium is a tough, fibrous protective sac that contains pericardial fluid. This fluid facilitates smooth movement of the heart muscle. The myocardium, the muscular wall of the heart, is the tissue that does the actual pumping. The endocardium is the thin membrane of tissue lining the inside of the heart.

Figure 9.2 illustrates the internal structures of the heart. A wall called the septum separates the two sides of the heart. Each side consists of two chambers: an atrium (anteroom), which holds the blood, and a ventricle, which pumps the blood. One-way valves at the entry to each chamber open only in response to pressure gradients, preventing backflow.

The right side of the heart pumps blood into the lungs, and the left side simultaneously pumps blood throughout the body. Figure 9.3 illustrates the blood flow in the heart. The atrioventricular (AV) valves separate the atria and ventricles. The right AV valve is the tricuspid, and the left AV valve is the bicuspid, or mitral valve. The AV valves open during the heart's filling phase, or diastole. This allows the ventricles to fill with blood. During the systole phase, when the heart pumps blood out of the ventricles, the valves close to prevent regurgitation of blood back into the atria.

The semilunar (SL) valves are located between the ventricles and the arteries. The pulmonic valve is in the right side of the heart, and the aortic valve is in the left side. They open during systole to allow ejection of blood from the heart.

The cardiac cycle, consisting of diastole and systole, is produced in response to an electrical current contained within specialized cells in the sinoatrial (SA) node located near the superior vena cava (Figure 9.4). Because the SA node has its own rhythm, it is known as the heart's "pacemaker."

During each cardiac cycle, unoxygenated red blood cells are pumped from the right side of the heart into the lungs for oxygenation. Simultaneously, the left side of the heart pumps oxygenated

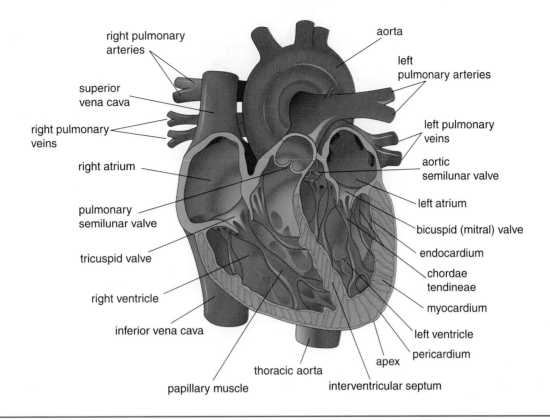

right pulmonary arteries

superior vena cava

right pulmonary veins

right atrium

pulmonary semilunar valve

tricuspid valve

right ventricle

inferior vena cava

papillary muscle

thoracic aorta

aorta

left pulmonary arteries

left pulmonary veins

aortic semilunar valve

left atrium

bicuspid (mitral) valve

endocardium

chordae tendineae

myocardium

left ventricle

pericardium

apex

interventricular septum

Figure 9.2   Internal Structures of the Heart

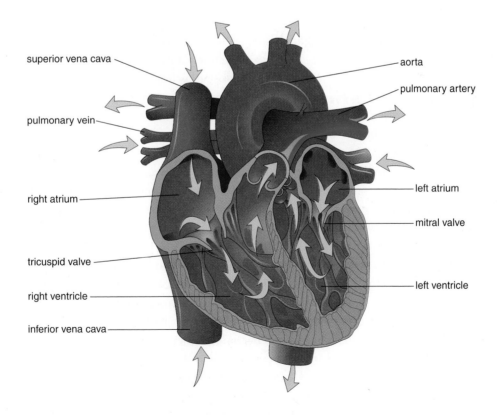

superior vena cava

pulmonary vein

right atrium

tricuspid valve

right ventricle

inferior vena cava

aorta

pulmonary artery

left atrium

mitral valve

left ventricle

Figure 9.3   Blood Flow in the Heart

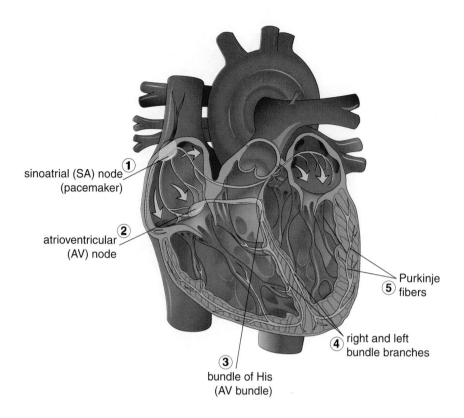

Figure 9.4   Electrical Current Flow in the Heart

blood into the body. The heart pumps between 4 and 6 liters of blood per minute throughout the body.

Physical Assessment

Cardiovascular assessment begins by noting the patient's vital signs. Abnormal respirations, blood pressure, and pulse can indicate heart disease. Other significant symptoms to note on examination include edema, pallor, and sweating (diaphoresis). A bluish color around the lips (circumoral cyanosis) and/or on the nail beds may indicate decreased oxygen. Clubbing of the fingers is a sign of chronic oxygen deficiency. Distention of the jugular veins in the neck is characteristic of right-sided heart failure. The examiner uses palpation to feel for the pulses and auscultation to listen for bruits or other abnormal sounds. Bruits in the carotid arteries may indicate occlusion of the carotid arteries.

The examiner may palpate the patient's chest for the point of maximal impulse (PMI). A complete assessment includes auscultation of the heart's sounds in four areas: at the apex, left sternal edge, aortic area, and pulmonary area. The start of systole, caused by the mitral and tricuspid valves closing, is noted as S1 (the first heart sound) and serves as the reference point for the other cardiac sounds. S2 (the second heart sound) represents the closure of the aortic and pulmonary valves. A third heart sound may be heard in children and is inconsequential; in adults S3 may indicate left ventricular failure. A fourth heart sound, S4, is abnormal and is caused by atrial hypertrophy.

The heart is examined with the patient in different positions to be sure that any murmurs or abnormal heart sounds are detected. Murmurs are described in relation to systole or diastole and the intensity of the sound is described on a scale of 1 to 6. For example, the physician may dictate "a grade two over six systolic ejection murmur," which is transcribed as 2/6 systolic ejection murmur. Other terms used to describe heart sounds include gallop, rub, click, musical, whistle, and thrill. The rhythm may be described as sinus rhythm, regular, and irregular. The rate may be described as bradycardic or tachycardic.

Diseases and Conditions

Heart disease can be divided into several major categories.

Coronary Artery Disease (Ischemic Heart Disease)

Ischemic heart disease, commonly called coronary artery disease (CAD), results when the coronary arteries are narrowed or occluded, preventing adequate blood, and therefore oxygen, from reaching the heart muscle. Ischemia causes chest pain (angina pectoris), and an acute ischemic event is a myocardial infarction (heart attack). The most common cause of occlusion is accumulation of plaque in the arterial lumen caused by high concentrations of lipids or lipoproteins in the blood, a condition called dyslipidemia. Stents may be placed to open occluded arteries, or bypass surgery may be performed to route blood around the blockage. Much effort is placed on preventing ischemic heart disease through diet, lifestyle changes, and medications to correct dyslipidemia.

Heart Failure

Heart failure is characterized by a weakening of the heart muscle, preventing adequate contraction. The most common form is congestive heart failure resulting in fluid accumulation, especially in the lungs and extremities (edema). Patients may experience acute weight gain, shortness of breath, and peripheral edema. Treatment includes diuretics to decrease fluid volume and reduce edema as well as ACE inhibitors to decrease systemic vascular resistance. Heart failure affects 5 million people in the United States, resulting in 12 to 15 million annual office visits and costing an estimated $31 billion annually.

Dysrhythmias

Dysrhythmias are characterized by slow heart rhythms (bradycardia), fast heart rhythms (tachycardia), or irregular heart rhythms. Dysrhythmias have several causes including electrical conduction problems (blocks), disturbances of the sinoatrial node (SA node), metabolic disturbance of electrolytes (sodium, potassium, calcium), muscle damage (infarction, hypertrophy, fibrosis), or reactions of the autonomic nervous system (vasovagal reaction). Atrial fibrillation is a common type of arrhythmia. Atrial fibrillation prevents adequate contraction of the ventricles, effectively stopping the pumping action of the heart. Patients may present with syncope (fainting), lightheadedness, dizzy spells, palpitations, or a sensation of a "skipped beat." Common treatments for arrhythmias include medication (antiarrhythmics), radiofrequency ablation of nodes, and pacemaker placement. Electrophysiology is the study of the "electrical" aspects of the heart that affect rate and rhythm.

Congenital Defects

Defects in structure cause a significant number of heart problems. Congenital malformations include tetralogy of Fallot, patent ductus arteriosus, atrioseptal defects, coarctation of the aorta, and valvular abnormalities. Most malformations are treated with surgery.

Valvular Disorders

Valvular disease interferes with the proper flow of blood into the chambers and arteries. Valves may be stenotic (narrowed), prolapsed (floppy), or weakened, allowing regurgitation (backflow) of blood. Valvular disorders may be congenital or acquired. The most common cause of mitral valve disease is rheumatic fever with cardiac involvement. Patients with mild or moderate valvular disease are treated with prophylactic antibiotics before invasive procedures and dental work to prevent bacteria from lodging in the defective valve, leading to endocarditis. Severe valvular disease may be treated with surgical placement of prosthetic valves.

Cardiomyopathies and Hypertensive Heart Disease

Cardiomyopathies include a group of diseases affecting the myocardium (causes other than ischemia, congenital, and valvular defects). Etiologies include genetic abnormalities, alcoholism, hypertension, and chemotherapy regimens. Cardiomyopathy may be classified as dilated, hypertrophic, or restrictive. One form of hypertrophic cardiomyopathy is a genetic disorder which manifests in late teens or early twenties resulting in an enlarged myocardium and is often the cause of sudden death in young, healthy athletes. Physical findings of cardiomyopathy may include left ventricular hypertrophy, diastolic dysfunction, increased jugular venous pressure, and cardiomegaly. The most common symptoms of cardiomyopathy are dyspnea, fatigue, and syncope, although there is a wide range of symptoms and treatments.

Infection and Inflammation

Specific tissues within or around the heart may become infected and/or inflamed. Myocarditis is inflammation of the heart valves and the myocardium. Endocarditis and pericarditis are inflammation of the inner and outer membranes of the heart. Patients may present with fever and flu-like symptoms and a physical exam commonly reveals a heart murmur. Pericardial effusion may be seen on echocardiogram. Infection may be caused by bacteria, virus, or fungi. Inflammation may be caused by infection, an autoimmune disorder, or a toxic reaction to medications.

Pulmonary Heart Disease (Cor Pulmonale)

In cor pulmonale (pool-mo-**nah**-ly), commonly called pulmonary heart disease, the heart is secondarily affected by disease which starts in the lungs. Chronic obstructive pulmonary disease causes increased resistance to blood flow through the lung tissue, putting backward pressure on the heart. The increased pressure creates a larger workload for the heart and eventually leads to heart damage and heart failure. Chronically decreased oxygen due to inefficient respiration can also affect the heart muscle. Treatment is primarily aimed at treating the underlying pulmonary disease.

Common Tests and Surgical Procedures

Tests for heart disease include those to assess risk and those to diagnose actual disease. Because ischemic heart disease, also known as coronary artery

disease (CAD), is a significant cause of morbidity and mortality in the United States, efforts have been focused on preventing occlusion of the coronary arteries, those vessels which supply blood to the heart muscle. Tests to determine *risk* of coronary artery disease include total cholesterol and the cholesterol fractions LDL, HDL, and VLDL. Maintaining the proper ratio of these cholesterol fractions reduces the formation of plaque that is known to narrow or occlude arterial vessels. Other laboratory tests used to assess risk include homocysteine, Lp(a) (lipoprotein A), highly sensitive CRP (hsCRP), and triglyceride levels.

Laboratory tests are also used to assess the status of *actual* heart damage or disease. A myocardial infarction is evaluated by measuring cardiac enzymes in the blood. Damaged heart muscle releases enzymes into the blood stream that can be measured. These include creatine kinase (CK-MB) and troponin I (TnI, TnT). Congestive heart failure is assessed by measuring brain natriuretic peptide (BNP) which is elevated when the left ventricle is damaged. Electrolytes (sodium, potassium, calcium, and chloride) are also important measures for monitoring disease.

In addition to laboratory tests, diagnosis of heart disease also relies upon invasive and noninvasive tests and imaging studies. Noninvasive tests include chest x-ray, electrocardiogram (ECG or EKG), echocardiogram, stress echocardiogram, multiple gated acquisition (MUGA) scan, Color flow Doppler, and continuous monitoring with a Holter monitor or event recorder. ECGs measure electrical impulses as they pass through the heart, and echocardiograms allow visualization of the movement of the heart walls and heart valves during rest and exercise (stress). Figure 9.5 shows the types of heart rhythms traced by an ECG. Transesophageal echocardiogram (TEE) is a minimally invasive test that is performed by placing the transducer in the esophagus and recording the movement of the heart.

The most common invasive test is cardiac catheterization, which is used to visualize the coronary arteries (angiography) and measure intracardiac pressures and contractility (ventriculogram). In this procedure, a catheter is passed through an incision usually made in the groin and threaded up through

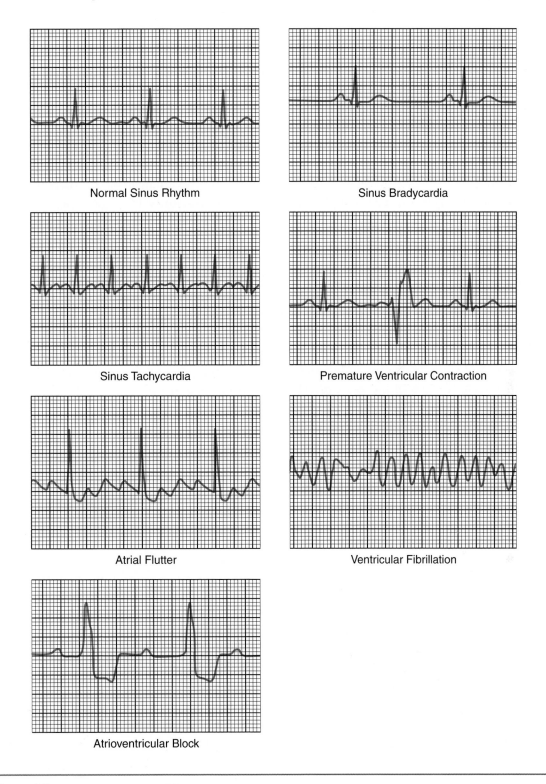

Normal Sinus Rhythm

Sinus Bradycardia

Sinus Tachycardia

Premature Ventricular Contraction

Atrial Flutter

Ventricular Fibrillation

Atrioventricular Block

Figure 9.5   Heart Rhythms in ECG Tracings

the femoral artery into the heart. Fluorescent dye is injected into the coronary arteries to allow visualization of the arteries and areas of occlusion. Often, a stent is placed during the catheterization procedure (called percutaneous coronary intervention or PCI). Stents force occluded arteries to open and remain open. Stents may contain drugs that "elute" (not to be confused with elude) into the bloodstream to prevent future blockage. When stents cannot be used to treat myocardial ischemia or infarction, bypass surgery is performed. A coronary artery bypass graft (CABG, pronounced "cabbage") uses veins and/or arteries from the leg (saphenous vein) or chest wall (internal mammary artery) to route blood from the aorta, around the blockage, and to the muscle tissue, thereby restoring oxygen to that area of the heart wall.

Patients with heart disease often take a battery of medications to reduce fluid volume (diuretics), increase contractile strength of the heart muscle (inotropics), control rhythm (antiarrhythmics), prevent clotting (anticoagulants), and to dilate blood vessels (nitroglycerin). Controlling blood pressure is integral to managing heart disease. Antihypertensives include ACE inhibitors, beta blockers, and calcium-channel blockers. Patients with valvular disease or atrial fibrillation may also be treated with anticoagulants (especially Coumadin) to prevent clots from forming in places where the blood pools or moves slowly. Prophylactic antibiotics are also given. Prevention and treatment of coronary artery disease includes medications to reduce cholesterol, such as statins.

Surgical procedures include pacemaker placement, coronary artery bypass grafting (CABG) and stent placement to open or bypass blocked arteries, valve repair or replacement, correction of congenital malformations, and radiofrequency node ablation to treat arrhythmias. In extreme cases, cardiac transplant is performed.

Terms Bank

These terms and abbreviations provide a foundation for the language and transcription skills you will develop in the following sections of this chapter. Terms marked with » will be included in the reports transcribed in the Building Transcription Skills section.

acyanotic »
(ay-sI-a-**not**-ik) (adj) pertaining to the absence of cyanosis (slightly bluish, grayish, slatelike, or dark purple discoloration of the skin due to a reduction of oxygenated blood

ambulation
(am-byoo-**lay**-shun) (n) walking or moving about

anastomosis
(a-**nas**-tO-mO-sis) (n) a natural or surgical connection between two blood vessels, spaces, or organs

aneurysm
(**an**-yoo-rizm) (n) bulging out of an arterial wall due to a weakness in the wall

angina pectoris
(**an**-ji-na / an-**jI**-na **pek**-tO-ris) (n) an attack of intense chest pain; also known as stenocardia

angiography »
(an-jee-**og**-ra-fee) (n) x-ray of blood vessels, usually after injecting a radiopaque substance

antiplatelet therapy
(anti-**playt**-let) (n) medications used to decrease platelet activity, reducing the likelihood of clot formation, especially in patients at risk for myocardial infarction

aorta »
(ay-**Or**-ta) (n) the main artery leaving the heart

aortic root »
(ay-**Or**-tik) (n) the opening of the aorta in the left ventricle of the heart

aortogram
(ay-**Or**-tO-gram) (n) x-ray of the aorta after injection of a radiopaque substance

arrhythmia
(a-**rith**-mee-a) (n) disturbance of normal rhythm; irregular heartbeat

arteriosclerosis
(ar-**teer**-ee-O-skler-**O**-sis) (n) hardening of the arteries

artery
(**ar**-ter-ee) (n) a vessel that carries blood away from the heart to other tissues throughout the body

ascending aorta
(n) the beginning section of the aorta, rising from the left ventricle of the heart to the arch

asymptomatic »
(ay-simp-tO-**mat**-ik) (adj) without symptoms

atelectasis »
(at-e-**lek**-ta-sis) (n) incomplete expansion of the lungs at birth or collapse of the adult lung

atherosclerosis
(**ath**-er-O-skler-**O**-sis) (n) buildup of fatty plaques inside arteries; a type of arteriosclerosis

atrial
(**ay**-tree-al) (adj) relating to the atrium

atrioventricular »
(**ay**-tree-O-ven-**trik**-yoo-lar) (adj) relating to both the atria (upper chambers) and the ventricles (lower chambers) in the heart, or blood flow between them

atrioventricular groove »
(n) a groove visible on the outside of the heart between the atria and the ventricles

atrium
(**ay**-tree-um) (n) one of the two upper chambers of the heart

attenuation
(a-ten-yoo-**ay**-shun) (n) process of weakening, such as the potency of a drug or the virulence of a disease-causing germ

auscultation »
(aws-kul-**tay**-shun) (n) process of listening for sounds produced in some of the body cavities to detect abnormal conditions

autologous »
(aw-**tol**-O-gus) (adj) indicating something that has its origin within an individual, especially a factor present in tissues or fluids

caliber
(**kal**-i-ber) (n) diameter of a tube or vessel, such as a blood vessel

capillary
(**kap**-i-layr-ee) (n) smallest type of blood vessels

cardiac tamponade
(**kar**-dee-ak tam-po-**nayd**) (n) compression of the venous return to the heart by fluid or blood in the pericardium

cardiomyopathy
(**kar**-dee-O-mI-**op**-a-thee) (n) disease of the heart muscle

cardioversion
(**kar**-dee-O-ver-zhun) (n) the conversion of an abnormal cardiac rhythm to a normal cardiac rhythm

catheter
(**kath**-e-ter) (n) a tube inserted into the body for removing or instilling fluids for diagnostic or therapeutic purposes

catheterization »
(**kath**-e-ter-I-**zay**-shun) (n) the insertion of a catheter

circumflex »
(**ser**-kum-fleks) (adj) bending around; describes anatomical structures that are shaped like an arc of a circle

collaterals »
(ko-**lat**-er-als) (n) accompanying, as side by side; blood vessels that branch from larger vessels

compressible »
(kom-**pres**-i-bl) (adj) pressed together; made more compact by or as by pressure

congestive heart failure »
(CHF) (kon-**jes**-tiv) (n) condition in which the heart is unable to pump adequate blood to the tissues and organs, often due to myocardial infarction

coronary bypass surgery
(**kOr**-o-nayr-ee) (n) vein grafts or other surgical methods are used to carry blood from the aorta to branches of the coronary arteries in order to increase the flow beyond a local obstruction

coronary cusp
(n) one of the triangular parts of a heart valve

cor pulmonale
(kore pool-mO-**nah**-ly) (n) pulmonary disease which causes backward pressure on heart and resulting heart damage due to resistance to blood flow through the lung tissue

cyanosis
(cI-a-n**O**-sis) (n) bluish discoloration of the skin and/or mucous membranes due to decreased amount of oxygen in the blood cells

deep vein (or venous) thrombosis »
(deep vayn throm-**bO**-sis) (n) a clump of various blood components in a blood vessel, forming an obstruction

defibrillator
(dee-**fib**-ri-lay-ter) (n) an agent, measure, or machine, e.g., an electric shock, that stops fibrillation of the ventricular muscle and restores the normal beat

diaphoresis »
(**dI**-a-f**O**-**ree**-sis) (n) profuse perspiration or sweating

diaphragm
(**dI**-a-fram) (n) the muscle that separates the thoracic (chest) and abdominal cavities

digoxin »
(di-**jok**-sin) (n) a heart stimulant

dilatation
(dil-a-**tay**-shun) (n) stretching or enlarging; dilation

distal »
(**dist**al) (adj) away from a center or point of reference; toward the far end of something

distally »
(**dis**-ta-lee) (adv) occurring farthest from the center, from a medial line, or from the trunk

Doppler »
(**dop**-ler) (n) a diagnostic instrument that emits an ultrasonic beam into the body

ductus arteriosus »
(**duk**-tus ar-ter-ee-**O**-sus) (n) blood vessel in the fetus connecting the pulmonary artery directly to the ascending aorta, thus bypassing the pulmonary circulation

dysfunction »
(dis-**funk**-shun) (n) abnormal or impaired function

dyslipidemia
(dis-lip-i-**dee**-mee-a)(n) abnormal ratios of high density lipoproteins (HDL), low density lipoproteins (LDL) and very low density lipoproteins (VLDL) in the blood

echocardiogram »
(ek-O-**kar**-dee-O-gram) (n) a sound-wave image of the heart's size, position, and motion

edema »
(e-**dee**-ma) (n) abnormal accumulation of fluid in intercellular tissue

ejection fraction
(e-**jec**-shun **frak**-shun) (n) the fraction of blood expelled from the ventricle after contraction, normally 50–60%

electrocardiogram »
(ee-**lek**-trO-**kar**-dee-**O**-gram) (n) a graphic record of electrical waves within the heart

elute
(ee-**loot**) to remove from a solid by gradually dissolving in fluid

embolism
(**em**-bO-lizm) (n) blockage of a blood vessel by an abnormal object, such as a clot

endocarditis
(**en**-dO-kar-**dI**-tis) (n) inflammation of the endocardium and/or the heart valves

endocardium
(en-dO-**kar**-dee-um) (n) inner lining of the heart

exudates »
(**eks**-oo-daytz) (n) accumulations of fluid in a cavity; matter that penetrates through vessel walls into adjoining tissues

femoral »
(**fem**-o-ral) (adj) relating to the thigh artery or bone, the femur

femoralis »
(fem-or-**awl**-is) (adj) pertaining to the femur, the longest and strongest bone in body, going from hip to knee

fibrinous »
(**fI**-brin-us) (adj) pertaining to, of the nature of, or containing fibrin (a whitish filamentous protein)

foramen ovale »
(fo-**ray**-men **O**-va-lay) (n) an oval opening through a bone or membrane; a hole normally found in the fetal heart that closes at birth

gestational age »
(ges-**tay**-shun-al aj) (n) age of a fetus or newborn, usually expressed in weeks since the onset of the mother's last menstrual period

gross
(grOs) (adj) visible to the naked eye

heart failure
(n) a cardiac syndrome resulting in a change of cardiac structure and function leading to a decrease in the ventricles' ability to properly fill or eject blood.

hemodynamic »
(**hee**-mO-dI-**nam**-ik) (adj) relating to the mechanics of blood circulation

hemostasis »
(**hee**-mO-stay-sis or hee-**mos**-ta-sis) (n) stopping bleeding either naturally through blood coagulation, mechanically (as with surgical clamps), or chemically (with drugs)

homocysteine
(ho-mO-**sis**-te-een) (n) a sulfur-containing amino acid homologous with cysteine; elevated levels in the blood are an independent risk factor for cardiovascular disease (cf homocystine)

hyperlipidemia
(hI-per-lip-i-**dee**-mee-a) (n) presence of excess lipids, especially cholesterol, in the blood

hypokinesis »
(**hI**-pO-ki-**nee**-sis) (n) decreased or slow motor reaction to stimulus

hypoperfusion »
(**hI**-pO-per-**fyoo**-zhun) (n) lower-than-normal passage of a liquid through an organ or body part

infarction »
(in-**fark**-shun) (n) formation of dead tissue as a result of diminished or stopped blood flow to the tissue area

inferior
(in-**fee**-ree-Or) (adj) lower; below; of lesser value

intimal
(**in**-ti-mal) (adj) relating to the innermost lining of a part, especially of a blood vessel; (n) intima

intravenous »
(IV) (**in**-tra-**vee**-nus) (adj) within or by way of a vein

ischemia »
(is-**kee**-mee-a) (n) decreased blood supply due to obstruction, such as narrowing of the blood vessels

lesion »
(**lee**-zhun) (n) general term for any visible, circumscribed injury to the skin; such as, a wound, sore, rash, or mass

mammary
(**mam**-a-ree) (adj) relating to the breast

millicuries
(**mil**-i-**kyoo**-rees) (n) a unit of radioactivity, abbreviated mCi

mitral »
(**mI**-tral) (adj) relating to the bicuspid or mitral valve of the heart, between the atrium and the ventricle on the left side of the heart

murmur
(**mer**-mer) (n) abnormal heart sound

myocardial »
(mI-O-**kar**-dee-al) (adj) relating to the myocardium, the heart muscle

obtuse »
(ob-**toos**) (adj) dull or blunt; not pointed or acute

occlusion »
(o-**kloo**-zhun) (n) blockage, such as coronary occlusion

orifice »
(**or**-i-fis) (n) mouth, entrance, or outlet of any aperture

oscilloscope
(o-**sil**-O-scOp) (n) an instrument which displays electrical oscillations (waves) on a screen

oximetry »
(ok-**sim**-e-tree) (n) measuring the amount of oxygen combined with the hemoglobin in a blood sample

pallor
(**pal**-or) (n) abnormal paleness of the skin; deficiency of color

palpitations
(pal-pi-**tay**-shuns) (n) stronger and more rapid heartbeats as felt by the patient; pounding or throbbing of the heart

parenteral
(pa-**ren**-ter-al) (adj) not through the digestive system, such as introduction of nutrients into the veins or under the skin

paroxysmal
(par-ok-**siz**-mal) (adj) relating to or recurring in paroxysms (sudden, severe attacks of symptoms or convulsions)

patent
(**pa**-tent) (adj) open; unblocked

pedal
(**ped**-al or **pE**dal) (adj) relating to the foot

pedicle »
(**ped**-i-kl) (n) the stem that attaches a new growth

pedunculated »
(pee-**dung**-Q-late-ed) (adj) possessing a stalk

perfusion »
(per-**fyoo**-zhun) (n) passing of a fluid through spaces

pericardial »
(per-i-**kar**-dee-al) (adj) surrounding the heart; relating to the pericardium

pericardial effusion
(per-i-**kar**-dee-al e-**fyoo**-zhun) (n) increased fluid in the pericardial sac

pericarditis »
(per-i-kar-**dI**-tis) (n) an inflammatory disease of the pericardium (tough outer layer of the heart wall and lining of the pericardial sac that surrounds the heart)

pericardium »
(per-i-**kar**-dee-um) (n) sac around the heart allowing movement without friction

peripheral vascular disease
(pe-**rif**-e-ral **vas**-kyoo-lar)(n) any disorder affecting the blood circulatory system, except the heart

phasic »
(**fay**-sic) (adj) pertaining to a phase, a stage of development

phlebitis »
(fle-**bI**-tis) (n) inflammation of a vein

phlebotomy
(fle-**bot**-O-mee) (n) incision into a vein for drawing blood

photon »
(**fO**-ton) (n) a unit of radiant energy or light intensity

pleural »
(**ploo**-ral) (adj) concerning the pleura (serous membrane that enfolds both lungs and is reflected upon the walls of the thorax and diaphragm)

popliteal »
(pop-**lit**-ee-al) (adj) concerning the posterior surface of the knee

precordial »
(pree-**kor**-dee-al) (adj) pertaining to the precordium (region of the chest over the heart)

prolapse »
(prO-**laps**) (n) dropping of an organ from its normal position, a sinking down

proximal »
(**prok**-si-mal) (adj) nearest the point of attachment, center of the body, or point of reference

proximally »
(**prok**-si-mal-lee) (adv) occurring nearest to the point of attachment, center of the body, or point of reference

radiopaque
(ray-dee-O-**payk**) (adj) opaque to x-rays or other radiation; an injection of a radiopaque dye or substance may be used to visualize areas of the body by x-ray

ramus »
(**ray**-mus) (n) branch, especially of a nerve or blood vessel

reflux »
(**ree**-fluks) (n) a return or backward flow

regurgitation »
(ree-**ger**-ji-**tay**-shun) (n) a backward flowing, as a backflow of blood through a defective heart valve or the bringing up of gas or undigested food from the stomach

retrograde »
(**ret**-rO-grayd) (adj) moving or going backward

rheumatic fever »
(roo-**mat**-ik **fee**-ver) (n) fever following infection with *Streptococcus* bacteria; may affect the joints, skin, and heart

saphenous vein »
(sa-**fee**-nus vayn) (n) either of two main veins in the leg that drain blood from the foot

scan
(n) scanning a tissue, organ, or system using a special apparatus that displays and records its image, such as computer tomography (CAT scan); the image so obtained

septal »
(**sep**-tal) (adj) pertaining to a dividing partition

septum »
(**sep**-tum) (n) a partition that separates a structure, as the two sides of the heart

sheath
(n) structure surrounding an organ, body part, or object

sinus rhythm
(**si**-nus **rith**-um) (n) normal cardiac rhythm

situs »
(**sI**-tus) (n) a position

stenocardia
(sten-O-**kar**-dee-a) (n) an attack of intense chest pain; also called angina pectoris

stenosis »
(ste-**nO**-sis) (n) narrowing or constriction of a passageway or opening, such as a blood vessel

sublingual
(sub-**ling**-gwahl) (adj) beneath the tongue

subxiphoid »
(sub-**zif**-oyd) (adj) below a sword-shaped structure, as the xiphoid process, a structure beneath the lowest portion of the sternum

systolic »
(sis-**tol**-ik) (adj) pertaining to systole, the part of the heart cycle in which the heart is in contraction

thermodilution
(**ther**-mO-di-**loo**-shun) (n) method of determining cardiac output; involves injecting a cold liquid into the bloodstream and measuring the temperature change downstream

thrombophlebitis
(**throm**-bO-fle-**bI**-tis) (n) inflammation of a vein with clot formation (thrombus)

thrombus »
(**throm**-bus) (n) blood clot attached to the interior wall of a vein or artery

tibia »
(tib-ee-a) (n) inner and thicker of the two bones of the human leg between the knee and the ankle

tibial »
(tib-ee-al) (adj) pertaining to the tibia

transesophageal »
(tranz-ee-sof-a-**jee**-al) (adj) pertaining to an abnormal opening between the trachea and esophagus

tomographic »
(tO-**mog**-ra-feek) (adj) referring to an x-ray technique which displays an organ or tissue at a particular depth

vena cava »
(**vee**-na **kav**-a) (n) one of the largest veins of the body; venae cavae (pl)

vascular
(**vas**-kyoo-lar) (adj) relating to the blood vessels

veno-occlusive »
(**vee**-nO O-**kloo**-siv) (adj) concerning obstruction of veins

venous »
(**vee**-nus) (adj) relating to a vein or veins

ventricle
(**ven**-tri-kl) (n) either of the two lower chambers of the heart

ventriculogram
(ven-**trik**-yoo-lO-gram) (n) an x-ray of the ventricles

ventriculography
(ven-trik-yoo-**log**-ra-fee) (n) x-ray visualization of heart ventricles after injection of a radiopaque substance

xiphoid
(**zif**-oyd) (adj) referring to the xiphoid process, the cartilage at the lower end of the sternum (breast bone); also spelled xyphoid

Abbreviations

ACE	angiotensin converting enzyme	K+	potassium
ACG	angiocardiography	LAD	left anterior descending coronary artery
AF or A fib	atrial fibrillation	LCA	left coronary artery
		LCF	left circumflex
AICA	anterior inferior communicating artery	LDL	low density lipoprotein
AS	aortic stenosis	LIMA	left internal mammary artery
ASD	atrial septal defect	LMCA	left main coronary artery
ASHD	arteriosclerotic heart disease	LPA	left pulmonary artery
AV	atrioventricular	MCL	midclavicular line
BBB	bundle-branch block	METs	metabolic equivalent of tasks
BMP	basic metabolic profile or panel	MI	myocardial infarction
BNP	brain natriuretic peptide	MPA	main pulmonary artery
Ca+	calcium	MR	mitral regurgitation
CABG	coronary artery bypass grafting	MS	mitral stenosis
CAD	coronary artery disease	MUGA	multiple gated acquisition (scan)
CC	cardiac catheterization	MVP	mitral valve prolapse
CCU	coronary care unit	Na+	sodium
CF	circumflex (artery)	OM	obtuse marginal [coronary artery]
CHF	congestive heart failure	PA	pulmonary artery
CK	creatine kinase	PAT	paroxysmal atrial tachycardia
CK-MB	creatine kinase myocardial band	PCI	percutaneous coronary intervention
CP	chest pain	PDA	posterior descending artery; patent ductus arteriosus
CPR	cardiopulmonary resuscitation		
CV	cardiovascular	PICA	posterior inferior communicating artery
CVA	cerebrovascular accident	PMI	point of maximal impulse
DVT	deep vein thrombosis	PVC	premature ventricular contraction
ECG or EKG	electrocardiogram	RAO	right anterior oblique (view)
		RCA	right coronary artery
EF	ejection fraction	RPA	right pulmonary artery
HDL	high density lipoprotein	SA	sinoatrial node
HF	heart failure	SFA	superficial femoral artery
hsCRP	highly sensitive C-reactive protein	SL	semilunar
HTN	hypertension	TEE	transesophageal echocardiogram
ICA	internal carotid artery	VLDL	very low density lipoprotein
IMA	internal mammary artery	VSD	ventricular septal defect
IV	intravenous		

Complete the following exercises, drawing on the information learned in the Exploring Cardiology section of this chapter and referencing the Terms Bank.

Exercise 9.1   Matching Sound and Spelling

The numbered list that follows shows the phonetic spelling of hard-to-spell words. Sound out the word and then write the correct spelling in the blank space provided. Check your answers in the Terms Bank or another appropriate reference.

1. **zif**-oyd _____

2. a-**rith**-mee-a _____

3. a-**nas**-tO-mO-sis _____

4. ni-**fed**-i-peen _____

5. lls-**in**-O-pril _____

6. lO-va-**stat**-in _____

7. **lee**-zhun _____

8. o-**kloo**-zhun _____

9. **an**-yoo-rizm _____

10. **vee**-nus _____

11. te-**ray**-zO-sin _____

12. pal-pi-**tay**-shuns _____

13. an-**jI**-na _____

14. ver-**ap**-a-mil _____

15. **cap**-tO-pril _____

Exercise 9.2   Recognizing Alike Words

Below is a list of frequently used words that look alike and/or sound alike. Study the meaning and pronunciation of each set of words, read the following sentences carefully, and then circle the word in parentheses that correctly completes the meaning.

BMP	(n) basic metabolic profile	**nitrate**	a salt of nitric acid; medication
BNP	(n) brain natriuretic peptide	**nitrite**	a salt of nitrous acid; found on urinalysis
corollary	consequence, result		
coronary	pertaining to the heart	**palpation**	examination by touching
		palpitation	rapid or fluttering heartbeat
effuse	(v) to flow out, emanate		
perfuse	(v) to spread about	**pedal**	(adj) relating to the foot
profuse	(adj) overabundant	**pedal**	(n) a foot-operated mechanism
		petal	(n) part of a flower
elude	(v) to avoid adroitly		
elute	(v) to remove from a solid by dissolving in fluid	**pericardial**	surrounding the heart
		precordial	in front of the heart
endocardial	within the heart	**plus**	increased by or added to
myocardial	relating to the heart muscle	**pulse**	regular, rhythmic beat
infra-	below or under	**recent**	(adj) not long ago
inter-	between	**resent**	(v) to be annoyed at
intra-	within		
		reinfected	infected again (as with an organism or pathogen)
instant	(adv) immediately		
in-stent	(adj) occurring within a stent	**reinjected**	injected again (as with a drug)

1. The patient's (interocular/intraocular) pressure was within normal limits.

2. A (recent/resent) blood pressure check reveals the patient to be hypertensive.

3. The posterior tibial (pluses/pulses) were 2+/4+.

4. The patient had 1+ (pedal/petal) edema.

5. The patient was given an (infection/injection) of amoxicillin (intramuscularly/intermuscularly).

6. Her urine shows no red cells, trace leukocytes, and positive (nitrates/nitrites).

7. The patient has no tenderness to deep (palpation/palpitation).

8. She is complaining of (palpations/palpitations) after drinking several cups of coffee.

9. His night sweats are so (perfuse/profuse) that he regularly soaks his pajamas.

10. His previous surgeries resulted in (pericardial/precordial) adhesions in various areas.

When transcribing dictation, the medical transcriptionist frequently needs to consider the situation when determining the word that correctly completes the sentence. From the list below, select the term that meaningfully completes each of the following statements.

ambulating	diaphoresis	ischemia
arrhythmia	dilatation	oximetry
artery	hemodynamic	prolapse
attenuation	infarction	proximal
catheter	intravenous	ventricular

1. If the patient had an MI, it means he or she had a myocardial _____.

2. The patient is _____ well with the use of a quad cane.

3. Due to dehydration, she will need _____ fluids.

4. The blockage was not in a main _____.

5. While my father was in the hospital, he was monitored by pulse _____.

6. The patient's ECG showed left _____ dysfunction.

7. After the surgery, he needed a transfusion to return him to his usual _____ state.

8. The patient's mitral valve _____ meant she needed to take an antibiotic whenever she had dental work done.

9. A vaccine gives you a (an) _____ of the disease.

10. He needed a Foley _____ inserted to collect the urine.

Exercise 9.4   Pairing Words and Meanings

From this list, locate the term that best matches each of the following definitions. Write the term in the space provided by each definition.

angiography	hypertension	stenosis
aorta	ischemia	thermodilution
atrium	myocardial	ventricle
diaphoresis	pericardial	
hemostasis	ramus	

1. concerning the middle layer of the heart walls   _____

2. branch of a nerve or blood vessel   _____

3. method of cardiac output determination   _____

4. study describing the blood vessels of the heart   _____

5. main trunk of the arterial system   _____

6. decreased blood supply to a given body part   _____

7. abnormal narrowing of a passageway or opening   _____

8. profuse sweating   _____

9. either of the two upper chambers of the heart   _____

10. cessation of bleeding   _____

Combine prefixes, root words, and suffixes from this list to create medical words that fit the following definitions. Fill in the blanks with the words you construct.

a-	no, without	sub-	beneath, under
brady-	slow	tachy-	swift, rapid
cardio-	heart	cor	heart
circum-	around	-cardia/o	heart
dia-	through, complete	-flect/-flex	bend
dynamo-	relating to force, energy	-function	work, action, operation
dys-	pain, improper, short	-gram	letter, picture, printout
electro-	current, conduction	-lingual	tongue
hemo-	blood, bleeding	-megaly	enlargement
hem/o-	relating to blood	-pathy	disease
intra-	within	-pnea	breathing, breath
myo-	muscle	-stasis	stopping, halting
organ/o	organ	-stolic	sent, sending
peri-	around, near	-ventricular	front, ventricle
pre-	before	-xiph-oid	sword-shaped
steno-	compressed		

1. rapid heartbeat _____

2. under the tongue _____

3. a squeezing pain in the heart _____

4. the stopping of bleeding _____

5. around the heart _____

6. shortness of breath _____

7. sending through (blood into heart) _____

8. bent around _____

9. condition characterized by a slow heartbeat _____

10. complete picture _____

11. within the heart _____

12. beneath the lower end of the sternum (breastbone) _____

13. before (in front of) the heart _____

14. relating to the force of the blood going through the heart _____

15. a picture (recording) of the electrical activity of the heart _____

Read the following report excerpts and look for errors in spelling, punctuation, plural vs. singular word forms, subject-verb agreement, complete sentences, pronoun-reference agreement, capitalization, and special punctuation marks such as quotation marks. Mark the corrections on this page and key the excerpts with all errors corrected. Save the documents as XXExercise09.06-1 and XXExercise09.06-2, using your initials in place of *XX* in the file names.

1.   Left heart catheterization and coronary angiography was performed via Judkins Technique using the rite femoral artery. hemodynamic recordings was made in the ascending aorta at rest.

    blood samples for oximetry were obtained from the pulmonary artery and ascending aorta. Repeat hemodynamic recordings were made on pull-back. The catheter was then withdrawn and direct pressure was applied to the right femoral artery. Both good hemostasis and petal pluses were obtained. the patient tolerated the procedure well and left the laboratory in satisfactory condition.

2.   The patent had no recurant chest pain throughout his admission her periferol adema improved somewhat but is still present.

Read this scenario carefully and then select the most appropriate response. Write an explanation for why you think your choice is the best answer.

You are transcribing a cardiology report on a patient with known congestive heart failure. The physician dictates "BNP 1262," although you are uncertain of the abbreviation. It also sounds like "BMP 1262." Your coworker, with 5 years of experience, tells you she always types "BMP." How can you resolve this problem?

a. Accept your coworker's advice and type BMP.

b. Leave the abbreviation blank.

c. After evaluating the meaning of both abbreviations, type BNP.

d. Type BMP and flag the report for the physician to review.

Best response: _____

Explanation: _____

_____

_____

_____

_____

You will apply the medical specialty and language information you learned in this chapter to transcription work in this section. After you learn the formatting recommendations of a radiology report, you will transcribe five reports related to three different patient studies.

Introducing the Radiology Report

The radiology report (Figure 9.6) is a description of the technique, findings, and interpretations of diagnostic procedures. Dictated by a radiologist after reviewing the films or test results, the report can focus on bone and joint films, soft tissue films, or special studies of the internal organs. The major diagnostic procedures include roentgenograms (basic x-rays), computerized tomography (CT) scans, magnetic resonance imaging (MRI) scans, nuclear medicine procedures such as thyroid scans and bone scans with an injection or infusion of radioactive contrast, and fluoroscopic examinations.

Required Headings/Content

Standard components of the radiology report include the test name (set like a heading in all capital letters), the reason for the study (indication), the technique used, the results of the test (findings), and the radiologist impression of the results. The radiology report will usually include the name of the physician who requested the test at the top of the report.

Refer to page 471 of Appendix A for a complete list of headings found in the radiology report template along with descriptions of the type of information found under each heading. Not every template heading will be included in every transcribed report.

Turnaround Time

The usual turnaround time is 12 to 24 hours or even less. However, some hospitals make a voice report available as soon as the radiologist dictates the report.

Preparing to Transcribe

To prepare for transcribing dictation, review the common cardiology terms and abbreviations in this chapter's Terms Bank. Then, study the format and organization of the model document shown in Figure 9.6, and key the model document, using the radiology report template on the Dictations and Templates CD as a starting point. Save the document as XXFigure09.06, using your initials in place of XX in the file name. Proofread the document by comparing it with the printed version. Categorize the types of errors you made, and document them on a copy of the Performance Comparison Chart. A template of this chart is available on the Dictations and Templates CD.

Transcribing Reports

Transcribe, edit, and correct each report in the following patient studies. Consult reference books for words or formatting rules that are unfamiliar.

As you work on the transcription assignment for this chapter, fill in the Performance Comparison Chart that you started when you keyed the model document. For at least three of the reports, categorize and document the types of errors you made. Answer the document analysis questions on the bottom of the chart. With continuous practice and assessment, the quality of your work will improve.

1" top and side margins

use left justification

PATIENT NAME:	Jim Andrews
MR #:	7093578
DOB:	12/23/XXXX
SEX:	Male
ROOM #:	804
REQUESTING PHYSICIAN:	Sondra Southward, MD
DATE:	01/12/20XX

ds

STRESS THALLIUM SCAN WITH REINJECTION ← test or x-ray name in all caps

ds

TECHNIQUE

At the time of peak exercise, 4 mCi of thallium-201 chloride was injected intravenously and exercise was continued for at least an additional minute. Single-photon emission computer tomographic study, as well as a planar LAO 45 image, was obtained immediately after exercise. The patient returned at least 3 hours later and was reinjected with 1 mCi of thallium-201 chloride. Thirty minutes later, a single-photon emission computer tomographic exam was obtained. The SPECT studies were reconstructed with images obtained in the short, horizontal, long, and vertical long axes. Comparison was made with standard data base, as well as bull's-eye plots. Images were evaluated on film, as well as on the computer console.

ds

FINDINGS

Images reveal some mild, fixed hypoperfusion of the inferior wall compared with the rest of the myocardium. This is probable on the basis of diaphragmatic attenuation. Heart appears smaller on stress than it does on redistribution imaging. Findings consistent with normal response to exercise.

ds

Quantitative analysis reveals several inconsistent areas of hypoperfusion. The inferior wall is relatively unremarkable on these plots.

ds

IMPRESSION

No evidence for stress-induced ischemia.

qs

____

J. Kronin, MD

ds

JK/XX

D: 01/12/20XX

T: 01/12/20XX

Figure 9.6 Radiology Report

Patient Study 9.A   Jim Andrews

The patient is a 63-year-old male who was admitted to the intensive care unit with chest pain radiating down to the left hand, diaphoresis, and pallor. During a routine checkup 2 months ago, his physical examination, blood work, and ECG were within normal limits.

REPORT 9.1   History and Physical

Use the Report0901.mp3 audio file and the history and physical template (History_and_Physical) when transcribing this report. This report will be introduced in Chapter 12, but the content is similar to the discharge summary studied in Chapter 8. Save the document as XXReport09.01, using your initials in place of *XX* in the file name.

If the patient's height is reported in feet and inches, the words feet and inches must be spelled out. Only metric units of measure may be abbreviated. When feet or inches are reported in a table, it is permissible to abbreviate, and an ending period is then necessary. Pounds and ounces must be similarly spelled out.

REPORT 9.2   Radiology Report

Use the Report0902.mp3 audio file and the radiology report template (Radiology_Report) when transcribing this report. Save the document as XXReport09.02, using your initials in place of *XX* in the file name.

Listen for these terms:
    LAO 45 image
    SPECT studies
    thallium-201 chloride

Radiology reports consist of language that is quite different from other medical/surgical language. This is a cardiac radiologic study which may be transcribed by the MT in either the cardiology or radiology department.

REPORT 9.3   Consultation Letter

Use the Report0903.mp3 audio file and the consultation letter template (Consultation_Letter) when transcribing this report. Save the document as XXReport09.03, using your initials in place of *XX* in the file name.

Set the dictator's job title under his signature line. The dictation includes instructions to indicate that enclosures are included with the letter. Therefore, set the word *Enclosures* as double-space (one blank line) below the dictator's and MT's initials. The consultation letter will be mailed with the radiology report transcribed as Report 9.2.

Patient Study 9.B

Chris Beltre

The patient is a 50-year-old male admitted for evaluation of coronary artery disease. His health history included a previous heart attack. During his last admission, the patient had severe chest pain and was diagnosed with acute anterior wall myocardial infarction. A cardiac catheterization showed severe left main coronary artery disease, and subsequent bypass surgery followed by a stress test showed persistent abnormalities at peak exercise. Cardiac catheterization was advised to evaluate the coronary disease and guide further therapy.

REPORT 9.4   Radiology Report

Use the Report0904.mp3 audio file and the radiology report template (Radiology_Report) when transcribing this cardiac catheterization report. Save the document as XXReport09.04, using your initials in place of *XX* in the file name.

This report will run onto a second page. This template will include a continued line in the first-page footer when a document extends onto a second page. If necessary, update the footer field by clicking F9 in the footer area of the document. Open the header and footer with the consecutive key combination Alt, V, H. Set the test name along with the patient's name and medical record number, the report's date, and the page number in the second-page header. Refer to Appendix B for more information.

Patient Study 9.C

Joshua Warren

Twenty-six-year-old Joshua Warren experienced mild chest pains while playing racquetball and subsequently was admitted to the emergency room. A treadmill stress test was ordered to determine the possibility of cardiovascular disease.

REPORT 9.5   Radiology Report

Use the Report0905.mp3 audio file and the radiology report template (Radiology_Report) when transcribing this treadmill stress test report. Save the document as XXReport09.05, using your initials in place of *XX* in the file name.

Use the template's headings when they are synonymous to the dictated headings, but transcribe additional headings and content as dictated.

Use figures for transcribing electrocardiographic chest leads and capital letters for waves and segments. The leads are V1 through V6 and aVL, aVR, and aVF. (It is also acceptable to transcribe the L, R, and F as subscript letters.) Waves include P, Q, R, S, T, and U and their combinations.

This female infant was born prematurely at approximately 24-1/2 weeks' gestation. Cardiovascular surgeons will perform a ductus arteriosus ligation to stabilize the baby's heart function.

REPORT 9.6   Operative Report

Use the Report0906.mp3 audio file and the operative report template (Operative_Report) when transcribing this report. Save the document as XXReport09.06, using your initials in place of *XX* in the file name.

Note that the overall point size will need to be reduced to allow the report to fit on one page. If needed, reduce some space above the signature line.

Junice Monroe is a 65-year-old woman who presented with symptoms of congestive heart failure and lung collapse. A CT scan and an echocardiogram revealed a cardiac tumor, which surgeons will remove.

REPORT 9.7   Operative Report

Use the Report0907.mp3 audio file and the operative report template (Operative_Report) when transcribing this report. Save the document as XXReport09.07, using your initials in place of *XX* in the file name.

Listen for these terms:
    atelectasis
    autologous
    foramen ovale
    Pacifico
    pedicle
    pledgeted
    trilobate

This dictator uses the word "trilobulated" which is not found in the dictionary. The correct term in this context is "trilobar" or "trilobate." It is not unusual for dictators to mispronounce words. It is always best to seek the correct spelling and pronunciation of the intended word, and if this is not possible, follow local guidelines for flagging such words or type them in quotation marks.

This report will continue onto a second page, so a first-page continued line and a second-page header will be needed. The template will include text in the first page footer and second page header, but you will need to update the fields. Use F9.

This 65-year-old man has a history of atherosclerosis and suffered a heart attack 3 years ago. He presented to the ER with chest pain, profuse sweating, and shortness of breath, which his nitroglycerin tablets had failed to relieve.

REPORT 9.8   Discharge Summary

Use the Report0908.mp3 audio file and the discharge summary template (Discharge_Summary) when transcribing this report. Save the document as XXReport09.08, using your initials in place of *XX* in the file name.

Match the template's order when transcribing the sections of the report. Note that the discharge diagnosis is at the top of the report. Also, transcribe the Physical Examination in list format, using the subheadings within the template.

Listen for these terms:
    BUN 21
    Dalmane
    Isordil
    Lasix
    Slow-K

Charles Bassinger is a 16-year-old patient who is suffering from pain in his right leg. Although this may be due to his recent diagnosis of leukemia, Mr. Bassinger is sent for a B-mode Doppler study to rule out DVT.

REPORT 9.9   Radiology Report

Use the Report0909.mp3 audio file and the radiology report template (Radiology_Report) when transcribing this Doppler study report. Save the document as XXReport09.09, using your initials in place of *XX* in the file name.

Use the template's headings when they are synonymous to the dictated headings.

Spell out nonmetric units of measurement and omit a comma between feet and inches.

Jennifer Malone is a pediatric patient who was diagnosed with a kidney tumor during childhood and was successfully treated using chemotherapy. However, as a result of the treatment, she has had a slight cardiac abnormality, which is being followed by the New York Cardiology Associates. The following dictations describe Jennifer's condition over several years.

REPORT 9.10 Radiology Report

Use the Report0910.mp3 audio file and the radiology report template (Radiology_Report) when transcribing this echocardiogram report. Save the document as XXReport09.10, using your initials in place of *XX* in the file name.

Use the template's headings when they are synonymous to the dictated headings.

Listen for these terms:
    D-ventricular looping
    intracardiac
    milliseconds
    pedunculated
    precordial
    situs solitus
    subxiphoid
    SVC

The provider will dictate information that is best set in columns. Use Word's Insert Table feature to transcribe this part of the report.

REPORT 9.11 Consultation Letter

Use the Report0911.mp3 audio file and the consultation letter template (Consultation_Letter) when transcribing this report. Save the document as XXReport09.11, using your initials in place of *XX* in the file name.

Listen for these terms:
    +60 degrees
    acyanotic
    AV
    grade 2/6
    hemodynamic
    QRS
    ST-T
    thrill
    Vasotec
    vibratory systolic murmur

Adjust the font size as needed to allow the letter to fit on one page.

Ten

Gastroenterology

Gastroenterology is the study of the digestive tract, liver, and pancreas. The digestive tract, also called the alimentary canal or gastrointestinal (GI) tract, is similar to a tube with openings at both ends. It includes the mouth, pharynx, esophagus, stomach, and small and large intestines. It also incorporates accessory organs: the salivary glands, teeth, liver, gallbladder, pancreas, and appendix. The physician who specializes in the GI tract is called a gastroenterologist. A rectosigmoid specialist (proctologist) studies diseases of the lower end of the digestive tract.

Objectives

» Identify the organs and components of the gastrointestinal system.

» Describe diseases and conditions that affect the gastrointestinal system.

» Recognize infectious organisms that affect the liver, stomach, and intestines.

» Define the four abdominal quadrants.

» Recognize laboratory tests and imaging studies used to diagnose gastrointestinal disease.

» Pronounce and correctly spell terminology related to gastroenterology.

» Transcribe dictation related to the medical specialty of gastroenterology.

» Describe a pathology report, including typical content, format, and turnaround time.

igestion, absorption, and elimination are the processes of the gastrointestinal tract. This complex system feeds the cells of the body, providing energy for cellular functions. As with the other systems of the body, the digestive system involves several organs and interacts with other body systems to carry out its vital functions. (See Figure 10.1)

Structure and Function

The mouth is the first organ of digestion. Food enters the body through the mouth, and the teeth masticate, or chew, to break the food into small particles. The salivary glands (parotid, submaxillary, and sublingual) located in the mouth secrete digestive juices and salivary enzymes, including amylase, at the rate of about 1.5 L per day. These substances begin the digestion process. As the food is swallowed, it passes through the pharynx into the esophagus by an involuntary process that causes the epiglottis to cover the tracheal opening. This prevents the aspiration of food into the airways. Esophageal peristalsis, or rhythmic muscle movements, cause the food to move down the esophagus, passing the lower esophageal sphincter (cardiac sphincter), and into the stomach. In

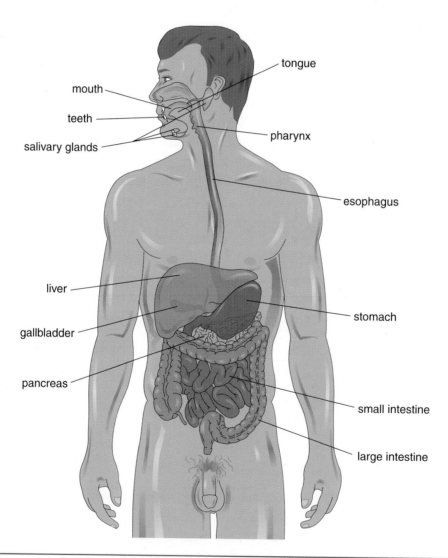

Figure 10.1 Organs of the Digestive System

order to prevent reflux into the esophagus, this sphincter closes tightly when the food enters the stomach.

In the stomach, hydrochloric acid is secreted by the gastric gland to further decompose the food particles. This highly acidic fluid is produced at the rate of about 2.5 L per day. Pepsin is secreted to begin the digestion of proteins. Additionally, intrinsic factor is produced and aids in the absorption of vitamin B_{12} in the ileum.

The pyloric sphincter acts as a two-way valve moving small, digested particles toward the small intestine and preventing large particles from entering too soon to allow proper absorption of nutrients. In the small intestine (Figure 10.2), the duodenum continues the digestive processes. There are several hormones and other regulators that control the secretions of the digestive system. Alkaline digestive juices flow into the intestine from the pancreas and neutralize the acid contents. Other digestive enzymes produced in the pancreas continue to break down the food. Trypsin, amylase, and lipase assist in the digestion of proteins, starches, and fats, respectively. The intestinal glands secrete mucus, which coats the lining of the intestine and protects it from erosion by the acidic juices.

Bile is secreted by the liver and stored in the gallbladder (Figure 10.3). When needed, the bile salts, cholesterol, and lecithin contained in the bile emulsify fatty substances into products that can be absorbed by the small intestine. At this point, peristalsis (the contractions of the intestine) causes the contents of the small intestine to be propelled into the colon, or large intestine (Figure 10.4).

Bacteria, known as normal flora, are present in the large intestine and play an important role in digestion, assisting with the absorption of bile salts and the further breakdown of waste products. *Escherichia coli,* or *E coli,* is one of the most common bacteria that normally occur in the intestines.

The final step of digestion is moving the waste material out of the body. As peristalsis propels waste products through the small intestine, the ileocecal valve opens, allowing some contents to enter the colon. Once waste has moved past the ileocecal valve, the valve closes to prevent the products from moving back into the small intestine. As the waste fills the colon and reaches the rectum, the rectum expands until there is an urge to defecate. The movement of waste from the rectum and out of the body can take up to three days, a period that allows for the resorption of fluid and electrolytes.

Stool, or feces, contains undigested foodstuffs, bacteria, water, and inorganic matter. The characteristic brown color is produced as bile is broken down by bacteria within the intestine. The fecal odor is caused by chemicals produced during digestion. The gastrointestinal tract contains gas from swallowed air and the action of intestinal bacteria. Gas expelled through the mouth is called a *belch, burp,* or *eructation;* gas expelled from the anus is called *flatus.*

Physical Assessment

Obtaining an accurate, complete patient history is probably the most important technique for the examiner. The patient is asked to describe any problems, starting from the mouth and teeth, and ending with a description of bowel habits. Diet and eating habits can suggest routines that could lead to the improper functioning of the GI organs. The mouth is inspected for proper moisture, teeth alignment, and any deviations in the structures. Next, the examiner may auscultate the abdomen from the epigastric area down to the suprapubic area, using a stethoscope and

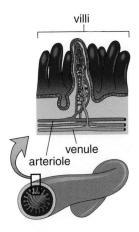

Figure 10.2 Cross Section of the Small Intestine

dividing the abdomen into four sections called quadrants (see Figure 10.5). Each quadrant is examined since different sounds might be heard in different areas. The physician then percusses (taps) all four quadrants, listening for the different sounds from the gas-filled mid-abdomen versus the denser spleen and liver. Lastly, the examiner palpates the abdomen from the suprapubic area up to the ribs, watching the patient for signs of pain, tenderness, or rebound tenderness, and palpating for masses, adenopathy, or organomegaly. Although it is customary to perform palpation before auscultation with other systems of the body, this is reversed in the examination of the abdomen since palpation could change the sound and pattern of gas within the intestine, and this could have an influence on the results of the examination.

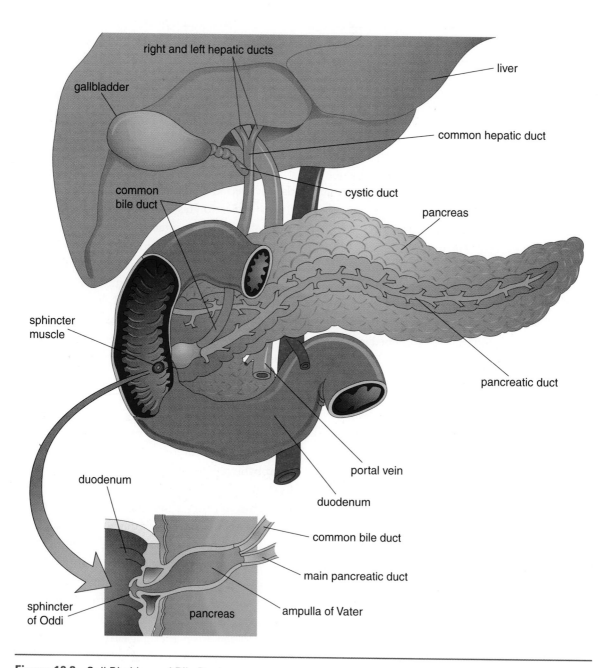

Figure 10.3 Gall Bladder and Bile Ducts

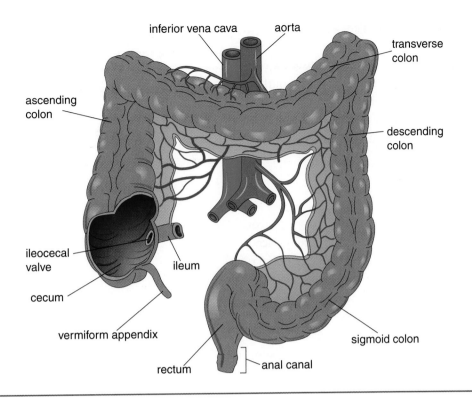

Figure 10.4 The Large Intestine

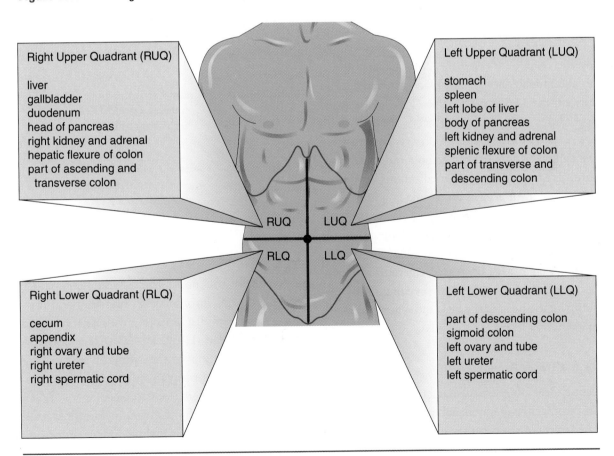

Right Upper Quadrant (RUQ)

liver
gallbladder
duodenum
head of pancreas
right kidney and adrenal
hepatic flexure of colon
part of ascending and
  transverse colon

Left Upper Quadrant (LUQ)

stomach
spleen
left lobe of liver
body of pancreas
left kidney and adrenal
splenic flexure of colon
part of transverse and
  descending colon

Right Lower Quadrant (RLQ)

cecum
appendix
right ovary and tube
right ureter
right spermatic cord

Left Lower Quadrant (LLQ)

part of descending colon
sigmoid colon
left ovary and tube
left ureter
left spermatic cord

Figure 10.5 Divisions of the Abdomen

Diseases and Conditions

There are a tremendous number of diseases that may affect the gastrointestinal tract, and an outline of those diseases is described in Table 10.1 and illustrated in Figure 10.6. Some of the most common disorders that you will encounter in transcription are described below.

Heartburn (GERD)

Heartburn, or acid reflux, referred to as gastroesophageal reflux disease (GERD, pronounced "gurd"), affects as much as 40% of the U.S. population. The symptoms are caused by the backflow of acidic stomach contents into the esophagus and posterior pharynx. Patients may complain of a burning sensation in the epigastrium, chest, or throat; the feeling of fluid in the throat; a sour taste; chronic cough; morning hoarseness that goes away after being out of bed for a while; and wheezing. The lower esophageal sphincter (LES) normally closes off the stomach, preventing stomach contents from regurgitating up into the esophagus. Some medications, alcohol, and cigarette smoking can relax or weaken the LES. A hiatal hernia or abdominal obesity can place increased pressure on the LES, causing it to "leak." Diagnostic procedures include esophagoscopy, barium swallow, and esophageal manometry, which measure the sphincter competence against increased pressure. Treatment involves medications to reduce the secretion of acid in the stomach and lifestyle changes. Medications include H_2 receptor antagonists (cimetidine) and proton pump inhibitors (Nexium). Lifestyle changes include diet modification, weight loss, decreased cigarette smoking, decreased alcohol intake, early evening meals, elevation of the head of the bed, and when necessary, hiatal hernia repair.

Peptic Ulcer Disease (PUD)

Peptic ulcer disease is characterized by lesions of the stomach and duodenal mucosa. Uncomplicated ulcer disease causes epigastric pain that is often relieved by eating, typically recurring two to four hours later. Two common causes include

Table 10.1

Areas of the Digestive Tract and Their Diseases

Area of GI Tract	Common Diseases
mouth and pharynx	candidiasis (thrush, moniliasis), herpetic stomatitis
esophagus	ulcers, infections, hiatal hernia, diverticula, cancer, gastroesophageal reflux disease, Schatzki ring, strictures, Zenker diverticulum, Mallory-Weiss tear, Barrett esophagus
stomach	gastric ulcers, tumors, gastritis, H pylori infection, GERD, cancer
duodenum	cancer, ulcers
liver	hepatitis, alcoholic liver disease, fatty liver, primary biliary cirrhosis, abscesses, tumors, parasites, cirrhosis, cancer
gallbladder	gallstones (cholelithiasis), cholangitis, choledocholithiasis
pancreas	acute and chronic pancreatitis, benign pseudocysts, malignant tumors
small intestine	tumors, Crohn disease, regional enteritis, terminal ileitis, cancer, hernia, appendicitis, celiac disease, malabsorption syndrome
colon	cancer, polyps, diverticular disease, ulcerative colitis, Crohn disease, irritable bowel syndrome
rectum	hemorrhoids, prolapse, cancer

chronic use of nonsteroidal antiinflammatory drugs (NSAIDs, pronounced "n-sades") and low-dose aspirin as well as infection with bacteria called *Helicobacter pylori* (H pylori). NSAIDs and aspirin promote ulceration of the stomach by blocking the production of protective prostaglandins. Progression of the ulcers leads to bleeding and possibly perforation of the stomach or intestinal wall. Testing for peptic ulcers includes upper endoscopy with small-bowel follow-through. *H pylori* can be detected using a urea breath test (in the physician's

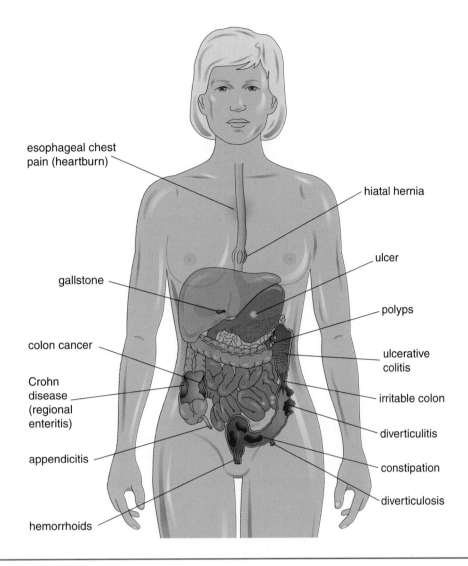

esophageal chest
pain (heartburn)

hiatal hernia

ulcer

gallstone

polyps

colon cancer

ulcerative
colitis

Crohn
disease
(regional
enteritis)

irritable colon

diverticulitis

appendicitis

constipation

diverticulosis

hemorrhoids

Figure 10.6 Common Diseases and Their Locations in the Digestive Tract

office) or a rapid urease test during endoscopy. Proton pump inhibitors, which reduce gastric acid, have been shown to promote healing of ulcers. Infection with *H pylori* is treated with proton pump inhibitors (e.g., Nexium), bismuth (Pepto-Bismol), and antibiotics.

Colitis

Antibiotic-associated colitis is an iatrogenic (result of medical treatment) infection caused by *Clostridium difficile* (sometimes spoken as "C dif"). This bowel infection is most common in the elderly or chronically ill patient and often acquired during hospitalization. Symptoms begin during or shortly after taking antibiotics for a different infection and

include left lower quadrant pain, diarrhea, greenish, foul-smelling stool, mucus in the stool, fever, and elevated white blood cell count. Diagnosis is made on the basis of a positive stool test for *C difficile* toxin. Treatment includes antibiotics such as metronidazole or vancomycin.

Crohn Disease

Crohn disease involves inflammation of the intestines, producing mucosal lesions called "skipping lesions," because they are not contiguous, and Peyer patches, which are aggregated lymphoid nodules. Chronic inflammation leads to fibrosis and stricture of the lumen, referred to as a "string sign" on barium enema. Symptoms include blood in the stool, abdominal pain, cramping, diarrhea, and ulceration. The etiology of Crohn disease is not known and there is no cure. Treatment involves antiinflammatory agents such as sulfasalazine as well as antibiotics such as metronidazole.

Ulcerative Colitis

Ulcerative colitis is also an inflammatory bowel disease characterized by diffuse mucosal inflammation involving the colon. It differs from Crohn disease in that it produces ulcerations in the mucosa of the colon. The hallmark symptom is bloody diarrhea with cramps, urgency, and tenesmus. Ulcerative colitis may be treated with the same medications as Crohn disease.

Diverticular Disease

Diverticular disease is characterized by the formation of bulging patches of intestinal mucosa that form outpockets. The presence of diverticula is called diverticulosis. The pockets trap bacteria and debris and are prone to infection and inflammation. Diverticulosis is common in the elderly, where it can be seen in 50% to 60% of individuals over 60 years of age. It is also common in younger individuals who eat a low-fiber diet or strain while stooling. Diverticulitis results when diverticula become infected. Left untreated, diverticulitis can lead to abscess, perforation of the bowel, or peritonitis. Chronic inflammation may cause the intestine to adhere to the bladder or other nearby tissues, causing fistulas to form. Symptoms of diverticulitis include abdominal pain, fever, increased white blood cell count, nausea, and vomiting. Diverticula may be visualized on an upper or lower GI study or a barium enema. Acute episodes of diverticulitis are treated with antibiotics, stool softeners, and a bland diet. After resolution, patients are encouraged to eat a high-fiber diet. A congenital anomaly of the GI tract causing a single diverticulum in the ileum is called Meckel diverticulum.

Cholecystitis and Cholelithiasis

Diseases of the gallbladder are extremely common and usually involve inflammation, referred to as cholecystitis, or the formation of stones in the gallbladder, called cholelithiasis. The stones may pass from the bladder into the bile ducts, referred to as choledocholithiasis, leading to obstruction of the ducts. Cholelithiasis is most common in females and is characterized by right upper quadrant pain that radiates to the scapula. Symptoms may also include nausea, vomiting, chills, fever, and jaundice. Laboratory tests show elevated liver enzymes (alkaline phosphatase, lactate dehydrogenase, and AST). Bilirubin levels may also be elevated. Stones may be visualized using ultrasonography. A HIDA scan (pronounced hy-da) is performed to visualize stones in the gallbladder and the ducts. Cholecystitis may be treated with antibiotics but commonly is treated with surgical removal of the gallbladder in a procedure called a cholecystectomy. Often this procedure is performed using a laparoscope and is referred to as a "lap chole" (laparoscopic cholecystectomy).

Cirrhosis

Cirrhosis of the liver involves replacement of functional liver tissue with fibrous, nonfunctioning tissue. Cirrhosis has many causes, but the most common are alcohol abuse and chronic viral infection. Because the liver plays a tremendous role in metabolism, detoxification, digestion, and coagulation, symptoms of extensive cirrhosis are far-reaching. Prominent symptoms include ascites (fluid accumulation in the peritoneal cavity), jaundice, and coagulopathies (blood clotting disorders). Because the circulation through the liver is also impaired, blood pressure in the portal vein elevates (portal hypertension). Increased pressure in the portal circulation results in esophageal varices. Death may result if the varices rupture and hemorrhage. Cirrhosis is not reversible and liver transplant may ultimately be required.

Hepatitis

Hepatitis is a general term referring to inflammation of the liver, but the term itself does not indicate the cause. Hepatitis may be infectious or noninfectious. Toxins, especially from poisonous mushrooms, and medications, most commonly acetaminophen (Tylenol), are the most common causes of noninfectious hepatitis. Viral infection accounts for the vast majority of infectious hepatitis cases.

Hepatitis produces hepatic cell destruction (necrosis), causing liver enzymes to spill out of the lysed cells into the blood stream. Measurement of liver enzymes (ALT, AST, GGT, alkaline phosphatase, LH) in the blood is used to assess liver damage, regardless of the etiology. Liver cells are the only human cell type capable of regenerating, so patients with self-limiting disease may fully recover.

With onset of viral hepatitis, the course and severity varies tremendously. Some cases go completely undetected (subclinical) while others are acute, fulminant, and cause death in a few days' time. Hepatic viruses are designated with uppercase letters: A, B, C, D, E, and G and abbreviated HAV, HBV, HCV, etc., respectively. Symptoms include anorexia, nausea, vomiting, jaundice, dark urine, clay-colored stool, hepatomegaly, right upper quadrant abdominal pain, fatigue, malaise, and fever. Laboratory studies show elevated alkaline phosphatase, increased liver enzymes (ALT, AST), elevated bilirubin, and increased PT and PTT. Viruses are difficult to culture, so laboratory studies to diagnose hepatitis A, B, and C look for specific antigens and antibodies in the patient's serum. The most common serological tests for hepatitis include anti-HAV (antibodies against hepatitis A), HB_sAg (hepatitis B surface antigen), and anti-HCV (antibodies to hepatitis C).

For the most part, treatment of hepatitis is supportive and directed at alleviating symptoms and correcting metabolic disturbances (coagulopathies, hypoglycemia, protein and electrolyte imbalances, renal failure) until the acute episode runs its course. Chronic cases of infectious hepatitis are treated with interferon alfa (note different spelling, alfa not alpha) and peginterferon.

Chronic, persistent viral hepatitis leads to cirrhosis and possibly hepatic carcinoma. Regardless of etiology, acute hepatic failure may ensue six weeks to six months after acute hepatitis and carries a poor prognosis. Acetaminophen overdose, accidental and suicidal, is now the most common cause of acute hepatic failure in the United States. Acetylcysteine is the antidote for acetaminophen overdose.

Common Tests and Surgical Procedures

Many of the diagnostic procedures in gastroenterology center on the use of the endoscope, which is a flexible tube with fiberoptics for visualizing the esophagus, stomach, intestinal tract, and related organs. Some of the common studies include esophagoscopy (esophagus), gastroscopy (stomach), colonoscopy (colon), flexible sigmoidoscopy, also called a "flex sig" (sigmoid colon), and anoscopy (anus). An endoscopic retrograde cholangiopancreatography (ERCP) is a specialized endoscopic test for visualizing the liver, gallbladder, and pancreatic ducts. To perform this test, an endoscope is passed through the stomach and into the biliary system via the sphincter of Oddi in the duodenum. During this procedure, the physician can examine and biopsy the liver, gallbladder, and pancreas.

X-rays are also used as diagnostic tools. A barium swallow, also called an upper GI series (UGI), delineates the structures in the throat, esophagus, stomach, and upper bowel (duodenum). The patient ingests barium, which is radiopaque, and then x-ray images are taken of the esophagus, stomach, and duodenum. Structures coated with barium appear white on the x-ray film. An upper GI with a small-bowel follow-through (SBFT) extends the upper GI series by taking x-rays at timed intervals while the barium migrates to the terminal ileum. A barium enema (BE), also referred to as a lower GI series, is performed by placing barium sulfate in the colon and then imaging the structures using x-rays. CT scans and ultrasound are also useful for imaging structures and organs in and around the GI tract. Two other tests, cholangiogram and HIDA scan, are used specifically to visualize the gallbladder and ducts.

Common surgical procedures include a Whipple operation to remove the pancreas and duodenum, an appendectomy to remove the appendix, hemorrhoidectomy to remove hemorrhoids, and gastrectomy to remove the stomach. A feeding tube is placed in a procedure called percutaneous endoscopic gastrostomy (PEG tube).

Common laboratory tests used to assess the gastrointestinal system include the liver enzymes ALT, AST, GGT, and alkaline phosphatase as well as pancreatic enzymes amylase and lipase. Total protein, albumin, total bilirubin, and indirect bilirubin are important tests for assessing liver function. A Hemoccult test, utilizing guaiac, is used to detect small amounts of blood in the stool to aid in the diagnosis of bleeding within the GI tract.

Terms Bank

These terms and abbreviations provide a foundation for the language and transcription skills you will develop in the following sections of this chapter. Terms marked with » will be included in the reports transcribed in the Building Transcription Skills section.

abdomen
(ab-**dO**-men/**ab**-dO-men) (n) that part of the body between the chest and the pelvis (the lower part of the trunk of the body)

achalasia
(ak-e-**lay**-zha) (n) failure to relax, especially a sphincter

adenocarcinoma »
(ad-en-O-**kar**-si-n**O**-ma) (n) malignant tumor of epithelial cells arising from the glandular structures which are a part of most organs of the body

adenopathy
(ad-e-**nop**-a-thee) (n) swelling or enlargement of the lymph nodes

adipose
(**ad**-i-pOz) (adj) fatty

albumin
(al-**byoo**-min) (n) a type of simple protein, varieties of which are widely distributed throughout the tissues and fluids

alimentary canal
(al-i-**men**-ter-ee ka-**nal**) (n) gastrointestinal tract; tubelike structure through which food passes and is digested and absorbed

anesthesia
(**an**-es-**thee**-zee-a) (n) absence of sensation, especially pain; usually applied to the medical technique of reducing or eliminating a person's sensation of pain to enable surgery to be performed

anesthetic
(**an**-es-**thet**-ik) (n) the medications used to produce anesthesia

angiodysplasia
(**an**-jee-O-dis-**play**-zee-a) (n) degenerative stretching or enlarging of the blood vessels in an organ

anorexia
(an-O-**rek**-see-a) (n) diminished appetite; aversion to food

anticholinergic
(an-tI-kO-lin-**er**-jik) (n) acting against an acetylcholine receptor; a class of drugs used to treat nausea

antiemetic
(**an**-ti-ee-**met**-ik) (n) pharmacologic agent used to decrease nausea and/or vomiting

aphagia
(a-**fay**-jee-a) (n) inability to swallow

aphthous stomatitis
(**af**-thus stO-ma-**tI**-tis) (n) small ulcers of the mucous membrane of the mouth

ascites
(a-**sI**-teez) (n) accumulation of fluid in the peritoneal cavity

Barrett esophagus
(**bair**-it ee-**sof**-a gus) (n) chronic peptic ulceration of the lower esophagus

benign
(bee-**nIn**) (adj) describing a mild illness or a nonmalignant tumor

bile
(bIl) (n) a thick, yellow-green-brown fluid secreted by the liver

bilirubin
(bil-i-**roo**-bin) (n) a red bile pigment, formed from hemoglobin during normal and abnormal destruction of erythrocytes

biopsy
(**bI**-op-see) (n) removal of a small amount of tissue and/or fluid from the body for microscopic examination; the specimen obtained

bulimia
(boo-**lim**-ee-a) (n) a chronic disorder involving repeated and secretive bouts of binge eating followed by self-induced vomiting, use of laxatives, or vigorous exercise in order to prevent weight gain

cachexia
(ka-**kek**-see-a) (n) a general weight loss and wasting occurring in the course of a chronic disease or emotional disturbance

caliber »
(**kal**-i-ber) (n) diameter of a tube or vessel; e.g., a blood vessel

carcinoma »
(kar-si-**nO**-ma) (n) malignant growth of epithelial cells that occurs in the linings of the body parts and in glands

cauterization »
(kaw-ter-i-**zay**-shun) (n) destroying tissue by burning for medical reasons

cecum »
(**see**-kum) (n) any part ending in a cul-de-sac; specifically the closed, pocket-like beginning of the large intestine in the lower right part of the abdomen

cholangiography »
(kO-lan-jee-**og**-ra-fee) (n) x-ray examination of the bile ducts

cholecystectomy »
(**kO**-lee-sis-**tek**-tO-mee) (n) excision of the gallbladder

cholecystitis
(**kO**-lee-sis-t**I**-tis) (n) inflammation or irritation of gallbladder, usually caused by the presence of gallstones

choledocholithiasis »
(kO-**led**-O-kO-lith-**I**-a-sis) (n) presence of calculi (stones) in the common bile duct

cholelithiasis »
(**kO**-lee-lith-**I**-a-sis) (n) formation or presence of gallstones in the gallbladder which may not cause any symptoms or perhaps only vague abdominal discomfort and intolerance to certain foods

cirrhosis »
(sir-**rO**-sis) (n) a chronic, degenerative disease of the liver

cirrhotic »
(sir-**rot**-ik) (adj) affected with cirrhosis

colonic »
(ko-**lon**-ic) (adj) pertaining to the colon

colostomy
(kO-**los**-to-mee) (n) surgical creation of an opening in the abdominal wall to allow material to pass from the bowel through that opening rather than through the anus

COX-2 inhibitor
(KOX too in-**hi**-bi-tor) (n) an agent which inhibits production of cyclooxygenase-2; a class of drugs used to treat pain, especially arthritis

Crohn disease »
(krOn) (n) chronic inflammatory condition affecting the colon and/or terminal part of the small intestine and producing frequent episodes of diarrhea, abdominal pain, nausea, fever, weakness, and weight loss

cryptitis »
(crip-**tI**-tis) (n) inflammation of a crypt or follicle

cyclooxygenase-2
(sI-**klO**-oks-i-jen-**ays**) (n) a prostaglandin produced by the body which promotes pain and inflammation.

cyst »
(sist) (n) a bladder or an abnormal sac containing gas, fluid, or a semi-solid material

cystic
(**sis**-tik) (adj) relating to a cyst

cystic duct
(n) the duct of the gallbladder which unites with the hepatic duct from the liver to form the common bile duct

dehydration »
(dee-hI-**dray**-shun) (n) extreme loss of water from the body tissues

Demerol »
(**dem**-err-all) (n) Brand name for meperidine, a narcotic analgesic

diathesis »
(dI-a-**thee**-sis) (n) unusual predisposition to certain disease conditions

digital »
(**dij**-i-tal) (adj) relating to or resembling a finger or toe

distention »
(dis-**ten**-shun) (n) the state of being stretched out or inflated

diverticulosis »
(**dI**-ver-tik-yoo-**lO**-sis) (n) presence of diverticula (pouches) in the intestinal tract

dyspepsia
(dis-**pep**-see-a) (n) imperfect digestion; epigastric discomfort

dysphagia
(dis-**fay**-jee-a) (n) difficulty swallowing

emetic
(e-**met**-ik) (n) pharmacologic agent used to induce vomiting and eliminate toxic substances

enteral
(**en**-ter-al) (adj) into or by way of the intestine

epigastric
(ep-i-**gas**-trik) (adj) related to or describing the area between the costal margins and the subcostal plane (top center of the abdomen)

epiploic »
(**ep**-i-**plO**-ik) (adj) relating to the omentum, a fold of peritoneum attached to the stomach and connecting it with the adjacent organs

epithelial
(ep-i-**thee**-lee-al) (adj) relating to or consisting of epithelium

epithelium »
(ep-i-**thee**-lee-um) (n) cell layers covering the outside body surfaces as well as forming the lining of hollow organs (e.g., the bladder) and the passages of the respiratory, digestive, and urinary tracts

eructation
(ee-ruk-**tay**-shun) (n) belching

esophageal varices
(ee-**sof**-i-**jee**-al **vair**-i-seez) (n) bulging, tortuous veins in the lower esophagus which are prone to ulceration and massive bleeding; caused by hypertension in the portal circulation.

esophagus
(ee-**sof**-a-gus) (n) the muscular canal that connects the pharynx and stomach

extravasation »
(eks-**trav**-a-**say**-shun) (n) a leakage of fluid (e.g., blood) to the tissues outside the vessel normally containing it, which may occur in injuries, burns, and allergic reactions

fecalith
(**fee**-ka-lith) (n) a hard mass consisting of impacted feces

fissure
(**fish**-ur) (n) a deep furrow, cleft, or slit; e.g., in the liver, lungs, ligaments, brain, or teeth

fistula »
(**fis**-tyoo-la) (n) abnormal opening or channel connecting two internal organs or leading from an internal organ to the outside. They are due to ulceration, a wound that does not heal, injury, or tumor

flatulence
(**flat**-yoo-lens) (n) presence of an excessive amount of gas in the stomach and intestines

flexure
(**flek**-sher) (n) a bend, as in an organ or structure

fungating »
(**fung**-gayt-ing) (adj) growing rapidly like a fungus, applied to certain tumors

gallbladder
(**gawl**-**blad**-er) (n) pear-shaped organ that is located on the lower surface of the liver and is a reservoir for bile until discharged through the cystic duct

gastritis
(gas-**trI**-tis) (n) inflammation of the gastric (stomach) mucosa

gastroenteritis
(**gas**-trO-en-ter-**I**-tis) (n) inflammation of the gastric mucosa and intestine

Gastrografin »
(Gas-tro-**graf**-in) (n) brand name for an oral contrast medium used for radiographic examination of the alimentary tract

gastroparesis
(gas-**trO**-pa-**ree**-sis) (n) weakness of gastric peristalsis causing delayed emptying of the stomach

gingiva
(**jin**-ji-va) (n) the gum; the tissue that attaches the teeth to the jaws

granuloma »
(gran-yoo-**lO**-ma) (n) a granular tumor or growth, usually of lymphoid and epitheloid cells

guaiac
(**gwI**-ak) (n) reagent used to test for occult blood

H₂ receptor antagonist
(an-**tag**-on-ist) (n) a class of drugs which blocks the action of histamine on H₂ receptors, preventing the release of hydrochloric acid. Cimetidine and ranitidine (Zantac) are the most common drug in this class.

hematemesis
(hee-ma-**tem**-e-sis) (n) vomiting of blood

hematochezia
(hee-ma-tO-**kee**-zee-a) (n) passage of bloody stools

hematocrit »
(**hee**-ma-tO-krit / **hem**-a-tO-krit) (n) centrifuge for separating solids from plasma in the blood; measure of the volume of red blood cells as a percentage of the total blood volume

hemorrhoid
(**hem**-a-royd) (n) varicose vein of anal opening

hemostasis »
(**hee**-mO-stay-sis / hee-**mos**-ta-sis) (n) cessation of bleeding either naturally through the blood coagulation process, mechanically (with surgical clamps), or chemically (with drugs)

hemostatic
(**hee**-mO-**stat**-ik) (adj) relating to procedure, device, or substance that stops flow of blood

hepatitis
(hep-a-**tI**-tis) (n) acute or chronic inflammation of the liver

hepatoduodenal »
(**hep**-at-O-doo-O-**dee**-nal) (adj) referring to the portion of the lesser omentum (fold of peritoneal tissue attaching and supporting the stomach and adjacent organs) between the liver and the duodenum

hepatomegaly
(hep-a-tO-**meg**-a-lee) (n) enlargement of the liver

hernia
(**her**-nee-a) (n) protrusion of an organ or part of an organ or other structure through the muscle wall of the cavity that normally contains it

hiatal »
(hI-**ay**-tal) (adj) pertaining to a hernia of part of the stomach into the opening in the diaphragm, through which the esophagus passes

homeostasis
(**hO**-mee-O-**stay**-sis) (n) equilibrium in the body with respect to various functions (e.g., temperature, heart rate) and to the chemical compositions of the fluids and tissues

hyperemesis
(hI-per-**em**-e-sis) (n) excessive vomiting

hyperemia »
(hI-per-**ee**-mee-a) (n) increased blood in part of the body, caused by inflammatory response or blockage of blood outflow

hyperemic »
(hI-per-**ee**-mik) (adj) showing hyperemia

ileostomy »
(**il**-ee-**os**-tO-mee) (n) surgical formation of an opening of the ileum (distal portion of the small intestine) onto the abdominal wall through which feces pass

ileum »
(**il**-ee-um) (n) the third portion of the small intestine, about 12 feet in length, extending from the junction with the jejunum to the ileocecal opening

ileitis »
(il-ee-**I**-tis) (n) inflammation of the ileum (lower-three-fifths of the small intestines)

ileus
(**il**-ee-us) (n) obstruction of the intestines

ilium
(**il**-ee-um) (n) the broad, flaring portion of the hip bone

infraumbilical »
(**in**-fra-um-**bil**-i-kal) (adj) below the umbilicus (navel)

intestine
(in-**tes**-tin) (n) the portion of the alimentary canal extending from the pyloric opening of the stomach to the anus (opening of the rectum)

intussusception
(**in**-tus-su-**sep**-shun) (n) taking up or receiving one part within another, especially the infolding of one segment of the intestine within another

lamina »
(**lam**-i-na) (n) thin membrane or plate-like structure, such as the two parts of a vertebra that join to hold the spinous process of the vertebra over the spinal cord (pl laminae)

laminar
(**lam**-i-nar) (adj) relating to lamina

laparoscope »
(**lap**-a-rO-skOp) (n) a device for observing the inside of an organ or cavity

lateral
(**lat**-er-al) (adj) relating to a side, away from the center plane; e.g., cheeks are lateral to the nose

leukocyte »
(**loo**-kO-sIt) (n) white blood cell

leukoplakia
(loo-kO-**play**-kee-a) (n) a precancerous change in a mucous membrane, such as the mouth or tongue

ligament

(**lig**-a-ment) (n) band of fibrous connective tissue that binds joints together and connects bones and cartilage

lobe

(lOb) (n) rounded part of an organ, separated from other parts of the organ by connective tissue or fissures

lumen »

(**loo**-men) (n) cavity, canal, or channel within an organ or tube; the space inside a structure

luminal »

(**loo**-min-al) (adj) related to the lumen of a tubular structure, such as a blood vessel

lymph

(limf) (n) a thin fluid that bathes the tissues of the body, circulates through lymph vessels, is filtered in lymph nodes, and enters the blood stream through the thoracic duct

lymphatic

(lim-**fat**-ik) (adj) relating to lymph

lymphoid »

(**lim**-foyd) (adj) resembling lymph or relating to the lymphatic system

lymphoma

(lim-**fO**-ma) (n) a general term for various types of tumors of the lymphatic system

malaise

(ma-**layz**) (n) a feeling of general discomfort or uneasiness, often the first indication of an infection or other disease

malignancy

(ma-**lig**-nan-see) (n) a cancer that is invasive and spreading

mastication

(mas-ti-**kay**-shun) (n) process of chewing food

melena »

(me-**lee**-na) (n) passage of dark, tarry stool

mucosal »

(myoo-**kO**-sal) (adj) concerning any mucous membrane

mucous »

(**myoo**-kus) (adj) having the nature of or resembling mucus

mucus

(**myoo**-kus) (n) viscous (sticky, gummy) secretions of mucous membranes and glands

nausea

(**naw**-zee-a; **naw**-zha) (n) inclination to vomit

nauseous

(**naw**-zee-us; **naw**-shus) (adj) causing nausea or feeling nausea

nodular

(**nod**-yoo-lar) (adj) small, firm, and knotty

obstipation

(ob-sti-**pay**-shun) (n) severe constipation

occult blood

(ok-**ult**) (n) blood in the stool in amounts too small to be seen but detectable with laboratory tests

opacification

(O-**pas**-i-fi-kay-shun) (n) clouding or loss of transparency, especially of the cornea or lens of the eye

organomegaly

(**Or**-ga-nO-**meg**-a-lee) (n) abnormal enlargement of an organ, particularly an organ of the abdominal cavity, such as the liver or spleen

palpable »

(**pal**-pa-bl) (adj) perceivable by touch

palpation

(pal-**pay**-shun) (n) technique of examination in which the examiner feels the firmness, texture, size, shape, or location of body parts

pancreas

(**pan**-kree-as) (n) gland lying behind the stomach that produces and secretes insulin, glucagon, and digestive enzymes

paracentesis

(pair-a-sen-**tee**-sis) (n) a procedure for withdrawing fluid from a body cavity, often referring to removal of fluid from the peritoneal cavity

parasite

(**par**-a-sIt) (n) an organism that lives on or in another and draws its nourishment therefrom

percutaneous »

(per-kyoo-**tay**-nee-us) (adj) through the skin

perforation

(per-fO-**ray**-shun) (n) abnormal opening or hole in a hollow organ

pericolonic »

(per-ee-ko-**lon**-ik) (adj) pertaining to the region around the colon

peristalsis

(per-i-**stal**-sis) (n) the movement of the intestine or other tubular structure, characterized by waves of alternate circular contraction and relaxation of the tube by which the contents are propelled onward

peritoneum

(per-i-tO-**nee**-um) (n) lining of the abdominal cavity

pharynx

(**far**-ingks) (n) throat; passageway for air from nasal cavity or larynx, and food from mouth to esophagus

pneumoperitoneum »

(**noo**-mO-per-i-ton-**ee**-um) (n) condition in which air or gas is collected in the peritoneal cavity

polyp »

(**pol**-ip) (n) a general descriptive term used with reference to any mass of tissue that bulges or projects outward or upward from the normal surface level

Prilosec »

(**pry**-low-sec) (n) Brand name for omeprazole, a gastric acid secretion inhibitor

proton pump inhibitor

(**prO**-ton) (n) a class of drugs which prevents the release of hydrochloric acid in the stomach; used to treat symptoms of hyperacidity (GERD, peptic ulcer disease)

proximal »

(**prok**-si-mal) (adj) nearest to a point of reference

pyrosis

(pI-**rO**-sis) (n) heartburn

reflux »

(**ree**-fluks) (n) abnormal backflow, as sometimes occurs with fluids in the esophagus or other body parts

regurgitation

(ree-gur-ji-**tay**-shun) (n) the return of gas or small amounts of food from the stomach

salivary gland
(**sal**-i-vayr-ee) (n) a gland that secretes saliva into the mouth

singultus
(sin-**gul**-tus) (n) hiccups

sigmoid colon
(**sig**-moyd **kO**-lon) (n) that part of the colon extending from the end of the descending colon to the rectum

sigmoidoscopy »
(**sig**-moy-**dos**-ko-pee) (n) the inspection of the rectum and colon via endoscope

sitz bath
(sitz) (n) immersion of only the peritoneum and buttocks

sphincter
(**sfingk**-ter) (n) a muscle that encircles a duct, tube, or opening in such a way that its contraction constricts the opening

sphincter of Oddi
(**sfingk**-ter of Od-**I**) (n) the sphincter which controls secretions from the liver, pancreas and gallbladder into the duodenum

splenomegaly
(sple-nO-**meg**-a-lee) (adj) enlargement of the spleen

steatorrhea
(stee-**a**-tO-**ree**-a) (n) presence of large amounts of fat in the stool caused by a failure to digest and absorb fat

sterile
(**ster**-il) (adj) free from living microorganisms

subcuticular »
(sub-kyoo-**tik**-yoo-lar) (adj) beneath the cuticle of epidermis

supine »
(soo-**pIn**) (adj) lying on the back

suprapubic
(soo-pra-**pyoo**-bik) (adj) above the pubic arch

tachycardia
(**tak**-e-**kar**-dee-a) (n) an abnormally rapid heart rate

tachycardic
(**tak**-e-**kar**-dik) (adj) relating to or suffering from an abnormally rapid heart rate

tenesmus
(te-**nez**-mus) (n) involuntary straining and the urge to defecate with little or no passage of stool

tracheostomy
(tray-kee-**os**-tO-mee) (n) a surgically created opening into the trachea (windpipe)

transmural »
(trans-**myoo**-ral) (adj) relating to the entire thickness of the wall of an organ

trocar »
(**trO**-kar) (n) sharply pointed surgical instrument used for aspiration or removal of fluids from cavities

ulcer
(**ul**-ser) (n) a break in skin or mucosal surface with erosion, loss of tissue, and accompanying inflammation

ulcerative colitis
(**ul**-ser-a-tiv kO-**lI**-tis) (n) a chronic disease characterized by ulcers in the colon and rectum

ultrasound
(**ul**-tra-sownd) (n) sound waves at very high frequencies used in the technique of obtaining images for diagnostic purposes

varices (plural of varix)
(**vair**-i-seez) (n) dilated, enlarged or tortuous veins

villi
(**vil**-I) (n) many tiny projections, occurring over the mucous membrane of the small intestine that accomplish the absorption of nutrients and fluids; villus (sing)

villous »
(**vil**-us) (adj) relating to villi

Abbreviations

a.c.	before meals
AFP	alpha fetoprotein
ALT	alanine aminotransferase
AST	aspartate aminotransferase
BaE or	
BE	barium enema
BCM	below costal margin
BM	bowel movement (bone marrow in oncology)
BX	biopsy
CRC	colorectal cancer
DCBE	double (air) contrast barium enema
EGD	esophagogastroduodenoscopy
ERCP	endoscopic retrograde cholangiopancreatoscopy
EtOH	ethanol (ethyl alcohol)
FAP	familial adenomatous polyposis
FBS	fasting blood sugar
FOBT	fecal occult blood test
GB	gallbladder
GE	gastroesophageal
GERD	gastroesophageal reflux disease
GGT	gamma-glutamyl transferase
GI	gastrointestinal
HAL	hyperalimentation
HAV	hepatitis A virus
HBV	hepatitis B virus
HCl	hydrochloric acid
HCV	hepatitis C virus

H&E	hematoxylin and eosin (stains for specimens on microscopic slides)
HNPCC	hereditary nonpolyposis colon cancer (Lynch syndrome)
H/O	history of
IBD	inflammatory bowel disease
IBS	irritable bowel syndrome
INR	international normalized ratio
IVC	intravenous cholangiography
LES	lower esophageal sphincter
LLQ	left lower quadrant
LRQ	lower right quadrant
LUQ	left upper quadrant
NG	nasogastric
n.p.o.	nothing by mouth
p.c.	after meals
p.p.	postprandial (after eating)
PTC	percutaneous transhepatic cholangiography
PUD	peptic ulcer disease
RLQ	right lower quadrant
R/O	rule out
RUQ	right upper quadrant
SBFT	small-bowel follow-through
TPN	total parenteral nutrition
UGI	upper gastrointestinal
ULQ	upper left quadrant
URQ	upper right quadrant

Complete the following exercises, drawing on the information learned in the Exploring Gastroenterology section of this chapter and referencing the Terms Bank.

Exercise 10.1   Matching Sound and Spelling

The numbered list that follows shows the phonetic spelling of hard-to-spell words. Sound out the word and then write the correct spelling in the blank space provided. Check your answers in the Terms Bank or other appropriate reference.

1. sir-**rO**-sis _____

2. a-**fay**-jee-a _____

3. ee-ruk-**tay**-shun _____

4. **pol**-ip _____

5. al-**byoo**-min _____

6. **af**-thus stO-ma-**tl**-tis _____

7. **in**-tus-su-**sep**-shun _____

8. ma-**lee**-na _____

9. **sfingk**-ter _____

10. ka-**kek**-see-a _____

11. me-**layz** _____

12. **flek**-sher _____

13. hee-ma-**tem**-e-sis _____

14. bil-i-**roo**-bin _____

15. **dI**-ver-tik-yoo-**lO**-sis _____

16. **il**-ee-um _____

Below is a list of frequently used words that look alike and/or sound alike. Study the meaning and pronunciation of each set of words, read the following sentences carefully, and then circle the word in parentheses that correctly completes the meaning.

aberrant	abnormal	**ileum**	the last part of the small intestine, between the jejunum and the large intestine
apparent	obvious, clear		
anesthesia	the loss of sensation of pain	**ileus**	obstruction of the intestines
anesthetic	the substance used to produce anesthesia	**ilium**	superior portion of the hipbone
		luminal	(adj) pertaining to a lumen (cavity or channel) within an organ or tube
cecal	pertaining to the cecum		
fecal	pertaining to feces	**Luminal**	trade name for anticonvulsant and sedative phenobarbital
thecal	pertaining to a sheath or capsule especially that encases a body part		
		mucous	(adj) having the nature of or resembling mucus
cite	(v) to quote or mention		
sight	(n) vision, view	**mucus**	(n) viscous (sticky, gummy) secretions of mucous membranes and glands
site	(n) location in the body		
dysphagia	difficulty swallowing		
dysphasia	difficulty speaking		
dyspnea	difficulty breathing	**reflex**	involuntary reaction or return
		reflux	abnormal backflow of fluid
hemostasis	cessation of bleeding		
hemostatic	pertaining to procedure, device, or substance that stops flow of blood		
homeostasis	steady state in the internal environment of the body		

1. After adequate (anesthesia/anesthetic) was documented, the cyst was incised.

2. Local (anesthesia/anesthetic) consisting of 1% lidocaine with epinephrine was infiltrated into the chest region.

3. After sutures were placed, good (hemostasis/homeostasis) was documented.

4. Colonoscopy was normal to the terminal (ileum/ilium).

5. The patient is to call if he notices yellow or green (mucous/mucus).

6. The (mucous/mucus) membranes are injected, with clear rhinorrhea.

7. I (cited/sighted) to the patient several reasons for quitting smoking.

8. The excision (cite/site) showed good healing.

9. Due to her (dysphagia/dysphasia/dyspnea) she has had little food intake over the past 24 hours.

10. Due to an (ileum/ileus) the patient was placed on total parenteral nutrition.

Exercise 10.3   Choosing Words from Context

When transcribing dictation, the medical transcriptionist frequently needs to consider the situation when determining the word that correctly completes the sentence. From the list below, select the term that meaningfully completes each of the following statements.

benign	fistula	malignancy
biopsy	hernia	palpable
cauterization	hyperemesis	pyrosis
Crohn disease	hyperemic	salivary glands
dehydration	laparoscope	supine

1. It was necessary to _____ the nodule to determine if it was malignant.

2. The homeless man was brought into the emergency room suffering from _____. He was started on IV fluids.

3. They found Mrs. Arnold lying _____ on her bed.

4. The patient had no _____ lymph nodes.

5. Mr. Johnson had a biopsy of the intestine that confirmed the diagnosis of _____.

6. Her tonsils are enlarged and mildly _____.

7. A _____ was passed through the abdominal wall to examine the peritoneal cavity.

8. If it is suspected that you have a _____, a biopsy may be performed.

9. _____ was used during the procedure to prevent excess bleeding.

10. There was a swelling on the face, particularly about the cheeks, which led to the diagnosis of obstruction of the _____.

11. Joseph had a _____ between the trachea and esophagus.

12. During her pregnancy, Mrs. Andrews suffered from _____ when lying down.

From this list, locate the term that best matches each of the following definitions. Write the term in the space provided by each definition.

adipose	epithelium	pancreas
cholecystectomy	extravasation	tachycardia
choledocholithiasis	gallbladder	tracheostomy
cirrhosis	lymph	
colostomy	lymphoma	

1. cell layers that cover the outside body surfaces and line the hollow organs   _____

2. a leakage of fluid from a vessel to the tissues outside it   _____

3. an abnormally rapid heart rate   _____

4. gland lying behind the stomach   _____

5. surgical creation of an opening through the abdominal wall into the colon   _____

6. excision of a gallbladder   _____

7. a chronic disease of the liver   _____

8. stone in the common bile duct   _____

9. fatty tissue   _____

10. a thin fluid that bathes the tissues of the body and is filtered in nodes before entering the blood stream   _____

Exercise 10.5   Creating Terms from Word Forms

Combine prefixes, root words, and suffixes from this list to create medical words that fit the following definitions. Fill in the blanks with the words you construct.

dys-	poor or bad; painful	**hemat/o**	blood
epi-	upon	**hepat/o**	liver
per-	throughout, completely	**stomat/o**	mouth
aden/o	glands	**cutaneous**	skin
carcin/o	cancer	**parotid**	glands by the ear
chol/e	bile	**peptic**	digestion
cyst/o	bladder	**-blast**	immature cell
enter/o	small intestine	**-emesis**	vomiting
gastr/o	stomach, abdomen	**-itis**	inflammation
gloss/o	tongue	**-oma**	tumor

1. through the skin _____

2. cancerous tumor _____

3. inflammation of the gallbladder _____

4. mumps (inflammation of the parotid gland) _____

5. swelling, redness, and pain in the mouth _____

6. malignant tumor in the glands _____

7. inflammation of the tongue _____

8. vomiting of blood _____

9. imperfection of digestion _____

10. malignant tumor in the liver _____

Read the following report excerpts and look for errors in format, usage, punctuation, capitalization, spelling, and mechanics. Mark the corrections on this page and key the excerpts with all errors corrected. Save the documents as XXExercise10.06-1 and XXExercise10.06-2, using your initials in place of *XX* in the file names.

1.   PROCEDURE The patient was placed on the operating table in the supine position. After satisfactory induction of general anesthesia, the abdomenal wall was prepared and drapped in the usual sterile fashion. Pneumoperitoneum was installed through a small infraumbilical excision and a Veress needle.

             Disection of the hepato-duodenal ligament was then commenced with identification of the cistic artery and the cystic duck.

             A percutaneous liver biopsy was preformed earlier in the procedure using a true-cut needle under the direct vision to the right lobe of the sliver. No bleeding was found from this sight later in the operation

             The abdomen was now copiously irritated through the lateral ports. The ports were now removed under direct vision.

2.   SPECIMEN:
A: ANTRUM B: GE JUNCTION

CLINICAL HISTORY:
H/O DYSPEPSIA
PROCEDURE – EGD & BX

PRE-OPERATIVE DIAGNOSIS:
R/O PUD

POST-OPERATIVE DIAGNOSIS:
REFLUX ESOPHAGITIS, GASTRITIS

GROSS DESCRIPTION:
Specimen is received in 2 Parts.
Part A is labelled "Antrum" and consists of 1 irregular piece of pink tan soft tissue measuring .4 x .3 x .3 cm. Entirly submitted in A1.

Part B is labelled GE Junction and consistes of 2 irregular pieces of pink tan soft tissue, each piece measuring .3 x.3 x .2 cm. Entirely submitted in B1.

DIAGNOSIS (Gross and Macroscopic):
PART A: ANTHRIUM BIOPSY. GASTRIC TISSUE WITH MILD CHRONIC INFLAMATION. NO HELICOBACTER ORGANISMS IDENTIFIED ON H&E.

PART B: GE JUNCTION BIOPSY. MULTIPLE PORTIONS OF SQUAMOUS MUCOSA WITH MILD CHRONIC INFLAMMATION WITH RARE INTRAMUCOSAL EOSINOPHILS CONSISTENT WITH REFLUX ESOPHAGITIS ORIGIN.

Exercise 10.7   Thinking Like a Professional

Read this scenario carefully and then select the most appropriate response. Write an explanation for why you think your choice is the best answer.

You work for a small community hospital in the transcription department. Your best friend's mother is admitted to the hospital for persistent headaches. Your friend is frantic and scared. She asks you to look up the results of her mother's MRI. What should you do?

a. Give the friend a verbal report but not a copy of the written report.

b. Explain that you cannot access her mother's records or discuss them with anyone.

c. Tell your friend you can only discuss results if her mother is present.

d. Have your friend sign a release so you will not be liable for release of information.

Best response: _____

Explanation: _____

_____

_____

_____

_____

You will apply the medical specialty and language information you learned in this chapter to transcription work in this section. After you learn the formatting recommendations of a pathology report, you will transcribe ten reports related to seven different patient studies.

Introducing the Pathology Report

The pathology report (Figure 10.7) is a diagnostic report describing the pathological or disease-related findings of a tissue sample taken during surgery, a biopsy, a special procedure, or an autopsy. Dictated by a pathologist, the report may also be called a biopsy report.

Required Headings/Content

The central information in a pathology report includes information about the specimens, the procedure completed to obtain the specimens, the gross description (the appearance of the specimen before it is prepared for microscopic study), the microscopic findings (cell- and blood-related), and the pathological diagnosis. Frequently, the gross descriptions of all the surgical specimens are dictated, transcribed, and given to the pathologist, who then dictates the microscopic descriptions. Once the microscopic descriptions are transcribed, the complete pathology reports are submitted to the pathologist for signature. Note that the pathology report is not the same as a laboratory report. The pathology report focuses on disease findings usually limited to tissue, while laboratory data usually concern body fluids.

Refer to page 471 of Appendix A for a complete list of headings found in the pathology report template along with descriptions of the type of information found under each heading. Not every template heading will be included in every transcribed report.

Turnaround Time

The expected turnaround time for a pathology report is generally 12–24 hours. However, in cases where a malignancy is suspected, the pathologist may render an opinion based on a frozen section of the specimen even before the patient is sutured, since more extensive surgery may be required.

Preparing to Transcribe

To prepare for transcribing dictation, review the common gastroenterology terms, drugs, and abbreviations presented in this chapter's Terms Bank. Then, study the format and organization of the model document shown in Figure 10.7, and key the model document, using the pathology report template on the Dictations and Templates CD as a starting point. Save the document as XXFigure10.07, using your initials in place of *XX* in the file name. Proofread the document by comparing it with the printed version. Categorize the types of errors you made, and document them on a copy of the Performance Comparison Chart. A template of this chart is available on the Dictations and Templates CD.

Transcribing Reports

Transcribe, edit, and correct each report in the following patient studies. Consult reference books for words or formatting rules that are unfamiliar.

As you work on the transcription assignment for this chapter, fill in the Performance Comparison Chart that you started when you keyed the model document. For at least three of the reports, categorize and document the types of errors you made. Answer the document analysis questions on the bottom of the chart. With continuous practice and assessment, the quality of your work will improve.

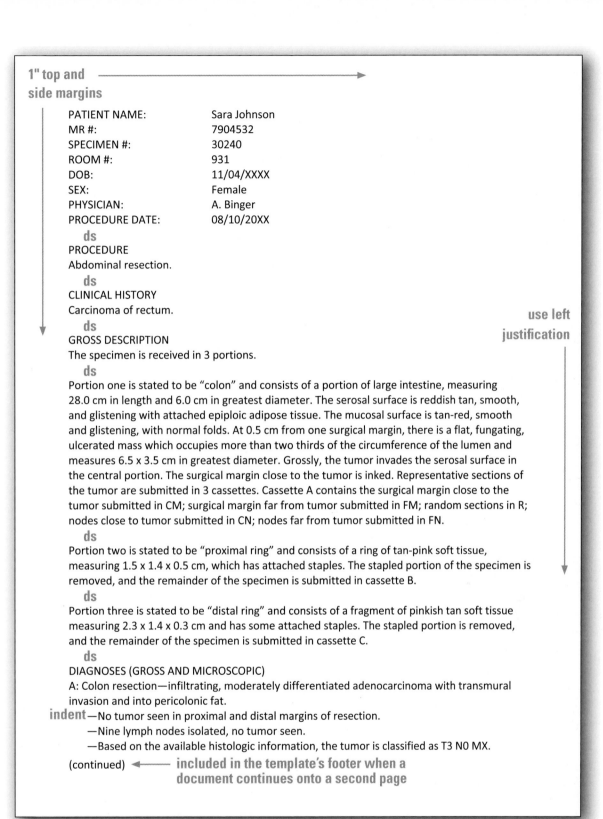

1" top and side margins

PATIENT NAME: Sara Johnson
MR #:   7904532
SPECIMEN #:   30240
ROOM #:   931
DOB: 11/04/XXXX
SEX: Female
PHYSICIAN: A. Binger
PROCEDURE DATE: 08/10/20XX

ds

PROCEDURE
Abdominal resection.

ds

CLINICAL HISTORY
Carcinoma of rectum.

ds

use left justification

GROSS DESCRIPTION
The specimen is received in 3 portions.

ds

Portion one is stated to be "colon" and consists of a portion of large intestine, measuring 28.0 cm in length and 6.0 cm in greatest diameter. The serosal surface is reddish tan, smooth, and glistening with attached epiploic adipose tissue. The mucosal surface is tan-red, smooth and glistening, with normal folds. At 0.5 cm from one surgical margin, there is a flat, fungating, ulcerated mass which occupies more than two thirds of the circumference of the lumen and measures 6.5 x 3.5 cm in greatest diameter. Grossly, the tumor invades the serosal surface in the central portion. The surgical margin close to the tumor is inked. Representative sections of the tumor are submitted in 3 cassettes. Cassette A contains the surgical margin close to the tumor submitted in CM; surgical margin far from tumor submitted in FM; random sections in R; nodes close to tumor submitted in CN; nodes far from tumor submitted in FN.

ds

Portion two is stated to be "proximal ring" and consists of a ring of tan-pink soft tissue, measuring 1.5 x 1.4 x 0.5 cm, which has attached staples. The stapled portion of the specimen is removed, and the remainder of the specimen is submitted in cassette B.

ds

Portion three is stated to be "distal ring" and consists of a fragment of pinkish tan soft tissue measuring 2.3 x 1.4 x 0.3 cm and has some attached staples. The stapled portion is removed, and the remainder of the specimen is submitted in cassette C.

ds

DIAGNOSES (GROSS AND MICROSCOPIC)
A: Colon resection—infiltrating, moderately differentiated adenocarcinoma with transmural invasion and into pericolonic fat.

indent —No tumor seen in proximal and distal margins of resection.
      —Nine lymph nodes isolated, no tumor seen.
      —Based on the available histologic information, the tumor is classified as T3 N0 MX.

(continued) ← included in the template's footer when a document continues onto a second page

Figure 10.7 Pathology Report

PATHOLOGY REPORT
PATIENT NAME: Sara Johnson
MR #: 7904532
PROCEDURE DATE: 08/10/20XX
Page 2

text and fields included in the second-page header in the template

ds
B: Proximal ring, segment—segment of large bowel with no evidence of malignancy.
ds
C: Distal ring, segment—segment of large bowel with no evidence of malignancy.

qs

_____

Nuri Bano, MD
Pathologist
ds
NB/XX
D: 08/10/20XX
T: 08/10/20XX

Figure 10.7   Pathology Report (Continued)

James Welton is a 34-year-old man who had eaten dinner and later complained of pain in his right side. He was nauseated and vomited several times during the evening and eventually was taken to the emergency department.

REPORT 10.1 Operative Report

Use the Report1001.mp3 audio file and the operative report template (Operative_Report) when transcribing this report. Save the document as XXReport10.01, using your initials in place of *XX* in the file name. Change the headings as needed to match the dictated content. However, if a template heading is appropriate, use it instead of the dictated heading. For example, use the template's Date of Surgery for the report's date. Consistency in report formats is important for locating information and managing electronic medical record data.

Listen for these terms:
Tru-Cut needle
Veress needle

According to *The Book of Style for Medical Transcription*, if a dictator lists more than one diagnosis or procedure, it is preferred to list and number them, even if the dictator does not indicate numbers.

The client will determine many aspects of transcribed reports style, including the order of the patient's names. For reports transcribed for this course, put the first name first, followed by the last name. Use this same order for physician names. Transcribe the names in this order even if the dictator says the last name first.

REPORT 10.2 Consultation Letter

Use the Report1002.mp3 audio file and the consultation letter template (Consultation_Letter) when transcribing this report. Save the document as XXReport10.02, using your initials in place of *XX* in the file name.

Listen for this drug name:
D5W Demerol

This report includes a reference to 0.45 NS, which means a 0.45% solution of normal saline. Since the dictator does not include the percent symbol, it should not be transcribed. Normal saline solution equals 0.9% sodium chloride (NaCl) and water, and half normal saline solution equals 0.45% (or 0.9% x ½ = 0.45%). Quartern normal saline equals 0.23% NaCl (or 0.9% x ¼ = 0.23%).

Sara Johnson is a 51-year-old woman who saw her physician after several weeks of intermittent constipation, abdominal distention, and bloody stools.

REPORT 10.3 Pathology Report

Use the Report1003.mp3 audio file and the pathology report template (Pathology_Report) when transcribing this report. Save the document as XXReport10.03, using your initials in place of *XX* in the file name.

Place the procedure name in the body of the report. Also, note that the dictated clinical diagnosis corresponds with the template's Clinical History heading.

This report includes a tumor classification based on the TNM system, which is a tumor classification system that will be described in more detail in Chapter 15. The classification should be transcribed as T3 N0 MX.

When transcribing measurements, try to visualize the actual size. If the size does not make sense in context, leave a blank or transcribe the number with a question mark or symbol indicating a possible error. The MT may also query the dictator. When using metric measure, it may be more difficult to imagine the actual size.

By convention, a zero after the decimal is not transcribed in dosages so that the amount is not mistakenly read as 10 times larger (e.g., 4.0 mg could be misread as 40 mg). An exception to this rule is made when the zero after the decimal is required to imply a more precise value. For example, potassium is reported to the tenth's place and the precision is required in this case, so potassium values are always reported with a decimal, even if the trailing decimal is a zero. Zeros should be retained when dictated and indicating a length or size. Do not transcribe the trailing zero if it is not dictated, as this will imply a degree of specificity that may not be intended by the dictator. However, the leading zero is transcribed (e.g., 0.5 cm compared to .5 cm) to prevent a 10-fold misinterpretation by overlooking the decimal.

When transcribing the specimen tissue description in this dictation, hyphenate the colors (and other words) that are equal, complimentary, or contrasting, such as *pink-tan*, *white-beige*, etc.

REPORT 10.4 Consultation Letter

Use the Report1004.mp3 audio file and the consultation letter template (Consultation_Letter) when transcribing this report. Save the document as XXReport10.04, using your initials in place of *XX* in the file name. Follow instructions for formatting an indented list.

This letter includes a tumor classification based on the TNM system. The classification should be transcribed as T3 N0 MX.

Patient Study 10.C — Jonathan Prince

Jonathan Prince is an 18-year-old young man who was diagnosed with Crohn disease one year prior to surgery. He had been doing well until last week when he began having intractable diarrhea, which required hospitalization for dehydration. He was given a presurgical barium enema and then sent to the operating room for a colostomy.

REPORT 10.5 Radiology Report of Barium Enema

Use the Report1005.mp3 audio file and the radiology report template (Radiology_Report) when transcribing this report. Save the document as XXReport10.05, using your initials in place of *XX* in the file name. Some changes will be needed to the dictated headings to correspond with the template's headings.

REPORT 10.6 Pathology Report of Colostomy Procedure

Use the Report1006.mp3 audio file and the pathology report template (Pathology_Report) when transcribing this report. Save the document as XXReport10.06, using your initials in place of *XX* in the file name.

Transcribe the letter designations for specimen portions in capitals (A, B, etc.) and the labels in quotation marks, for example, "15-cm ileostomy."

In the Gross Description section of the report, treat each portion description as a separate paragraph.

Patient Study 10.D — David Dronen

David Dronen is a 52-year-old man who has been evaluated in the emergency department for severe abdominal pain.

REPORT 10.7 Radiology Report of Flexible Sigmoidoscopy

Use the Report1007.mp3 audio file and the radiology report template (Radiology_Report) when transcribing this report. Save the document as XXReport10.07, using your initials in place of *XX* in the file name. Use the appropriate report headings, even when a heading is not dictated.

Patient Study 10.E — Mary Gonzales

Mary Gonzales is a 64-year-old woman with a long history of anemia. She was admitted to the hospital for tests to determine the cause of chest pain and dark, tarry stools.

REPORT 10.8 Discharge Summary

Use the Report1008.mp3 audio file and the discharge summary template (Discharge_Summary) when transcribing this report. Save the document as XXReport10.08, using your initials in place of *XX* in the file name.

Listen for these words:
  guaiac-negative
  Prilosec
  Xanax

Correct any dangerous abbreviations.

Patient Study 10.F

Jonathan Areade

Jonathan Areade complained of sharp pain in the right upper quadrant. He went to the emergency department, and on physical exam he was found to have jaundice and right upper quadrant tenderness.

REPORT 10.9 Pathology Report

Use the Report1009.mp3 audio file and the pathology report template (Pathology_Report) when transcribing this report. Save the document as XXReport10.09, using your initials in place of *XX* in the file name.

Format the listed procedures as a numbered list, even though the dictator does not dictate numbers.

Patient Study 10.G

Ronald Forest

Ronald Forest is a 70-year-old gentleman who was found to have occult blood in his stool on routine examination. An abdominal CT scan revealed a mass in the colon.

REPORT 10.10 Pathology Report

Use the Report1010.mp3 audio file and the pathology report template (Pathology_Report) when transcribing this report. Save the document as XXReport10.10, using your initials in place of *XX* in the file name.

Eleven

Obstetrics and Gynecology

Obstetrics is the specialty concerned with the management of women's health during pregnancy, childbirth, and the three to six weeks following delivery. Gynecology is the study of the diseases of the female, particularly of the genital, urinary, and rectal organs. The practice of obstetrics and gynecology is usually done by the same physician, who is referred to as a gynecologist and/or obstetrician.

Objectives

» Identify the organs and structures of the female reproductive system.

» Describe sexually transmitted diseases and their causative agents.

» Define the three phases of a female's reproductive life and the stages of the menstrual cycle.

» Recognize common procedures for diagnosis and treatment of gynecologic disorders.

» Pronounce and correctly spell terminology related to obstetrics and gynecology.

» Transcribe dictation related to the medical specialties of obstetrics and gynecology.

» Describe a labor and delivery report including typical content, format, and turnaround time.

The joint specialty of obstetrics and gynecology has an acronym for its name: OB-GYN (pronounced letter by letter, O-B-G-Y-N, or as O-B-Gin). Recently, there have been separations in this specialty. There are physicians who only see patients during their prenatal (before birth), antenatal (after birth), and parturition (birth) periods. Other physicians deal only with high-risk pregnancies, that is, with women who have illnesses during pregnancy or who have fetuses that are considered at risk for problems in utero or at parturition. A patient might see a fertility specialist to deal with problems of infertility. The field also includes nurse-midwifery specialists. In addition to specialists, some family and general practitioners also deliver babies, provide well-woman exams, and perform gynecologic/obstetric procedures.

Structure and Function

The female is born with a lifetime supply of eggs, or ova. These 30,000 to 40,000 eggs exist in an undeveloped form within the ovaries, which are almond-shaped glands located in the pelvic cavity on either side of the uterus (Figure 11.1). The uterus is a pear-shaped muscular organ that has a narrow neck called the cervix; a body, or corpus; and the fundus, which is the uppermost part. The uterus is surrounded by the peritoneum and is held in the pelvic cavity by ligaments. The cornua are the upper lateral portions of the uterus from which the oviducts, or fallopian tubes, extend. The fallopian tube, ligaments, and ovary are collectively called the (right and left) adnexa. The lumen of the fallopian tube is contiguous with the uterine cavity. At the distal end of each fallopian tube is the infundibulum, which is a broad, funnel-like ending with finger-like extensions called fimbriae.

The menstrual cycle occurs in response to the stimulation of hormones. The very first time menstruation occurs is known as menarche. Follicle-stimulating hormone (FSH) and luteinizing hormone (LH) are released by the pituitary gland located in the brain (see Chapter 14). With each menstrual

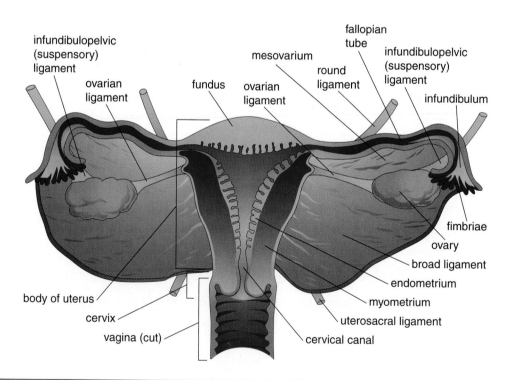

Figure 11.1 Internal Female Genitalia

cycle, these hormones cause several ova to ripen into follicles. During this follicular (or preovulatory) phase, one of the ripening follicles becomes dominant and is referred to as the graafian follicle. This follicle enlarges and moves toward the surface of the ovary. The surface of the ovary ruptures, releasing the egg, or oocyte, into the pelvic cavity. The fimbriae sweep the oocyte into the fallopian tube.

The discharge of the oocyte from the ovary is referred to as ovulation and occurs about halfway through the menstrual cycle. This may be accompanied by some pain, called mittelschmerz, in the lower groin area as well as some vaginal discharge. If the oocyte is met by a spermatozoon, the male reproductive cell, conception takes place, usually occurring within a fallopian tube. After releasing the egg from the ovary, the graafian follicle becomes yellow and is referred to as the corpus luteum (yellow body). During the second half of the menstrual cycle, called the luteal phase, the corpus luteum secretes progesterone, which promotes the thickening of the uterine lining in preparation for implantation of an egg. Fertilization of the egg produces human chorionic gonadotropin (hCG), which maintains the corpus luteum, thereby promoting implantation of the fertilized egg. If conception does not occur, hCG is not produced, and the corpus luteum degenerates. The degenerated corpus luteum causes a drop in progesterone, which causes the endometrium to begin to thin out and slough the blood-rich layer. This blood flow is called menstruation and occurs approximately every 28 days during the reproductive life of the woman.

The menstrual cycle continues until the woman reaches menopause, defined as cessation of menstruation for six months. The average age of menopause is about 50 years. The time period (months or even years) leading up to and immediately following menopause is called perimenopause and is characterized by fluctuating hormone levels. At menopause, hormone production diminishes, causing vaginal atrophy and dryness, breast changes, loss in bone density, and vascular changes. The changes in hormone levels cause menopausal symptoms that may include hot flushes (sudden sensation of heat, often accompanied by profuse sweating), psychologic changes, and changes in sleep patterns.

Physical Assessment

The physician begins the assessment of the female reproductive system by examining the external organs. The breasts are the first part of the assessment. Observation includes size, shape, deformities, markings (such as nevi), nipples, and areolar tissue (Figure 11.2). The breasts are then palpated

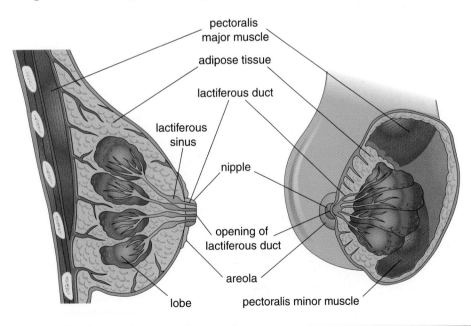

Figure 11.2 Structure of the Female Breast

for texture, masses, or abnormalities. The abdomen is examined as described in Chapter 10, Gastroenterology.

The external genitalia (Figure 11.3), or vulva, include the mons pubis, labia majora, labia minora, clitoris, vestibule of the vagina, Skene or vestibular glands, and Bartholin glands. The physician inspects the genitalia, noting the urinary meatus, the anus, and the vulva.

Following the external inspection, the physician performs a digital examination. A rectal exam is often included, and if stool is present, a guaiac test may be performed to test for occult blood. A speculum (Figure 11.4) is usually inserted into the vagina to provide a wider opening for the visual exam of the cervix, fornices, and vaginal walls.

Next, the physician completes a bimanual ("two hands") exam by inserting one or two fingers of a gloved and lubricated hand into the vagina and placing the other hand on the patient's abdomen (Figure 11.5). This procedure allows the physician to assess the size, shape, and position of the uterus along with any masses or tenderness. The physician also notes any cervical motion tenderness.

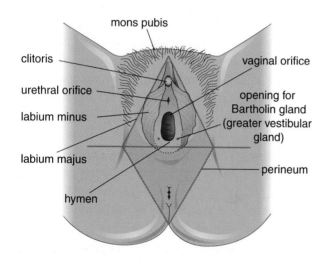

Figure 11.3   External Female Genitalia

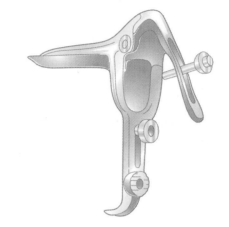

Figure 11.4   Vaginal Speculum

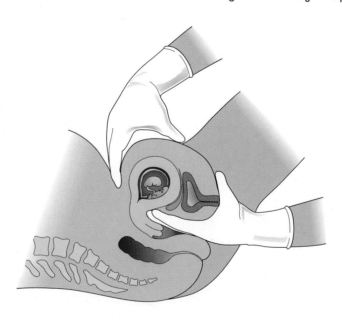

Figure 11.5   Bimanual Method of Palpating the Internal Genitalia

Diseases and Conditions

Along with cancers of the breast, uterus, ovaries, and cervix, common diseases of the female reproductive system include fibrocystic breast disease, endometriosis, fibroids, polycystic ovary syndrome (PCOS), abnormal uterine bleeding (AUB), dysfunctional uterine bleeding (DUB), pelvic inflammatory disease (PID), and sexually transmitted diseases (STD).

Fibroids, also known as leiomyomas, are the most common benign tumors in women. They consist of smooth muscle and fibrous connective tissue. They are classified by their location within the uterus (intramural, subserosal, or submucous). On palpation, the uterus may be enlarged and irregularly contoured. The enlarged uterine cavity increases the mucosal surface, increasing uterine bleeding during menstruation (menorrhagia). Fibroids may interfere with conception. Treatment, when necessary, is typically myomectomy.

Endometriosis is a benign condition in which there is aberrant endometrial tissue growing outside the uterine wall. Symptoms associated with endometriosis include extreme menstrual pain, abnormal bleeding, infertility, and dyspareunia. Surgery and/or hormonal therapy to cause atrophy of the endometrium may be necessary to treat endometriosis.

Sexually transmitted diseases (STD) are those infections (bacterial, protozoan, and viral) that are passed from one person to another during sexual contact. Human papillomavirus (HPV) is a sexually transmitted disease that causes genital warts. HPV infection can now be prevented by a vaccination marketed under the trade name Gardasil. An increased risk of cervical cancer is associated with certain types of HPV infection; therefore, frequent Pap smears are indicated. Other STDs include gonorrhea (*Neisseria gonorrhea*), syphilis (*Treponema pallidum*), chlamydia (*Chlamydia trachomatis*), trichomoniasis (*Trichomonas vaginalis*), and herpes (herpes simplex virus). The most devastating and life-threatening STD is human immunodeficiency virus (HIV), which is the causative agent of acquired immunodeficiency syndrome (AIDS).

Pelvic inflammatory disease (PID) is an inflammatory condition of the pelvic cavity that may be localized or spread throughout the reproductive organs. Also called acute salpingitis, the disease is usually caused by a bacterial agent such as gonococci or staphylococci and results in vaginal discharge, pain, and tenderness. Other symptoms include fever, pain on movement of the cervix and/or palpation of the adnexa. PID is treated with the appropriate antibiotic therapy.

Vaginitis, or inflammation of the vaginal tissue, is often caused by *Candida albicans* or *Gardnerella vaginalis*. Changes in vaginal pH, which normally occur during the menstrual cycle, may cause a disturbance of the normal vaginal flora, leading to an overgrowth of one of these two microorganisms. Chemical irritation from douches and retention of a diaphragm or tampon may also lead to vaginitis.

Polycystic ovary syndrome (PCOS) is a common cause of infertility. It is characterized by cysts on the ovaries and increased androgens. Masculinization symptoms caused by increased androgens include acne, deep voice, increased body hair (hirsutism), and increased insulin levels.

Abnormal or dysfunctional uterine bleeding (AUB or DUB) is caused by disruption of normal hormonal control of the menstrual cycle and is most common in perimenopausal women. If hormonal treatment fails, a dilatation and curettage (D&C), endometrial ablation (destruction of the endometrial lining), or hysterectomy may be required.

Disorders during pregnancy include hyperemesis gravidarum (excessive vomiting during pregnancy), miscarriage, preterm labor (labor causing dilation and effacement of the cervix before the 37th week of pregnancy), gestational hypertension, and gestational diabetes. Preeclampsia is characterized by hypertension, proteinuria, and edema, commonly occurring after the 20th week of gestation. Placenta previa (placental implantation partially or completely covering the cervical os) and abruptio placentae (premature detachment of placenta) are two potentially life-threatening conditions of pregnancy.

Common Tests and Surgical Procedures

Blood tests commonly employed by the gynecologist include CBC, especially to evaluate hemoglobin levels in cases of abnormal uterine bleeding, iron levels, and thyroid hormones (TSH, T_3, and T_4). Other hormone levels evaluated include FSH, LH, progesterone, estrogen, and testosterone. Pregnancy is confirmed by measuring human chorionic gonadotropin (hCG) levels in the blood or urine.

During pregnancy, it is important to determine the ABO blood type of the mother as well as the Rh status (Rh positive or Rh negative). An Rh-negative mother will produce antibodies directed against the Rh antigen if the fetus is Rh positive. The first pregnancy may not be affected by the antibodies, but fetuses in subsequent pregnancies may suffer erythroblastosis fetalis (lysis of red blood cells due to antibodies against Rh antigens on the surface of red blood cells). Rh-negative mothers are treated with RhoGAM to prevent the formation of Rh antibodies.

The most common test performed during the gynecologic examination is the Papanicolaou (Pap) smear, which is a cytologic test to screen for cervical cancer. The Bethesda System (TBS), a standardized system for reporting Pap smears, is based on narrative reporting of descriptive diagnoses using clinically relevant cell findings. Pap smears showing cervical intraepithelial neoplasia (CIN), which is a precancerous condition, are graded according to the following scale:

CIN-1: mild dysplasia

CIN-2: moderate dysplasia

CIN-3: severe dysplasia

Colposcopy is performed when there is an abnormal Pap smear. The colposcope is inserted into the cervix allowing visualization of the abnormal tissue. Biopsies are taken to provide tissue for diagnosis. Cone biopsy (conization), which removes an inverted cone of tissue from the cervix, is performed for the removal of premalignant cells.

Dilatation and curettage (D&C) is a surgical procedure performed to obtain endometrial or endocervical tissue for cytologic examination and to control abnormal uterine bleeding. The cervix is dilated and a curette is used to obtain uterine scrapings.

Hysterectomy is the surgical procedure to remove the cervix and uterus. A hysterectomy with removal of the fallopian tubes and ovaries is known as a total hysterectomy with bilateral salpingo-oophorectomies.

Sonograms are commonly used to assess the pelvic and abdominal structures and are especially useful in pregnancy because the sound waves are not harmful to the developing fetus. Hysteroscopy, which uses an endoscope to visualize the interior of the uterus, is used to diagnose fibroids and endometriosis as well as assess the uterine cavity for other signs of disease or malformation. Laparoscopy involves passing a scope through the abdominal wall to assess the abdominopelvic cavity.

C-section (cesarean section) is the surgical delivery of a baby through the abdominal wall. A C-section is carried out in cases of ineffective labor, cephalopelvic disproportion, fetal distress, breech presentations, multiple births, and infections in the mother. This type of delivery accounts for approximately 20-25% of all deliveries.

Mastectomy is the surgical removal of a breast, usually because of a cancerous tumor. The removal of only the tumor and minimal surrounding tissue is called a lumpectomy.

A mammogram is a radiographic image of the breast. It can detect abnormalities that cannot be palpated. Breast MRI studies are gaining in popularity and are helping to further evaluate suspicious findings on x-ray.

Apgar score is used to quickly evaluate the newborn infant immediately after birth. It is usually performed twice within the first 10 minutes after delivery. A numerical value between 0 and 2 is assigned to each of five categories: heart rate, respiratory effort, muscle tone, response to stimulation, and skin color. Scores are added together and a score of 8-10 indicates the best possible condition.

Terms Bank

These terms and abbreviations provide a foundation for the language and transcription skills you will develop in the following sections of this chapter. Terms marked with ≫ will be included in the reports transcribed in the Building Transcription Skills section.

adenocarcinoma ≫
(**ad**-e-nO-kar-si-**nO**-ma) (n) a malignant adenoma arising from a glandular organ

adenopathy ≫
(ad-e-**nop**-a-thee) (n) swelling or enlargement of any gland, especially the lymph nodes

adenosis ≫
(ad-e-**nO**-sis) (n) any disease of a gland, especially of a lymphatic gland

adhesion
(ad-**hee**-zhun) (n) the union of opposing surfaces, especially opposing surfaces of a wound in the abdominal cavity

adipose ≫
(**ad**-i-pOz) (adj) containing fat

adnexal ≫
(ad-**nek**-sal) (adj) relating to appendages or accessory parts of an organ

adrenarche
(**ad**-ren-ar-kee) (n) the beginning of hormonal activity that leads up to puberty and the associated sexual development

amenorrhea
(a-men-O-**ree**-a) (n) stoppage or absence of menses

amniocentesis
(**am**-nee-O-sen-**tee**-sis) (n) taking a sample of amniotic fluid

amnion ≫
(**am**-nee-on) (n) the inner of the fetal membranes; a thin transparent sac that holds the fetus

anovulation
(an-ov-yoo-**lay**-shun) (n) absence of egg production or release from the ovary

anovulatory ≫
(an-**ov**-yoo-la-tOr-ee) (adj) not accompanied by production of or discharge of an ovum (egg) or suppressing ovulation

anteflexion
(an-te-**flek**-shun) (n) the abnormal position of an organ that is bent forward over itself

Apgar score
(n) scoring system to assess newborn's physical condition

axilla ≫
(**ak**-sil-a) (n) the armpit

axillary node ≫
(**ak**-sil-ayr-ee nOd) (n) any of the lymph glands of the armpit that help to fight infection in the neck, chest, and arm area

biopsy
(**bI**-op-see) (n) the sampling of tissue and/or fluid from the body for microscopic study; the specimen obtained

Braxton Hicks sign
(n) irregular contractions of the uterus after the first trimester of pregnancy

breech presentation ≫
(n) fetal position in which the feet or buttocks appear first in the birth canal

calcification
(**kal**-si-fi-**kay**-shun) (n) a hardening of tissue resulting from the formation of calcium salts within it

carcinoma ≫
(kar-si-**nO**-ma) (n) a malignant growth of epithelial cells

cautery ≫
(**kaw**-ter-ee) (n) a means of destroying tissue by electricity, freezing, heat, or corrosive chemicals

centimeter
(**sen**-ti-mee-ter) (n) unit of measurement; one hundredth of a meter; approximately 0.4 inches

cephalad ≫
(**sef**-a-lad) (adv) toward the head

cerclage ≫
(sair-**klazh**) (n) procedure to encircle tissues with a ligature, wire, or loop

cervical
(**ser**-vi-kal) (adj) relating to a neck, or cervix, especially the neck (cervix) of the uterus

cervix ≫
(**ser**-viks) (n) the neck or part of an organ resembling a neck, such as the cervix of the uterus

chromosome
(**krO**-mO-sOm) (n) the structure in the cell nucleus that transmits genetic information; consists of a double strand of DNA in the form of a helix; there are normally 46 in humans

colostrum
(kO-**los**-trum) (n) the first milk secreted after childbirth

colposcopy
(kol-**pos**-ko-pee) (n) examination of the tissues of the vagina and cervix with a lighted instrument that magnifies the cells

condyloma
(kon-di-**lO**-ma) (n) warty growth in the genital area

cornual
(**kor**-noo-al) (adj) relating to a horn-shaped structure, as in the cornual area of the uterus

cribriform ≫
(**krib**-ri-form) (adj) perforated with small holes of uniform size; (n) a polyporous structure

cul-de-sac
(kool-de-**sak**) (n) a blind pouch

culdoscopy
(kool-**dos**-kO-pee) (n) introduction of an endoscope through the posterior vaginal wall

curettage
(koo-re-**tahzh**) (n) scraping of an interior of a cavity, usually to remove growths or tissue

cyanosis
(cI-a-**nO**-sis) (n) condition in which the skin and/or mucous membranes turn blue due to decreased amount of oxygen in the blood cells

decelerations »
(dee-cel-er-**ay**-shunz) (n) decreases in speed or rate (of contractions)

dysgerminoma »
(dis-jer-mi-**nO**-ma) (n) a rare cancerous ovarian tumor

dysmenorrhea »
(dis-men-Or-**ee**-a) (n) painful menstruation

dyspareunia
(dis-pa-**roo**-nee-a) (n) painful sexual intercourse

ectopic pregnancy
(ek-**top**-ik) (n) pregnancy in which a fertilized ovum is implanted outside the uterus, often in a fallopian tube

edema
(e-**dee**-ma) (n) excessive accumulation of fluid in tissues, especially just under the skin or in a given cavity

effacement
(ee-**fays**-ment) (n) thinning of the cervix just before or during labor

emesis
(**em**-e-sis) (n) retching; throwing up

endocervical »
(en-dO-**ser**-va-cal) (adj) pertaining to the lining of the canal of the cervix uteri

endometrium
(**en**-dO-**mee**-tree-um) (n) lining of the womb, composed of three layers and shed during menstruation

endometrial »
(en-do-**mee**-tree-al) (adj) pertaining to the mucous membrane lining of the uterus

engorged
(en-**gorjd**) (adj) filled to the limit of expansion

epidural »
(ep-i-**doo**-ral) (adj) located over or under the dura

episiotomy »
(e-peez-ee-**ot**-O-mee) (n) incision of perineum to facilitate delivery and prevent laceration (jagged tear)

epithelial »
(ep-i-**thee**-lee-al) (adj) pertaining to or composed of epithelium, the layer of cells forming the epidermis of the skin and the surface layer of mucous and serous membranes

estradiol »
(es-tra-**dI**-ol) (n) a hormone produced by the ovary; often used to treat menopausal symptoms

eversion
(ee-**vur**-zhun) (n) turning out or inside out

excrescence
(eks-**kres**-ens) (n) abnormal projection or outgrowth; such as a wart

fallopian tubes
(fa-**lO**-pee-an) (n) passageways from ovaries to uterus

fascia »
(**fash**-ee-a) (n) fibrous connective tissue that supports and sheathes soft organs and muscles

fetal distress
(**fee**-tal) (n) life-threatening condition affecting the fetus

fibroid
(**fI**-broyd) (adj) composed of fibers or fibrous tissue

fibrosis »
(fI-**brO**-sis) (n) a condition marked by thickening and scarring of connective tissue

fundus
(**fun**-dus) (n) the bottom or base of an organ; the part farthest from the opening; fundi (pl)

genital
(**jen**-i-tal) (adj) relating to reproduction or the organs of reproduction

genitalia
(jen-i-**tay**-lee-a) (n) male or female reproductive organs, especially the external ones

gestation »
(jes-**tay**-shun) (n) the intrauterine development of an infant; pregnancy

gonorrhea
(gon-O-**ree**-a) a contagious disease usually affecting the genitourinary tract; transmitted chiefly by sexual intercourse; caused by *Neisseria gonorrhea*

graafian follicle
(**graf**-ee-an) (n) a mature follicle on the ovary in which an oocyte matures and is released at ovulation

gravida »
(**grav**-i-da) (n) a pregnant woman; may be used in combination with a number or prefix to indicate the number of pregnancies and their outcome

histiocytes »
(**his**-tee-O-sItz) (n) cells present in loose connective tissues

homeostasis »
(**hO**-mee-O-**stay**-sis/**hO**-mee-**os**-ta-sis) (n) equilibrium in the internal environment of the body, such as temperature and electrolyte balance

hypermenorrhea
(**hI**-per-men-O-**ree**-a) (n) lengthy or heavy menses; menorrhagia

hypomenorrhea
(**hI**-pO-men-O-**ree**-a) (n) decreased menses

hysterectomy
(his-ter-**ek**-tO-mee) (n) surgical removal of the uterus

immunohistochemistry »
(**im**-yoo-nO-**his**-tO-**kem**-is-tree) (n) special techniques used on cells to identify certain characteristics, especially the presence of specific antigens

incised »
(in-**sIzd**) (v) cut with a knife

Indocin »
(in-**doe**-sin) (n) Brand name for indomethacin, an analgesic non-steroidal anti-inflammatory drug

infundibulopelvic »
(in-fun-**dib**-yoo-lO-**pel**-vik) (adj) relating to or located in the infundibulum (the end of the fallopian tube farthest from the uterus) and the pelvis

in situ »
(in **sI**-too) (adj, adv) in position; at the original location, or site

intraductal
(adj) inside a duct

intramural
(in-tra-**myoo**-ral) (adj) within the wall of a cavity

intrauterine »
(in-tra-**yoo**-ter-in) (adj) within the uterus

introitus »
(in-**trO**-i-tus) (n) an opening or entrance into a canal or cavity, such as the vagina

inversion
(in-**vur**-shun) (n) reversal of position, as upside down or inside out

knuckle
(**nuk**-l) (n) a finger joint; an abnormal kink or loop

laparotomy »
(lap-a-**rot**-O-mee) (n) a surgical incision made into the abdominal wall

leiomyoma
(lI-O-mI-**O**-ma) (n) benign tumor arising from smooth muscle

leukemia
(loo-**kee**-mee-a) (n) production of abnormal white blood cells; a type of cancer of the blood

lochia
(**lO**-kee-a) (n) vaginal discharge occurring after childbirth

loop
(n) a curve or bend forming a complete or almost complete oval or circle

loupe
(loop) (n) a magnifying lens

lumbar »
(**lum**-bar) (adj) pertaining to the part of the back between the thorax and pelvis

lymphatic »
(lim-**fat**-ik) (adj) relating to or resembling lymph or lymph nodes

lymphocyte »
(**lim**-fO-sIt) (n) a subgroup of white blood cells produced in lymphatic tissue. Lymphocytes normally make up 22-28% of peripheral white cells.

lymphocytic
(lim-fO-**sit**-ik) (adj) relating to or characteristic of lymphocytes

mammogram »
(**mam**-O-gram) (n) x-ray of the breast

meconium »
(mee-**kO**-nee-um) (n) first bowel movement of a newborn, which are thick, sticky, greenish to black and composed of bile pigments and gland secretions

mediolateral »
(**mee**-dee-O-**lat**-er-al) (adj) relating to the middle and side of a structure

menarche »
(me-**nar**-kee) (n) the initial menstrual period

menometrorrhagia
(**men**-O-mee-trO-**ray**-jee-a) (n) excessive menstrual bleeding or bleeding between menstrual periods

menopause
(**men**-O-pawz) (n) the end of a woman's reproductive period of life and cessation of menses

menorrhagia »
(men-O-**ray**-jee-a) (n) prolonged or heavy menses; hypermenorrhea

menorrhalgia
(men-O-**ral**-jee-a) (n) painful menstruation or pelvic pain accompanying menstruation

menses »
(**men**-seez) (n) monthly flow of bloody fluid from the uterus

menstruation
(men-stroo-**ay**-shun) (n) the discharge of a bloody fluid from the uterus at regular intervals during the life of a woman from puberty to menopause

mesosalpinx »
(**mez**-O-**sal**-pinks) (n) free end of the broad ligament which supports the fallopian tubes

metastatic »
(met-a-**stat**-ic) (n) pertaining to metastasis (movement of cells, especially cancer cells, from one part of the body to another)

metrorrhagia
(mee-trO-**ray**-jee-a) (n) bleeding from the uterus between menstrual periods

multipara
(mul-**tip**-a-ra) (n) a woman who has given birth to two or more children

necrosis »
(ne-**crO**-sis) (n) dead areas of tissue or bone surrounded by healthy parts

nodule »
(**nod**-yool) (n) a small mass, distinct from surrounding tissue

nuchal
(**noo**-kal) (adj) relating to the nape or back of the neck

nulligravida »
(nul-i-**grav**-i-da) (n) a woman who has never been pregnant

nulliparous
(nul-**ip**-a-rus) (adj) a woman who has not had a child

occiput »
(**ok**-si-put) (n) the back part of the skull

oligohydramnios »
(**ol**-i-gO-hI-**dram**-nee-os) (n) abnormally small amount of amniotic fluid

oligomenorrhea »
(**ol**-i-gO-men-O-**ree**-a) (n) infrequent or very light menstrual bleeding

omental
(O-**men**-tal) (adj) relating to the omentum

omentum

(O-**men**-tum) (n) fold of peritoneal tissue attaching to and supporting the stomach and intestines

oophorectomy

(O-of-Or-**ek**-tO-mee) (n) surgical removal of one or both ovaries

organomegaly

(**Or**-ga-nO-**meg**-a-lee) (n) abnormal enlargement of an organ, particularly an organ of the abdominal cavity, such as the liver or spleen

palpate »

(**pal**-payt) (v) to examine by touch; to feel

para

(**par**-a) (n) a woman who has given birth to one or more children; the term may be used in combination with a number or prefix to indicate how many times a woman has given birth

pelvic »

(**pel**-vik) (adj) relating to or located near the pelvis

pendulous »

(**pen**-ju-lus) (adj) loosely hanging

perineum »

(per-i-**nee**-um) (n) the external region between the urethral opening and the anus, including the skin and underlying tissues

peritoneal »

(per-i-tO-**nee**-al) (adj) relating to the peritoneum

Pfannenstiel incision

(**fahn**-in-shteel) (n) a transverse incision made just above the pubes

Pitocin »

(pi-**tO**-sin) (n) Brand name for oxytocin, a synthetically produced, naturally-occurring hormone

peritoneum »

(per-i-tO-**nee**-um) (n) lining of the abdominal cavity

polycystic »

(pol-ee-**sis**-tik) (adj) having or consisting of many cysts

preeclampsia

(pree-ee-**klamp**-see-a) (n) development of hypertension, proteinuria and/or edema during pregnancy

primipara

(prE-**mip**-ah-ra) (n) a woman who has had one pregnancy that produced a living infant

pyelogram

(**pI**-el-O-gram) (n) x-ray of the kidney and ureters; usually a radiopaque dye is injected into the patient to show the outline of the kidney and associated structures

rectovaginal »

(**rek**-tO-**vaj**-i-nal) (adj) relating or located near the rectum and vagina

retraction

(ree-**trak**-shun) (n) the act of pulling back

sac

(sak) (n) pouch

sentinel node »

(**sen**-ti-nal nOd) (n) an enlarged, supraclavicular lymph node infiltrated with cancer cells that have metastasized from an obscurely located primary cancer

sonometer

(**son**-O-mee-ter) (n) a bell-shaped instrument used to measure hearing

speculum »

(**spek**-yoo-lum) (n) instrument for examination of canals

squamous »

(**skway**-mus) (adj) covered with scale-like cells

station

(**stay**-shun) (n) the degree of descent of the presenting part of the fetus, measured in relation to the ischial spines of the maternal pelvis and reported in negative to positive numbers

supine

(soo-**pIn**) (adj) lying on the back

Tanner staging

(n) method of indicating the sexual development of a child or adolescent

thelarche

(thee-**lar**-kee) (n) the beginning of breast development in girls

thyroid

(**thI**-royd) (n) a gland in the neck that secretes thyroid hormone

thyromegaly »

(thI-rO-**meg**-a-lee) (n) enlargement of the thyroid gland

TORCH

acronym for toxoplasmosis, other infections, rubella, cytomegalovirus infection, and herpes simplex. A TORCH titer is performed on pregnant women to assess their immune status.

transverse »

(trans-**vers**) (adj) lying at right angles to the long axis of the body; crosswise

ureter »

(**yoo**-re-ter) (n) the tube that carries urine from the kidney to the bladder

uterine »

(**yoo**-ter-in/**yoo**-ter-In) (adj) relating to the uterus (the female reproductive organ where the fertilized egg develops before birth; the womb)

vertex »

(**ver**-teks) (n) the crown or top of the head

vesicouterine »

(**ves**-i-kO-**yoo**-ter-in) (adj) pertaining to the urinary bladder and uterus

vortex »

(**vor**-teks) (n) whirlpool; resembling a whirlpool

vulva »

(**vul**-va) (n) external female genital organs; vulvae (pl)

vulvar

(**vul**-var) (adj) relating to the vulva

xeromammogram »

(**zeer**-O-**mam**-o-gram) (n) type of x-ray of the breast

Abbreviations

AB, Ab	abortion		GYN	gynecology
AIDS	acquired immune deficiency syndrome		hCG	human chorionic gonadotropin
AUB	abnormal uterine bleeding		HIV	human immunodeficiency virus
BBT	basal body temperature		HPV	human papilloma virus
BCP	birth control pill(s)		HRT	hormone replacement therapy
BSO	bilateral salpingo-oophorectomy (removal of both ovaries and fallopian tubes)		HSG	hysterosalpingography
			IUD	intrauterine device
BTL	bilateral tubal ligation (sterilization by cutting or cauterizing the fallopian tubes)		LEEP	loop electrosurgical excision procedure
			LH	luteinizing hormone
CIN	cervical intraepithelial neoplasia		LMP	last menstrual period
CPD	cephalopelvic disproportion		NB	newborn
CS,	cesarean section		OB	obstetrics
C-section			Pap	Papanicolaou
D&C	dilatation and curettage		PCOS	polycystic ovary syndrome
DHEAS	dehydroepiandrosterone sulfate		PID	pelvic inflammatory disease
DOB	date of birth		PMP	previous menstrual period
DUB	dysfunctional uterine bleeding		STD	sexually transmitted disease
EDC	estimated date of confinement		TAH	total abdominal hysterectomy
FEKG	fetal electrocardiogram		TAH/BSO	total abdominal hysterectomy with bilateral salpingo-oophorectomy
FHR	fetal heart rate			
FHT	fetal heart tones		TBS	The Bethesda System
FSH	follicle-stimulating hormone		TSH	thyroid stimulating hormone
FTND	full term, normal delivery		UC	uterine contractions
FTNSVD	full term, normal spontaneous vaginal delivery		VH	vaginal hysterectomy
GC	gonococcus (gonorrhea)		VBAC	vaginal birth after cesarean section

Building Language Skills

Complete the following exercises, drawing on the information learned in the Exploring Obstetrics and Gynecology section of this chapter and referencing the Terms Bank.

Exercise 11.1   Matching Sound and Spelling

The numbered list that follows shows the phonetic spelling of hard-to-spell words. Sound out the word and then write the correct spelling in the blank space provided. Check your answers in the Terms Bank or other appropriate reference.

1. e-peez-ee-**ot**-O-mee _____

2. kol-**pos**-ko-pee _____

3. **krO**-mO-sOm _____

4. a-men-O-**ree**-a _____

5. kon-di-**lO**-ma _____

6. **graf**-ee-an _____

7. jes-**tay**-shun _____

8. his-ter-**ek**-tO-mee _____

9. **kyoo**-re-**tahzh** _____

10. in **sl**-too _____

11. mul-**tip**-a-ra _____

12. gon-O-**ree**-a _____

13. **men**-O-**rah**-jee-a _____

14. **ol**-i-gO-men-O-**ree**-a _____

15. per-i-**nee**-um _____

Below is a list of frequently used words that look alike and/or sound alike. Study the meaning and pronunciation of each set of words, read the following sentences carefully, and then circle the word in parentheses that correctly completes the meaning.

amenorrhea	absence of menses for three months or more	**elicit**	(v) to bring out
		illicit	(adj) illegal
dysmenorrhea	painful menstruation		
hypermenorrhea	prolonged or heavy menses	**eminent**	prominent, famous, standing out
hypomenorrhea	diminished menses	**imminent**	about to occur
oligomenorrhea	infrequent or scant menstrual bleeding		
		foul	offensive
		fowl	bird
an ovulatory	adjective, describing one who ovulates	**leap**	to jump
anovulatory	not ovulatory	**LEEP**	acronym for loop electrosurgical excision procedure
Apgar	a grading system for assessing newborn infants	**menometrorrhagia**	
			irregular or excessive bleeding during menses and between menses
APGAR	acronym for adaptation, partnership, growth, affection, and resolve; a family assessment instrument	**menopause**	cessation of reproductive period of life and cessation of menses for at least one year
bimanual	using two hands, a method for examining the pelvic area	**menorrhagia**	prolonged or heavy menses
by manual	using the hands	**menorrhalgia**	painful menstruation or pelvic pain accompanying menstruation
colposcopy	examination of vagina and cervix using an endoscope		
culdoscopy	introduction of endoscope through posterior vaginal wall	**perineum**	external region between the urethral opening and the anus
		peritoneum	lining of the abdominal cavity
continual	regular or frequent	**thorough**	complete, meticulous
continuous	ceaseless; uninterrupted in time	**through**	nonstop, straight, finished, by way of
cornea	outer protective layer of the eye		
cornua	plural of cornu; horn		
decent	(adj) appropriate, conforming to acceptable behavior		
descent	(n) downward movement, lowering		

1. The patient denies use of (elicit/illicit) drugs.

2. Palpation of the area did not (elicit/illicit) pain.

3. She had a (continual/continuous) menstruation that lasted more than four weeks.

4. The patient seemed anxious to get (thorough/through) the physical examination.

5. The (decent/descent) of the laparoscope into the suprapubic area proceeded with minimal discomfort to the patient.

6. The patient has (amenorrhea/dysmenorrhea) with menses but Advil usually controls the pain.

7. Hypermenorrhea and (menorrhagia/menorrhalgia) mean the same thing.

8. Noting that the birth of the baby seemed (eminent/imminent), the nurse paged the obstetrician.

9. Dysmenorrhea and (menorrhagia/menorrhalgia) mean the same thing.

10. The end of one's reproductive life phase is called (menopause/menses).

Exercise 11.3   Choosing Words from Context

When transcribing dictation, the medical transcriptionist frequently needs to consider the situation when determining the word that correctly completes the sentence. From the list below, select the term that meaningfully completes each of the following statements.

adhesions	hypomenorrhea	menses
carcinoma	introitus	para
dysmenorrhea	lymphocyte	peritoneum
genital	mammogram	uterine
gravida	menopause	

1. Her previous abdominal surgery resulted in extensive _____, especially between the bowel and uterus.

2. Mrs. Jones states she has severe cramping at the time of her _____.

3. She has a condyloma on her external _____ area.

4. The _____ is found at the entrance of the vagina.

5. Her blood count revealed an increased _____ count, possibly indicating a viral infection.

6. Since the patient is 48 years old, her lack of menses is most likely due to _____.

7. The hysterectomy was performed after the biopsy revealed a _____.

8. Mrs. Green is a (an) _____ 2, para 1, and presents to the birthing center today in active labor.

9. The _____ contractions increased steadily until the baby was delivered.

10. After the tumor was removed from the abdominal wall, the _____ was washed.

Exercise 11.4   Pairing Words and Meanings

From this list, locate the term that best matches each of the following definitions. Write the term in the space provided by each definition.

adrenarche	endometriosis	nulligravida
amenorrhea	hysterectomy	oligomenorrhea
anovulation	intramural	preeclampsia
calcification	menarche	
edema	menses	

1. absence of egg release from an ovary   _____

2. within the wall of a cavity   _____

3. changes that occur at puberty   _____

4. hypertension and proteinuria during pregnancy   _____

5. a hardening of tissue from formation of calcium   _____

6. ectopic uterine tissue   _____

7. excessive amount of fluid in body tissues   _____

8. first menstrual period   _____

9. a woman who has never conceived a child   _____

10. monthly flow of blood from the uterus   _____

Exercise 11.5   Creating Terms from Word Forms

Combine prefixes, root words, and suffixes from this list to create medical words that fit the following definitions. Fill in the blanks with the words you construct.

a-	without; absence	**son/o**	sound waves
dys-	difficult, painful	**thyr/o**	thyroid
hepat/o	liver	**germin**	germinal tissue
hyster/o	uterus	**-algi/o**	pain
lei/o	smooth	**-ectomy**	cutting out, removal
mamm/o	breast	**-gram**	record
mast/o	breast	**-itis**	inflammation
men/o	(month) menses	**-megaly**	enlargement
my/o	muscle	**-oma**	tumor
olig/o	little	**-rrhagia**	unusual or excessive flow (discharge)
oophor/o	ovary		
organ/o	liver, spleen	**-rrhea**	flow, discharge
salping/o	tube		

1. removal of fallopian tubes _____

2. very large thyroid gland _____

3. inflammation of the ovary _____

4. menstruation _____

5. benign tumor arising from smooth muscle tissue _____

6. rare ovarian malignant tumor that causes pain _____

7. x-ray of breast _____

8. radiographic image of the uterus and fallopian tubes _____

9. removal of ovary _____

10. removal of breast _____

11. ultrasound image/record _____

12. absence of menses _____

13. scanty menstrual flow _____

14. excessive menstrual flow _____

15. painful menstruation _____

Exercise 11.6   Proofreading Review

Read the following report excerpts and look for errors in punctuation, spelling, plural vs. singular word forms, subject-verb agreement, incomplete sentences, and modifier placement. Mark the corrections on this page and key the excerpts with all errors corrected. Save the documents as XXExercise11.06-1 and XXExercise11.06-2, using your initials in place of *XX* in the file names.

1. Increased density is again seen in the upper outer quadrants bilaterally, unchanged and consistent with fibroglandular tissue. Neither breasts demonstrates evidence of architectural distortion, clustered microcalcifications, skin thickening or retraction.

2. The patient was placed on the operating table in the supine position under satisfactory general endotracheal anesthesias. A #14 foley cathether was inserted. The abdomen was then prepped with betadine scrub and solution and was drapped in the usual sterile manner.

Exercise 11.7   Thinking Like a Professional

Read this scenario carefully and then select the most appropriate response. Write an explanation for why you think your choice is the best answer.

The physician dictates what sounds like Synthroid 175 mg, but a conversation in the background partially obscures the dictation and you are not sure of the dose. What should you transcribe?

---

a. Transcribe what you think you hear and let the physician correct it if it is wrong.

b. Transcribe Synthroid 175 mcg.

c. Transcribe 0.175 mg.

d. Leave the dosage blank.

Best response: _____

Explanation: _____

_____

_____

_____

_____

You will apply the medical specialty and language information you learned in this chapter to transcription work in this section. After you learn the formatting recommendations of the labor and delivery report, you will transcribe nine reports related to nine different patient studies.

Introducing the Labor and Delivery Report

As its title suggests, the labor and delivery report (Figure 11.6) summarizes the procedures used in the delivery of a baby. Although most are brief reports, those describing a delivery that requires the physician's surgical intervention—for example, delivery by forceps—can be as extensive as an operative report.

Required Headings/Content

Although no specific headings are required, the labor and delivery report includes headings similar to those in an operative report. Usually dictated are the preoperative and postoperative diagnoses, the title and date of the procedure, the indications for the procedure, and the actual description of the procedure.

Refer to page 472 of Appendix A for a complete list of headings found in the labor and delivery report template along with descriptions of the type of information found under each heading. Not every template heading will be included in every transcribed report.

Turnaround Time

Generally, labor and delivery reports should be transcribed within 24 hours after dictation. However, this guideline varies among hospitals.

Preparing to Transcribe

To prepare for transcribing dictation, review the common obstetrics and gynecology terms, drugs, and abbreviations presented in this chapter's Terms Bank. Then, study the format and organization of the model document shown in Figure 11.6, and key the model document, using the labor and delivery template on the Dictations and Templates CD as a starting point. Save the document as XXFigure11.06 using your initials in place of *XX* in the file name. Proofread the document by comparing it with the printed version. Categorize the types of errors you made, and document them on a copy of the Performance Comparison Chart. A template of this chart is included on the Dictations and Templates CD.

Transcribing Reports

Transcribe, edit, and correct each report in the following patient studies. Consult reference books for words or formatting rules that are unfamiliar.

As you work on the transcription assignment for this chapter, fill in the Performance Comparison Chart that you started when you keyed the model document. For at least three of the reports, categorize and document the types of errors you made. Answer the document analysis questions on the bottom of the chart. With continuous practice and assessment, the quality of your work will improve.

PATIENT NAME: Jung-Ah Wang
PHYSICIAN: Alexandra Mateo, MD
DATE OF PROCEDURE: 10/21/20XX
    ds

PREOPERATIVE DIAGNOSIS
Arrest of descent.
    ds

POSTOPERATIVE DIAGNOSIS
Single viable female infant.
    ds

NAME OF PROCEDURE
Indicated low forceps delivery.
    ds

ANESTHESIA
Epidural.
    ds

INDICATIONS
This is a 33-year-old gravida 1, para 0, who pushed greater than 2 hours and then consented to epidural anesthesia. She pushed for 1 more hour and pushed the baby to +2 station and consented for assisted vaginal delivery.
    ds

PROCEDURE
After adequate epidural anesthesia, the patient was placed in stirrups and was prepared and draped in the usual sterile fashion. The cervix was again examined and noted to be completely dilated, completely effaced. The pelvis was noted to be adequate. The estimated fetal weight was approximately 8 pounds. Position of the infant was noted to be right occiput posterior. The station was noted to be +2.
    ds

The bladder was drained with a red Robinson catheter. Simpson forceps were then soaked in Betadine solution and the posterior blade was carefully placed, with the opposite hand protecting the vaginal side wall. The same procedure was repeated on the opposite site. Correct blade placement was then verified x2. A midline episiotomy was then performed. With adequate maternal expulsive efforts, a viable female infant was delivered over a midline episiotomy. A vigorous cry was noted on the perineum. Inspection of the infant noted correct blade placement. The baby was bulb suctioned on the perineum and passed off to the awaiting pediatricians, given Apgar scores of 9 and 10. Weight of the infant was 3762 g. Cord pH was obtained, arterial 7.29, venous 7.33.
    ds

The vagina was inspected for lacerations and there were none. The cervix and rectum were intact. The midline episiotomy was then reapproximated with a 2-0 Vicryl suture. The placenta was easily removed followed by vigorous fundal massage, and intravenous Pitocin was given.

(continued)

Figure 11.6   Labor and Delivery Report

LABOR AND DELIVERY REPORT
PATIENT NAME: Jung-Ah Wang
DATE OF PROCEDURE: 10/21/20XX
Page 2

second page
running head

Uterine tone was noted to be firm. After delivery of the infant at 0234, both mother and infant were doing well.
        ds
COMPLICATIONS
There were no complications.

        qs

_____
Alexandra Mateo, MD
        ds
AM/XX
D: 10/21/20XX
T: 10/22/20XX

Figure 11.6 Labor and Delivery Report (Continued)

Felicia Stallward is a 25-year-old woman who had leukemia as a young child and presently complains of irregular menstruation. She is seen by the gynecologist.

REPORT 11.1 Consultation Letter

Use the Report1101.mp3 audio file and the consultation letter template (Consultation_Letter) when transcribing this report. Save the document as XXReport11.01, using your initials in place of *XX* in the file name.

Listen for these abbreviations and terms:
> DHEAS (dehydroepiandrosterone sulfate)
> rectovaginal
> TSH (thyroid-stimulating hormone)

This letter will include information related to a physical exam, and this section should be transcribed in paragraph form. After the physical exam narrative, this letter will include two internal headings. Transcribe the headings as dictated, and set them flush left in all capital letters.

Rosemary Barnes discovered a lump in her left breast when she was performing her monthly breast self-examination. She was seen in the gynecologist's office immediately. She was sent to the surgeon for examination and excision of the mass.

REPORT 11.2 Pathology Report

Use the Report1102.mp3 audio file and the pathology report template (Pathology_Report) when transcribing this report. Save the document as XXReport11.02, using your initials in place of *XX* in the file name.

Use the pathology report template (Pathology_Report.dot) for this report.

Listen for this term:
> fibroglandular

Remember that a clinical diagnosis is synonymous to a clinical history in the context of this report.

Jung-ah Wang is a 33-year-old woman who was admitted to the hospital to deliver her first child. She has had an unproductive labor and has agreed to an assisted vaginal delivery with forceps.

REPORT 11.3 Labor and Delivery Report

Use the Report1103.mp3 audio file and the labor and delivery report template (Labor_and_Delivery_Report) when transcribing this report. Save the document as XXReport11.03, using your initials in place of *XX* in the file name.

It is important to apply the template headings as much as possible in order to organize the important details in the transcribed report. Although the provider does not dictate the Anesthesia and Complications headings, your transcribed report should include them. Details regarding estimated blood loss are not dictated.

Gravida refers to the number of times a woman has been pregnant. Para indicates the number of deliveries after the 20th week of gestation. A woman who has been pregnant five times (two term infants, one premature infant, one abortion, and one miscarriage) may be described in several different ways, all of which are acceptable:

"The patient is gravida five, para three." (transcribed gravida 5, para 3)

"The patient is G five, P three." (transcribed G5, P3)

"The patient is gravida five, para three, aborta two." (transcribed gravida 5, para 3, aborta 2)

"The patient is G five, P three, AB two [or A two]." (transcribed G5, P3, AB 2 [or A2])

The physician may also use TPAL terminology, listing numbers in an order that correlates with the following designations: T = term infants, P = premature infants, A = abortions or miscarriages, L = living children.

Thus, if the dictator says, "The patient is gravida five, para two one two three" or "obstetric history two one two three," you would key: The patient is gravida 5, para 2-1-2-3 or Obstetric history: 2-1-2-3.

Some physicians use the military style for expressing time. For example, in this report, the dictator notes that the infant was delivered at "zero two thirty-four," which means 2:34 a.m., and which should be transcribed as 0234. See Chapter 4 for more information on transcribing time expressions.

Mary Ewing is an 18-year-old female who has experienced intermittent abdominal pain for several weeks. She was seen by her physician, and, at that time, there were no significant findings. Three weeks ago, she found that her waist had significantly increased in size. She also had continued abdominal pain and had some vomiting for the past several days. She returned to her physician who palpated a mass in the lower abdomen and referred her to the surgeon.

REPORT 11.4 Operative Report

Use the Report1104.mp3 audio file and the operative report template (Operative_Report) when transcribing this report. Save the document as XXReport11.04, using your initials in place of *XX* in the file name.

Listen for these terms:
  infundibulopelvic
  mesosalpinx

Within this report, the provider will dictate information related to the estimated blood loss and the operation's complications within the body of the report. Transcribe these important details under the appropriate headings in the template.

This report demonstrates the difficulty in hearing numbers correctly when two numbers are dictated consecutively. Although it sounds like the dictator is using 22-0 silk sutures, silk sutures are not available in 22-0. The dictator is stating the number of sutures using 2-0 silk. Listen carefully to correctly transcribe the numbers.

There are times when a report is dictated by someone other than the person signing the report. For example, a resident may dictate a report for a physician. For these cases, *Dictated by:* and the person's name should be transcribed directly following the report body but before the signature line. The initials at the bottom of the report should correspond.

Gena Martin is a 21-year-old woman who was admitted to the hospital in labor with her first child. When tests indicated fetal distress, Gena agreed to undergo a cesarean section.

REPORT 11.5 Operative Report

Use the Report1105.mp3 audio file and the operative report template (Operative_Report) when transcribing this report. Save the document as XXReport11.05, using your initials in place of *XX* in the file name.

Listen for these terms:
  DeLee suctioned
  vancomycin

Be sure to correct any dangerous abbreviations.

Patient Study 11.F   Marta Valdez

Marta Valdez is a 22-year-old woman who is pregnant with twins. With her previous pregnancy, she developed cervical dilation at 20 weeks of gestation, which required cervical cerclage. Her obstetrician has recommended cervical cerclage with this pregnancy to prevent premature labor and delivery.

REPORT 11.6 Operative Report

Use the Report1106.mp3 audio file and the operative report template (Operative_Report) when transcribing this report. Save the document as XXReport11.06, using your initials in place of *XX* in the file name.

Physicians may use clock terminology to indicate areas on a circular surface. In this report, for example, the dictator describes the placement of a 5 mm Mersilene band at the "6 o'clock position" and the "2 o'clock" position of the cervix. Transcribe these expressions using figures and the word "o'clock" (6 o'clock and 2 o'clock).

Listen for these terms:
amnion
Indocin
Sims elevator
Trendelenburg position
Unasyn

Be sure to correct any dangerous abbreviations.

Patient Study 11.G   Amy Bataglia

Amy Bataglia is a 21-year-old pregnant woman who was admitted to the hospital in labor. She has received her prenatal care in the medical center's OB clinic and is known to have a breech malpresentation with oligohydramnios. In consultation with her physician, she has agreed to a cesarean section.

REPORT 11.7 Operative Report

Use the Report1107.mp3 audio file and the operative report template (Operative_Report) when transcribing this report. Save the document as XXReport11.07, using your initials in place of *XX* in the file name.

Listen for these terms:
cul-de-sac
Kocher clamp
Mauriceau-Smellie-Veit maneuver
Metzenbaum scissors
oligohydramnios
Pfannenstiel incision

In this dictation, the physician uses the made-up word "exteriorized." It is used by the dictator to describe the bringing of the uterus to the exterior. There would be no appropriate way that the MT could rewrite this sentence. Therefore, exteriorized is used in the final transcription.

Be sure to correct any dangerous abbreviations.

This is the pathology report of a 68-year-old female who had an exploratory laparotomy with hysterectomy to remove a large pelvic mass.

REPORT 11.8 Pathology Report

Use the Report1108.mp3 audio file and the pathology report template (Pathology_Report) when transcribing this report. Save the document as XXReport11.08, using your initials in place of *XX* in the file name.

Listen for the following terms:

    debulking
    endomyometrium
    endosalpingosis
    lap = laparotomy
    mucinous
    müllerian
    multicystic
    multiloculated
    omentectomy
    omentum
    papillae
    RPMI
    supracervical

If a dictator uses a trailing zero in a measurement, include it in the transcribed report. Do not add a trailing zero if it is not dictated.

This pathology report is from a 31-year-old female who underwent a partial mastectomy, sentinel node biopsy with axillary node dissection.

REPORT 11.9 Pathology Report

Use the Report1109.mp3 audio file and the pathology report template (Pathology_Report) when transcribing this report. Save the document as XXReport11.09, using your initials in place of *XX* in the file name.

Listen for these terms:

    adenosis
    cribriform
    fibrofatty
    homogeneous
    in situ
    micrometastases
    pancytokeratin
    subcapsular

Urology and Nephrology

Urology is the study of the urinary tract in both sexes and the genital tract in the male. Nephrology is the science related to the structure and function of the kidney. Because the systems are interdependent, the specialties are often considered together in medical studies. The subspecialists concerned with the urinary system are the urologist and the nephrologist.

Objectives

» Identify the organs and structures of the male reproductive system.

» Identify the organs and structures of the male and female urinary systems.

» Describe the function of the kidneys and bladder.

» Recognize diagnostic and laboratory tests used to evaluate the urinary system.

» Pronounce and correctly spell terminology related to the male reproductive systems and the male and female urinary systems.

» Transcribe dictation related to the medical specialties of urology and nephrology.

» Describe a history and physical report, including typical content, format, and turnaround time.

The urinary system consists of those organs and related structures that produce urine and eliminate it from the body: the kidneys, ureters, bladder, and urethra (Figure 12.1). The body must have a proper balance of fluids and electrolytes to sustain life. Electrolytes (primarily sodium, potassium, and chloride) are charged particles dissolved in the intracellular, extracellular, and intravascular compartments. The urinary system regulates the fluid and electrolyte balance within the body by filtration, reabsorption, and secretion. The urinary system is also responsible for transporting and excreting chemical and metabolic wastes from the body. Although there are other avenues by which the body eliminates wastes, such as sweat and stool, urine is the primary transporter of metabolic byproducts. The kidneys also play a key role in maintaining blood pressure through the secretion of antidiuretic hormone (ADH). Erythropoietin, also secreted by the kidneys, is a hormone that stimulates the bone marrow to produce red cells.

Structure and Function

The body houses two kidneys, each a few centimeters to the right and left of the thoracic vertebrae. A thin capsule surrounds each kidney to protect and separate it from the abdominal cavity. Renal arteries branching off the aorta provide the blood supply.

The outer portion of the kidney is called the cortex; the inner portion is called the medulla. Within the kidney are approximately one million nephrons (Figure 12.2), which do the actual work of the kidney. Blood that is to be filtered enters the kidney through the renal artery, which branches into progressively smaller arterioles then capillaries. The capillaries are lined with a basement membrane designed to filter blood. A cluster of capillaries is called a glomerulus. Each glomerulus is surrounded by a Bowman capsule, which forms the beginning of the collecting tubule. The tubule is divided into four parts: a proximal convoluted tubule, the loop of Henle, a distal convoluted tubule, and a collecting tubule.

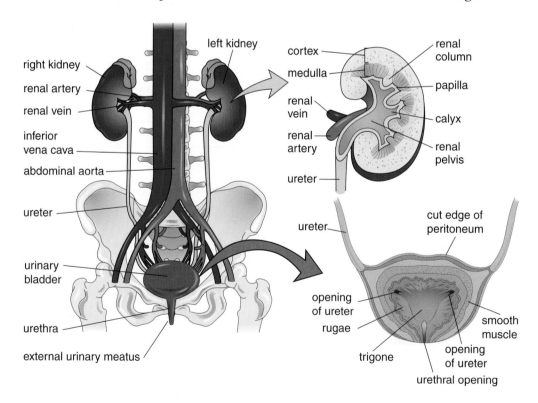

Figure 12.1 The Urinary System

As blood flows through the glomerulus, fluid filters out through the walls of the glomerular capillary tufts. This filtrate is composed of water, glucose, wastes, and electrolytes. As the filtrate travels through the tubule, electrolytes and water are reabsorbed or excreted as necessary to adjust the urine and electrolyte concentrations (conserve or eliminate sodium or potassium and concentrate the urine to prevent dehydration). The remaining fluid that reaches the kidney pelvis is urine.

From the renal pelvis, the urine travels through the ureters and into the bladder by peristaltic waves occurring about one to five times per minute. The bladder is lined with smooth muscle, which adapts to the slow filling and does not usually produce the sensation to void until there is approximately 200 to 300 mL of urine. The external urethral sphincter is a muscle that is under voluntary control, which is learned in early childhood. When there is a desire to urinate, the sphincter is relaxed. This allows the bladder muscles to contract and expel urine through the urethra and out the urinary meatus.

Women are seen by the gynecologist for many urogenital problems but may be referred to a urologist for chronic bladder problems. Men usually are seen by the urologist for problems with the urogenital system, which include the male sexual organs. While male sexual dysfunction may be treated by the urologist, male infertility may be managed by an infertility specialist. Figure 12.3 depicts the structures of the male urogenital anatomy.

The testes are contained in the scrotum. They are made of coils called seminiferous tubules. The hormone testosterone, responsible for male secondary sexual characteristics, is produced by the testes. The seminiferous tubules also produce spermatozoa (sperm). Over these tubules is the epididymis, where sperm migrate and mature.

When the penis is stimulated, it fills with blood and becomes erect. Sperm travels from the epididymis through the vas deferens by smooth muscle contractions. The sperm mixes with fluid secreted by the prostate gland, which is located at the base of the bladder. This alkaline substance, called semen, protects the sperm from the acidic environment of the male urethra and the female vagina. During ejaculation, semen passes through the urethra. The sphincter at the base of the bladder closes during ejaculation to prevent urine from exiting and semen from entering the bladder.

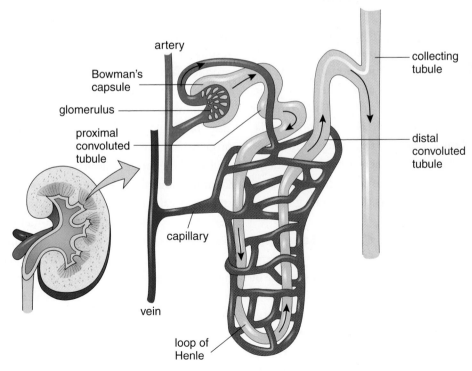

Figure 12.2 Structure of the Nephron

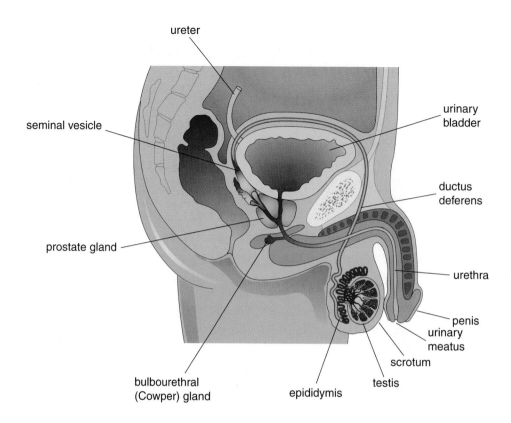

ureter

seminal vesicle

urinary
bladder

ductus
deferens

prostate gland

urethra

penis
urinary
meatus

scrotum

bulbourethral
(Cowper) gland

testis

epididymis

Figure 12.3 Male Urogenital System

Physical Assessment

Assessment of the urinary system is done by evaluating the patient's medical history and laboratory findings. The physical examination usually is secondary. The examiner asks about the color, odor, frequency, and volume of urine. The examiner queries for symptoms such as dysuria, nocturia, oliguria, polyuria, urgency, frequency, continence or incontinence, and characteristics of the urine stream. The male physical exam includes a digital rectal exam (DRE) to assess the prostate gland.

Diseases and Conditions

Diseases and pathology are described by the area of the urinary system involved. Common conditions affecting the kidney include renal failure, glomerulonephropathy, polycystic disease, acute tubular necrosis (ATN), nephrolithiasis, and hydronephrosis. Renal failure is categorized as prerenal (problems outside the kidney causing reduced blood flow coming into the kidney), intrarenal (conditions within the kidney), and postrenal (obstructions preventing outflow of urine). Renal failure results in decreased excretion of metabolic waste products (uremia) and fluid imbalances, which can lead to serious and life-threatening complications.

Nephrotic syndrome refers to a group of diseases of the glomerular apparatus that cause plasma proteins to cross the glomerular membrane and spill into the urine. Glomerulonephritis, which is inflammation of the glomeruli, is often a result of streptococcal infection due to accumulation of antigen-antibody complexes in the glomeruli. Immune complexes associated with systemic lupus erythematosus (SLE), scleroderma, and other autoimmune disorders may also cause glomerulonephritis.

Kidney stones (nephroliths) cause a painful condition called nephrolithiasis. Stones, also called urinary calculi, usually consist of calcium oxalate or calcium phosphate but may also be composed of uric acid. Calculi lodge in the renal pelvis and/or the ureters and bladder, obstructing the flow of urine.

Obstructions may cause painful spasms called renal colic. An obstruction can cause urine to accumulate in the kidney or ureters, leading to hydronephrosis. If the stones cannot be passed, the physician may perform lithotripsy to break up the calculi.

Bladder disorders may manifest by a loss of urinary control causing urgency, frequency, and/or incontinence. Cystitis (bladder inflammation and/or infection) may be characterized by dysuria, pyuria, and urinary frequency.

Disorders of the prostate gland have an effect on urination because the prostate gland sits at the base of the bladder and surrounds the prostatic urethra. Prostatitis (inflammation and/or infection of the prostate) may cause urgency and frequency, dysuria, and possibly urinary obstruction. Benign prostatic hypertrophy (BPH) is a nonmalignant hyperplasia of the prostate and is quite common in older men. Symptoms include decreased urinary stream caliber and force, hesitancy, interrupted stream, dribbling, or urine retention.

Common Tests and Surgical Procedures

A urinalysis is the most common test performed to evaluate the kidneys and bladder. Urine samples are collected in two ways:

- Clean-catch urine: the urinary meatus is cleaned with an antiseptic and the urine is collected midstream in a sterile container
- Catheterized specimen: a sterile, flexible tube (catheter) is inserted through the meatus into the bladder and the urine is collected in a sterile receptacle

A urinalysis (UA) has two components: the chemical analysis, and the microscopic analysis. The chemical analysis (sometimes called a dipstick test) tests for specific gravity, pH, glucose, protein, hemoglobin, leukocyte esterase, nitrites, urobilinogen, and ketones. The microscopic analysis examines the urine for formed elements such as red or white cells, epithelial cells, crystals, casts, and microorganisms. The color and clarity of the urine is also noted as part of the urinalysis.

Prostate specific antigen (PSA) level in the blood is used to assess the prostate. An elevated PSA level for a prolonged period of time indicates the possibility of prostate cancer.

Urea and creatinine are the major end products of protein metabolism. These two metabolites are only excreted through the kidneys, so serum levels are used to evaluate kidney function. A creatinine clearance test measures creatinine excretion in a urine specimen collected over at least 12 hours, but usually 24 hours, as well as the plasma level of creatinine on the same day. These values are used to calculate an estimated glomerular filtration rate (GFR). A more exact method to determine the filtration rate is through a nuclear scan (nuclear GFR).

Blood urea nitrogen (BUN) is a blood test that measures the blood level of urea. In kidney disease, the BUN results will be elevated, indicating the kidneys' inability to excrete urea properly.

Imaging tests to evaluate the urinary tract include KUB (x-ray of kidneys, ureters, bladder) and IVP (intravenous pyelogram). A cystometrogram (CMG) evaluates the bladder filling capacity and strength of contractions. A voiding cystourethrogram (VCUG) is performed to evaluate the function of the kidneys, urethra, and bladder. Contrast is instilled in the bladder and various x-rays are taken while the patient voids.

Lithotripsy and ureteroscopy are performed in order to crush and/or capture kidney stones within the kidney and/or within the ureter. Noninvasive treatment of ureteral stones, called expulsive therapy, can be accomplished using calcium channel blockers (with or without corticosteroids) and/or an alpha-blocker. These calcium channel blockers directly relax the "colicky" smooth muscle in the distal ureter and help to expel the stone.

Orchidopexy is a surgical procedure performed to correct an undescended testicle. A vasectomy is a surgical procedure used as a method of birth control in which the vas deferens is bisected in order to prevent sperm from entering the semen. Transurethral resection of the prostate (TURP) may be required to remove the prostate in cases of cancer or refractory hypertrophy.

Terms Bank

These terms and abbreviations provide a foundation for the language and transcription skills you will develop in the following sections of this chapter. Terms marked with » will be included in the reports transcribed in the Building Transcription Skills section.

auscultation »
(aws-kul-**tay**-shun) (n) process of listening for sounds produced in some of the body cavities, especially chest and abdomen, in order to detect abnormal conditions

Bactrim »
(**back**-trim) (n) brand name for co-trimoxazole, a sulfonamide antibiotic

biliary »
(**bil**-ee-ayr-ee) (adj) relating to bile or the gallbladder and its ducts

biopsy
(**bI**-op-see) (n) the removal of tissue and/or fluid from the body for microscopic examination; the specimen obtained

bulbar »
(**bul**-bar) (adj) bulb-shaped or relating to the medulla oblongata in the brain

calculus
(**kal**-kyoo-lus) (n) stone; a hard stone-like mass formed in the body; calculi (pl)

carotid »
(ka-**rot**-id) (n) paired arteries (right and left) that arise from the aorta and provide the principal blood supply to the head and neck

catheter
(**kath**-e-ter) (n) a tube inserted into the body for removing or instilling fluids for diagnostic or therapeutic purposes

cerebrospinal »
(**ser**-a-brO-**spI**-nal, se-**ree**-brO-**spI**-nal) (adj) referring to the brain and spinal cord

cystitis »
(sis-**tI**-tis) (n) inflammation of the urinary bladder

cortex »
(**kor**-tex) (n) the outer layer of an organ, such as the kidney, as distinguished from the inner portion, or medulla

cystoscopy »
(sis-**tos**-ko-pee) (n) examination of the inside of the urinary bladder with a lighted instrument inserted through the urethra

cystostomy »
(sis-**tos**-tO-mee) (n) surgical creation of an opening in the bladder

dilation »
(dI-**lay**-shun) (n) expansion of an organ or vessel

diltiazem »
(dil-**tie**-a-zem) (n) a generic calcium channel blocker, used for hypertension

diuretic
(dI-yoo-**ret**-ik) (n) an agent that increases the excretion of urine

dysuria
(dis-**yoo**-ree-a) (n) difficult or painful urination

edema »
(e-**dee**-ma) (n) excessive accumulation of fluid in tissues, especially just under the skin or in a given cavity

edematous
(e-**dem**-a-tus) (adj) having edema

electron
(ee-**lek**-tron) (n) a subatomic particle with a negative charge

encephalopathy »
(en-sef-a-**lop**-a-thee) (n) any dysfunction of the brain

endocapillary »
(**en**-dO-**cap**-i-layr-ee (n) within one of the tiny blood vessels

endoscope »
(**en**-dO-skOp) (n) a lighted instrument for examining the inside of a body cavity or organ

enuresis
(en-yoo-**ree**-sis) (n) bed-wetting; involuntary urination, especially at night in bed

epididymis
(ep-i-**did**-i-mis) (n) one of a pair of long, coiled ducts in the scrotum; they carry and store spermatozoa between the testes and ductus deferens

epispadias
(ep-i-**spay**-dee-as) a malformation in which the urinary meatus is on the upper surface of the penis

epithelial »
(ep-i-**thee**-lee-al) (adj) relating to or composed of epithelium

epithelium
(ep-i-**thee**-lee-um) (n) cell layers covering the outside body surfaces as well as forming the lining of hollow organs (such as the bladder) and the passages of the respiratory, digestive, and urinary tracts

extrahepatic
(eks-tra-he-**pat**-ik) (adj) unrelated to or located outside the liver

exudative »
(eks-yoo-**day**-tiv) (adj) pertaining to any fluid that has exuded out of a tissue or its capillaries

fascia
(**fash**-ee-a) (n) a thin layer of fibrous connective tissue that supports soft organs and covers structures such as muscles; fasciae (pl)

fetoprotein »
(fee-tO-**prO**-teen) (n) antigen (substance or organism that produces an antibody) naturally present in the fetus and sometimes present in adults with certain cancers

flank
(flaynk) (n) the fleshy part of the side between the ribs and the hip bone

fossa »
(**fos**-a) (n) channel or shallow depression; fossae (pl)

fundus »
(**fun**-dus) (n) the bottom or lowest parts of a sac or hollow organ; fundi (pl)

gastroesophageal »
(**gas**-trO-ee-soph-a-**jee**-al) (adj) related to both stomach and esophagus

genital
(**jen**-i-tal) (adj) relating to reproduction or the organs of reproduction

genitalia
(**jen**-i-**tay**-lee-a) (n) the genitals; male or female reproductive organs, especially the external ones

glomerulus »
(glO-**mayr**-yoo-lus) (n) a cluster of capillaries at the beginning of each nephron (the functional unit of the kidney); glomeruli (pl)

hematuria
(hee-ma-**too**-ree-a) (n) presence of blood in the urine

hemorrhagic »
(hem-O-**raj**-ik) (adj) relating to or experiencing a hemorrhage

histology »
(his-**tol**-O-jee) (n) a science of tissues, including their cellular composition and organization

hyperglycemic »
(**hI**-per-glI-**see**-mic) (adj) pertaining to or characterized by hyperglycemia, an abnormally large concentration of glucose in the circulating blood

hyperplasia »
(hI-per-**play**-see-a) (n) increase in size of a tissue or organ due to an increase in the number of cells (not including tumor formation)

hyperplastic
(hI-per-**plas**-tik) (adj) relating to hyperplasia

hypospadias
(hI-pO-**spay**-dee-as) (n) a malformation in which the urinary meatus is on the ventral side of the penis, proximal to its normal glanular position

idiopathic
(**id**-ee-O-**path**-ik) (adj) of unknown cause; describes a disease for which no identifiable cause can be determined

idiopathy
(id-ee-**op**-a-thee) (n) any disease of unknown cause

inguinal »
(**ing**-gwin-al) (adj) pertaining to the region of the groin

interstitial »
(in-ter-**stish**-al) (adj) relating to or located in the space between tissues, such as interstitial fluid

intrahepatic »
(**in**-tra-he-**pat**-ik) (adj) within the liver

kidneys
(**kid**-neez) (n) a pair of bean-shaped organs near the spinal column that filter blood and produce urine

levator
(le-**vay**-ter / le-**vay**-tOr) (n) muscle that lifts or raises the body part to which it is attached

lithotomy
(li-**thot**-O-mee) (n) surgical removal of a stone, especially from the urinary tract

lithotripsy »
(**lith**-O-trip-see) (n) procedure using a laser to break apart stones (calculi)

lumen »
(**loo**-men) (n) cavity, canal, or channel within an organ or tube; lumina or lumens (pl)

lymphadenitis
(lim-**fad**-e-**nI**-tis) (n) inflammation of one or more lymph nodes

lymphadenopathy »
(lim-fad-e-**nop**-a-thee) (n) any disorder of lymph nodes or of the lymphatic system

meatus
(mee-**ay**-tus) (n) a passage or channel, especially with an external opening

microscopy
(mI-**kros**-kO-pee) (n) use of a microscope to magnify and examine objects

micturition
(n) (mik-choo-**rish**-un) urination

mitotic »
(mI-**tot**-ik) (adj) pertaining to mitosis, a type of cell division in which a cell divides into two genetically identical daughter cells

mucosa »
(myoo-**kO**-sa) (n) mucous membrane

neoplasm
(**nee**-O-plazm) (n) any abnormal growth of tissue, usually malignant; tumor

nephrectomy »
(ne-**frek**-tO-mee) (n) surgical removal of a kidney

nephrolithiasis
(**nef**-rO-li-**thI**-a-sis) (n) presence of stones (calculi) in the kidney(s)

nephrolithotomy
(**nef**-rO-li-**thot**-O-mee) (n) surgical incision into a kidney to remove stones (calculi)

nephron
(**nef**-ron) (n) the functional unit of the kidney that filters the blood

nephrostomy
(ne-**fros**-tO-mee) (n) surgical creation of an opening in the kidney for drainage

nocturia
(nok-**too**-ree-a) (n) frequent urination during the night

nodular
(**nod**-yoo-lar) (adj) containing or resembling nodules; having small, firm, knotty masses

obturator
(**ob**-too-ray-tor) (n) device or body structure that closes up or covers an opening

orchidopexy »
(Or-ki-**dop**-eks-ee) (n) surgical procedure in which an undescended testicle is sutured into place; also orchiopexy

orchiectomy »
(Or-kee-**ek**-tO-mee) (n) surgical removal of one or both testes

orchiocele
(**Or**-kee-O-seel) (n) scrotal hernia; tumor of a testis

papilledema »
(pa-pill-e-**dee**-ma) (n) edema and inflammation of the optic nerve at its point of entrance into the eyeball

pendulous
(**pen**-ju-lus) (adj) loosely hanging

perineum
(**per**-i-**nee**-um) (n) the external region between the vagina and the anus in women and between the scrotum and the anus in men

polydipsia »
(pol-ee-dip-**see**-a) (n) excessive thirst

polyphagia »
(pol-ee-**fay**-jee-a) (n) eating abnormally large amounts of food at a meal

polyuria »
(pol-ee-**yoo**-ree-a) (n) excessive urinary output

prostate gland
(**pros**-tayt) (n) a gland located at the base of the bladder and surrounding the beginning of the urethra in the male

prostatic »
(pros-**tat**-ik) (adj) relating to the prostate gland

proteinaceous »
(**prO**-tee-**nay**-shus / **prO**-tee-i-**nay**-shus) (adj) relating to or resembling proteins

proteinuria
(prO-tee-**noo**-ree-a) (n) presence of abnormally large amounts of protein in the urine

proximal »
(**prok**-si-mal) (adj) nearest to a point of reference or center of the body

renal »
(**ree**-nal) (adj) related to the kidney

renal failure
(**ree**-nal) (n) inability of the kidneys to function

retinopathy »
(re-ti-**nop**-a-thee) (n) any disorder of the retina

rhabdomyosarcoma »
(**rab**-dO-**mI**-O-sar-**kO**-ma) (n) highly malignant tumor developing from striated muscle cells

sclerotic »
(sklee-**rot**-ic) (adj) pertaining to or affected with sclerosis, a condition that shows hardness of tissue resulting from inflammation, mineral deposits, or other causes

sonography »
(so-**nog**-ra-fi) (n) ultrasonography; use of high-frequency sound waves to produce an image of an organ or tissue

steroid
(**steer**-oyd) (n) any of a large number of similar chemical substances, either natural or synthetic; many are hormones; produced mainly in the adrenal cortex and gonads

stress incontinence
(stres in-**kon**-ti-nens) (n) inability to retain urine under tension, such as sneezing or coughing

suprapubic »
(soo-pra-**pyoo**-bik) (adj) above the pubic bones

testicular »
(tes-tik-yoo-lar) (adj) related to the testes, a pair of male gonads or sex glands that produce sperm and secretes androgens

thyromegaly »
(thI-rO-**meg**-a-lee) (n) enlargement of the thyroid gland

transaminase »
(trans-**am**-i-nays) (n) an enzyme that catalyzes transamination, the transfer of an animo group from one compound to another or the transposition of an animo group within a single compound

transperineal »
(trans-per-i-**nee**-al) (adj) across or through the perineal region between the urethral opening and the anus, including the skin and underlying tissues

transurethral »
(trans-yoo-**ree**-thral) (adj) through the urethra, such as a surgical procedure

trochanteric »
(trO-kan-**ter**-ik) (related to a trochanter, either of the two bony processes below the neck of the femur)

ureter »
(yoo-**ree**-ter / **yoo**-ree-ter) (n) either of a pair of tubes that carry urine from the kidney to the urinary bladder

ureteral »
(yoo-**ree**-te-ral) (adj) relating to the ureters

urethra »
(yoo-**ree**-thra) (n) a tube that drains urine from the bladder to the outside

ureteroscopy »
(n) procedure to pass a ureteroscope up through the bladder into the ureter to inspect the ureteral lumen

urethroscopy »
(yoo-ree-**thros**-ko-pee) (n) an examination of the inside of the urethra with a urethroscope, a lighted instrument

vesical »
(**ves**-i-kul) (adj) referring to the bladder or gallbladder

vesicle »
(**ves**-i-kl) (n) blister; small, raised skin lesion containing clear fluid

viscera

(**vis**-er-a) (n) main internal organs within the trunk of the body, especially those in the abdominal cavity

visceral »

(**vis**-er-al) (adj) relating to or located near the viscera

vasectomy »

(va-**sek**-tO-mee) (n) excision of a portion of the vas deferens, in association with prostatectomy or to produce sterility

visceromegaly »

(**vis**-er-O-**meg**-a-lee) (n) generalized enlargement of the abdominal organs

visualization

(**vich**-oo-al-I-**zay**-shun) (n) the act of viewing an object, especially the picture of a body structure as obtained by x-ray study

Abbreviations

ADH	antidiuretic hormone	K	potassium
AGN	acute glomerulonephritis	KUB	kidneys, ureters, bladder (x-ray)
ATN	acute tubular necrosis	Na	sodium
BPH	benign prostatic hypertrophy	PD	peritoneal dialysis
BUN	blood urea nitrogen (lab test)	PE	physical exam
Cl	chloride	PSA	prostate specific antigen
CMG	cystometrogram	RP	retrograde pyelogram
CVA	costovertebral angle	SLE	systemic lupus erythematosus
cysto	cystoscopy	TUR	transurethral resection (bladder or prostate)
DRE	digital rectal exam	TURP	transurethral resection of the prostate
ESRD	end-stage renal disease	UA or	
ESWL	extracorporeal shock-wave lithotripsy	U/A	urinalysis
GFR	glomerular filtration rate	UPJ	ureteropelvic junction
GU	genitourinary	UTI	urinary tract infection
HEENT	head, ears, eyes, nose, throat	UVJ	ureterovesical junction
hpf	high-power field	VCUG	voiding cystourethrogram
I&O	intake and output	VDRL	Venereal Disease Research Laboratory (test for syphilis)
IVP	intravenous pyelogram		
JVD	jugular venous distention		

Complete the following exercises, drawing on the information learned in the Exploring Urology and Nephrology section of this chapter and referencing the Terms Bank.

Exercise 12.1   Matching Sound and Spelling

The numbered list that follows shows the phonetic spelling of hard-to-spell words. Sound out the word, then write the correct spelling in the blank space provided. Check your answers in the Terms Bank or other appropriate reference.

1. dis-**yoo**-ree-a _____

2. pol-ee-**yoo**-ree-a _____

3. lim-**fad**-e-**nI**-tis _____

4. nok-**too**-ree-a _____

5. **rab**-dO-**mI**-O-sar-**kO**-ma _____

6. **prO**-tee-**noo**-ree-a _____

7. **nef**-rO-li-**thot**-O-mee _____

8. ep-i-**did**-i-mis _____

9. Or-kee-**ek**-tO-mee _____

10. **kal**-kyoo-lus _____

11. **prO**-tee-**nay**-shus _____

12. ep-i-**thee**-lee-um _____

13. ne-**fros**-tO-mee _____

14. **Or**-kee-O-seel _____

15. **pros**-tayt _____

Below is a list of frequently used words that look alike and/or sound alike. Study the meaning and pronunciation of each set of words, read the following sentences carefully, and then circle the word in parentheses that correctly completes the meaning.

addition	counting, increase	**hole**	opening
edition	issue of a publication	**whole**	total, complete
creatine	high-energy phosphate	**mitotic**	related to mitosis
creatinine	product excreted in urine that is an indicator of kidney function	**mycotic**	related to fungus
		perianal	around the anus
cystoscopy	inspection of the bladder interior using a cystoscope	**perineal**	pertaining to the perineum
cystostomy	creation of an opening into the urinary bladder	**perineum**	area between the anus and genitalia
		peritoneal	pertaining to the peritoneum
dilatation	synonym of dilation	**peritoneum**	area in the abdomen
dilation	expansion of an organ or vessel		
dilution	a substance that has been diluted (liquid has been added)	**seen**	noticed, viewed
		scene	sight, background, display of emotion
do	to perform	**states**	(n) government units of land
due	owing	**states**	(v) expresses, says
		status	(n) rank, condition
efflux	given off, as in a stream		
reflux	a flowing back	**to**	toward, through
		too	also, additionally
ethanol	drinking alcohol	**two**	numerical unit, a pair
ethenol	vinyl alcohol		
farther	(adv) refers to physical distance		
father	(n) male parent		
further	(adv) additional, extra, greater		
further	(v) to advance, to help		

1. A tracheostomy establishes a (hole/whole) into the trachea.

2. Are you going to the medical conference with them (to/too/two)?

3. He lives (farther/further) from the hospital than I do.

4. If you have (farther/further) questions about the medical procedure, please call.

5. The ambulance arrived on the (scene/seen) within a few minutes.

6. The lesion was (to/too/two) small to be seen by the naked eye.

7. The patient is (states/status) post hysterectomy.

8. We went (to/too/two) the anatomy lecture yesterday.

9. With the (addition/edition) of hydrochlorothiazide, her blood pressure is now under good control.

10. The pupils were (dilated/diluted) on exam.

Exercise 12.3   Choosing Words from Context

When transcribing dictation, the medical transcriptionist frequently needs to consider the situation when determining the word that correctly completes the sentence. From the list below, select the term that meaningfully completes each statement.

catheter	meatus	renal failure
endoscope	neoplasm	steroid
genitalia	pendulous	urethra
hematuria	proximal	vesicle

1. When we saw Mr. Johnson in our office, his exam revealed a blood pressure of 210/100, ascites, and pitting pedal edema. He was admitted to the hospital immediately with the diagnosis of impending _____.

2. The _____ was inserted, and the urinary collection totaled only 50 mL in the first hour.

3. The catheter could not be passed through the _____ urethra.

4. The IV catheter was placed _____ to the antecubital fossa.

5. There was an oozing _____ on the abdomen where the incision had been made.

6. It was decided to place Mr. Arnold on _____ therapy to decrease the allergic reaction.

7. After the Foley catheter was removed, the patient had a small amount of gross _____, which cleared with the next void.

8. In our differential diagnosis, we considered an infectious process versus a (an) _____.

9. Pelvic exam revealed normal female _____.

10. During the procedure, the _____ was repositioned several times to obtain different views.

11. The urinary catheter was inserted through the _____ in order to obtain the specimen.

12. There was a blockage in the _____, thus preventing urine from exiting the meatus.

Exercise 12.4   Pairing Words and Meanings

From this list, locate the term that best matches each of the following definitions. Write the term in the space provided by each definition.

edema	perineum	transurethral
epididymis	proteinuria	viscera
fascia	sonography	
idiopathic	suprapubic	

1. pertains to an operation performed through the urethra _____

2. region between the urethral opening and the anus _____

3. presence of large amounts of protein in the urine _____

4. abnormal collection of fluid in spaces between cells _____

5. fibrous connective tissue that supports soft organs _____

6. tightly coiled duct that carries sperm _____

7. a disease for which no cause can be determined _____

8. main internal organs within body cavities _____

9. use of ultrasound to produce an image _____

10. the area above the pubis _____

Exercise 12.5   Creating Terms from Word Forms

Combine prefixes, root words, and suffixes from this list to create medical words that fit the following definitions. Fill in the blanks with the words you construct.

dys-	painful	**path/o**	disease
extra-	outside	**ren/i (o)**	pertaining to kidney
intra-	inside	**ureter/o**	ureter
aden/o	gland	**urethr/o**	urethra
cyst/o	bladder or sac	**ur/o**	urine
hem/o (ato)	blood	**-ectomy**	removal, incision
hepat/o	liver	**-gram**	recording; x-ray
hydr/o	water	**-ia/sis**	condition of
lith/o	stone, calcification	**-ic**	pertaining to
lymph/o	clear, thin fluid	**-itis**	inflammation
meat/o	passageway	**-lith**	stone, calcification
nephr/o	kidney	**-osis**	condition of
noct	night	**-pexy**	repair
orchi/o (do)	testicle		

1. removal of the kidneys _____

2. difficult, painful urination _____

3. related to the liver _____

4. blood in the urine _____

5. disease of the lymph glands _____

6. urination during the night _____

7. inflammation of the urethra _____

8. removal of a testicle _____

9. inflammation of the kidney _____

10. outside of the liver _____

11. condition of having kidney stones _____

12. repair of a testicle _____

13. inflammation of the bladder _____

14. x-ray procedure to view the bladder _____

Read the following report excerpt and look for errors in capitalization, word use, punctuation, spelling, meaning, and format. Mark the corrections on this page and key the excerpt with all errors corrected. Save the document as XXExercise12.06, using your initials in place of *XX* in the file name.

SUBJECTIVE

56-year-old middle eastern male who is seen in follow up for a elevated PSA, recent pylonephritis and microscopic hematuria. He has been referred to urology and will see them in 2 weeks. Today, he says he has occasional mild burning with urination but the disuria has overall improved. He denies any flake or abdominal pain, nausea or vomiting.

OBJECTIVE

Routine laboratory was done at his last visit. His PSA was 14.3. He says that in the past his highest PSA was 6, and that was roughly six months ago. He had a transureteral resection of the prostrate in 2002. Other laboratories: A CBC showed a platelet count of 124,000. Hemoglobin 14.9. MCV 92. Chemistry profile within normal limits, including renal function.

ASSESSMENT

1. Resolved pyelonephritis.

2. Elevated PSA with a patient history of benign prostatic hypotrophy raises the question of possible prostate cancer.

PLAN

1. Will give another 7-day course of Bactrim to insure that the urinary track infection is resolved by the time of his Urology appointment in two weeks.

2. Patient is to call if he has any worsening of his symptoms.

Read this scenario carefully and then select the most appropriate response. Write an explanation for why you think your choice is the best answer.

You are transcribing an MRI report of the abdomen. The reason (indication) for the test is to rule out a mass in the right kidney. Throughout the report, the radiologist dictates findings for the left kidney. What should you do?

---

a. Change the results to match the indication for the test, which is to evaluate the right kidney. All references should be changed to *right*.

b. Leave all references to right or left blank and flag the report for review.

c. "Left" was mentioned three times in the body of the report and "right" was only dictated once (in the indication), so change the report so that all results reflect the left kidney.

d. Transcribe the report exactly as dictated.

Best response: _____

Explanation: _____

_____

_____

_____

_____

You will apply the medical specialty and language information you learned in this chapter to transcription work in this section. After you learn the formatting recommendations of the history and physical report, you will transcribe nine reports related to nine different patient studies.

Introducing the History and Physical Report

When a patient enters a healthcare system, the physician or examiner generates a comprehensive document called a history and physical (H&P) report (Figure 12.4). This report focuses on the patient's medical and social history and the illness or complaint that prompted the person to seek medical attention. The primary purpose of the history and physical is to provide the information the physician needs to make a diagnosis and choose the appropriate care and treatment for the patient. The MT transcribes the H&P report to provide a written documentation for the chart.

Required Headings/Content

As the title of the report suggests, there are two main sections: (1) a complete history, including the current medical problem; and (2) the results of the physical examination performed by the physician. For the entire report, The Joint Commission requires these headings: Chief Complaint, History of Present Illness, Review of Systems, Physical Examination, and Impression. Individual hospitals and physicians, however, may expand the headings beyond these basic requirements. Medical transcriptionists need to be aware of the specific format the employer prefers.

Refer to page 466 of Appendix A for a complete list of headings found in the history and physical report template along with descriptions of the type of information found under each heading. Not every template heading will be included in every transcribed report.

The healthcare provider frequently documents the actual words used by the patient in describing the subjective data. This information may be included in a history and physical report in the Chief Complaint (CC) or History of Present Illness (HPI). If both sections are dictated, the Chief Complaint section is usually a brief summary statement and the History of Present Illness section includes a longer explanation. The history and physical report will also usually include objective data, organized through review of available clinical information, such as vital signs, measurements, laboratory tests, x-ray findings, and so on, which have been performed before admission and for which results are known.

Despite the variety of subheadings, most physicians follow the same order when dictating the report, including more or less, depending on the complexity of the patient's complaint. As with any report, it is important to utilize the standard headings and transcribe the information in the template's standard order, even if the provider dictates the information in a different order.

History In the history section of the report, several variations or subheadings are possible, including details of the present illness, past medical history, surgical history, and social history. Details may focus on habits and risk factors.

The Past Medical History section begins by listing the patient's past or ongoing illnesses not specifically related to the current illness. A history of pregnancies and deliveries is recorded for a female.

Social History is another subheading that may be included. This subsection describes social habits such as alcohol use, smoking history, occupation, recreational interests, home environment, marital status, and sexual history. This information helps the interviewer develop an understanding of the patient as an individual and as a member of a family and a community.

Information on the health of the patient's parents, siblings, and grandparents may follow as a separate *Family History* section. These data can point to the possibility of genetic traits or diseases.

Review of Systems   The Review of Systems section is a question-and-answer review of all the body systems conducted by the healthcare provider. The review is in cephalocaudal order—from head to foot. This is a list of symptoms reported by the patient or the person accompanying the patient and should not be confused with the physical examination, which lists findings observed by the examiner. The following lists the subheadings and the type of information that may be included in this section of the report.

- Skin: Lesions, rashes, itching, moles, eruptions, changes to nails or hair.
- Head: Headaches, dizziness.
- Eyes: Visual problems, glaucoma, conjunctivitis, discharge, use of glasses.
- Ears: Earaches, hearing loss, discharge, dizziness, fainting, ringing in the ears, pain.
- Nose, Sinuses: Discharges, sense of smell, colds, allergies, nosebleeds.
- Mouth and Throat: Condition of teeth, dental history, difficulty in swallowing, hoarseness, tonsillectomy.
- Neck: Thyroid, movement of neck.
- Breasts: Lumps or masses, history of cysts, tenderness, discharge.
- Respiratory: Shortness of breath, cough with or without production of sputum or blood.
- Cardiac: Increased heart rate, angina, or chest pain.
- Gastrointestinal: Appetite, indigestion, difficulty swallowing, vomiting, changes in weight, stool history, jaundice, gallbladder problems.
- Genitourinary: Pain on urination, blood in urine, frequency, incontinence, urgency, sexually transmitted diseases.
- Gynecologic: Menarche, menstrual history, discharges, contraceptive use, obstetric history, painful menses.
- Musculoskeletal: Pain, stiffness, limitation of movement, fractures.
- Peripheral Vascular: Cold feet, pain when walking, pallor, numbness, varicose veins.
- Neurologic: Numbness, dizziness, fainting, pain, paralysis, difficulty walking, falling, convulsions.
- Hematologic: Easy bruising, history of clotting disorders, history of anemia.
- Endocrine: History of diabetes, frequent urination, increased thirst, difficulties with temperature regulation, excessive sweating.
- Psychiatric: Mood swings, anxiety.

Physical Examinations   A complete physical exam (PE) is usually performed after the history is recorded. This is arranged in cephalocaudal order, beginning with the visible areas of the body. Four basic procedures are included in the exam:

1. Inspection: looking at the body.
2. Palpation: feeling various parts and organs.
3. Percussion: listening to the sounds produced when a particular region is tapped using the hands or a small hammerlike tool.
4. Auscultation: listening to body sounds.

After noting general appearance, height, weight, age, race, nutritional state, and possibly emotional status (euphoric, lethargic, distracted, alert, oriented, agitated, flat affect), the physician dictates vital signs and then a description of findings on the rest of the body, similar to those described for the Review of Systems section. For a detailed review of the subheadings within the Physical Examination section, refer to page 467 of Appendix A.

Impression and Plan   A final section in the history and physical report is the Impression section (sometimes dictated as the Diagnosis, Differential, or Assessment), which lists many possibilities to explore or rule out. The plan of care is often dictated as a numbered list, written in order of most important to least important, or as a random list. It will include recommendations for further studies and treatment and followup.

Turnaround Time

The history and physical examination should be completed, dictated, and transcribed within the first 24 hours of admission as an inpatient. If a complete exam has been performed within 30 days before admission, such as in a physician's office, a copy of this report is placed in the patient's medical record and—in some hospitals—no new exam is required (provided no changes have occurred or provided changes that have occurred are noted in the medical record at the time of admission).

Preparing to Transcribe

To prepare for transcribing dictation, review the common urology and nephrology terms, drugs, and abbreviations presented in the Terms Bank section of this chapter. Study the format and organization of the model document shown in Figure 12.4, and key the model document, using the history and physical template on the Dictations and Templates CD as a starting point. Save the document as XXFigure12.04 using your initials in place of XX in the file name. Proofread the document by comparing it with the printed version. Categorize the types of errors you made, and document them on a copy of the Performance Comparison Chart. A template of this chart is included on the Dictations and Templates CD.

Transcribing Reports

Transcribe, edit, and correct each report in the following patient studies. Consult reference books for words or formatting rules that are unfamiliar.

As you work on the transcription assignment for this chapter, fill in the Performance Comparison Chart that you started when you keyed the model document. For at least three of the reports, categorize and document the types of errors you made. Answer the document analysis questions on the bottom of the chart. With continuous practice and assessment, the quality of your work will improve.

PATIENT NAME: Raymond Cheever
MR #:   93-22-17
PHYSICIAN: Harry Washington, MD
DATE: 07/10/20XX

ds

CHIEF COMPLAINT
Severe pain in the left hip.

ds

HISTORY OF PRESENT ILLNESS
The patient is a 57-year-old white male who is admitted from the emergency department with hypertension, hyperglycemia, and greater trochanteric bursitis. The patient has been under treatment for greater trochanteric bursitis with Lortab and Naprosyn. He returns today because of increasing left hip pain. In the emergency room, he was noted to be significantly hypertensive and hyperglycemic. He is unaware of having a history of either.

PAST MEDICAL HISTORY
Negative.

SURGICAL HISTORY
Tonsils and adenoids removed in early childhood.

SOCIAL HISTORY
The patient does not smoke at present. He stopped smoking 6-7 years ago; he smoked an average of a pack per day for many years. He denies ethanol use. He is married. He has 2 children who are alive and in good health. He works as a plant manager for a chemical company.

FAMILY HISTORY
His mother is alive and in good health. His father is deceased secondary to complications of black lung and asthma. He has 2 brothers and 1 sister. He thinks his sister has a history of hypertension.

ALLERGIES
No known allergies.

CURRENT MEDICATIONS
1. Lortab 7.5 mg daily.
2. Naprosyn 375 mg daily.

REVIEW OF SYSTEMS
A full review of systems was negative. He states that his weight has been stable in the past year. He denies polyuria, polydipsia, or polyphagia.

PHYSICAL EXAMINATION
GENERAL: Well-developed, well-nourished male in no acute distress.
VITAL SIGNS: Blood pressure 200/104. Repeat, after rest and pain medication, was 170/96. The pulse was 72. Respiratory rate was 18 and labored. Patient refused to be weighed at this time because of pain.

(continued)

Figure 12.4 History and Physical Report

HISTORY AND PHYSICAL
PATIENT NAME: Raymond Cheever
MR #: 93-22-17
DATE: 07/10/20XX
Page 2

ds

HEENT: Pupils were somewhat constricted, but fundi were visualized minimally. No hypertensive retinopathy, exudates, hemorrhages, or papilledema was noted. Oral examination revealed no ulcerations, erosions, or masses.
NECK: Supple, without lymphadenopathy. The carotid upstrokes were brisk and equal bilaterally, without bruits. Thyroid nonpalpable.
THORAX AND LUNGS: Chest was clear to auscultation in all fields.
CARDIOVASCULAR: Regular rate and rhythm, without murmurs, thrill, gallop, or click.
ABDOMEN: Nontender, nondistended, without masses, organomegaly, guarding, tenderness, or rebound.
EXTREMITIES: No clubbing, cyanosis, or edema. Peripheral pulses were intact, with good upstrokes. Palpation of the left hip did reveal tenderness, although the patient did report it was much improved after analgesia.

LABORATORY DATA
Review of the Chem-7 revealed a blood sugar of 201. His urinalysis revealed greater than 1000 glucose. CBC revealed a hemoglobin of 16.3 and a hematocrit of 50, white count was 14.7, platelets were 291,000; differential was essentially within normal limits.

IMPRESSION
1. Marked hypertension.
2. Asymptomatic hyperglycemia with glycosuria.
3. Left greater trochanteric bursitis.

PLAN
1. Admit.
2. Orthopedic consultation.
3. Endocrinology consultation.
4. Cardiology consultation.

qs

_____
Harry Washington, MD

HW/XX
D: 07/10/20XX
T: 07/11/20XX

Figure 12.4 History and Physical Report (Continued)

Patient Study 12.A   Alice Castanza

Alice Castanza is a 5-year-old child whose mother noticed that Alice's stomach appeared to be larger than usual. Alice had no complaints of pain, but her mother took her to the pediatrician, who was able to palpate an abdominal mass. She was sent for x-rays, lab work, and other tests. A surgical procedure was performed to remove a tumor and the right kidney. Alice was diagnosed with a Wilms tumor, a malignant tumor of the kidney, treated by surgery and chemotherapy.

REPORT 12.1 Radiology Report

Use the Report1201.mp3 audio file and the radiology report template (Radiology_Report) when transcribing this report. Save the document as XXReport12.01, using your initials in place of *XX* in the file name.

Listen for these words:
   echogenicity
   extrahepatic
   intrahepatic

The dictation will not include the Findings heading, but include it in the transcribed report.

The clinical data included in this report is the actual data seen on the sonogram. The radiologist uses this information to form an impression, which is documented in the report.

Patient Study 12.B   Melissa Perlman

Melissa Perlman is a 3½-year-old child who was healthy until June of (last year) when she developed tonsillitis. The throat culture was negative for strep. In July, her mother noted that her diapers were not wet for 1 whole day and she was edematous. She was taken to the pediatrician and, after testing, was diagnosed with renal failure.

REPORT 12.2 Pathology Report

Use the Report1202.mp3 audio file and the pathology report template (Pathology_Report) when transcribing this report. Save the document as XXReport12.02, using your initials in place of *XX* in the file name. Use the template's Procedure Date for the dictated "date of operation."

Listen for these words:
   circumferential
   glomerulosclerosis
   hypercellularity
   mitotic
   proteinaceous
   pseudocrescents
   visceral

PAS (periodic acid Schiff) is a stain that is applied to tissue slices that have been affixed to a microscope slide. The stain attaches to polysaccharides within cells. PAS stain is applied to kidney biopsy tissue to visualize the glomerular basement membrane. PAS is dictated as individual letters, not as an acronym.

The word *minute* is dictated as "mI-**noot**," meaning very small.

Jonathan Blondell is a 35-year-old male who was having difficulty voiding for about 2 weeks. He saw his internist, who diagnosed a urinary tract infection. After treatment for several days, Jonathan continued to have pain on urination and blood in the urine. He was referred to the urologist for further evaluation.

REPORT 12.3 Operative Report

Use the Report1203.mp3 audio file and the operative report template (Operative_Report) when transcribing this report. Save the document as XXReport12.03, using your initials in place of *XX* in the file name. Use the dictated hospital number as the patient's medical record number. Use the template's Name of Operation heading for the dictated Operation heading, but change the heading to the plural form because there are multiple operations dictated. Also, place the Anesthesia section according to the template and use the template's Procedure heading for the dictated Findings and Procedure heading.

Listen for these instrument names:
> #20-French 2-way tube
> #24-French 3-way catheter with 5 mL balloon
> Vim-Silverman needle

Listen for these terms:
> rhabdomyosarcoma
> transperineal
> transurethral
> urethroscopy

Make sure you correct the dangerous abbreviation that is dictated in this report.

The overall type size of the report may need to be reduced slightly to fit the report on one page.

Raymond Cheever is a 57-year-old male who is admitted from the emergency department with hypertension, hyperglycemia, and greater trochanteric bursitis. He came to the emergency department because of increasing left hip pain and was unaware of his hypertension and hyperglycemia.

REPORT 12.4 History and Physical

Use the Report1204.mp3 audio file and the history and physical report template (History_and_Physical) when transcribing this report. Save the document as XXReport12.04, using your initials in place of *XX* in the file name. Use the dictated hospital number as the patient's medical record number. Within the physical exam section use the report's subheading Thorax and Lungs for the dictated subheading Chest.

The report will extend on to a second page. This template will include a continued line on the first page footer when the document extends onto the second page. If necessary, update the footer field by clicking F9 in the footer area of the document. Open the header and footer with the consecutive key combination Alt, V. H. The second-page header will include jump fields, as well as a page field. Review Appendix B for formatting help.

Note the use of the word ethanol for alcohol.

Polyuria, polydipsia, and polyphagia are the triad of symptoms usually associated with diabetes mellitus. Because the patient is hyperglycemic, the dictator notes specifically in the Review of Systems section that the patient has not experienced the triad of symptoms that often accompanies hyperglycemia.

Dennis Chang is a 9-month-old male who was well until 2 weeks ago when his parents noticed that his left testicle was enlarged. The pediatrician referred the Changs to Dr. Roland Browne, a urologist, who scheduled a biopsy.

REPORT 12.5 Consultation Letter

Use the Report1205.mp3 audio file and the consultation letter template (Consultation_Letter) when transcribing this report. Save the document as XXReport12.05, using your initials in place of *XX* in the file name.

Numbers dictated with a metric unit should be transcribed with a decimal and not a fraction. In this report, transcribe the head circumference with a decimal.

The Institute for Safe Medication Practices advises against the use of the symbols > (greater than) and < (less than) because they are often misread. In this letter, the dictator directs the MT to use the less than symbol. The transcription should use words, not the symbol.

Although trailing zeros are considered unsafe, within this dictation, two amounts are provided with trailing zeros. In this instance, it is appropriate to transcribe these trailing zeros as they indicate a level of accuracy.

The abbreviation hCG stands for human chorionic gonadotropin hormone, which is a marker for germ cells. The abbreviation is appropriate within the transcribed report.

The letter "m" in front of IU means "milli." Since IU (International Units) is on the list of dangerous abbreviations, the correct form to be transcribed is milliunits.

The dictation file includes instruction to copy the letter to two places, a file and a physician. Set a tab after the cc: to allow the stacked file name and physician name to align. Set the tab so the space from cc: is similar to a single space.

This letter will extend onto a second page. Although a continued line is not required on the first page, the patient's name, the date of the letter, and the page number will be needed in the running header field of the second page. See Appendix B for information about working with the templates.

William Booth has an appointment for his annual physical. Since he lives in an out-state area and was once treated by this urologist for a prostate problem, he continues to have his annual checkup with the urologist.

REPORT 12.6 History and Physical

Use the Report1206.mp3 audio file and the history and physical report template (History_and_Physical) when transcribing this report. Save the document as XXReport12.06, using your initials in place of *XX* in the file name. Use the dictated patient's number as the medical record number.

Listen for this term:

visceromegaly

In order to create consistency between transcribed reports, default to the template's headings, both in regard to order and content. For example, in this dictation the dictator will indicate the patient's allergies *after* the current medications and this order should be reversed, according to the template. Also, use the template's subheadings within the Physical Examination section. For example, when the dictator says "CNS," which stands for central nervous system, use the Neurologic subheading from the template instead. Other changes will need to be made to the dictated headings to align with the template's headings.

Listen for a dangerous abbreviation and be sure to correct it in the transcribed report.

Marc Bario is a 32-year-old male who was admitted through the emergency department with a history of 6 hours of acute ureteral colic on the right side. Subsequent testing revealed a large stone in his right ureter.

REPORT 12.7 History and Physical

Use the Report1207.mp3 audio file and the history and physical report template (History_and_Physical) when transcribing this report. Save the document as XXReport12.07, using your initials in place of *XX* in the file name. Use the template's headings order and content in the transcribed report. Within the Physical Examination section, use the Pelvic subheadings for the dictated Genitalia heading.

Listen for these terms:
    costovertebral angle
    jugular venous (JV) distention
    ureterovesical (UV) junction

Some institutions prefer drug allergies to be typed in all caps to bring attention to this critical piece of data. Allergies may also be typed in bold font. Choose either all caps or bold (but not italic or underlined) according to client specifications. For this report, transcribe penicillin in all caps.

This dictation will include several abbreviations. They should be transcribed as dictated. The exception is in the impression section. Only key the unabbreviated term when the meaning is known or obvious based on the content.

The report's point size may need to be reduced to allow the content to fit on one page.

Sandra Davis is a 78-year-old woman who was recently hospitalized for a herpes infection. Two days after she was discharged, she was brought to the emergency room with a possible stroke and subsequently was admitted to the hospital for tests and treatment.

REPORT 12.8 Discharge Summary

Use the Report1208.mp3 audio file and the discharge summary template (Discharge_Summary) when transcribing this report. Save the document as XXReport12.08, using your initials in place of *XX* in the file name. Several changes will need to be made to the dictated headings to best utilize the template's headings.

Listen for these terms:
  bilateral ureteral lithiasis
  ceftazidime
  clindamycin
  diltiazem-CD
  DSS
  Nephro-Vite

Although the dictator is identified at the top of the report, do not include the dictator's name in the report's heading. Rather, only include it in the signature line.

The term non-insulin-dependent diabetes mellitus is used in this report. The American Diabetes Association recommends dropping the use of this phrase (non-insulin-dependent) in favor of *type 2 diabetes mellitus*, but physicians still commonly dictate *non-insulin-dependent*. For this exercise, transcribe as dictated.

When dictating a list of medications, dictators often do not dictate the units of measure (e.g.: mg, mEq, g). Client preference determines whether or not the units are transcribed when not dictated. If missing units are transcribed, the units *must be confirmed* using a reliable reference. For this exercise, use your references to transcribe the missing units of measure.

Be alert that many caregivers will pronounce ceftazidime as ceftazidine with an "n" sound at the end of the word instead of an "m" sound.

Be sure to correct any unsafe abbreviations found within this report.

This will be a two-page report, so a continued line on the first page and a second-page header will need to be included in the transcription file. See Appendix B for formatting information.

Rishera is a 24-month-old girl referred for evaluation and treatment of a left upper abdominal mass noted on recent examination consistent with a renal tumor.

REPORT 12.9 Operative Report

Use the Report1209.mp3 audio file and the operative report template (Operative_Report) when transcribing this report. Save the document as XXReport12.09, using your initials in place of *XX* in the file name.

Listen for these terms:
- #2-0 PDS sutures
- ballotable
- contiguous
- electrocautery
- fascial
- Gerota fascia
- Para-aorta
- PICU (may be dictated as Pick-U, or each letter may be said individually)
- prepubertal
- splenocolic ligaments
- tenotomy scissors

In the dictation, the dictator does not indicate headings for Past Medical History, Review of Systems, or Physical Examination, but the report content implies these headings are needed. Include them in the transcribed report, following the template for the H&P report. Include subheadings within the Physical Examination section and edit the transcribed content to follow the listed style of this type of report.

According to guidelines set by The Joint Commissions, an H&P report should be filed before an operative report is done and thus *before* an operative report is created. In spite of this rule, this operative report includes H&P information.

Since the passage of the Health Insurance Portability and Accountability Act (HIPAA), medical transcriptionists are taking care to avoid including personally identifiable information within the body of a report. Therefore, the patient's name has been replaced in the model answer by "the patient."

Make sure you correct the dangerous abbreviation that is dictated in this report.

The names given for the assistant and the anesthetist do not include the physician's first names. Since these doctors are not included in the current list of physicians, transcribe only their last names. List the anesthetist under the assistant.

Transcribe the estimated blood loss under the appropriate template heading.

This report will print on three pages, and appropriate continued lines and page headings will need to be included.

chapter

Thirteen

Orthopedics

Orthopedics is the field of medicine concerned with diseases, injuries, and deformities of the musculoskeletal system, which includes the joints, muscles, and the fibrous connective tissue surrounding the bones and joints. Specialists in orthopedic medicine are orthopedists, who may also be skilled orthopedic surgeons. Due to the complexity of problems within the musculoskeletal system, orthopedic surgeons may further specialize in one anatomic area such as hip, knee, shoulder, foot, hand, or spine.

Objectives

» Identify major muscles, bones, joints, and tendons that make up the musculoskeletal system.

» Understand the function of muscles, bones, joints, and tendons.

» Differentiate common types of bone fractures.

» Recognize various signs and maneuvers used to assess reflexes and test for nerve impairment.

» Pronounce and correctly spell terminology related to orthopedics.

» Transcribe dictation related to orthopedics.

» Describe an emergency department report, including typical content, format, and turnaround time.

The musculoskeletal system (Figures 13.1 and 13.2) enables the body to move. It also provides support and protection for body organs. Within the bone is the bone marrow, which has the equally important responsibility of producing blood cells, a process called hematopoiesis. Bones are responsible for storing calcium and phosphorus. There are 206 named bones in the human body.

Structure and Function

Bone is the major tissue component of the musculoskeletal system. A complex type of calcified connective tissue, bone is made up of approximately 95 percent organic material and about 5 percent inorganic minerals.

The center of the bone is called the medullary cavity, which contains the bone marrow (Figure 13.3). The marrow looks like blood that has gritty and fatty particles in it. All bones of the body contain marrow. However, blood cells are formed mostly in the long bones and flat bones (iliac bones).

An extensive vascular system feeds the bones and moves blood cells in and out of the bone marrow (Figure 13.4). Osteocytes are bone cells embedded throughout the bone and are responsible for maintaining the matrix. Osteoclasts are constantly reabsorbing bone tissue to be replaced by new osteoblasts, which mature into osteocytes. This cycle occurs throughout the life of a healthy individual in response to physical activity, weight-bearing, and hormonal stimuli.

A periosteal layer of cells forms the covering of bone. This is a dense, fibrous membrane that contains the nerves, blood, and lymph vessels. The periosteum is the attachment point for muscles, ligaments, and tendons.

The long bones, like the humerus in the arm or the femur in the leg, are divided into the distal and proximal epiphyses (singular: epiphysis) on each end, and the diaphysis, the shaft or long section in the middle. The epiphyses are formed of spongy bone necessary to maintain growth, while the diaphysis is composed of compact bone that provides support. The articular cartilage on the end of the epiphyses provides the cushioning effect in the joints.

Flat bones provide protection for internal organs and wide surfaces for muscle attachment. The skull bones and sternum are flat bones. Short bones have a core of spongy, or cancellous, bone surrounded by a layer of compact tissue. These bones are small and have an irregular shape, as in the wrists and phalanges. The irregular bones, such as the vertebrae and bones of the ear, do not fit into any one category.

Joints are the articulations that allow bones to move. There are three major classifications: diarthroses are freely movable joints, amphiarthroses are slightly movable joints, and synarthroses are immovable joints. To allow free movement, synovial fluid is secreted into each joint cavity as a lubricant (Figure 13.5). Ligaments connect bones to each other and add strength and stability to joints.

Muscles function to maintain posture, stabilize joints, provide movement, and generate heat. There are three types of muscle cells: skeletal, smooth, and cardiac. Each type has a different appearance under the microscope and has a particular function. Tendons attach the fleshy part of the muscle to the bones. A point of tendon attachment is called an insertion.

Skeletal muscle covers the skeleton. It is the only muscle type that is under our voluntary control. It is also called striated muscle because of its striped appearance. There are several parts of skeletal muscle as shown in Figure 13.6. Myofibrils, the long thin threads of muscle fiber, actually do the work, or movement, in the skeletal muscle.

Smooth muscle lines the walls of the body's organs, such as the stomach and small intestines. Cardiac muscle is involved with the heart's conduction system and the heartbeat. Both of these muscle groups are under involuntary control.

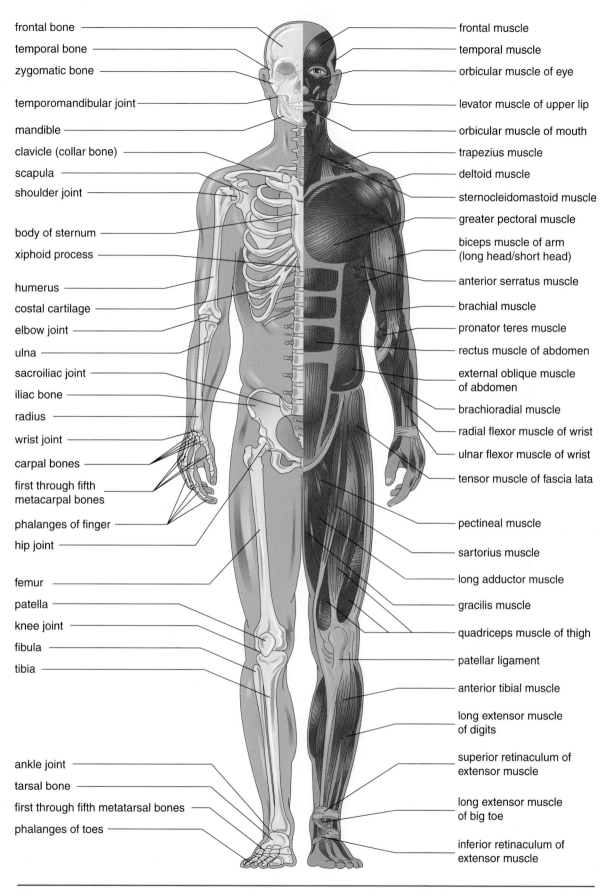

frontal bone

temporal bone

zygomatic bone

temporomandibular joint

mandible

clavicle (collar bone)

scapula

shoulder joint

body of sternum

xiphoid process

humerus

costal cartilage

elbow joint

ulna

sacroiliac joint

iliac bone

radius

wrist joint

carpal bones

first through fifth
metacarpal bones

phalanges of finger

hip joint

femur

patella

knee joint

fibula

tibia

ankle joint

tarsal bone

first through fifth metatarsal bones

phalanges of toes

frontal muscle

temporal muscle

orbicular muscle of eye

levator muscle of upper lip

orbicular muscle of mouth

trapezius muscle

deltoid muscle

sternocleidomastoid muscle

greater pectoral muscle

biceps muscle of arm
(long head/short head)

anterior serratus muscle

brachial muscle

pronator teres muscle

rectus muscle of abdomen

external oblique muscle
of abdomen

brachioradial muscle

radial flexor muscle of wrist

ulnar flexor muscle of wrist

tensor muscle of fascia lata

pectineal muscle

sartorius muscle

long adductor muscle

gracilis muscle

quadriceps muscle of thigh

patellar ligament

anterior tibial muscle

long extensor muscle
of digits

superior retinaculum of
extensor muscle

long extensor muscle
of big toe

inferior retinaculum of
extensor muscle

Figure 13.1 Anterior View of the Musculoskeletal System

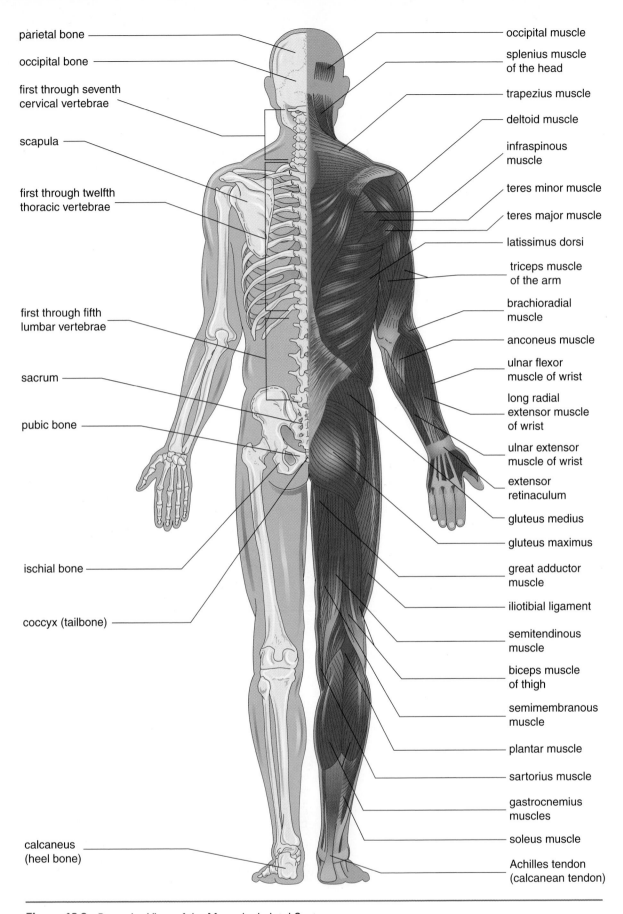

parietal bone

occipital bone

first through seventh
cervical vertebrae

scapula

first through twelfth
thoracic vertebrae

first through fifth
lumbar vertebrae

sacrum

pubic bone

ischial bone

coccyx (tailbone)

calcaneus
(heel bone)

occipital muscle

splenius muscle
of the head

trapezius muscle

deltoid muscle

infraspinous
muscle

teres minor muscle

teres major muscle

latissimus dorsi

triceps muscle
of the arm

brachioradial
muscle

anconeus muscle

ulnar flexor
muscle of wrist

long radial
extensor muscle
of wrist

ulnar extensor
muscle of wrist

extensor
retinaculum

gluteus medius

gluteus maximus

great adductor
muscle

iliotibial ligament

semitendinous
muscle

biceps muscle
of thigh

semimembranous
muscle

plantar muscle

sartorius muscle

gastrocnemius
muscles

soleus muscle

Achilles tendon
(calcanean tendon)

Figure 13.2   Posterior View of the Musculoskeletal System

Physical Assessment

The patient who sees the orthopedist is usually suffering from a fracture, an acute pain episode, or chronic pain. The physician will begin the examination by assessing the patient's standing and walking movements. Posture, movement of the extremities, and any signs of pain (facial grimace is the giveaway) will be noted. The orthopedist will ask about the history of the pain, the beginning of the pain, any precipitating events, and any injuries. Information about activities, sports, sleeping habits, and lifestyle as well as limitations on activities of daily living (ADLs) as a result of the pain will be noted in the medical record.

The examination will include full range of motion activities and strength assessments for each muscle group. Obvious malformations, such

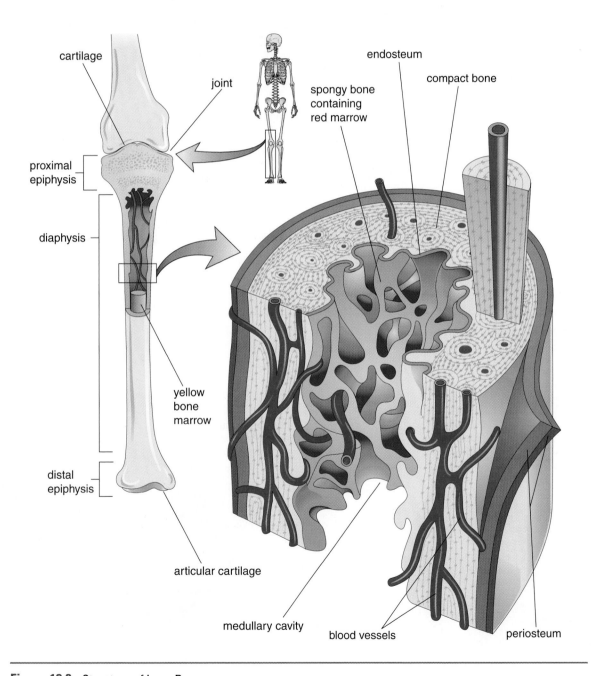

Figure 13.3 Structure of Long Bones

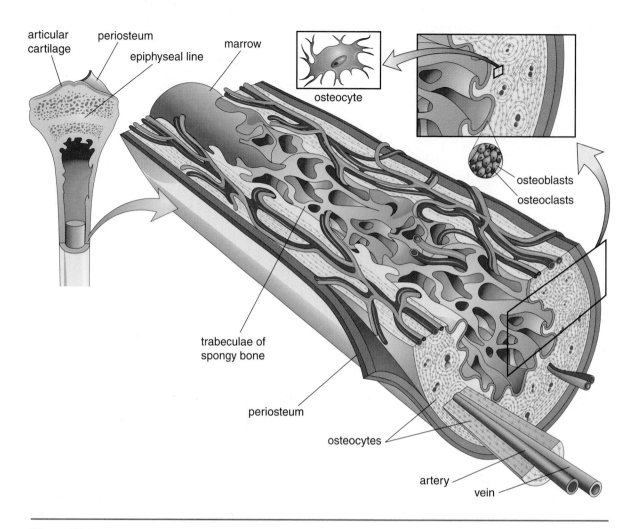

Figure 13.4 Microscopic View of Bone

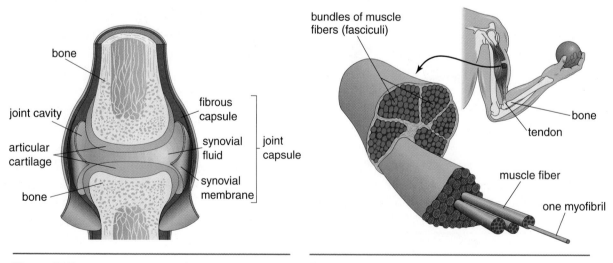

Figure 13.5 Diarthrotic (Synovial) Joint

Figure 13.6 Structure of Skeletal Muscle

as scoliosis or kyphosis, will be noted. Asymmetry may be an indication of an abnormality. Joints will be examined for swelling, redness, warmth, and tenderness on palpation. Because of the interrelationship of the nervous system with the musculoskeletal system, the physician will test reflexes, gait, and other related areas. Common tests and maneuvers performed by an orthopedist include Lhermitte (head flexion), straight-leg raise (nerve root irritation in the low back), Spurling (cervical nerve root impingement), Lasègue (sciatica), Neer impingement (shoulder), Phalen and Tinel (carpal tunnel), drawer sign (knees), Babinski (lower limb reflexes), and Homans (DVT).

Diseases, Conditions, and Injuries

For young people, a bone fracture may precipitate the first visit to the orthopedist. Terminology used to describe fractures is listed in Table 13.1. Inflammatory joint diseases or stress injuries are likely reasons for adults to seek medical help from an orthopedist. Osteoarthritis, for example, is a degenerative disease characterized by pain, swelling, and a loss of flexibility in the area where cartilage is worn away. It affects mostly weightbearing joints and is the main reason for total hip joint replacement surgery. Rheumatoid arthritis is an autoimmune disorder and is discussed in Chapter 16.

Sprains and strains are common injuries involving muscles, ligaments, and tendons. A sprain is an injury to a ligament due to excessive forces on a joint. A strain refers to stretching or tearing of a muscle or its tendon. Physicians use the acronym RICE to help patients remember how to initially treat injuries: rest, ice, compression, and elevation. Common sports injuries treated by orthopedists include lateral and medial epicondylitis (elbow), medial meniscal tears (knee), anterior cruciate ligament (ACL) tears (knee), and rotator cuff tears (shoulder).

Another frequent disorder is herniated intervertebral disks (herniated nucleus pulposus), which occurs most often in patients between 20 and 45 years of age and is more common in men.

Table 13.1

Fractures

Fracture Type	Description
open or compound	a fracture that causes the bone to break through the skin
comminuted	a fracture that creates more than 2 fragments (splintered)
spiral	a fracture resulting from twisting a bone
transverse	a break running across the bone at a right angle to the long axis of the bone
greenstick	an incomplete break caused by bending the bone
compression	fractures in a vertebral body
avulsion	injury that causes a tendon or ligament to tear away from the bone, taking a piece of bone with it

Some 90 percent of intervertebral herniations occur in the L4-L5 or L5-S1 spinal interspaces, the areas experiencing the greatest amount of motion. Degenerative disk disease (DDD) is an age-related disease of the intervertebral disks that results in diminished space (cushion) between the vertebral bodies and narrowing of the neural foramen, which is the opening through which nerves exit the spinal canal. Narrowed spaces result in compression of nerve roots, inflammation due to irritation of nerves, and pain. Physical therapy, pharmaceutical muscle relaxers, heat, cold compresses, and NSAIDs (nonsteroidal anti-inflammatory drugs) are the most common treatment modalities for back pain. More intense pain may be treated with narcotics, such as Vicodin. Treatment for chronic back pain may include lumbar epidural steroid injections (LESI) to reduce inflammation caused by pressure on the nerve roots. If all conservative measures have failed, surgical removal of intervertebral disks (spinal fusion) may bring relief or reduction of back pain.

A common work-related orthopedic injury is carpal tunnel syndrome (CTS), which results from pressure on the median nerve passing through the wrist to the hand. Carpal tunnel syndrome is one of many occupational injuries caused by repetitive motions or incorrect ergonomics. Plantar fasciitis is the most common cause of heel pain in adults, occurring more frequently in women than men. It is characterized by heel pain that occurs with the first steps in the morning and diminishes with walking. Treatment consists of rest, stretching, strengthening, shoe modifications, NSAIDs, and ice therapy.

Osteoporosis, or fragile bones, is a common disease in older women. Characterized by the loss of bone mass, osteoporosis results in porous and brittle bones that break easily. Osteoporosis is a serious concern in the elderly, as fractures heal slowly and require prolonged immobilization, leading to decubitus ulcers, venous stasis, congestive heart failure, and life-threatening pneumonia.

Septic arthritis refers to a microbial infection of a joint. Osteomyelitis is an inflammation of bone and/or bone marrow often caused by infectious organisms. Infections in the bones and joints are often difficult to treat, requiring a prolonged course of antibiotics.

Common Tests and Surgical Procedures

X-rays are commonly performed to diagnose fractures, dislocations, arthritis, and other conditions affecting bones and joints. MRIs are especially helpful for diagnosing tendon and ligament injuries. A reduction is performed to put a fractured bone back into alignment. Closed reduction refers to the repair of a fracture by manipulation, casting or cast application, and splinting. Open reduction involves a surgical procedure to correct the alignment. Open reduction and internal fixation (ORIF) utilizes metal pins, screws and/or plates to hold the bone in alignment during healing.

Arthrography produces a radiograph taken after injection of a radiopaque dye into a joint, such as the knee or shoulder. The x-ray outlines the joint. Arthrocentesis is a procedure to obtain synovial fluid for examination in the laboratory. Usually this is performed if infection is suspected. Arthroscopy allows the physician to look inside a joint, most often the knee, using an instrument called an arthroscope.

Blood tests that are helpful in orthopedics include the CBC (to check for infection, anemia, and tumor markers) and alkaline phosphatase, an enzyme that appears in higher concentrations in the blood as a result of bone injury or destruction. Hip and knee replacement procedures constitute a large portion of orthopedic surgeries.

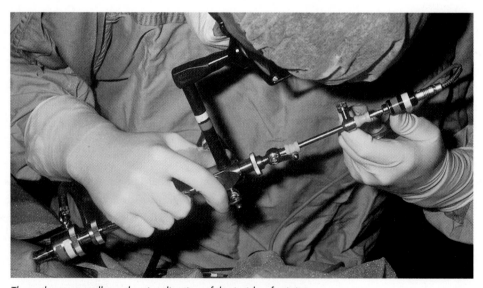

The arthroscope allows the visualization of the inside of a joint.

These terms and abbreviations provide a foundation for the language and transcription skills you will develop in the following sections of this chapter. Terms marked with » will be included in the reports transcribed in the Building Transcription Skills section.

abduction
(ab-**duk**-shun) (n) movement of a leg or arm away from the middle of the body

adduction
(ad-**duk**-shun) (n) movement of a leg or arm toward the middle of the body

ankylosis
(**ang**-ki-**lO**-sis) (n) stiffening or rigidity of a joint either as a result of a disease process or from surgery

ankylotic
(ang-ki-**lot**-ik) (adj) relating to or having ankylosis

apophyseal
(a-pO-**fiz**-ee-al) (adj) relating to or having an apophysis

apophysis »
(a-**pof**-i-sis) (n) a projection or outgrowth of a bone

arteritis
(**ar**-tur-**I**-tis) (n) inflammation of one or more arteries

arthralgia
(ar-**thral**-jee-a) (n) joint pain

arthritis
(ar-**thrI**-tis) (n) inflammation of one or more joints

arthroplasty »
(**ar**-thrO-plas-tee) (n) surgical repair of a joint; creation of a new joint

articulation
(ar-tik-yoo-**lay**-shun) (n) the connecting of bones as a joint

asepsis
(a-**sep**-sis) (n) lack of germs; a state of sterility; methods used to create or maintain a sterile environment

aseptic
(a-**sep**-tik / ay-**sep**-tik) (adj) sterile; being without infection or contamination

calcaneus
(kal-**kay**-nee-us) (n) heel bone; calcanei (kal-**kay**-nee-I) (pl)

callous
(**kal**-us) (adj) pertaining to or resembling callus

callus
(**kal**-us) (n) thickened skin that develops at points of pressure or friction; the bony deposit which develops around the broken ends of bone during healing

carpal
(**car**-pal) (adj) relating to a carpus, a bone in the wrist

carpal tunnel
(**kar**-pul **tun**-nul) (n) where the median nerve and flexor tendons pass through the wrist

cervical »
(**ser**-vi-kal) (adj) relating to a neck or cervix

chondral
(**kon**-drul) (adj) relating to cartilage

chondritis
(kon-**drI**-tis) (n) inflammation of cartilage

chondromalacia
(**kon**-drO-ma-**lay**-shee-a) (n) softening of cartilage

claudication
(klaw-di-**ka**-shun) (n) limping; painful cramps in calf of leg due to poor blood circulation

clavicle
(**klav**-i-kl) (n) clavicula; collar bone

clavicula
(kla-**vik**-yoo-la) (n) clavicle; collar bone

condyle
(**kon**-dil) (n) the rounded projecting end of a bone where ligaments are attached

Coumadin »
(**coo**-mah-din) (n) Brand name for warfarin, an agent to prevent blood clots

crepitus »
(**krep**-i-tus) (n) grating sound or vibration made by movement of fractured bones (bone fragments); crepitation

dactylomegaly
(dak-til-O-**meg**-a-lee) (n) abnormal enlargement of one or more fingers or toes

degenerative »
(di-**jen**-er-a-tiv) (adj) relating to or causing deterioration or worsening of a condition

diaphysis
(dI-**af**-i-sis) (n) shaft of a long bone

distal »
(**dis**-tal) (adj) farthest from the center from a medial line, or from the trunk

distraction
(dis-**trak**-shun) (n) a force applied to body parts to separate bony fragments or joint surfaces

edema
(e-**dee**-ma) (n) excessive accumulation of fluid in tissues, especially just under the skin or in a given cavity

edematous »
(e-**dem**-a-tus) (adj) having edema

epiphyseal
(ep-i-**fiz**-ee-al) (adj) relating to an epiphysis

epiphysis
(e-**pif**-i-sis) (n) end of a long bone, separated by cartilage from the shaft until the bone stops growing when the shaft and end are joined

eversion
(ee-**vur**-zhun) (n) turning out or inside out

exacerbation »
(eg-zas-er-**bay**-shun) (n) aggravation of symptoms or increase in the severity of a disease

extension
(eks-**ten**-shun) (n) a motion of an extremity which reduces the angle of the joint (straightening)

facial
(**fay**-shul) (adj) relating to the face

fascia
(**fash**-ee-a) (n) fibrous connective tissue that supports soft organs and encloses structures such as muscles; fasciae (pl)

fascial
(**fash**-ee-al) (adj) relating to fascia

fasciitis
(fa-see-**I**-tis) (n) inflammation of the fascia

femoral
(**fem**-o-ral) (adj) relating to the thigh bone or femur

flexion »
(**flek**-shun) (n) the act of bending or the condition of being bent, in contrast to extending

foramina »
(for-**ray**-mi-na) (n) apertures or perforations through a bone or a membrane structure; plural of foramen

foramen »
(fO-**ray**-men) (n) hole or opening, especially in a bone or membrane

fracture
(**frak**-chur) (v) to break; (n) a broken bone

girdle »
(**ger**-dl) (n) a zone or belt

hemarthrosis
(**hee**-mar-**thrO**-sis/**hem**-ar-**thrO**-sis) (n) accumulation of blood in a joint

hematoma »
(hee-ma-**tO**-ma) (n) a tumor or swelling that contains blood

hemodynamic »
(**hee**-mO-dI-**nam**-ik) (adj) relating to the physical aspects of the blood circulation

hemostasis »
(**hee**-mO-**stay**-sis) (n) arrest of bleeding or of circulation

hepatic »
(he-**pat**-ik) (adj) pertaining to the liver

humeral »
(hyoo-mer-al) (adj) pertaining to the humerus, the upper bone of arm extending from the elbow to the shoulder joint where it articulates with the scapula

humerus »
(**hyoo**-mer-us) (n) the long bone of the upper arm

ischium
(**is**-kee-um/**ish**-ee-um) (n) bone upon which body rests when sitting; fuses with the ilium and pubis to form the pelvis; ischia (**is**-kee-a) (pl)

kyphosis
(kI-**fO**-sis) (n) abnormal curving of the spine causing a hunchback

Le Fort
(n) classification system for facial fractures

lipping
(**lip**-ing) (n) excessive growth in a liplike shape at the edge of a bone

lordosis
(lOr-**dO**-sis) (n) abnormal curving of the spine causing a swayback

malleolus »
(ma-**lee**-O-lus) (n) either of the two bumplike projections on each side of the ankle; malleoli (pl)

metatarsal »
(**met**-a-**tar**-sal) (adj) relating to a metatarsus; (n) a metatarsal bone

metatarsus
(**met**-a-**tar**-sus) (n) any of the five long bones of the foot between the ankle and the toes

necrosis
(ne-**krO**-sis) (n) death of some or all of the cells in a tissue

necrotic
(ne-**krot**-ik) (adj) relating to or undergoing necrosis

neural »
(**noo**-ral) (adj) relating to nerves or the nervous system

odontoid process »
(O-**don**-toyd **pros**-es) (n) the toothlike projection from the upper surface of the second cervical vertebra on which the head rotates

osseous
(**os**-ee-us) (adj) bony; resembling bone; osteal

osteal
(**os**-tee-ul) (adj) bony; resembling bone; osseous

ostealgia
(os-tee-**al**-jee-a) (n) pain in a bone

osteophyte
(**os**-tee-O-fIt) (n) a bony outgrowth; projection or bone spur

osteoporosis
(os-tee-O-pO-**rO**-sis) (n) abnormal loss of bone tissue, causing fragile bones that fracture easily

ostial
(**os**-tee-ul) (adj) relating to any opening (ostium)

parietal
(pa-**rI**-e-tal) (adj) relating to the walls of a body cavity

plantar
(**plan**-tar) (adj) relating to the undersurface (sole) of the foot

prosthesis
(pros-**thee**-sis) (n) artificial replacement for a diseased or missing part of the body, such as artificial limbs; prostheses (pl)

proximal »
(**prok**-si-mal) (adj) nearest the point of attachment, center of the body, or point of reference

radiograph
(**ray**-dee-O-graf) (n) an image produced through exposure to x-rays

residual
(re-**zid**-yoo-al) (adj) related to a residue which is left behind

rheumatoid
(**roo**-ma-toyd) (adj) resembling rheumatism, with pain, inflammation, and deformity of the joints

rigidity
(ri-**jid**-i-tee) (n) stiffness; inflexibility

Salter-Harris
(sawl-ter har-is) (n) classification system for epiphysial plate injuries

scapula »
(**skap**-yoo-la) (n) a large, triangular, flattened bone lying over the ribs

sclerosis »
(sklee-**rO**-sis) (n) hardening or induration of an organ or tissue, especially that due to excessive growth of fibrous tissue

scoliosis
(skO-lee-**O**-sis) (n) abnormal curvature of the spine to one side

sphincter »
(**sfingk**-ter) (n) circular muscle constricting an orifice

spinous »
(**spI**-nus) (adj) pertaining to or resembling a spine, a short, sharp process of bone

splenic »
(**splen**-ik) (adj) referring to the spleen

spondylitis
(spon-di-**lI**-tis) (n) inflammation of one or more vertebrae

sprain
(n) injury to a joint by overstretching the ligaments; (v) to injure a joint and sometimes the nearby ligaments or tendons

sternocleidomastoid »
(**ster**-nO-**klI**-dO-**mas**-toyd) (n) one of two muscles arising from the sternum and the inner part of the clavicle

strain
(n) injury, usually to muscle, caused by overstretching or overuse; (v) to injure muscles by overstretching or overuse

subluxation
(n) (sub-luk-**sA**-shun) incomplete dislocation of a joint

synovial fluid
(si-**nO**-vee-al **floo**-id) (n) protective lubricating fluid around joints

tarsal
(**tar**-sal) (adj) relating to a tarsus, a bone in the midfoot

tibia
(**tib**-ee-a) (n) the larger bone of the lower leg; shin bone

transverse »
(trans-**vers**) (adj) at right angles to the long axis of the body or an organ; crosswise; side to side

trochanter
(trO-**kan**-ter) (n) one of the projections at the upper end of the femur (thigh bone)

vertebral »
(ver-**tee**-bral) (adj) relating to a vertebra or the vertebrae

Vistaril »
(**viss**-ta-rill) (n) Brand name for hydroxyzine, used for the treatment of anxiety and nausea

Abbreviations

ACL	anterior cruciate ligament	HP	hemipelvectomy
ADLs	activities of daily living	ID	internal development (ortho)
AE	above-elbow (amputation)	IS	intracostal space
AK	above-knee (amputation)	KD	knee disarticulation
AP	anteroposterior	L1, etc.	lumbar vertebrae
AROM	active range of motion	LESI	lumbar epidural steroid injection
BE	below the elbow (amputation)	MCP joint	metacarpophalangeal joint
BK	below the knee (amputation)	MRI	magnetic resonance imaging
C1, etc.	cervical vertebrae	MTP joint	metatarsophalangeal joint
CDH	congenital dislocation of the hip	NSAID	nonsteroidal anti inflammatory drug
CTS	carpal tunnel syndrome	OA	osteoarthritis
DDD	degenerative disk disease	ORIF	open reduction and internal fixation
DIP joint	distal interphalangeal joint	ortho	orthopedics
DJD	degenerative joint disease	PIP joint	proximal interphalangeal joint
DOS	date of service	PROM	passive range of motion
DVT	deep venous thrombosis	RICE	rest, ice, compression, and elevation
EMG	electromyography	ROJM	range of joint motion
ER	emergency room	ROM	range of motion
FROJM	full range of joint motion	S1, etc.	sacral vertebrae
FROM	full range of motion	SD	shoulder disarticulation
fx	fracture	T1, etc.	thoracic vertebrae
HD	hip disarticulation	TENS	transcutaneous electric nerve stimulation
HNP	herniated nucleus pulposus (disk)	THA	total hip arthroplasty

Complete the following exercises, drawing on the information learned in the Exploring Orthopedics section of this chapter and referencing the Terms Bank.

Exercise 13.1   Matching Sound and Spelling

The numbered list that follows shows the phonetic spelling of hard-to-spell words. Sound out each word and then write the correct spelling in the blank space provided. Check your answers in the Terms Bank or other appropriate reference.

1. **os**-ee-us _____

2. **kon**-drO-ma-**lay**-shee-a _____

3. kal-**kay**-nee-us _____

4. **krep**-i-tus _____

5. trO-**kan**-ter _____

6. ang-ki-**lO**-sis _____

7. kl-**fO**-sis _____

8. kla-**vik**-yoo-la _____

9. dl-**af**-i-sis _____

10. kon-**drl**-tis _____

11. pa-**rl**-e-tal _____

12. **os**-tee-O-flt _____

13. **is**-kee-um/**is**-shee-um _____

14. skO-lee-**O**-sis _____

15. **hyoo**-mer-us _____

16. **dak**-til-O-**meg**-a-lee _____

17. ang-ki-**lot**-ik _____

18. spon-di-**ll**-tis _____

19. **roo**-ma-toyd _____

20. os-tee-**al**-jee-a _____

Below is a list of frequently used words that look alike and/or sound alike. Study the meaning and pronunciation of each set of words, read the following sentences carefully, and then circle the word in parentheses that correctly completes the meaning.

abduction	to move an extremity away from the midline of the body	**fibers**	thin structures
adduction	to move an extremity toward the midline of the body	**fibrose**	to form fibrous tissue
		fibrosis	reparative or reactive tissue
		fibrous	composed or containing fibers
affect	(n) emotional or psychological disposition	**flanges**	projecting borders or edges
affect	(v) to influence or alter	**phalanges**	bones of the fingers or toes
affective	(adj) pertaining to emotions	**graft**	an implant of tissue or a substitution for an organ or body part that is taken from one part to another
effect	(n) result		
effect	(v) to bring about, accomplish		
effective	(adj) producing the desired result	**graph**	a diagram or chart
accept	(v) to take	**H&P**	history and physical
except	(prep) other than; with exclusion of	**HNP**	herniated nucleus pulposus
except	(v) to leave out	**of**	(prep) indicating possession or origin
checkup	(n) an examination of the health of an individual	**off**	(adj) gone, absent
		off	(adv) apart, away, below
check up	(v) to investigate	**osteal**	(adj) bony
facial	relating to the face	**ostial**	(adj) relating to an orifice
fascia	fibrous connective tissue that supports soft organs and encloses structures such as muscles; fasciae (pl)	**sprain**	(v) to injure a joint
		sprain	(n) traumatic injury to a joint
		strain	(v) to injure a muscle
fascial	relating to fascia	**strain**	(n) injury to a muscle
		weak	(adj) feeble, delicate
		week	(n) a period of seven successive days

1. She complains of feeling (weak/week) and tired.

2. She has had flu symptoms for approximately 1 (weak/week).

3. The medication (affected/effected) her bladder control.

4. As steroids were gradually tapered (of/off), the patient's strength returned.

5. The new medication was (affective/effective) in reducing inflammation.

6. The patient acknowledged the instruction and (accepted/excepted) the plan.

7. Mr. Braccia's pain was diagnosed as originating in the (osteal/ostial) tissue of the hip.

8. The patient displayed a flat (affect/effect).

9. During her gymnastics class, the patient jumped off the balance beam and (sprained/strained) her ankle.

10. The skin exam was unremarkable (accept/except) for a small lesion on the left cheek.

Exercise 13.3   Choosing Words from Context

When transcribing dictation, the medical transcriptionist frequently needs to consider the situation when determining the word that correctly completes the sentence. From the list below, select the term that meaningfully completes each of the following statements.

aseptic	edematous	prosthesis
cervical	hemostasis	radiograph
chondritis	kyphosis	residual
crepitus	necrosis	tibia
degenerative	neural	

1. It was necessary for Mr. Jones to have a(n) _____ after the amputation.

2. The _____ of the chest showed pneumonia.

3. Although there was considerable necrosis of the tumor after the chemotherapy, there was some _____ tumor.

4. The boy suffered a fractured _____ after he fell off his bicycle.

5. The legs were _____ because the woman was in heart failure.

6. The pain was in the _____ region of the back.

7. When he opened the sterile package, he used a(n) _____ technique.

8. He had _____ of the thoracic spine, which caused pain when he stood too long.

9. The pathology report showed _____ tissue taken from the brain.

10. After the radiation treatments, there was considerable _____ at the tumor site.

11. A clamp was applied in order to assure _____ during the surgery.

12. Dr. Jones heard the _____ as the fractured bones rubbed when Jane attempted to walk.

Exercise 13.4   Pairing Words and Meanings

From this list, locate the term that best matches each of the following definitions. Write the term in the space provided by each definition.

apophysis	femoral	odontoid process
distal	foramen	osteoporosis
epiphysis	malleolus	proximal
fascia	metatarsus	synovial sarcoma

1. a bone of the foot   _____

2. a malignant tumor   _____

3. loss of bone tissue   _____

4. a small projection or outgrowth on a bone   _____

5. toothlike projection that serves as pivot point
    when head turns   _____

6. end portion of a long bone   _____

7. a hole or opening in a bone or membrane   _____

8. fibrous, connective tissue that supports small organs   _____

9. a bumplike projection on the ankle bone   _____

10. pertaining to the thigh bone   _____

11. nearest to the center of the body   _____

12. farthest from the center of the trunk   _____

Exercise 13.5 Creating Terms from Word Forms

In the following exercise, combine prefixes, root words, and suffixes to create medical words that fit the definitions below. Fill in the blanks with the words you construct.

ankyl/o-	crooked, fusion, stiffness	**oste/o-**	bone
arthr/o-	joint	**por/o-**	cavity, passage
articul/o-	joint	**spondyl/o-**	vertebra
chondr/o-	cartilage	**tend/o-;**	tendon
dia-	through	**tendin/o-**	
epi-	on, in addition to	**tarsus**	instep of foot
kyph/o-	humped	**-arthria**	condition involving the ability to articulate
lord/o-	bent		
meta-	after, beyond	**-itis**	inflammation
muscul/o	muscle	**-osis**	condition
myel/o	bone marrow or spinal cord	**-physis**	bone portion; growth
my/o-	muscle	**-phyte**	outgrowth
necro/o-	death		

1. abnormal loss of bone tissue _____

2. end of long bone, secondary bone _____

3. inflammation of vertebra _____

4. tissue death _____

5. convexity of spine; swayback _____

6. inflammation of bone and marrow _____

7. bone between ankle and toes _____

8. inflammation of spinal cord _____

9. shaft of long bone _____

10. hunchback, curved spine _____

11. growth zone of long bone _____

12. bony outgrowth _____

13. condition of crooked, stiff bones _____

14. inflammation of the joint _____

Exercise 13.6   Proofreading Review

Read the following report excerpt and look for errors in punctuation, plural vs. singular word forms, subject-verb agreement, complete sentences, and the use of numbers. Mark the corrections on this page and key the excerpt with all errors corrected. Save the document as XXExercise13.06, using your initials in place of *XX* in the file name.

> ADMISSION DATE: August 5/XX
>
> Jonathan is states post rite baloney amputation for synoviale sarcoma he is without
>
> complaints and is ambulating with his below knee prosthesis quiet well. His abdomen
>
> is soft and non-tender. there are no mass. The incisor is well heeled. The right thigh
>
> skin graph sight is clean. Their is no palpable mass and there is no open wound. If he
>
> experiences pain, he is to take one Vicodin p.o. q four to six hours.

Exercise 13.7   Thinking Like a Professional

Read this scenario carefully and then select the most appropriate response. Write an explanation for why you think your choice is the best answer.

> You are working as an independent contractor for a transcription service. You have just sat down to work and have downloaded a full day's worth of transcription, which is due by 5 p.m. You receive a call from school that your child has fallen and possibly broken his arm. How should you proceed?

a. Go immediately to the emergency department to have your son's arm evaluated and plan to complete the work as soon as you return home.

b. Delete the work from your queue before leaving to pick up your son.

c. Call your employer or client and explain the situation and let them decide how to handle the jobs you have downloaded.

d. Finish the work as fast as you can and then go pick up your son.

Best response: _____

Explanation: _____

_____

_____

_____

_____

You will apply the medical specialty and language information you learned in this chapter to transcription work in this section. After you learn the formatting recommendations of the emergency department report, you will transcribe eight reports related to six different patient studies.

Introducing the Emergency Department Report

Because emergency department cases can range from simple injuries to life-threatening traumas, emergency department reports (Figure 13.7) can likewise vary from short chart notes to lengthy, complex reports. The latter may include the results of laboratory studies, x-ray films, and ECGs, along with operative procedures and the results from detailed physical examinations. Common procedures in the emergency department include endotracheal intubation, insertion of chest tubes and nasogastric tubes, catheterization of the bladder, placement of central venous catheters, and suturing of wounds.

Transcribing emergency department reports presents challenges usually not encountered with other medical specialties. For example, sometimes a dictation may be incomplete or interrupted because the physician may have been handling several complex cases, including some that were life-threatening. This factor may also lead to inconsistencies in the dictation, which should be pointed out to the physician for correction. Refer to page 472 of Appendix A for a complete list of headings found in the emergency department report template along with descriptions of the type of information found under each heading. Not every template heading will be included in every transcribed report.

Required Headings/Content

The Joint Commission mandates no specific headings. However, reports typically include chief complaint, history of present illness, physical examination, ED (or ER) course, laboratory data and/or diagnostic studies, diagnosis, condition at discharge, and treatment plan. The Joint Commission does require ED physicians to record the patient's time of arrival, time seen by the physician, and the time of discharge or transfer. Sometimes the physician dictates these times; otherwise, the information is included in another part of the medical record.

Turnaround Time

Rapid turnaround is required for emergency department reports since frequently the patient is admitted to the hospital and the information is vital for continued treatment. The ideal turnaround time is one to two hours, although critical cases may require that transcription is completed within an hour of dictation.

Preparing to Transcribe

To prepare for transcribing dictation, review the common orthopedics terms, drugs, and abbreviations presented in this chapter's Terms Bank. Study the format and organization of the model document shown in Figure 13.7 and key the model document, using the emergency department report template on the Dictations and Templates CD as a starting point. Save the document as XXFigure13.07 using your initials in place of *XX* in the file name. Proofread the document by comparing it with the printed version. Categorize the types of errors you made, and document them on a copy of the Performance Comparison Chart. A template of this chart is included on the Dictations and Templates CD.

Transcribing Reports

Transcribe, edit, and correct each report in the following patient studies. Consult reference books for words or formatting rules that are unfamiliar.

As you work on the transcription assignment for this chapter, fill in the Performance Comparison

Chart that you started when you keyed the model document. For at least three of the reports, categorize and document the types of errors you made. Answer the document analysis questions on the bottom of the chart. With continuous practice and assessment, the quality of your work will improve.

1" top and side margins

PATIENT NAME: Alex Cavara
MR #:   510-879-21
DOV: 09/05/20XX

HISTORY OF PRESENT ILLNESS
This 27-year-old Hispanic male was admitted today following a motor vehicle accident. The patient was the unrestrained driver of a vehicle which struck a tree at approximately 40 miles per hour. The patient had a momentary loss of consciousness and appeared confused at the scene. He complained of immediate head and neck pain. Paramedics transported the victim in full spine precautions.
ds

PHYSICAL EXAMINATION
HEENT: The patient had a 5 x 8 cm hematoma of the left forehead and several small facial lacerations. The pupils were slow to respond but equal and round. The teeth were not broken. There were no intraoral lacerations. Pharynx was clear.
NECK: On examination the patient noted pain in the right arm with left lateral flexion-rotation-compression maneuvers to the neck. There was profound hematoma along the course of the sternocleidomastoid muscle. Cervical flexion-extension maneuvers were limited. There was gross crepitus on palpation of the spinous processes of C5, C6, and C7.
THORAX AND LUNGS: The lungs were clear to auscultation.
CARDIOVASCULAR: Showed regular rate and rhythm and no murmurs.
ABDOMEN: Mildly tender diffusely, but without signs of splenic or hepatic trauma.
PERIPHERAL VASCULAR: Distal pulses were intact, and the fingers were warm and well perfused.
EXTREMITIES: There was an obvious spiral oblique fracture of the right humeral shaft with marked malangulation and shortening.
ds

DIAGNOSIS
Major polytrauma and major skeletal injuries secondary to motor vehicle accident.
ds

CONDITION ON DISCHARGE
The patient is hemodynamically stable at the present time.
ds

PLAN
The patient will be admitted to the orthopedic surgical unit and taken immediately to surgery for internal fixation of his fractures. His hemodynamic status will be carefully monitored over the next few hours. Chest x-ray and labs will be followed serially.

qs

_____
Jill McKensie, MD
ds
JM/XX
D: 09/05/20XX
T: 09/05/20XX

Figure 13.7 Emergency Department Report

Roberta Flagner is a 51-year-old woman who was complaining of back pain, particularly around the upper spine. The pain radiates toward the left arm from the shoulder blade. She went to see her physician, Joseph White, MD, who referred her to an orthopedist, Samuel Larchmont, MD.

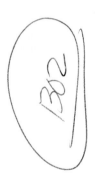

REPORT 13.1 Radiology Report

Use the Report1301.mp3 audio file and the radiology report template (Radiology_Report) when transcribing this report. Save the document as XXReport13.01, using your initials in place of *XX* in the file name.

DOS stands for date of service. Transcribe using the appropriate heading at the top of the report. Include the template's Findings heading, even though the actual heading is not dictated.

To find the name of a joint, muscle, ligament, tendon, or bone, reference a medical dictionary or specialty word book, looking first under the noun (joint, muscle, ligament, and so on). This also applies to surgical terms as there are many specialized names for the screws, nails, plates, and wires used to repair fractures.

A neural foramen (pl. foramina) is an opening or aperture between vertebral bodies which allows a nerve to exit the spinal canal. The term is often dictated as if it were a single word (neuroforamen), but the correct terminology is two separate words.

REPORT 13.2 Consultation Letter

Use the Report1302.mp3 audio file and the consultation letter template (Consultation_Letter) when transcribing this report. Save the document as XXReport13.01, using your initials in place of *XX* in the file name.

This report includes the abbreviation ROJM. The dictator uses the full term, followed by the abbreviation the first time it is used. In subsequent references, he uses just the abbreviation.

Steve Gatlin is a 28-year-old man who cut his left index finger with a carving knife and came to the emergency department for treatment.

REPORT 13.3 Emergency Department Report

Use the Report1303.mp3 audio file and the emergency department report template (Emergency_Dept_Report) when transcribing this report. Save the document as XXReport13.03, using your initials in place of *XX* in the file name.

Some of the dictated headings will be similar to, but not exactly the same as the template's headings. Use the template's headings. For example, use the abbreviation DOV instead of the dictated "date of ED visit" at the top of the report.

Remember, a numeral should not begin a sentence. Edit the sentence under the Assessment to avoid starting the sentence with the numeral 4. (Spelling out numerals at the beginning of a sentence is also acceptable. If accompanied by a unit of measure, spell that out also. Ex: 4 cm – Four centimeters)

Mrs. Arlene Elvin was walking through the Brookfield Natural History Museum when she tripped on a slanted floor board and twisted her foot. She felt immediate pain and was assisted by her husband and the security guard to a seat. The museum nurse brought a wheelchair, and ice was applied. Mrs. Elvin was taken to the Brookfield Emergency Department where she was diagnosed with a fracture of the foot.

REPORT 13.4 Radiology Report

Use the Report1304.mp3 audio file and the radiology report template (Radiology_Report) when transcribing this report. Save the document as XXReport13.04, using your initials in place of *XX* in the file name.

Transcribe the report using the template's headings. In this report, clinical information is synonymous to the indication or the reason that the test is being done. Also, not all dictated punctuation should be transcribed.

For reports transcribed in this text, set the patient's first name first rather than setting the last name first, even if the dictator indicates a different order. Similarly, set the physician's first name (or initial) first. Because Dr. Trish is not listed on the physician directory, it is appropriate to transcribe her first name initial rather than the full first name.

REPORT 13.5 Discharge Summary

Use the Report1305.mp3 audio file and the discharge summary template (Discharge_Summary) when transcribing this report. Save the document as XXReport13.05, using your initials in place of *XX* in the file name.

Use the template's Discharge Instructions and Discharge Medications headings for the information dictated under the Disposition heading.

Patient Study 13.D   Alex Cavara

Alex Cavara is a 27-year-old man who was brought to the emergency room by ambulance following a car accident in which he ran into a tree while driving approximately 40 miles per hour. He suffered a momentary loss of consciousness and complained of immediate head and neck pain.

REPORT 13.6 Emergency Department Report

Use the Report1306.mp3 audio file and the emergency department report template (Emergency_Dept_Report) when transcribing this report. Save the document as XXReport13.06, using your initials in place of *XX* in the file name.

Listen for these terms:
malangulation
sternocleidomastoid muscle

The term *flexion-rotation-compression maneuvers* requires hyphens, as shown.

In this report, you will hear the dictator mention "spine precautions," which refers to a protocol for transferring patients with possible spinal cord injuries. A cervical collar is applied to the neck, and the patient is immobilized on a back board.

This report includes a Physical Examination section. Use the template's subheadings, even if they are not dictated. The order of the subheadings should match the template's order, not the order dictated.

Patient Study 13.E   Ivy Haines

Ivy Haines is a 72-year-old with a history of chronic, progressive left hip pain for the past 25 years. She has been admitted to the hospital for left total hip arthroplasty.

REPORT 13.7 History and Physical

Use the Report1307.mp3 audio file and the history and physical report template (History_and_Physical) when transcribing this report. Save the document as XXReport13.07, using your initials in place of *XX* in the file name.

Use the template's heading content and order to guide your transcribing of the dictated report. Many providers will dictate out of order and MTs are expected to place the information under the appropriate heading.

In the Physical Examination section, you will hear the term "normocephalic," which means the head is normal in shape and size.

This report will continue onto a second page, and a *continued* line and second-page header will be needed.

Jan Stanley is a 36-year-old woman with a history of juvenile rheumatoid arthritis. In 1990 she had bilateral total knee replacements with good results. In the past few years, however, she has experienced increasing left hip pain and was recently admitted to the hospital for a left total hip replacement.

REPORT 13.8 Discharge Summary

Use the Report1308.mp3 audio file and the discharge summary report template (Discharge_Summary) when transcribing this report. Save the document as XXReport13.08, using your initials in place of *XX* in the file name.

Where synonymous to the dictated headings, use the template's headings. Add headings and sections as needed as you transcribe this report. Because the dictator's name is included in the signature line, do not include this physician's name at the top of the report.

Note the difference in abduction and adduction. One way to distinguish adduction and abduction is to remember that adduction means "toward," as if "adding" to the body, whereas abduction means to "take away" or "move away" from the body. Recognizing the difficulty in distinguishing the sounds of these two words, the dictator may dictate the first two letters individually, such as "a-b duction" and "a-d duction."

Fourteen

Neurology and Psychiatry

Neurology is the study of the nervous system—the body's communication network. The nervous system serves to conduct the impulses and signals that drive all bodily functions. The organs of the nervous system consist of the brain, the spinal cord, and nerves. The physician who treats diseases of the nervous system is the neurologist. A neurosurgeon performs surgery on organs of the nervous system. This chapter includes terms used in psychiatry. This field of practice is separate from neurology.

Objectives

» Identify and understand anatomy and major components of the neurologic system.

» Describe diseases affecting the neurologic system.

» Describe the major psychiatric disorders.

» Recognize classes of pharmaceuticals used in the treatment of neurologic and psychiatric disorders.

» Recognize standardized tests used to evaluate learning and behavior.

» Pronounce and correctly spell terminology related to neurology and psychiatry.

» Transcribe dictation related to neurology and psychiatry.

» Describe a neuropsychological evaluation report, including typical content, format, and turnaround time.

The nervous system is probably the most complicated system in the human body. Think of it as the body's Internet, an information superhighway that activates and controls all bodily functions and receives and processes stimuli from the outside world. The most powerful computers in the world cannot match the complexity of the human brain and the supporting components of the nervous system.

Structure and Function

The human nervous system is divided into the central nervous system (CNS), which includes the brain and spinal cord, and the peripheral nervous system (PNS), which connects the spinal cord to the nerve, sensory, and muscle fibers (Figure 14.1). The PNS is further divided into the somatic nervous system (SNS) and the autonomic nervous system (ANS). The somatic nervous system is under the voluntary control of the individual. It innervates muscles that control voluntary movement.

The autonomic nervous system (ANS) produces the involuntary actions of the body, such as the heartbeat and digestion (Figure 14.2). There are two subdivisions of the ANS: the sympathetic and parasympathetic nervous systems, which function as opposites. The hormones norepinephrine and acetylcholine, also opposites, mediate these responses. Most notably these two are responsible for the "fight or flight" response. At the first sign of fear, the sympathetic nerve fibers prepare the body to fight and move quickly by increasing the heart rate, constricting peripheral blood vessels to move more blood to the heart and skeletal muscles, dilating the pupils for better vision, slowing down peristalsis, and increasing energy production. The parasympathetic nervous system, by contrast, includes the nerves that function during quiet, nonstressful times.

The brain sends feedback to the endocrine system, which responds with the appropriate hormones. This combined system is known as the neuroendocrine system. The cerebrum (Figure 14.3) is the portion of the brain that generates thought through the cerebral cortex, which is the gray matter. Folds, or gyri, increase the brain's surface area, increasing the amount of brain tissue that will fit within the skull. The brain is divided into two functional sides, the left and right hemispheres. The left brain, which controls muscles on the right side of the body, is involved with reasoning and language, as required for science and math. The right brain, which controls the muscles on the left side of the body, is responsible for imagination, insight, and artistic and musical abilities.

The cerebellum is located below the posterior portion of the cerebrum. It consists of the right and left cerebral hemispheres. The hemispheres are further divided by the brain's fissures, or crevices, called sulci. The brain stem is the continuation of the cervical segment of the spinal cord, which consists of bundles of nerve fibers and nuclei. Figure 14.4 shows the sections of the brain and the functions they control. Figure 14.5 is a sagittal section of the brain that shows structures involved in endocrine and sensory function.

The neuron (Figure 14.6) is the basic structural cell of the nervous system. Another class of cells called the neuroglia is supporting cells. The parts of a neuron include the soma (body), dendrites (branches leading toward the center of the soma), and an axon (a branch leading away from the soma). The soma contains the DNA for the cell. The dendrite is a tree-like area that receives signals from other neurons and sensory cells. The axon transmits signals away from the cell body and passes these signals to other neurons. Many of the axons are surrounded by a myelin sheath that protects the axon and accelerates impulses through it.

Communication between two neurons occurs when an electrical signal is converted into a chemical signal. These chemicals, called neurotransmitters, cross the synapse, a minuscule space between neurons, and cause the next neuron to become electrically excited. The signal proceeds through the nerve pathway at nearly unfathomable speed.

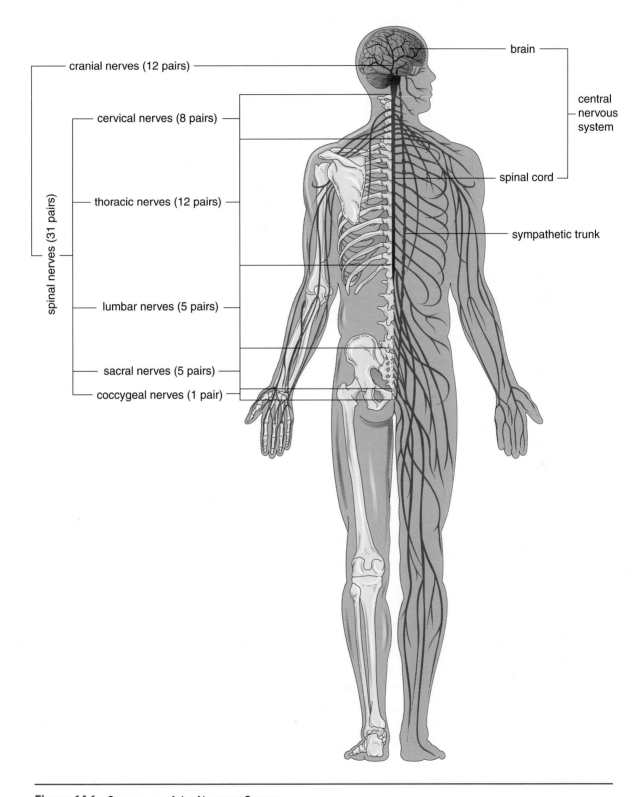

cranial nerves (12 pairs)

cervical nerves (8 pairs)

thoracic nerves (12 pairs)

spinal nerves (31 pairs)

lumbar nerves (5 pairs)

sacral nerves (5 pairs)

coccygeal nerves (1 pair)

brain

central
nervous
system

spinal cord

sympathetic trunk

Figure 14.1 Structures of the Nervous System

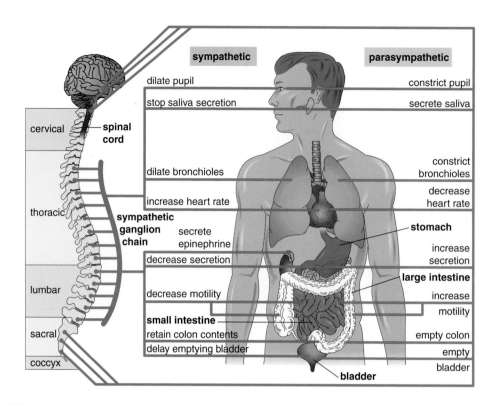

sympathetic

dilate pupil
stop saliva secretion

cervical — **spinal cord**

dilate bronchioles

increase heart rate

thoracic — **sympathetic ganglion chain**

secrete epinephrine

decrease secretion

lumbar

decrease motility

small intestine

sacral

retain colon contents

delay emptying bladder

coccyx

parasympathetic

constrict pupil
secrete saliva

constrict bronchioles

decrease heart rate

stomach

increase secretion

large intestine

increase motility

empty colon

empty bladder

bladder

Figure 14.2 Autonomic Nervous System

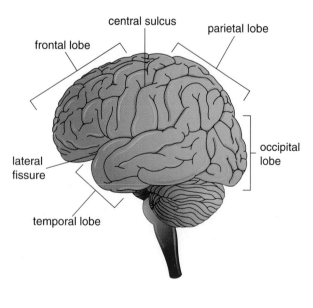

central sulcus
parietal lobe
frontal lobe

occipital lobe

lateral fissure

temporal lobe

Figure 14.3 The Cerebrum

Physical Assessment

Neurologic diseases have presenting symptoms ranging from paralysis, numbness, shaking, and weakness to gait disturbances, recurring headaches, seizures, and syncope (fainting). Using both direct and indirect methods, a neurological exam typically includes assessment of mental status, the twelve cranial nerves, sensation, coordination, and reflexes.

Much of the mental status exam is assessed throughout the patient interview and physical exam. The physician will note the patient's alertness, overall appearance, responsiveness to questions, appropriateness of answers, attention span, ability to carry on a conversation, thought content, mood, orientation with respect to time (time of day, date, season, year), person (identification of self, family, and friends), and place (location, city, and state). A more extensive mental status exam might also include assessment of intellectual function, memory, the patient's fund of knowledge (also called fund of information), judgment, and insight into their illness and its possible causes. The

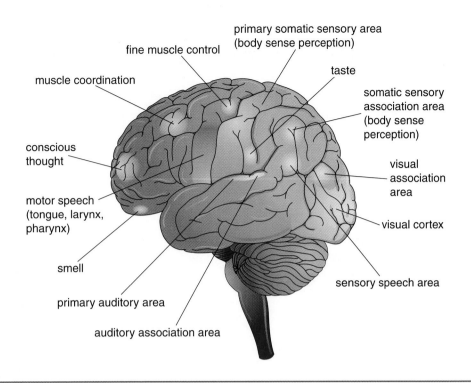

Figure 14.4 Functional Areas of the Cerebral Cortex

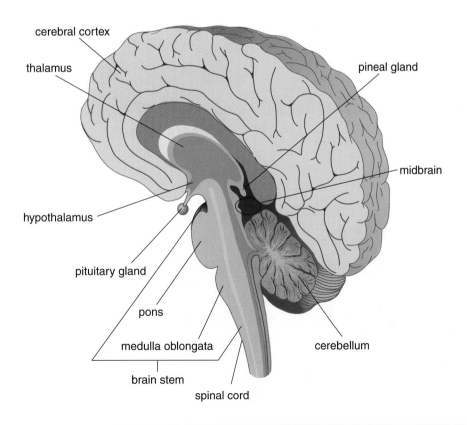

Figure 14.5 Sagittal Section of the Brain

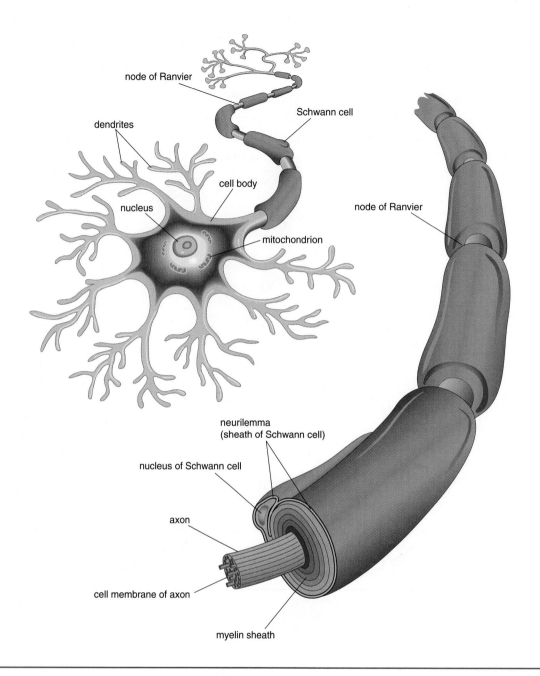

node of Ranvier

dendrites

Schwann cell

cell body

nucleus

node of Ranvier

mitochondrion

neurilemma
(sheath of Schwann cell)

nucleus of Schwann cell

axon

cell membrane of axon

myelin sheath

Figure 14.6 Neuron (Nerve Cell)

patient's state of consciousness is assessed in a range from alert to comatose. The Glasgow coma scale is used to assess consciousness, especially in cases of severe trauma. The affect, or mood, is described using words such as hyperactive, euphoric, hostile, agitated, or flat. A general assessment of intellect involves asking the patient to perform simple mathematical calculations, defining familiar vocabulary, and describing recent, intermediate, or past events (a test of memory).

Motor and sensory deficits are also evaluated. Weakness, paralysis, or atrophy of muscles are indicators of motor-nerve impairment. Sensory nerves are tested by feel (touch and gentle pinpricks), temperature (heat, cold), vibration perception, and limb position (proprioception). The reflexes are examined by tapping a reflex hammer over the tendons and watching for the contraction of the appropriate muscle. Reflexes tested include the biceps, triceps, patellar, Achilles tendon, and plantar. When the plantar surface is stimulated, the normal response is plantar flexion of all the toes (often described as "downgoing"); an abnormal response is known as a Babinski sign and consists of dorsiflexion of the great toe and spreading of the other toes. Results of the tendon reflex assessment are recorded as shown in Table 14.1.

A patient's behavior is evaluated by assessing the state of dress, appropriateness of language, gestures, facial expressions, and attentiveness to the examiner. Speech is an important part of the neurologic examination. It shows coordination of thought with appropriate muscle movements and function of the cranial nerves.

The cerebellum is the center for balance and muscle coordination. There are several tests that the physician uses to assess this function. Balance is tested by observing gait. If there is any abnormality, a cerebellar disorder is suggested. The Romberg is a test for sensory equilibrium. A positive Romberg test means the patient loses balance with eyes closed and feet together. The finger-to-nose test assesses coordination by checking for "past-pointing" in which the patient brings the fingertip beyond the nose. The physician will test for muscle strength and range of motion and observe for involuntary body movements such as tics, twitches, and tremors.

Table 14.1

Tendon Reflex Assessment

Test Result	Meaning
0	no response
1+	diminished response
2+	normal response
3+	more brisk than average response
4+	hyperactive response (hyperreflexia)

Neurological Diseases and Conditions

Cerebrovascular disease describes a group of disorders caused by mild to severe interruption of blood flow to the brain, including cerebral arteriosclerosis (most commonly atherosclerosis), aneurysm, thrombosis, and embolism. A transient ischemic attack (TIA) occurs when there is a brief decrease in blood flow to an area of the brain, resulting in a temporary loss of neurologic function. A cerebrovascular accident (CVA), commonly known as a stroke, results from impaired cerebral blood supply caused by hemorrhage, embolism, or thrombosis. A stroke typically results in permanent neurological damage and may result in paresis, paralysis, aphasia, and/or seizures.

Epilepsy is a disorder marked by unpredictable bursts of excessive neuronal discharge (called a seizure). Seizures can occur at any age and often follow a stroke or head injury, but in many cases the etiology is never known. An aura such as a particular smell, a flash of light, or a particular feeling, may occur just before the seizure. This is known as the preictal phase—allowing the individual to anticipate a seizure. During the actual seizure, called the ictal phase, the person may or may not lose consciousness. Some seizures may cause loss of bowel and/or bladder control. Following the seizure, the postictal phase is characterized by tiredness and/or sleepiness. Many patients are treated very successfully with anticonvulsants, such as phenobarbital and phenytoin (Dilantin).

Neurologists also treat patients suffering from chronic and/or severe headaches. Migraine headaches result from vascular spasm and include symptoms of head pain, nausea with vomiting, vertigo, and photophobia. Acute attacks may be lessened in duration and intensity using ergotamines (Cafergot), or analgesics combined with caffeine, taken at the first sign of an oncoming headache. Patients with frequent migraines are prescribed prophylactic medications called triptans, such as Imitrex or Frova.

Attention deficient disorder (ADD) is characterized by a lack of attention, organization, and impulse control. ADD may be accompanied by hyperactivity, in which case it is called attention deficit hyperactivity disorder (ADHD). ADD or ADHD is usually diagnosed in early childhood but often persists into adulthood. Symptoms include underachievement in school, hyperactivity with short attention span, obsessive-compulsive behaviors, and tics. Both forms of the disorder are treated paradoxically with stimulants, such as amphetamines (Dexedrine) and methylphenidate (Ritalin).

Parkinsonism usually begins in middle age. It is a defect of the extrapyramidal tract, especially in the basal ganglia. Classic motor disturbances include tremor, flat facial expression, stooping posture, balance and walking disturbances, bradykinesia, excessive salivation, speech difficulties, and immobility. Anticholinergic medications, such as Sinemet (levodopa and carbidopa), are used to treat the symptoms of Parkinson disease, but no treatment has been shown to prevent progression of the disease.

Peripheral neuropathy involves nerves of the upper and/or lower extremities. Symptoms include paresthesia, loss of sensation, weakness, depressed or absent tendon reflexes, and pain. In the United States, the most common cause of peripheral neuropathy is diabetes mellitus. Worldwide, a common cause is leprosy. Peripheral neuropathy is rarely reversible, but symptoms can be lessened with medication, especially Neurontin.

Brain tumors, both malignant and benign, are another frequent neurologic affliction. Tumors, also referred to as space-occupying lesions, either destroy or compress brain tissue and vary in aggressiveness. The most common brain tumors are metastatic tumors, not primary brain tumors, which have spread from another area, such as the breast or lung. Primary spinal cord tumors may be benign or malignant and occur one-tenth as frequently as brain tumors. Two major types of primary brain tumors are gliomas and neurofibromas.

Alzheimer disease results from structural changes in the brain, the exact cause of which is unknown. Patients experience a gradual loss of cognitive function that ends with total disability and death. Many therapies have been developed that will slow the progression of the disease and help patients cope with the symptoms, but there is

no cure. Other disorders addressed by a neurologist include multiple sclerosis, characterized by scattered patches of demyelination of nerve cells, and Bell palsy, a temporary, unilateral paresis or paralysis of facial muscles due to demyelination of the 7th cranial nerve. Tourette syndrome, an inherited disorder that causes motor and phonic tics, may also be diagnosed and followed by a neurologist. As with many neurological disorders, cures are rarely possible, although many will spontaneously remit. Treatment most often focuses on alleviation of symptoms.

Psychiatric Diseases and Conditions

The field of psychiatry encompasses knowledge of the nervous system as well as the effects that are seen throughout the body when there are abnormalities. There are subspecialists in this field, including those who specialize in geriatrics, sports, children, and adolescents, to name a few.

Classification of psychiatric disorders can be found in the *Diagnostic and Statistical Manual of Mental Disorders* (DSM-IV). This reference includes names of the disorders and the symptomatology for each disorder. It is an important reference for mental health professionals.

There are many disorders that are seen within the field of psychiatry. Affective disorders include depression and bipolar disorder. These types of disorders are characterized by feelings of unworthiness, profound sadness, guilt, apathy, and hopelessness. Often there is a loss of interest and pleasure in taking part in usual activities. There may be a slowing of physical activity or the opposite with a display of agitation. There may be alterations in sleeping, eating, and libido.

Depression is one of the most common problems seen in the general practitioner's office with an estimated 12.1 hours per week being spent on direct care. The person suffering from depression may complain of muscle pain, headaches, nausea, chest pain, shortness of breath, and fatigue, which are all common complaints associated with various other diseases or problems.

Anxiety disorders may develop during childhood, adolescence, or young adulthood. The most common disorder is generalized anxiety disorder (GAD), which is seen most commonly in middle or older adulthood.

The person with bipolar disorder, also called manic-depressive illness, suffers from shifts in mood, energy, and functional ability—ranging from severe depression through mania.

Treatment for patients with anxiety and/or depression includes tricyclics, such as amitriptyline; monoamine oxidase inhibitors (MAOIs), such as Nardil and Parnate; selective serotonin reuptake inhibitors (SSRIs), which include Prozac and Zoloft; and others. Lithium and some anticonvulsant medications are used to treat bipolar disorder.

Patients suffering from chronic, intractable major depression may be treated with electroconvulsive therapy (ECT). This procedure produces a grand mal seizure and subsequent neurotransmission changes that may change the affect. Any interventions should be supported by some form of psychotherapy.

Posttraumatic stress disorder (PTSD) is also treated by psychiatrists. Patients who have experienced life-threatening or life-changing trauma may show symptoms of PTSD immediately or several months or years after the event. Symptoms of PTSD go beyond the usual period of posttraumatic grief and recovery. Examples of patients at risk for PTSD include war veterans and persons who experience child or sexual abuse. PTSD is characterized by chronic depression, emotional detachment, nightmares, insomnia, memory loss, and anxiety. Patients may develop drug or alcohol addiction.

Substance abuse and dependence cross all gender, racial, social, and economic boundaries. It may include alcohol and/or drug abuse, dependency, and withdrawal.

Many psychiatric patients are at risk of suicide. Suicidal ideation means that there is a thought of committing suicide. This includes patients with depression, bipolar disorder, schizophrenia, or an organic brain disorder that includes psychosis or a personality disorder. Patients may establish a pattern of self-injury as a way to handle feelings of anger, anxiety, or substance abuse.

Common Tests and Surgical Procedures

Both neurology and psychiatry use standardized tests, some written and some oral, to evaluate the patient's cognitive, physical, and mental condition. Table 14.2 lists common tests used to assess patients as well as the characteristics being evaluated. Many standardized tests report results in percentiles, which compare the patient's performance to similar "normal" patients. Results are also expressed as to the degree of difference, or deviation, when compared to the mean or average. Results may be

Table 14.2

Common Standardized Tests Used in Neurological and Psychological Evaluations

Test Name	Characteristic Assessed
Stanford-Binet Intelligence Scale	Intelligence
Bender Visual Motor Gestalt Test	Visuospatial and visuomotor function
Rorschach Test (inkblot test)	Attitudes, emotions, and personality
Minnesota Multiphasic Personality Inventory-2 (MMPI-2)	Broad range of personality and social/interpersonal skills
Wechsler Adult Intelligence Scale (WAIS)	General intelligence
Wechsler Memory Scale, Third Edition (WMS-III)	Learning, memory, and working memory
Peabody Picture Vocabulary Test, Third Edition (PPVT-III)	Receptive vocabulary and verbal ability
Boston Naming Test	Aphasia
Beck Depression Inventory	Depression
Thematic Apperception Test (TAT)	Interpersonal conflicts
Achenbach Child Behavior Checklist	Behavioral problems
Piers-Harris Children's Self-Concept Scale	Self-perception

expressed as 1 or 2 standard deviations (1 SD or 2 SD), with 2 SD being further (more different) from the mean (typical or average).

Many procedures and studies give insight into the nervous system without requiring surgery or invasive techniques. Magnetic resonance imaging (MRI) is used extensively to visualize the brain or spinal cord. A contrast medium, usually gadolinium, is used to enhance or outline the structures. Magnetic resonance angiography (MRA) is used to assess arteries for stenosis and aneurysm, especially those within the head and neck. The computerized axial tomography (CT or CAT) scan uses x-rays to image structures as a series of thin "slices" that are reconstructed into 2-dimensional images. Positron emission tomography (PET) is an imaging technology that uses a gamma ray detector and an injection of sugar molecules tagged with a radioisotope (called FDG) to visualize metabolic activity within tissues. Cells with increased metabolic activity, such as cancer cells, take up the tagged sugar molecules in higher concentrations than normal cells. Tissues are then scanned for increased gamma ray activity, indicating cells with increased metabolic activity. Single photon emission computed tomography (SPECT) uses very similar technology as PET scans but uses technetium as the tracer molecule (instead of FDG). CT scans provide structural information while PET and SPECT provide functional (i.e., metabolic) information about the tissues being evaluated. Newer technology combines CT and PET techniques to convey structural and functional information simultaneously.

Myelography produces an x-ray picture of the spinal cord after injection of a radiopaque dye. This procedure has largely been replaced by newer, less invasive tests.

Electroencephalography (EEG) produces a graphic recording of the electrical activities of the brain, similar to an electrocardiogram (ECG) for the heart. Electrodes are placed on the scalp to detect and record brain impulses. This test assists in the diagnosis of epilepsy.

Nerve conduction velocity (NCV) studies are used to measure the speed at which impulses travel through nerves, especially the peripheral nerves. Slower velocities are indicative of nerve damage, demyelination, or nerve blocks. Electromyography (EMG) studies are often performed at the same time as nerve conduction studies. Electrodes in the form of needles are placed in the muscle and the patient is instructed to contract the muscle. This test measures the muscle's strength and ability to respond to nerve impulses.

Lumbar puncture (LP), or spinal tap, is performed by inserting a small-gauge needle between the vertebrae into the spinal canal. This test is used to measure the pressure within the spinal canal and to withdraw cerebrospinal fluid (CSF) for analysis in the laboratory. Medications can be injected directly into the CSF through the needle.

Stereotactic surgery is a method of locating a precise area of the brain using a 3-dimensional measurement. This operation is performed by a highly skilled neurosurgeon. Laminectomy can be performed by a neurosurgeon or an orthopedic surgeon. It involves excision of a portion of the vertebral body to relieve pressure on spinal nerves.

Trephination is performed by making a bur hole into the skull to decrease intracranial pressure.

Terms Bank

These terms and abbreviations provide a foundation for the language and transcription skills you will develop in the following sections of this chapter. Terms marked with » will be included in the reports transcribed in the Building Transcription Skills section.

abduction »
(ab-**duk**-shun) (n) the lateral movement of a limb away from the median plane of the body

adenopathy »
(a-den-**op**-a-thee) (n) swelling and morbid change in lymph nodes

agnosia
(ag-**nO**-see-a) (n) unable to perceive or recognize sensory stimuli

agraphia
(a-**graf**-ee-a) (n) impairment of the ability to write

akinesis
(ay-kI-**nee**-sis) (n) an extrapyramidal disorder causing a loss of power to perform voluntary movements

amnesia
(am-**nee**-zee-a) (n) a disturbance of long-term memory; total or partial inability to recall past experiences

angiography
(an-jee-**og**-ra-fee) (n) an x-ray taken after a radiopaque dye is given to visualize the vessels

anticonvulsant »
(**an**-tee-kon-**vul**-sant) (n) a therapeutic agent that prevents seizures

aphasia
(a-**fay**-zee-a) (n) difficulty with using and understanding words

aphonia
(a-**fO**-nee-a) (n) loss of the voice as a result of disease or injury

arachnoid
(a-**rak**-noyd) (n) the middle of the three membranes covering the brain; it is a delicate fibrous membrane, resembling a cobweb

astereognosis
(a-**steer**-ee-og-**nO**-sis) (n) loss of the ability to judge the form of an object by touch

asymmetry »
(ay-**sim**-e-tree) (n) lack of symmetry of parts or organs on opposite sides of body

ataxia
(a-**tak**-see-a) (n) muscular incoordination

atrophy
(**at**-rO-fee) (n) a decrease in size of a part or organ; a wasting away of tissue as a result of disuse, radiation therapy, surgery, disease

aura »
(**aw**-ra) (n) a sensation, as of light or warmth, that may precede an attack of migraine or a seizure

auscultation »
(aws-kul-**tay**-shun) (n) act of listening through a stethoscope to body sounds, including lungs, heart, and abdomen

axial »
(**ak**-see-al) (adj) situated in or relating to an axis

Babinski reflex »
(bab-**in**-skeez **ree**-fleks) (n) an extension or moving of the big toe upward or toward the head, with the other toes fanned out and extended when the sole of the foot is stimulated

Brudzinski sign
(n) in meningitis, if a leg is passively flexed, a similar movement occurs in the other leg; if the neck is passively flexed, the legs also flex

bruit »
(**broo**-ee/broot) (n) an adventitious sound of venous or arterial origin heard on auscultation

causalgia
(kaw-**zal**-jee-a) (n) burning pain, usually associated with peripheral nerve damage

central nervous system (CNS)
(n) portion of the nervous system consisting of the brain and spinal cord

cephalalgia
(**sef**-al-**al**-jee-a) (n) headache

cerebellar
(ser-e-**bel**-ar) (adj) relating to the cerebellum, the part of the brain concerned with the coordination and control of voluntary muscular activity

cerebrospinal
(**ser**-e-brO-spI-nal/se-**ree**-brO-spI-nal) (adj) relating to the brain and spinal cord

cerebrovascular »
(**ser**-e-brO-**vas**-kyoo-lar) (adj) relating to the blood vessels of the brain, especially to pathological changes

Chvostek sign
(**khvosh**-teks) (n) an abnormal spasm of facial muscles when the facial nerve is tapped lightly

clonus »
(**klO**-nus) (n) abnormal condition in which a skeletal muscle alternately contracts and relaxes

concussion
(kon-**kush**-un) (n) an injury of a soft structure, as the brain, resulting from a blow or violent shaking

coprolalia
(kOp-rO-**lay**-lee-a) (n) involuntary utterance of obscene words, often seen in Tourette syndrome

corneal »
(**kor**-nee-al) (adj) the clear, transparent, anterior portion of the fibrous coat of the eye composing about one-sixth of its surface

coronal »
(ka-**rO**-nal) (adj) pertaining to a corona, a structure resembling a crown

cortex
(**kOr**-teks) (n) an outer part of an organ, such as the brain

cortical
(**kOr**-ti-kal) (adj) relating to a cortex

craniotomy »
(cray-nee-**ot**-O-mee) (n) surgical opening into the skull, performed to control bleeding, remove tumors, relieve pressure inside the cranium, or insert electrodes for diagnosis

cranium
(**kray**-nee-um) (n) the bony skull that holds the brain

cyanosis »
(sI-a-**nO**-sis) (n) bluish discoloration of the skin and mucous membranes, occurring when the oxygen in the blood is sharply diminished, as in carbon monoxide poisoning

decompression
(**dee**-kom-presh-un) (n) removal of bone to relieve pressure

delusion
(dee-**loo**-zhun) (n) belief in something in spite of incontrovertible evidence

dementia
(dee-**men**-shee-a) (n) a general mental deterioration due to organic or psychological factors

Dexedrine »
(**dex**-a-dreen) (n) brand name for dextroamphetamine, a CNS stimulant

diffuse »
(di-**fyoos**) (adj) spreading, scattered

Dilantin »
(dill-**ann**-tin) (n) brand name for phenytoin, used for the prevention and management of seizures

diplopia »
(di-**plO**-pee-a) (n) double vision

dorsum »
(**dOr**-sum) (n) the back or posterior surface of a part

dural »
(**doo**-ral) (adj) pertaining to the dura mater, the outer membrane covering the spinal cord and brain

dura mater
(**doo**-ra **may**-ter/**mah**-ter) (n) the outermost of the three membranes surrounding the brain and spinal cord; it is tough and fibrous

dyseidetic »
(dis-I-**det**-ik) (adj) inability to visualize and recall objects (words) previously seen

dyslexia »
(dis-**lek**-see-a) (n) impairment of ability to read in which letters and words are reversed

dysphonetic »
(dis-fO-**net**-ik) (adj) inability to connect sounds to objects (words)

dysphoria
(dis-**fOr**-ee-a) (n) mood characterized by anxiety, depression, discontent

echolalia
(ek-O-**lay**-lee-a) (n) involuntary repetition of a word or sentence just spoken by another person

electrophoresis »
(ee-lek-trO-fO-**ree**-sis) (n) the movement of charged suspended particles through a liquid medium in response to changes in an electric field; for example, a hemoglobin electrophoresis measures the types of hemoglobin in the blood

encephalopathy
(en-**sef**-a-**lop**-a-thee) (n) disease or dysfunction of the brain

encopresis »
(en-cO-**pree**-sis) (n) inability to control bowel movements, fecal incontinence

epilepsy
(**ep**-i-lep-see) (n) convulsive disorder

epileptiform »
(ep-i-**lep**-ti-fOrm) (adj) having the form of epilepsy

erythema »
(er-i-**thee**-ma) (n) abnormal redness of the skin resulting from dilation of the capillaries, as occurs in sunburn

euthymic
(yoo-**thI**-mik) (adj) characterized by moderation of mood

exotropia »
(ek-sO-**trO**-pee-a) (n) outward turning of one eye relative to the other

extensor »
(eks-**ten**-ser, eks-**ten**-sOr) (n) muscle that, when flexed, causes extension of a joint or straightening of an arm or leg

extraocular »
(eks-tra-**ok**-yoo-lar) (adj) outside the eye

fissures
(**fish**-urz) (n) deep grooves in the brain

flexor »
(**flek**-ser, **flek**-sOr) (n) muscle that bends a joint

fundus
(**fun**-dus) (n) that part of the interior of the eyeball exposed to view through the ophthalmoscope; fundi (pl)

funduscopic »
(fun-dus-**skop**-ik) (adj) the examination of the ocular fundus with an ophthalmoscope

gadolinium »
(gad-O-**lin**-ee-um) (n) a rare earth metallic element

ganglion
(**gang**-glee-on) (n) a group of nerve cell bodies located in the peripheral nervous system

Glasgow coma scale
(**glas**-gO/**glaz**-gO) (n) a clinical scale to assess impaired consciousness; assessment includes motor responsiveness, verbal performance, and eye opening

glial cells
(**glee**-al sels) (n) cells of the nervous system with functions other than transmitting signals

glove-stocking anesthesia
(**an**-es-**thee**-see-a) (n) glove or gauntlet anesthesia is loss of sensation in the hand; stocking anesthesia is loss of sensation in the area covered by a stocking

grand mal (seizure)
(grahn mal) (n) generalized tonic-clonic seizure

hallucination
(ha-**loo**-si-**nay**-shun) (n) the sensory perception (see, hear, smell, or taste) of something that does not actually exist or has not actually occurred

hematocrit
(**hee**-ma-tO-krit, **hem**-a-tO-krit) (n) a measure of the packed cell volume of red cells

hemiparesis »
(hem-ee-pa-**ree**-sis, hem-ee-**par**-e-sis) (n) muscular weakness of one half of the body

hemoglobin
(hee-mO-**glO**-bin) (n) the iron-containing pigment of the red blood cells

hepatosplenomegaly »
(**hep**-a-tO-**meg**-a-lee, hee-**pat**-O-**meg**-a-lee) (n) enlargement of both liver and spleen

hippocampus
(hip-O-**kam**-pus) (n) structure within the brain

hydrocephalus
(hI-drO-**sef**-a-lus) (n) an excessive accumulation of fluid in the brain

hyperesthetic »
(hI-per-es-thet-ik) (adj) characterized by acute sensitivity to pain or other stimuli

hyperreflexia
(**hI**-per-ree-**flek**-see-a) (n) a condition marked by exaggerated deep tendon reflexes

hypometabolism
(**hI**-pO-me-**tab**-O-lizm) (n) lowered metabolism

hypnotic
(hip-**not**-ik) (n) an agent which brings on sleep

ichthyosis »
(ik-thee-**O**-sis) (n) condition in which the skin is dry and scaly, resembling fish skin

ictal »
(**ik**-tal) (adj) referring to the onset of a seizure

icteric »
(ik-**ter**-ik) pertaining to jaundice

interictal
(in-ter-**ik**-tal) (adj) between seizures

ischemia
(is-**kee**-mee-a) (n) decreased blood supply due to obstruction, such as narrowing of the blood vessels

lethargy
(**leth**-ar-jee) (n) state of sluggishness, stupor, unresponsiveness

lobectomy »
(lO-**bek**-tO-mee) (n) surgical procedure in which a lobe is removed (thyroid, brain, liver, and lungs are divided into lobes)

lymphadenopathy »
(**lim**-phad-e-**nop**-a-thee) (n) disease of the lymph nodes

mania
(**may**-nee-a) (n) a psychiatric disorder characterized by restlessness, euphoria, grandiosity, and poor judgment with symptoms of insomnia, rapid speech, and distractibility

medulla oblongata
(me-**dool**-a ob-long-**gah**-ta) (n) the lowest part of the brain, connecting to the spinal cord; contains the cardiac, vasomotor, and respiratory centers of the brain

meninges
(me-**nin**-jeez) (n) membranes covering the brain and spinal cord

meningitis
(men-in-**jI**-tis) (n) inflammation of the membranes of the brain or spinal cord

meningocele
(me-**ning**-gO-seel) (n) protrusion of the brain or spinal cord through a defect in the skull or spinal column

mesial
(**mee**-zee-al; **mes**-ee-al) (adj) situated toward the midline of the body or the central part of an organ or tissue (also called medial)

myasthenia gravis
(mI-as-**thee**-nee-a **grav**-is) (n) a chronic progressive muscular weakness, beginning usually in the face and throat, due to a defect in the conduction of nerve impulses

nausea
(**naw**-zee-a, **naw**-zha) (n) an inclination to vomit

neoplastic »
(nee-O-**plas**-tik) (adj) pertaining to the nature of new, abnormal tissue formation; usually refers to cancer

neuralgia
(noo-**ral**-jee-a) (n) pain of a severe, throbbing, or stabbing character along the course of a nerve

neurapraxia
(noor-a-**prak**-see-a) (n) loss of conduction in a nerve without structural degeneration

neurasthenia
(noor-as-**thee**-nee-a) (n) a condition, commonly accompanying or following depression, characterized by fatigue believed to be brought on by psychological factors

neurilemma
(noor-i-**lem**-a) (n) a cell that enfolds one or more axons of the peripheral nervous system

neuron
(**noor**-on) (n) nerve cell; the morphological and functional unit of the nervous system, consisting of the nerve cell body, the dendrites, and the axon

neuropathy »
(noo-**rop**-a-thee) (n) disorder affecting the cranial or spinal nerves

nuchal »
(**noo**-kal) (adj) pertaining to the neck, or nucha (nape of neck)

nystagmus
(nis-**tag**-mus) (n) involuntary, rhythmic oscillation of the eyeballs

palsy »
(**pawl**-zee) (n) an abnormal condition characterized by partial paralysis

paresthesia
(par-es-**thee**-zee-a) (n) an abnormal sensation of tingling, prickling, burning

parietal
(pa-**rI**-e-tal) (adj) relating to the inner walls of a body cavity; a section (lobe) of the brain

peripheral nervous system
(per-**if**-er-al) (n) portion of nervous system that connects the CNS to other body parts

perseveration
(per-sev-er-**ay**-shun) (n) an uncontrollable, persistent thought

petit mal
(pe-**tee** mahl) (n) a type of seizure characterized by a brief blackout of consciousness with minor rhythmic movements, seen especially in children

phobia
(**fO**-bee-a) (n) an unfounded fear that invokes a state of panic

phonation »
(fO-**nay**-shun) (n) process of uttering vocal sounds

pia mater
(**pI**-a **may**-ter / **pee**-a **mah**-ter) (n) the innermost of the three membranes surrounding the brain and spinal cord; it carries a rich supply of blood vessels

pineal gland »
(**pin**-ee-al) (n) small, cone-shaped gland in the brain thought to secrete melatonin

pituitary gland
(pi-**too**-i-tayr-ee) (n) gland suspended from the base of the hypothalamus

plantar »
(**plan**-tar) (adj) relating to the undersurface (sole) of the foot; a reflex

plexus
(**plek**-sus) (n) a network of intersecting nerves and blood vessels or of lymphatic vessels

polyneuropathy
(**pol**-ee-noo-**rop**-a-thee) (n) a disorder involving two or more peripheral nerves

postictal »
(pOst-**ik**-tal) (adj) relating to the period following a seizure

pronator »
(**prO**-nay-ter, **prO**-nay-tOr) (n) muscle that moves a part into the prone position

proprioception »
(**prO**-pree-O-**sep**-shun) (n) sensation due to receiving stimuli from muscles, tendons, or other internal tissues which provides a sense of movement and position of the body

proton »
(**prO**-ton) (n) a positively charged particle that is a fundamental component of the nucleus of all atoms; used in radiotherapy

psychosomatic
(**sI**-kO-sO-**mat**-ik) (adj) relating to the influence of the mind upon the functions of the body

quadriceps »
(**kwah**-dri-seps) (adj) four-headed, as a quadriceps muscle; one of the extensor muscles of the legs

quadriparesis
(kwod-ri-pa-**ree**-sis) (n) paralysis of both arms and both legs

radiculopathy
(ra-**dik**-yoo-**lop**-a-thee) (n) disease of the spinal nerve roots

refractory »
(ree-**frak**-tO-ree) (adj) obstinate, stubborn; resistant to ordinary treatment

reticulocyte »
(re-**tik**-yoo-lO-sIt) (n) a red blood cell containing a network of granules representing an immature stage in development

retina
(**ret**-i-na) (n) a 10-layered, delicate nervous tissue membrane of the eye that receives images of external objects and transmits visual impulses through the optic nerve to the brain

Romberg
(**rom**-berg) (n) a simple test to assess for loss of proprioception wherein the patient stands with feet apart and then closes their eyes

sagittal »
(**saj**-i-tal) (adj) relating to a line from front to back in the middle of an organ or the body

sciatica
(sI-**at**-i-ka) (n) pain in the lower back and hip radiating down the back of the thigh into the leg, usually due to herniated lumbar disk

sclera »
(**skleer**-a) (n) a tough white fibrous tissue that covers the so-called white of the eye

shunt »
(shunt) (v) to turn away from; to divert

sickle cell anemia
(**sik**-l sel a-**nee**-mee-a) (n) hereditary blood disease in which abnormal hemoglobin causes red blood cells to become sickle-shaped, fragile and nonfunctional, leading to many acute and chronic complications

somatization
(**sO**-mat-I-**zay**-shun) (n) a condition in which a person expresses psychological needs through physical symptoms

sphenoidal »
(sfee-**noy**-dal) (adj) concerning the sphenoid bone

subdural hematoma
(sub-**doo**-ral hee-ma-**tO**-ma / hem-a-**tO**-ma) (n) an accumulation of blood under the dura mater surrounding the brain

syncopal
(**sin**-kO-pal) (adj) relating to fainting

syncope
(**sin**-ko-pee) (n) fainting

temporal »
(**tem**-po-ral) (adj) pertaining to the temple of the head or the corresponding lobe of the brain

thecal
(**thee**-kal) (adj) referring to a covering or enclosure

thrombosis
(throm-**bO**-sis) (n) condition in which a blood clot forms within a blood vessel

uvula »
(**yoo**-vyoo-la) (n) small, fleshy mass hanging from the soft palate in the mouth

ventricle »
(**ven**-tri-kl) (n) either of the two lower chambers of the heart; areas of the brain that produce and drain cerebrospinal fluid (CSF)

Abbreviations

ADD	attention deficit disorder	LP	lumbar puncture
ADHD	attention deficit hyperactivity disorder	MAOI	monoamine oxidase inhibitor
ALS	amyotrophic lateral sclerosis	MMPI-2	Minnesota Multiphasic Personality Inventory-2
ANS	autonomic nervous system		
AVM	arteriovenous malformation	MRA	magnetic resonance angiography
CAT, CT	computerized axial tomography	MRI	magnetic resonance imaging
CBT	cognitive behavioral therapy	MS	multiple sclerosis
CNS	central nervous system	NCV	nerve conduction velocity
CP	cerebral palsy	OCD	obsessive-compulsive disorder
CSF	cerebrospinal fluid	OD	(drug) overdose
CVA	cerebrovascular accident	PD	Parkinson disease
DSM-IV	*Diagnostic and Statistical Manual of Mental Disorders, Fourth Edition*	PET	positron emission tomography
		PNS	peripheral nervous system
DTR	deep tendon reflex	PPVT-III	Peabody Picture Vocabulary Test, Third Edition
ECT	electroconvulsive therapy		
EEG	electroencephalogram or electroencephalography	PTSD	posttraumatic stress disorder
		SNS	somatic nervous system
EMG	electromyography	SPECT	single photon emission computed tomography
FDG	^{18}F-fluoro-2-deoxyglucose fluorodeoxyglucose		
		SSRI	selective serotonin reuptake inhibitor
FSIQ	full scale intelligence quotient	TIA	transient ischemic attack
GAD	generalized anxiety disorder	TAT	Thematic Apperception Test
HNP	herniated nucleus pulposus	WAIS	Wechsler Adult Intelligence Scale
LOC	loss of consciousness	WMS-III	Wechsler Memory Scale, Third Edition

Building Language Skills

Complete the following exercises, drawing on the information learned in the Exploring Neurology and Psychiatry section of this chapter and referencing the Terms Bank.

Exercise 14.1   Matching Sound and Spelling

The numbered list that follows shows the phonetic spelling of hard-to-spell words. Sound out the word and then write the correct spelling in the blank space provided. Check your answers in the Terms Bank or other appropriate reference.

1. **sin**-ko-pee _____

2. ra-**dik**-yoo-**lop**-a-thee _____

3. **naw**-zee-a/**naw**-zha _____

4. **noor**-on _____

5. me-**nin**-jeez _____

6. noor-as-**thee**-nee-a _____

7. a-**fay**-zee-a _____

8. noo-**ral**-jee-a _____

9. pe-**tee** mahl _____

10. **sI**-kO-sO-**mat**-ik _____

11. me-**ning**-gO-seel _____

12. pi-**too**-i-tayr-ee _____

13. **ser**-e-brO-**spl**-nal/se-**ree**-brO-**spl**-nal _____

14. a-**tak**-see-a _____

Below is a list of frequently used words that look alike and/or sound alike. Study the meaning and pronunciation of each set of words, read the following sentences carefully, and then circle the word in parentheses that correctly completes the meaning.

acetic	sour		**gait**	manner of walking
acidic	pertaining to acid		**gate**	entrance or opening in a wall or fence
ascitic	a fluid that accumulates in the abdominal cavity			
			ictal	relating to a seizure
affect	to influence (v)		**icterus**	jaundice
affect	(n) the emotional feeling, tone, and mood attached to a thought, including its external manifestations		**pair**	(n) two, couple
			pare	(v) peel, scrape
			pear	(n) fruit
effect	(v) to bring about like, to effect a change; (n) cause and effect		**radical**	(adj) aimed at the origin of a disease or condition; complete, as in surgical excision
afferent	toward the center		**radicle**	(n) a nerve or vessel branch that joins others to form larger vessels or nerves
efferent	away from the center			
anesthetic	an agent that blocks pain receptors			
asthenic	loss of energy		**recession**	the withdrawal of a part from its normal position
esthesic	pertaining to the perception of pain		**resection**	the cutting out of a portion of an organ
esthetic (aesthetic)	pertaining to one's appearance			
cereal	grain		**regression**	a return to an earlier condition
serial	referring to a series		**remission**	partial or total disappearance of a disease
clench	(n) fist, vise		**repression**	restraint
clench	(v) close tightly			
clinch	(v) confirm, ensure		**their**	(possessive pronoun) belonging to
conscience	(n) the sense of right and wrong		**there**	(adv) in that place
conscious	(adj) aware		**they're**	(contraction) they are
crises	(n, pl) turning points		**tic**	spasmodic jerk of a muscle or group of muscles or a quirk in speech
crisis	(n, sing) turning point			
cue	a prompt or signal		**tick**	insect; sound of a clock
queue	a waiting line; an area for persons or things waiting		**workup**	(n) an intensive diagnostic study
			work up	(v) to produce by mental or physical work
fecal	relating to feces			
thecal	relating to a sheath			

1. Because he did not take good care of his teeth, he now has (recession/regression/repression) of the gums.

2. He is suffering jaw pain because of frequent teeth (clenching/clinching).

3. Within two hours of surgery, the patient became (conscience/conscious).

4. I used a (pair/pare/pear) of tweezers to remove the splinter.

5. The surgeon had to (pair/pare/pear) the nerve from the bone.

6. She is suffering from situational depression precipitated by several (crisis/crises) in her life.

7. After experiencing severe trauma to the lower spine, the patient underwent (radical/radicle) surgery.

8. (Their/There/They're) children are both in college now.

9. The patient's (effect/affect) changed due to the side (effect/affect) of the medication.

10. We are thankful his leukemia is now in (remission/repression).

11. The patient was asked to walk down the hall and back in order to assess his (gate/gait).

Exercise 14.3   Choosing Words from Context

When transcribing dictation, the medical transcriptionist frequently needs to consider the situation when determining the word that correctly completes the sentence. From the list below, select the term that meaningfully completes each of the following statements.

atrophy	cranium	parietal
cerebellar examination	funduscopic	plantar
cerebrovascular	hemiparesis	postictal
clonus	interictal	ventricle

1. The brain is found within the _____.

2. There was marked _____ after the stroke.

3. The _____ section of the brain was affected by the cerebrovascular accident.

4. The neurologic exam was normal, including _____ flexion, a negative Babinski sign.

5. Increased intracranial pressure can be visualized by _____ examination with the ophthalmoscope.

6. _____ is best performed by having the patient walk down the hallway to see if there is any ataxia.

7. The radiation therapy caused a small amount of _____ of the parietal area of the brain.

8. Between seizures, the woman had a (an) _____ period where she slept for a few minutes.

9. There was a blockage of the right _____ in the brain caused by a cystic lesion, most likely benign.

10. The 72-year-old man had a (an) _____ accident which caused him to have left-sided hemiparesis.

11. The patient had marked _____ of the left arm as an effect of the cerebral palsy.

12. The _____ phase of his seizures is always determined by his deep sleep.

Exercise 14.4   Pairing Words and Meanings

From this list, locate the term that best matches each of the following definitions. Write the term in the space provided by each definition.

cerebrovascular	hyperreflexia	syncope
cyanosis	perseveration	uvula
euthymic	sagittal	
hemifacial	somatization	

1. expression of psychological needs through physical symptoms _____

2. the plane from front to back in the middle of an organ or body _____

3. small structure hanging from soft palate in mouth _____

4. fainting caused by decreased blood flow to the brain _____

5. exaggeration of deep tendon reflexes _____

6. bluish discoloration of skin resulting from diminished supply of oxygen in blood _____

7. affecting half of the face _____

8. persistence of a thought _____

9. pertaining to blood vessels of brain _____

10. having moderate mood _____

Exercise 14.5   Creating Terms from Word Forms

Combine prefixes, root words, and suffixes from this list to create medical words that fit the following definitions. Fill in the blanks with the words you construct.

a-	without, lacking	**myel/o**	spinal cord
dys-	bad, difficult	**ventricul/o**	ventricle
hemi-	half, slight	**neur/o**	nerve
para-	beside, abnormal; alongside	**ictal**	onset, as in a stroke or seizure
phono-	sound, speech	**-algia**	pain
poly-	two or more, many	**-ia**	condition
thym-	emotion	**-itis**	inflammation
cephal/o	head	**-kines/i**	motion
cerebell/o	cerebellum	**-lepsy**	seizure
cerebr/o	cerebrum	**-otomy**	incision
crani/o	cranium	**-paresis**	minor paralysis
encephal/o	brain	**-plegia**	paralysis

1. partial paralysis _____

2. inflammation of brain tissue _____

3. head pain _____

4. paralysis of the lower extremities _____

5. condition characterized by a lack of ability to move _____

6. condition characterized by a loss of speech _____

7. inflammation of large number of nerves _____

8. condition characterized by difficult emotions (depression) _____

9. paralysis on one side _____

10. inflammation of spinal cord _____

11. cutting into the skull _____

12. incision into the ventricle of the brain _____

Read the following emergency department report excerpt and look for errors in punctuation, word use, capitalization and spelling. Even though some of the abbreviations are acceptable, do not allow any abbreviations except in the ED Course heading. Mark the corrections on this page and key the excerpt with all errors corrected. Save the document as XXExercise14.06 using your initials in place of *XX* in the file name.

CC

LOC, drug OD.

HPI

The patient is a 40-year-old female who was found blue in the face and unconscious by family this am. This occurred approximately 10 to 15 minutes after she had injected a line of Heroin intravenously. Reportedly, her son started cardio pulmonary resuscitation and she gasped for breath. Fire department arrived and administered Naloxone.

The patient now complains of headache. She reports that she has not used heroin for several months. The family reports that she does heroin 4 to 5 times per week.

PMH

Seizure disorder, epilepsy since childhood.

SOCIAL HISTORY

Intravenous drug addict for ten years.

CURRENT MEDICATIONS

No known drug allergies.

Percocet for migraine headaches, dilantin, and phenobarbital.

PHYSICAL EXAMINATION

GENERAL: A well-developed, well-nourished caucasian female in no acute distress, awake, alert, oriented. HEENT: Pupils equal, round, and reactive to light and accommodation; extraocular muscles intact. Speech clear. THORAX AND LUNGS: Respirations unlabored. Clear to percussion and auscultation. HEART: Regular rate and rhythm. NEUROLOGIC: She follows instructions appropriately and moves all extremities. Deep tendon reflexes are symmetric.

ED COURSE

The patient was examined as above. She will be observed for another hour, and if she maintains her present level of consciousness, plan to discharge to home with appropriate instructions.

DIAGNOSIS

Heroin overdose. The patient is to be referred to the mental health unit for addition counseling. She should continue with her dilantin and phenobarbital and follow up with her family medical doctor.

Exercise 14.7   Thinking Like a Professional

Read this scenario carefully and then select the most appropriate response. Write an explanation for why you think your choice is the best answer.

You are working for a company that has a policy governing the number of blanks that can be left in a document. You have been assigned to a new dictator who practices a medical specialty you have never transcribed before. You have exceeded the number of blanks allowed in several reports. What should you do?

a. Request help from your co-workers.
b. Choose reports from dictators that you are familiar with and leave the new dictator for someone else.
c. Transcribe the reports, leaving out phrases that would have blanks, especially those phrases that do not seem relevant to the overall report.
d. Continue to leave blanks where necessary and send the chart to a QA editor for review, prior to it going back to the facility to be placed in the patient's chart.

Best response: _____

Explanation: _____

_____

_____

_____

_____

Building Transcription Skills

You will apply the medical specialty and language information you learned in this chapter to transcription work in this section. After you learn the formatting recommendations of the neuropsychological evaluation report, you will transcribe seven reports related to seven different patient studies.

Introducing the Neuropsychological Evaluation

Neuropsychological evaluation reports (Figure 14.7) contain information on patients seen in a clinic or hospital setting. A psychologist or neurologist dictates the report. The purpose of the report is to document a patient's history, mental status, assessment, and previous treatment to assist with planning care and treatment. The language on these reports includes terms related to neuropsychological development, human behavior, and treatment.

Required Headings/Content

Typically, the information is provided in narrative format. Content includes a history of the present illness followed by the findings of both physical and neurologic examinations. The dictator may omit report headings. Sometimes, only neurologic information is included, along with the results of specific developmental and neurologic tests. Because this type of report is fairly specialized, it is not included in Appendix A. Headings should be transcribed as dictated.

Turnaround Time

If the patient is admitted to a hospital, the report is usually dictated and transcribed within the first 24 hours of admission. In clinic settings, the report may be dictated and transcribed within 48 hours.

Preparing to Transcribe

To prepare for transcribing dictation, review the common neurology and psychiatry terms, drugs, and abbreviations presented in this chapter's Terms Bank. Study the format and organization of the model document shown in Figure 14.7, and key the model document, using the neuropsychological evaluation report template on the Dictations and Templates CD as a starting point. Save the document as XXFigure14.07 using your initials in place of XX in the file name. Proofread the document by comparing it with the printed version. Categorize the types of errors you made, and document them on a copy of the Performance Comparison Chart. A template of this chart is included on the Dictations and Templates CD.

Transcribing Reports

Transcribe, edit, and correct each report in the following patient studies. Consult reference books for words or formatting rules that are unfamiliar.

As you work on the transcription assignment for this chapter, fill in the Performance Comparison Chart that you started when you keyed the model document. For at least three of the reports, categorize and document the types of errors you made. Answer the document analysis questions on the bottom of the chart. With continuous practice and assessment, the quality of your work will improve.

1" margins and left justification

PATIENT NAME: Aaron Rightman
DOB: 08/30/20XX
DOV: 07/10/20XX

double-space

The patient, age 7 years 10 months, was seen for a pediatric neurological assessment on July 10. The parents were the informants. The reason for this visit was for a "second opinion." The patient has been diagnosed as having a learning disability with an attention deficit disorder.

At 2 years of age it was noted that the patient had articulation difficulties and delayed expressive language. He was given speech therapy. At 3 years of age he was placed in a preschool program for the handicapped. He had no problems socially and began to do well. At that time the school recommended that he attend a regular nursery school. The patient was enrolled in the synagogue nursery school at the age of 4. He soon developed encopresis. The parents characterized the patient's school experiences as being "a disaster." He began to exhibit poor attention, anger, and hostility. When he reached the age of 5, he was placed in a day school, which was also attended by his friends from nursery school. By this time he was "already viewed as a bad child by the other children."

The patient recently completed 2nd grade at the day school. There he received tutoring on a one-to-one basis. He was also seen by a learning disability expert twice a week. He had speech and language therapy 1/2 hour per week. He is still reading below grade level.

In March, the patient had a neurobehavioral evaluation. It was noted that the patient was "functioning within the high average range perceptually and in the very superior range verbally." However, there was a 22-point disparity between his verbal and nonverbal abilities. He did best when he "was able to communicate verbally." His cognitive strengths included "word fluency and word knowledge, practical knowledge, common sense, and paper/pencil skills. Cognitive weaknesses included shifting of mental set, visual discrimination, visual searching, nonverbal deductive reasoning, and analysis/synthesis." The evaluators thought that the patient did have an attention deficit hyperactivity disorder, and they noticed that he was a child with "poor phonological awareness, was unable to process certain sounds quickly enough, and encountered problems holding language sounds in short-term memory and manipulating them in active working memory. It is hard for him to break words down into their component sounds and re-blend them or try to substitute a new sound for an existing one in a word."

Family history reveals that the father has reading problems. A paternal uncle has ADD. A paternal cousin is in a special education class and is said to have a learning disability and ADD. The mother's cousin has ADD. There is no family history of tics or obsessive-compulsive habits. There are 3 siblings: a 12-year-old and a 4-year-old are doing well. The brother, who is 10, has mild learning difficulties and ADHD symptoms.

The patient entered the examining room while his parents waited outside. He appeared to be anxious about the exam since there were 3 other observers in the room with me. Initially, he

(continued)

Figure 14.7 Neuropsychological Evaluation Report

NEUROPSYCHOLOGICAL EVALUATION
PATIENT NAME: Aaron Rightman
DOV: 07/10/20XX
Page 2

was very subdued and almost sad. However, he answered questions appropriately and showed no evidence of an activity disturbance. He is poorly oriented to left and right on himself and in space. When he copied geometric forms, he exhibited visual/motor integration difficulties, putting "ears" on the diamond figure. When he was given the Boder test for dyslexia, he had marked trouble spelling words which are in his sight vocabulary. From the screening test, he seemed to me to have a combination of dyseidetic-dysphonetic difficulties.

His height of 130 cm was in the 80th percentile, his weight of 26.6 kg was in the 60th percentile, and his head circumference of 52 cm was in the 50th percentile.

Head and neck were benign. Lungs were clear to percussion and auscultation. Heart: Regular sinus rhythm, no murmurs. Abdomen: Soft and nontender. Liver and spleen not palpable. Genitalia: Testes in scrotal sac. Tanner 1. Skin revealed mild ichthyosis over the dorsum of his legs. Skeletal was negative. There were no dysmorphic features.

On neurological exam, the patient's head was of normal shape. He had a single whorl on the right. He tracked well. He did not have difficulty with rapidly moving his tongue from side to side. He could not isolate the tongue movement from movement of his jaw. The remainder of the cranial nerves were normal. Visual fields by confrontation were normal. Vision and hearing were grossly normal. The tone of his muscles was normal. Fine and gross coordination was normal. Deep tendon reflexes were physiologic. Plantars were flexor. There was no clonus. He had some immature overflow phenomena and a slightly positive Prechtl sign. He is right-handed. He held a pencil well.

In summary, the patient has many symptoms of minimal cerebral dysfunction, which is probably on a genetic basis. These symptoms include: (1) a learning disability, primarily involving reading, which grossly appears to be the dyseidetic-dyskinetic type; (2) an attention deficit hyperactivity disorder, which is responding well to Dexedrine; (3) a vocal tic, which may be a precursor to developing Tourette syndrome; and (4) immature motor signs, as noted on the Prechtl and overflow phenomena. I think that the patient's regression 6 months ago may reflect overt depression, which may still be present.

Therapeutically speaking, I think the parents are doing everything possible to help this young man. There is no question that he belongs in a psychotherapeutic relationship. I am assuming that the tricyclic antidepressant is being given for his depressive symptoms. (The parents think that this is helping.) The Dexedrine is effective for the ADHD symptoms. Personally, if his weight

(continued)

Figure 14.7 Neuropsychological Evaluation Report (Continued)

NEUROPSYCHOLOGICAL EVALUATION
PATIENT NAME: Aaron Rightman
DOV: 07/10/20XX
Page 3

loss continues, I would suggest not using the sustained release form but, rather, giving him a dose in the morning, at noon, and at 4 p.m., and this should be given before meals.

I told the parents that they should not put too much stress on the patient's academic learning, but look for activities where he might be successful, which would make him feel good about himself. I also told them that I would discuss the patient's case with Dr. Balla, a research educator who is utilizing a specific therapy for children who have problems with auditory processing. I promised to send the reports of the neuropsychological evaluation and my reports to Dr. Balla to see if she would be interested in seeing the patient.

qs

_____

Lawrence Trent, MD
Professor of Pediatrics
ds
LT/XX
D: 07/10/20XX
T: 07/11/20XX
ds
cc: Dr. L. Balla

Patient Study 14.A

Brian T. Brendon

Brian Brendon is a 31-year-old patient who was diagnosed with a pineal region tumor a year prior to this visit. He had suffered dizzy spells, difficulty walking, and headaches for a month prior to his diagnosis. He was referred to Dr. Stone, who placed a ventricular shunt in the right ventricle to relieve the increased pressure caused by the tumor. He was then treated with chemotherapy and cranial irradiation. He is having an MRI of the brain as a followup study at the completion of his therapy.

REPORT 14.1 MRI Brain Scan

Use the Report1401.mp3 audio file and the radiology report template (Radiology_Report) when transcribing this report. Save the document as XXReport14.01, using your initials in place of *XX* in the file name.

Listen for these terms:
- T1 weighted images
- T2 techniques

Remember to set the test name in all capital letters and use the template's internal headings, even if they are not dictated. At the top of the report, delete the headings without dictated content.

Patient Study 14.B

Michelle Kuvell

Michelle Kuvell is a 7-year-old girl diagnosed with a brain tumor arising in the brainstem. She has been treated with radiation therapy and chemotherapy. She is visiting the neurologist for continuing followup in the office.

REPORT 14.2 Consultation Letter

Use the Report1402.mp3 audio file and the consultation letter template (Consultation_Letter) when transcribing this report. Save the document as XXReport14.02, using your initials in place of *XX* in the file name.

This transcribed letter will include internal headings similar to those found in previously transcribed reports. Set each dictated heading in all capital letters followed by a single hard return.

Review the appropriate formats for ranges that are presented as fractions.

Transcribe the radiation therapy dosages as 120 cGy and 6480 Gy.

Michael Wright is a 40-year-old male with a history of complex partial seizures for the past 23 years. Although he is taking Dilantin and Mysoline, his seizures have occurred more frequently in recent months. He was admitted to the hospital for evaluation and subsequently underwent a left anterior temporal lobectomy.

REPORT 14.3 Discharge Summary

Use the Report1403.mp3 audio file and the discharge summary template (Discharge_Summary) when transcribing this report. Save the document as XXReport14.03, using your initials in place of *XX* in the file name.

Listen for these terms and drug names:

> Decadron taper
> depth electrodes
> semiology
> sphenoidal
> Vicodin

Use the template's headings instead of the similar but slightly different dictated headings. There will be a dictated heading that will need to be added to the template's headings. The dictator's names should appear under the standard signature line, not at the top of the report.

Seven-year-old Aaron Right-man has been diagnosed previously as having a learning disability with an attention deficit disorder. His parents have requested an evaluation and a second opinion by Dr. Lawrence Trent.

REPORT 14.4 Neuropsychological Evaluation

Use the Report1404.mp3 audio file and the neuropsychological evaluation template (Neuropsychological_Eval) when transcribing this report. Save the document as XXReport14.04, using your initials in place of *XX* in the file name. This report is formatted in paragraph style with no internal headings.

Listen for these abbreviations and terms:

ADD (attention deficit disorder)
ADHD (attention deficit hyperactivity disorder)
Boder test
clonus
dyseidetic-dysphonetic difficulties
encopresis
Prechtl sign
Tourette syndrome
whorl

To ensure patient privacy, remember to change the patient's name to "the patient" if the name is dictated in the body of a report. This policy applies to names of family members as well.

The provider will include some punctuation in his dictation. Avoid using dashes, even if requested, and instead, use a colon.

Set the numbered list of symptoms in a run-in paragraph style to save space.

Joe Drinkowski is a 21-year-old man who has been experiencing episodes of involuntary contractions of his right arm followed by involuntary "shaking" of his legs. There are no other symptoms of seizures.

REPORT 14.5 History and Physical

Use the Report1405.mp3 audio file and the history and physical template (History_and_Physical) when transcribing this report. Save the document as XXReport14.05, using your initials in place of *XX* in the file name.

Listen for these terms:

hyperesthetic
pronator drift
proprioception
pseudoseizure

Within the Physical Examination section, the physician dictates characteristics of the HEENT using separate headings. Use the individual headings rather than the HEENT heading. Reference the headings from the Review of Systems section of the template as needed.

Tanisha Wilder is a 14-year-old child who has a history of sickle cell anemia. She has had multiple admissions for sickle cell crises and other complications related to sickle cell. She was admitted to the hospital with a history of confusion, lethargy, and inability to speak clearly.

REPORT 14.6 Discharge Summary

Use the Report1406.mp3 audio file and the discharge summary template (Discharge_Summary) when transcribing this report. Save the document as XXReport14.06, using your initials in place of *XX* in the file name.

Listen for these terms and drug names:
    Hib and Pneumovax vaccine
    penicillin V potassium
    reticulocyte

Note that a primary physician name is supplied in the patient information section, but another physician has dictated the report.

Bryan Charles is a 5-year-old boy who has been diagnosed with a recurring primary brain sarcoma. He has had chemotherapy, a bone marrow transplant, and radiation therapy following surgery. His parents brought him to the Institute for the Study of Child Development for a neuropsychological evaluation.

REPORT 14.7 Neuropsychological Evaluation

Use the Report1407.mp3 audio file and the neuropsychological evaluation template (Neuropsychological_Eval) when transcribing this report. Save the document as XXReport14.07, using your initials in place of *XX* in the file name.

As with other reports, set the main headings in all capital letters followed by a single hard return. Transcribe the headings dictated. Set the Test Administered and Results subheadings in all capital letters, followed by a colon and run-in text.

Test results for the Stanford-Binet Intelligence Scale should be transcribed in columnar form, using a Word table. List the subtests in the first column, the SAS (Standard Age Score) in the second column, and the percentile rank in the third column. The test includes four subtests (verbal reasoning, abstract/visual reasoning, quantitative reasoning, and short-term memory) and a composite score. Each subtest is further divided into parts, the names of which should be indented.

Fifteen

Hematology-Oncology

Hematology is the field of medicine devoted to diagnosing and treating diseases of the blood and blood-forming tissues. Oncology is the study and treatment of cancer. The subspecialties of hematology and oncology are often combined in one practice. The physician who specializes in these areas is called a hematologist-oncologist.

Objectives

» Identify major components of blood and describe their function.

» Explain the importance of the ABO and Rh antigen systems in blood transfusions.

» Describe diseases affecting red blood cells and white blood cells.

» Define coagulopathy and hemophilia.

» Differentiate between the major forms of cancer.

» Describe various treatment modalities for cancer.

» Define tumor staging and the TNM system.

» Pronounce and correctly spell terminology related to hematology and oncology.

» Transcribe dictation related to hematology and oncology.

» Describe an outpatient visit note, including typical content, format, and turnaround time.

The word *hematology* is derived from the Greek word *haima,* for blood. The term cancer was first used by the Greek physician Hippocrates as a metaphor for the spreading tendency of the disease. He compared metastases to the tentacles of a crab. Cancer is Latin for "crab." Cancer is indeed frightening because of the destruction it causes within the body. Though life-threatening, many adult cancers and a vast majority of pediatric cancers are curable today.

Structure and Function

Blood cells are produced in the bone marrow in a process called hematopoiesis. Bone marrow is found in the center of bones, particularly flat bones and long bones. Hematopoiesis begins with a pluripotent stem cell, which is capable of becoming any type of blood cell. The types of blood cells and the phases of differentiation and maturation are illustrated in Figure 15.1.

Blood has many components (Figure 15.2). The major kinds of blood cells are white blood cells and red blood cells. These cells are suspended in the plasma portion of blood, which also contains proteins, such as albumin, immunoglobulins, and fibrinogen. Blood provides a vehicle for the transport of nutrients, gases, hormones, electrolytes, and cellular waste products. Table 15.1 lists blood cells by their type and function. White cells are primarily responsible for defending the body against foreign intrusion. The normal immune system has the ability to differentiate self from non-self. Autoimmune diseases result when the immune system erroneously identifies "self" as foreign and launches an attack to destroy the "foreign" tissue. Platelets are not actually cells but are fragments of cytoplasm released from megakaryocytes in the bone marrow. Platelets play a key role in repairing vascular injury by providing a "plug" and preventing hemorrhage.

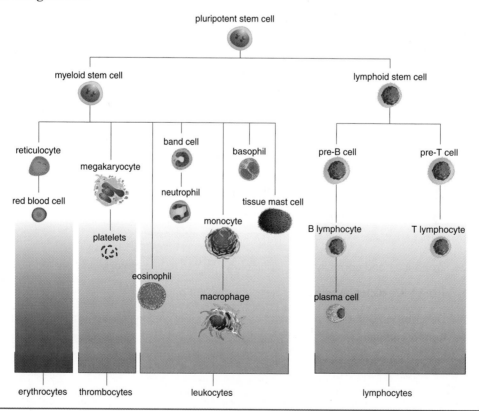

Figure 15.1 Hematopoiesis Tree

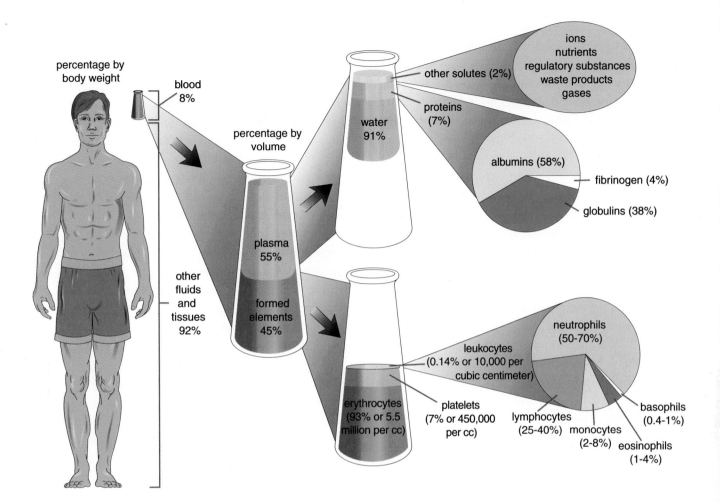

Figure 15.2 Components of Blood

The red blood cell's main function is to carry oxygen from the lungs to the tissues and then exchange the oxygen for carbon dioxide, a metabolic end-product. Red cells return carbon dioxide to the lungs to be exhaled. In addition, the outer surface of red blood cells contain blood group antigens, called agglutinins. Although there are many blood group antigen systems, the two most significant are ABO and Rh. The presence or absence of these antigens is a major factor in blood typing. Blood typing is done to determine the specific blood type the person has inherited from both parents.

Within the ABO system, there are four possible blood types: A, B, AB, and O. Individuals whose red cells carry only one antigen, A, are considered type A; those whose red cells carry antigen B are categorized as type B; and individuals carrying neither

Table 15.1

Cell Type Function

Cell Type	Function
red blood cells (RBCs)	carry oxygen to cells
white blood cells (WBCs)	fight invading substances such as bacteria and viruses
neutrophils	ingest bacteria and foreign cells
eosinophils	defend against parasites and participate in allergic responses
basophils	release histamine
lymphocytes	produce antibodies (B), participate in cellular immunity (T)
monocytes	transform into macrophages in the tissues
platelets	promote blood clotting after injury

antigen are called group O. A small group of people have type AB blood, which means their red cells have both the A and B antigens.

Red blood cells may also carry Rh antigens. People who carry the Rh antigen are called Rh positive. Those who do not are Rh negative. This designation is added to the blood type. Thus, a person with type O blood who is found to be Rh-negative would be classified as O negative. Normally, a specific antibody is formed after exposure to the corresponding antigen. The ABO blood group antigens are unique in that antibodies against other blood group antigens develop without exposure to the antigen itself. For example, a person with type A blood will have antibodies to the B antigen even though they have never been transfused with type B blood. The innate presence of A and B antibodies requires blood typing and cross-matching of donor and recipient red cells before a blood transfusion. Rh antibodies form in an Rh-negative individual in response to exposure to Rh-positive blood. This is a significant issue in obstetrics, especially when an Rh-negative mother carries a second child that is Rh positive.

One method of blood typing is the slide test (Figure 15.3) in which a drop or two of the patient's blood is placed on each end of a slide. Anti-A serum is added to one end and anti-B to the other. If antigen is present in either of the samples, agglutination (cell clumping) will occur, indicating the blood type. A "type and cross" is performed before transfusing blood. In addition to determining the blood type of the recipient and donor (called typing), the cells and serum of each are mixed (called a cross-match) to confirm compatibility.

If a person is given a blood transfusion of an incompatible blood type, a dangerous hemolytic transfusion reaction could occur. Antibodies attach to their corresponding antigen on the red cell membrane which "tags" the red cell for destruction by components of the immune system. Table 15.2 lists the occurrence of the various blood types in the population, the agglutinins present in each, and the type(s) of donor blood needed for safe (compatible) transfusions.

Coagulation factors, a group of plasma proteins, along with platelets are responsible for sealing vascular injuries and preventing excessive bleeding. When platelets come in contact with vascular endothelium, which is exposed when a vessel is injured, they release chemicals that trigger coagulation (Figure 15.4). Many factors control the delicate balance between clot formation

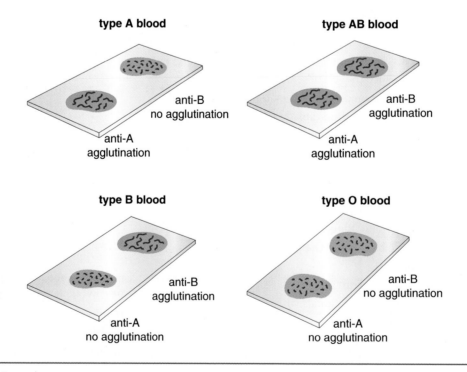

type A blood

anti-B
no agglutination

anti-A
agglutination

type AB blood

anti-B
agglutination

anti-A
agglutination

type B blood

anti-B
agglutination

anti-A
no agglutination

type O blood

anti-B
no agglutination

anti-A
no agglutination

Figure 15.3 Blood Typing Based on the Principle of Agglutination

Table 15.2

Blood Types and Transfusions

Blood Type	Agglutinins in Plasma	Frequency of Occurrence	Safe Transfusions (May Receive)
type A	anti-B	40%	types A, O
type B	anti-A	10%	types B, O
type AB	none	4%	types A, B, AB, O (universal recipient)
type O (universal donor)	anti-A, anti-B	45%	type O
Rh positive	none	85%	should receive Rh-positive blood but may receive Rh-negative blood if necessary
Rh negative	anti-D	15%	may receive only Rh-negative blood

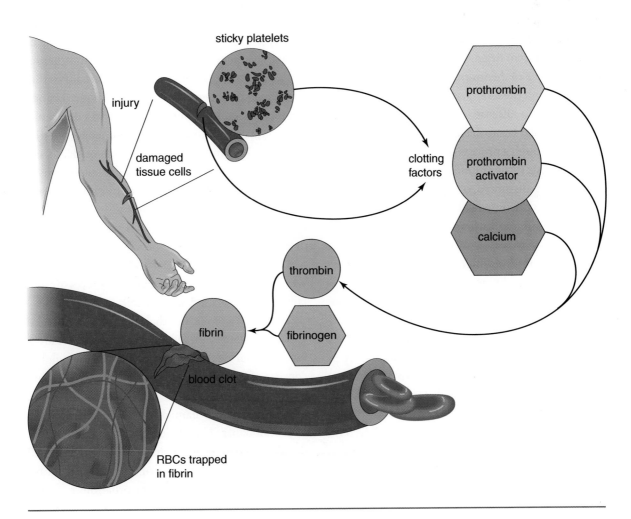

Figure 15.4 Blood Clotting Cascade

and clot dissolution. Ideally, clots should form and then dissolve as the tissue is repaired, but at times, clots dislodge and travel through the blood stream to the lungs (pulmonary embolism) or brain (stroke). Clots may also improperly form within the coronary arteries, especially arteries already narrowed by cholesterol plaque, inducing a myocardial infarction. Disorders of the clotting system are called coagulopathies, which include hypercoagulation disorders (increased tendency to form clots) and hemophilia (an inherited defect causing uncontrolled bleeding).

The lymph system includes the spleen and the thymus as well as a network of lymph nodes connected by lymph vessels. Microorganisms, other foreign cells, damaged or destroyed cells, as well as cancerous cells move from the intercellular spaces into the lymphatic vessels and on to clusters of lymph nodes where many immune processes take place. Lymph nodes often become enlarged as a result of the immune system's activity. The lymphatic system drains into the blood circulation so byproducts of the immune system can be eliminated through the liver and kidneys.

Cancer is a disease resulting from a loss of normal cellular control. Normally, tissues are rejuvenated through a process of cell division (mitosis) and apoptosis (programmed cell death). In cancer, the process is disrupted, often resulting in a mass of tissue due to uncontrolled mitosis and/or delayed apoptosis. Another cardinal feature of cancer cells is the ability to metastasize, or move from the primary tissue to a different part of the body or tissue type (e.g., breast cancer cells often metastasize to the liver and brain). Normal cells cannot invade or flourish in tissue types other than their own. Cancer cells usually do not carry out their original function. Instead, they invade and overtake normal cells and prevent normal function. There are three main methods for cancer cells to metastasize: (1) by direct extension to surrounding structures; (2) through the lymphatic system; or (3) via the blood system, which is called hematogenous spread.

Physical Assessment

The patient who presents to the hematology-oncology (heme-onc) specialist may be nervous, upset, and often quite ill. The referring physician may have already ordered blood tests that have suggested a blood dyscrasia, hemoglobinopathy, or cancer. Prior x-rays and/or scans may have indicated the possibility of a solid tumor. Sometimes specific symptoms send the person to the hematologist-oncologist. A detailed review of systems and a complete physical examination are essential to planning the patient's care.

Hematologic Diseases and Conditions

Anemia is an extremely common hematologic disorder, defined as a decrease in the red cell number or the hemoglobin concentration. Anemias may result from decreased red cell production or increased red cell loss and/or destruction (hemolysis). There are several red cell abnormalities that cause increased hemolysis. These include osmotic fragility, hereditary spherocytosis, and a deficiency of the glucose-6-phosphate dehydrogenase (G6PD) enzyme. The most common cause of decreased red cell production is iron deficiency, often caused by poor dietary intake of iron-rich foods. Chronic blood loss (e.g., abnormal uterine bleeding or an occult bleed, often from the GI tract) may result in anemia as well as B_{12} or folic acid deficiency. Aplastic anemia is a life-threatening disorder in which the bone marrow becomes hypoplastic and fails to produce adequate red cells.

Sickle cell anemia and thalassemias are inherited hemoglobinopathies, which are disorders caused by abnormal hemoglobin molecules. Hemoglobin consists of four chains of amino acids (called globin chains) wrapped around four heme molecules. Globin chains are named with the letters of the Greek alphabet. Under decreased oxygen tension, the globin chain changes shape, forcing the red cell into a sickle shape instead of the typical concave disk. Exercise, high altitudes, or situations resulting in decreased oxygen may cause a sickle cell crisis, as shown in Figure 15.5. Sickled cells become trapped in capillaries, causing swelling in the joints, especially in the distal extremities, as well as congestion within internal organs. The misshapen red cells are easily destroyed, and the increased red cell destruction results in anemia.

Thalassemia is common among individuals of Mediterranean, black, or Asian descent. There are many forms of thalassemia, but all are characterized by impaired synthesis or absence of one or both globin chains. Symptoms may be undetectable, mild or severe, depending on the type of mutation.

Immune (idiopathic) thrombocytopenic purpura (ITP) is characterized by petechiae and ecchymoses as a result of a low platelet count. ITP in children often follows a viral illness and may be self-limiting. Adult-onset ITP is more typically chronic. In ITP, antibodies attach to platelets, targeting them for splenic macrophage destruction.

Thrombosis is the formation or presence of clots inside blood vessels, which may lead to blockage and subsequent infarction of the tissues supplied by the vessel. There are various types of thromboses, including deep venous, cerebral, coronary, pulmonary, placental, and compression. Thrombosis may result from injury to a vessel or from pooling of blood in the deep veins of the legs as a result of decreased mobility, such as occurs when traveling in planes or during bedrest after surgery.

Patients with hypercoagulation disorders are especially susceptible to deep venous thrombosis, which may lead to pulmonary embolism or stroke. On the other hand, patients with hemophilia cannot adequately form clots and are at risk for life-threatening hemorrhage. Hemophilia is an inherited disorder characterized by a deficiency of either factor VIII (hemophilia A) or factor IX (hemophilia B, also called Christmas disease). Treatment includes infusion of the deficient coagulation factor.

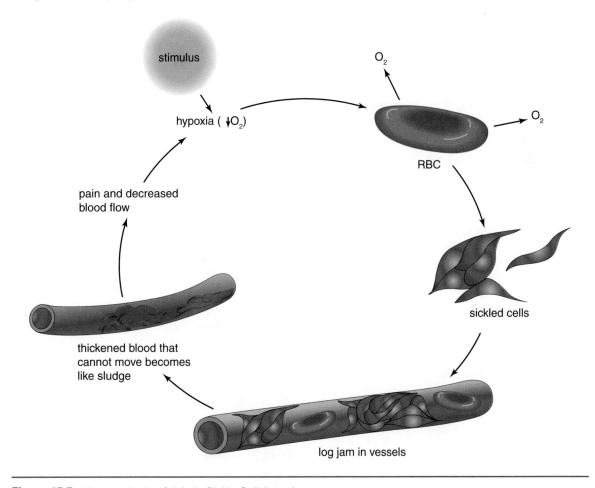

Figure 15.5 Vasoocclusive Crisis in Sickle Cell Anemia

Oncologic Diseases and Conditions

Cancers are classified into two major categories: hematologic cancers and solid tumors. Hematologic cancers involve the blood-forming tissues and include lymphomas, leukemias, and multiple myeloma. Solid tumors include sarcomas and carcinomas. Sarcoma describes cancers of the connective tissues, such as muscle, blood vessels, and bone. Carcinomas are subdivided into adenocarcinomas (originating in surface linings of the glands) and squamous cell, or epidermoid, carcinomas (originating in epithelium of a non-glandular nature, such as the surface of the skin or the membranes of the respiratory tract).

Some 90 percent of cancers are solid tumors; 10 percent are hematologic tumors. The leading causes of cancer deaths in adults are lung cancer, colorectal cancer, prostate cancer, and breast cancer. In children, the most prevalent type of hematologic cancer is leukemia, and brain tumors are the most common solid tumor.

Common Tests, Surgical Procedures, and Treatment Regimens

Methods for treating cancers depend on the specific type of cancer. For solid tumors, the staging or classification is most important for prognosis and treatment. Several classification systems are used, depending on the body area affected. For example, Dukes staging is used for colon cancer and Jewett staging is used for bladder cancer. The TNM (tumor, node, metastasis) system is commonly used to describe the extent of disease:

T (T1–T4) Classifies the extent of the primary tumor
N (N0–N3) Indicates extent of regional lymph node involvement
M (M0–M1) Indicates presence (M1) or absence (M0) of distant metastasis

Solid tumors are removed surgically if the tumor is resectable. Debulking, or surgical reduction in the size of a tumor that cannot be completely removed, may be performed to improve the outcome of chemotherapy or if the size of the tumor is causing life-threatening problems. Neoadjuvant therapy is chemotherapy given before debulking. Another widely used treatment is radiation therapy, which involves directing a radiation beam toward the cancer to rearrange the cellular DNA and kill the cell.

The word *chemotherapy* means chemical therapy and can refer to any pharmacologic agent; however, the term usually refers to the chemical treatment of cancer. Cytotoxic and antimetabolic agents kill rapidly dividing cells, including cancer cells, hair cells, cells of the mucous membranes, and blood cells. Many of the side effects and toxicities associated with chemotherapeutic agents are due to the collateral destruction of normal cells. Chemotherapy agents are usually given in combinations, called regimens or protocols, and are named with initials and acronyms. The generic name and the brand name may be used to form the acronym. The list includes in Table 15.3 some of the most common chemotherapy treatment regimens.

Hormone therapy (e.g., tamoxifen and leuprolide) and enzymes (e.g., asparaginase) are also used for cancer treatment as well as immunotherapy, also called biotherapy or biological response modifier therapy (BRM). Using recombinant DNA technology, monoclonal antibodies are produced that are directed at specific antigens on the surface of cancer cells. The antibodies attach to the antigens, triggering the immune system to destroy the cell. Examples of monoclonal antibody (MAB) therapies include Herceptin (trastuzumab) and Rituxan (rituximab). Another form of immune therapy uses vaccines (e.g., Melacine to treat melanoma) to induce the patient's immune system to create antibodies against the cancerous cells, thereby tagging the cancer cells for destruction.

This always-changing field is a challenge for the practitioner, the transcriptionist, and the patient. Researchers all over the world continue to try to find a cure for all cancers. Scientists continue to pursue treatments using recombinant DNA technology and biotherapy as well as studying the influence of the mind-body connection, or neuropsychoimmunology. Many new agents, particularly in the field of oncology, are on what is called the "fast track" for FDA approval so these important agents can be available to the public more quickly. Despite great advances in the treatment of cancer, early detection is still the best weapon against cancer. Recommended periodic screening methods include breast self-exam (BSE), mammography, prostate exam, sigmoidoscopy, and colonoscopy. In addition, certain markers in the blood can predict persons at risk for specific cancers. Those with known genetic risks should be watched closely for the earliest signs of cancer.

Table 15.3

Common Chemotherapy Treatment Regimens

Regimen Name	Drugs Prescribed	Regimen Name	Drugs Prescribed
BL	bicalutamide (Casodex), leuprolide (Lupron)	HiDAC ("high dak")	high dose Ara-C
CAF	cyclophosphamide, Adriamycin (doxorubicin), 5-fluorouracil	ICE	carboplatin, etoposide, efosfamide
CAVE	cyclophosphamide, Adriamycin (doxorubicin), vincristine, etoposide	MACOP-B	("may-cop-B") methotrexate, Adriamycin (doxorubicin), cyclophosphamide, Oncovin (vincristine), prednisone, bleomycin
Carbo-Tax	carboplatin, paclitaxel		
CHOP	("chop") cyclophosphamide, hydroxydaunomycin (Adriamycin), Oncovin (vincristine), prednisone	MOPP	("mop") mechlorethamine (or methotrexate), Oncovin (vincristine), prednisone, procarbazine
CytaBOM	cytarabine, bleomycin, Oncovin (vincristine), methotrexate	ProMACE	prednisone, methotrexate, leucovorin, Adriamycin (doxorubicin), cyclophosphamide, etoposide
DCTER ("doctor")	dexamethasone, cytosine arabinoside, thioguanine, etoposide, rubidomycin		
DECAL	daunomycin, etoposide, cyclophosphamide, Ara-C, L-asparaginase	VAD	vincristine, Adriamycin (doxorubicin), dexamethasone
		VC	vinorelbine, cisplatin
FAM	5-fluorouracil, Adriamycin (doxorubicin), mitomycin C		

Terms Bank

These terms and abbreviations provide a foundation for the language and transcription skills you will develop in the following sections of this chapter. Terms marked with ›› will be included in the reports transcribed in the Building Transcription Skills section.

additive
(**ad**-i-tiv) (n) a substance which is added in small quantities to improve the qualities of the original

adenopathy
(ad-e-**nop**-a-thee) (n) swelling or enlargement of any gland, especially the lymph nodes

adjuvant
(**ad**-joo-vant) (n) therapy given to enhance another therapy's effect such as giving chemotherapy before surgical therapy

agglutination
(a-gloo-ti-**nay**-shun) (n) the process in which cells group or clump together, especially as a response to a specific antibody; commonly used in blood typing

allogeneic
(al-O-je-**ne**-ik) (adj) describing tissues or cell types that are from different individuals belonging to the same species; describing individuals of the same species

alpha fetoprotein
(al-fa fee-tO-**prO**-teen) (n) a protein normally produced during the 12th to 15th week of gestation and may also appear in the serum of patients with embryonal carcinomas or carcinoma of the GI tract (stomach, colon, pancreas) or the lung

anaphylactic ››
(**an**-a-fi-**lak**-tik) (adj) describing an allergic hypersensitivity reaction of the body to a substance

apoptosis
(ap-O-**tO**-sis / ap-op-**tO**-sis) (n) a cell fragmenting into pieces which are phagocytosed by other cells; programmed cell death

asparaginase ››
(as-**par**-a-ji-nays) (n) an antineoplastic agent derived from the bacterium *Escherichium coli*

autologous
(aw-**tol**-o-gus) (adj) describing a transplantation where the tissue graft is taken from the same individual receiving it

bilateral
(bI-**lat**-er-al) (adj) affecting or relating to two sides

BRCA 1 and 2 genes
("braka 1" and "braka 2") (n) acronym for two genes associated with increased risk of breast and ovarian cancer

capillary fragility
(**kap**-i-layr-ee) (n) used in a test to determine the presence of vitamin C deficiency or thrombocytopenia; pressure is applied to the arm, and then the number of petechiae (representing broken capillaries) in a small area are counted

capsular ››
(**cap**-soo-lar) (adj) pertaining to a sheath of continuous enclosure around an organ or structure

carcinoma
(kar-si-**nO**-ma) (n) a malignant tumor of epithelial cells

cellular
(**sel**-yoo-lar) (adj) composed of or derived from cells

cellular immunity
(n) immunity which is based on the T cells recognizing the antigen itself, rather than the presence of an antibody; cell-mediated immunity

coagulation
(kO-ag-yoo-**lay**-shun) (n) process of blood clotting

coagulopathy
(kO-ag-yoo-**lop**-a thee) (n) a disorder affecting the blood's ability to clot correctly

collagen ››
(**kol**-le-jen) (n) the gelatin or sticky substance of skin, bone, cartilage, ligaments, and connective tissue

craniotomy ››
(kray-nee-**ot**-O-mee) (n) surgical incision into the skull, performed to control bleeding, remove tumors, relieve pressure inside the cranium, or insert instruments for diagnosis

debulking
(n) a surgical procedure to remove part of a tumor which otherwise cannot be completely excised

dysuria ››
(dis-**yoo**-ree-a) (n) painful or difficult urination, symptomatic of numerous conditions (e.g., cystitis; urethritis; infection in urinary tract)

ecchymosis ››
(ek-im-**O**-sis) (n) reddish or purplish flat spot on the skin; a bruise; ecchymoses (pl)

embryo
(**em**-bree-O) (n) in humans, the developing prenatal child from conception to the end of the second month

embryonal
(**em**-bree-O-nal) (adj) relating to an embryo; in an early stage of development

emesis ››
(**em**-e-sis) (n) vomiting; may be of gastric, systemic, nervous, or reflex origin

eosinophil
(ee-O-**sin**-O-fil) (n) a type of white blood cell readily stained with eosin

erythrocyte ››
(e-**rith**-rO-sIt) (n) mature red blood cell

erythromycin »
(ee-rith-rO-**mI**-sin) (n) antibiotic used to treat infections caused by a wide variety of bacteria and other microorganisms

fibrinogen
(fi-**brin**-O-jen) (n) a substance in the blood plasma that can be converted into fibrin to produce blood clotting

fibrosis »
(fI-**brO**-sis) (n) abnormal formation of fibrous tissue

follicle »
(**fol**-i-kl) (n) pouch-like cavity, such as a hair follicle in the skin enclosing a hair, or a graafian follicle

follicular »
(fo-**lik**-yoo-lar) (adj) pertaining to a follicle or follicles (a small secretory sac or cavity [pouchlike cavity, as that in the skin enclosing a hair])

fundus
(**fun**-dus) (n) the bottom or base of an organ; the part farthest from the opening

gallium
(**gal**-ee-um) (n) a rare metal; a gallium scan after an infusion of gallium provides a better view of lymphatic tissue

granuloma »
(gran-yoo-**lO**-ma) (n) a mass of tissue consisting of many newly growing capillaries formed during the healing process; growth may be due to injury, infection, or inflammation

hemangioma
(he-**man**-jee-**O**-ma) (n) a congenital benign tumor consisting of a mass of blood vessels

hematopoiesis
(**hee**-ma-tO-poi-**ee**-sis) (n) the process by which red and white blood cells and platelets are formed

hemoglobinopathy
(**hee**-mO-glO-bi-**nop**-a-thee) (n) a hereditary disorder characterized by the synthesis of abnormal hemoglobin molecules

hemolysis
(hee-**mol**-i-sis) (n) the destruction of red blood cells which leads to the release of hemoglobin

hemophilia
(hee-mO-**fil**-ee-a) (n) a hereditary disorder caused by a deficiency of one or more clotting factors causing increased tendency to hemorrhage

hemorrhage
(**hem**-o-rij) (n) loss of a large amount of blood quickly, either externally or internally

hyperdiploid »
(**hI**-per-**dip**-loyd) (n) an individual organism or cell that has one or more extra chromosomes; (adj) relating to such an individual or cell

inguinal
(**ing**-gwi-nal) (adj) relating to or located in the groin area (where the abdomen and thighs join)

karyotype
(**kar**-ee-O-tIp) (n) chromosomal makeup of a cell; often displayed as chromosome pairs arranged by size

laparotomy
(lap-a-**rot**-O-mee) (n) a surgical procedure in which an incision is made into the abdominal wall

leukemia »
(loo-**kee**-mee-a) (n) production of abnormal white blood cells; a type of cancer of the blood

lumbar
(**lum**-bar) (n) relating to the lower back, between the ribs and pelvis

lymphadenitis
(**lim**-fad-e-**nI**-tis) (n) inflammation of one or more lymph nodes

lymphadenopathy »
(lim-fad-e-**nop**-a-thee) (n) any disorder of lymph nodes or of the lymphatic system

lymphatic
(lim-**fat**-ik) (adj) relating to or resembling lymph or lymph nodes

lymphoblastic »
(lim-fO-**blas**-tik) (adj) relating to or resembling lymphoblasts, immature white blood cells

lymphocyte »
(**lim**-fO-sIt) (n) white blood cell that produces antibodies

mediastinal »
(**mee**-dee-as-**tI**-nal) (adj) relating to the space in the chest cavity between the lungs that contains the heart, aorta, esophagus, trachea, and thymus

metastasis
(me-**tas**-ta-sis) (n) spread of a tumor from its site of origin to distant sites

monoclonal antibody
(mon-O-**klO**-nal **an**-tee-bod-ee) (n) an antibody produced by a cloned cell that is biologically engineered to create a specific antibody directed against a particular antigen

morphology
(mOr-**fol**-O-jee) (n) the shape and structure of an organism or body part

necrosis »
(ne-**krO**-sis) (n) death of some or all of the cells in a tissue

neutropenia
(noo-trO-**pee**-nee-a) (n) a condition characterized by decreased neutrophils in the peripheral blood

neutrophil
(**noo**-trO-fil / **noo**-trO-fIl) (n) the most common type of mature white blood cell; its primary function is phagocytosis; granular leukocyte

orchiectomy
(Or-kee-**ek**-tO-mee) (n) surgical removal of one or both testes

organomegaly »
(**Or**-ga-nO-**meg**-a-lee) (n) abnormal enlargement of an organ, particularly an organ of the abdominal cavity, such as the liver or spleen

palliative
(**pal**-ee-a-tiv) (adj) describes a treatment that minimizes symptoms but does not cure the disease

parenchyma »
(pa-**reng**-ki-ma) (n) the functional or specific tissue of an organ, not including supporting or connective tissue

pelvis
(**pel**-vis) (n) the bones in the lower portion of the trunk of the body; the bones between the spine and legs

petechial »
(pee-**tee**-kee-al / pee-**tek**-ee-al) (adj) relating to or having petechiae, tiny reddish or purplish spots on the skin from broken capillaries

phagocytosis
(**fag**-O-sI-**tO**-sis) (n) the process in which a cell engulfs and destroys bacteria, foreign particles, cellular debris, and other cells

platelet »
(**playt**-let) (n) disc-shaped, small cellular element in the blood that is essential for blood clotting

pluripotential
(**ploo**-ree-pO-**ten**-shal) (adj) not having a fixed or defined potential development. White blood cells are developed from a single pluripotential cell which is capable of differentiating into the various types of white cells

poikilocytosis
(**poy**-ki-lO-sI-**tO**-sis) (n) having poikilocytes (abnormal and irregularly shaped red blood cells) in the blood

porphyrins
(**pOr**-fi-rinz) (n) a group of pigmented compounds essential to life; for example, hemoglobin contains the heme porphyrin

pruritus »
(proo-**rI**-tus) (n) itching skin condition

purpura »
(**pur**-poo-ra) (n) any of several bleeding disorders in which the escape of blood into tissues below the skin causes reddish or purplish spots

radiology
(rA-dE-**ol**-O-jE) (n) the field of study involving ionizing radiation, ultrasound, nuclear imaging techniques, and radioisotopes to create medical images for the diagnosis and treatment of disease

scirrhous
(**skir**-us) (adj) describing or resembling a hard, fibrous, malignant tumor

sclerosis »
(skle-**rO**-sis) (n) condition characterized by hardening of a tissue or organ, resulting from inflammation and mineral deposits

scrotal
(**skrO**-tal) (adj) relating to the scrotum

scrotum
(**skrO**-tum) (n) the pouch of skin containing the testes, the male reproductive glands

sequela
(see-**kwel**-a) (n) an abnormal condition resulting from a disease; sequelae (see-**kwel**-ee) (pl)

serous
(**seer**-us) (adj) relating to or having a watery consistency

sessile
(**sess**-il) (adj) attached directly at the base; not on a stalk

sonography
(so-**nog**-ra-fi) (n) ultrasonography; use of high-frequency sound waves to produce an image of an organ or tissue

splenectomy
(sple-**nek**-tO-mee) (n) surgical removal of the spleen

squamous
(**skway**-mus) (adj) scaly; covered with or consisting of scales

staphylococcemia
(**staf**-i-lO-kok-**see**-mee-a) (n) the presence of staphylococci (bacterial microorganisms) in the blood

suppuration
(**sup**-yu-**ray**-shun) (n) the production or discharge of pus

testicular
(tes-**tik**-yoo-lar) (adj) relating to the testes, the male reproductive glands

thrombocytopenia »
(**throm**-bO-sI-tO-**pee**-nee-a) (n) an abnormal decrease in platelets in the blood, resulting in bleeding and easy bruising

thalassemia
(thal-a-**see**-mee-a) (n) an inherited disorder characterized by abnormal synthesis of one or both of the globin chains that combine to form hemoglobin

thrombocytopenic »
(**throm**-bO-sI-tO-**pee**-nik) (adj) relating to thrombocytopenia

thrombosis »
(throm-**bO**-sis) (n) the formation, development, or existence of a blood clot, or thrombus, within the vascular system

tumor
(**too**-mor) (n) abnormal mass of tissue; neoplasm

tympanic »
(tim-**pan**-ik) (adj) pertaining to the middle ear or tympanic cavity

yolk sac
(**yOk** sak) (n) a membranous sac surrounding the food yolk in the embryo

Abbreviations

Hematology

AHF	antihemophilic factor VIII
AHG	antihemophilic globulin factor VIII
ANC	absolute neutrophil count
baso	basophil
CBC	complete blood count
DIC	disseminated intravascular coagulation
diff	differential
DNA	deoxyribonucleic acid
DVT	deep venous thrombosis
eos	eosinophil
ESR	erythrocyte sedimentation rate
G6PD	glucose-6-phosphate dehydrogenase
hCG	human chorionic gonadotropin (tumor marker for germ cells)
HCT, Hct	hematocrit
HGB, Hgb	hemoglobin
ITP	immune (idiopathic) thrombocytopenic purpura
LDH	lactate dehydrogenase
lymphs	lymphocytes
MCH	mean corpuscular hemoglobin
MCHC	mean corpuscular hemoglobin concentration
MCV	mean corpuscular volume
mono	monocyte
plts or PLT	platelets
PMN	polymorphonuclear leukocyte
polys	polymorphonuclear neutrophils
PT	prothrombin time
PTT	partial thromboplastin time
RBC	red blood cell
sed rate	sedimentation rate (also known as erythrocyte sedimentation rate)
segs	segmented neutrophils
WBC	white blood cell

Oncology

AFP	alpha-fetoprotein (tumor marker for liver and germ cells)
ALL	acute lymphocytic leukemia (lymphoblastic)
AML	acute myeloid leukemia
ANLL	acute nonlymphoblastic leukemia
APL, APML	acute promyelocytic leukemia
BCE	basal cell epithelioma
BM	bone marrow (or bowel movement)
BMA	bone marrow aspiration
BMT	bone marrow transplant
BRM	biological response modifier
BSE	breast self-exam
bx	biopsy
CA	cancer, carcinoma
CA-125	ovarian carcinoma antigen (tumor marker for ovary)
CEA	carcinoembryonic antigen (tumor marker for colon, lung, breast, others)
cGy	centigray
CLL	chronic lymphocytic leukemia
CML	chronic myelocytic leukemia
DES	diethylstilbestrol
FAB	French-American-British (classification system for leukemia)
Gy	gray
HD	Hodgkin disease (also referred to as Hodgkin lymphoma)
MAB	monoclonal antibody
PSA	prostate specific antigen (tumor marker for prostate)
RT	radiation therapy
TNM	tumor, nodes, metastasis (refers to tumor staging)

Building Language Skills

Complete the following exercises, drawing on the information learned in the Exploring Hematology-Oncology section of this chapter and referencing the Terms Bank.

Exercise 15.1   Matching Sound and Spelling

The numbered list that follows shows the phonetic spelling of hard-to-spell words. Sound out each word and then write the correct spelling in the blank space provided. Check your answers in the Terms Bank or other appropriate reference.

1. ek-im-**O**-sis _____

2. **fag**-O-sl-**tO**-sis _____

3. **ses**-il _____

4. **pal**-ee-a-tiv _____

5. lim-**fat**-ik _____

6. me-**tas**-ta-sis _____

7. pol-ee-**mor**-fO-**noo**-klee-ar _____

8. loo-**kee**-mee-a _____

9. a-gloo-ti-**nay**-shun _____

10. **skir**-us _____

11. **hem**-o-rij _____

12. **skway**-mus _____

13. **lim**-fO-slt _____

14. **krO**-mik _____

15. **staf**-i-lO-kok-**see**-mee-a _____

Below is a list of frequently used words that look alike and/or sound alike. Study the meaning and pronunciation of each set of words, read the following sentences carefully, and then circle the word in parentheses that correctly completes the meaning.

acetic	(adj) pertaining to acetic acid or vinegar	**generic**	(adj) nonspecific, nontrademark
acidic	(adj) acid-forming	**genetic**	(adj) hereditary
ascitic	(adj) watery, albumin- and glucose-containing	**incidence**	occurrence, rate of occurrence
		incidents	multiple occurrences
advice	(n) opinion given	**instance**	example, sample
advise	(v) to counsel, to give advice	**knot**	(n) lump, bump; measurement of nautical speed
anergy	(n) impaired ability to react to certain antigens	**naught**	(adj) zero
		not	(adv) a negative response
energy	(n) capacity to do work	**presence**	(n) attendance
basal	(adj) basic, elemental, forming the base	**presents**	(n) gifts
		presents	(v) displays, appears
basil	(n) herb used in cooking	**prostate**	(n) male gland
for	(prep) as; to	**prostrate**	(adj) lying face down
fore	(adj) front; near		
four	(adj) the number "4"		
free radical	(n) an atom or group of atoms carrying an unpaired electron and no charge		
radical	(adj) going to the root of the cause		
radicle	(n) small root of a nerve or vessel		

1. I (adviced/advised) the patient to return in one week.

2. Medical papers always use the (generic/genetic) name for drugs.

3. The patient (presence/presents) with a two-week history of headaches.

4. I gave the patient (advice/advise) regarding proper diet and exercise.

5. The pathology report states that the lesion is a (basal/basil) cell carcinoma.

6. The patient appears depressed and is complaining of lack of (anergy/energy) and insomnia.

7. The patient had breast cancer, requiring a (radical/radicle) mastectomy.

8. The patient was cautioned regarding greasy, spicy, and (acetic/acidic) foods.

9. The (prostate/prostrate) was smooth and without nodules.

10. When the ambulance arrived, she was found (prostate/prostrate) on her bathroom floor.

11. This is another (incidence/incidents/instance) of a disorder that is increasing in (incidence/incidents/instance).

Exercise 15.3   Choosing Words from Context

When transcribing dictation, the medical transcriptionist frequently needs to consider the situation when determining the word that correctly completes the sentence. From the list below, select the term that meaningfully completes each of the following statements.

carcinoma	leukemia	pelvis
embryo	lumbar	petechiae
emesis	lymphadenopathy	platelet
hemorrhage	parenchyma	sclerosis

1. The most common childhood malignancy is _____.

2. The patient had a low _____ count, which caused him to bleed profusely after the phlebotomy.

3. Mr. Smith had a hepatic _____, which required chemotherapy.

4. There was _____ of the vein after the chemotherapeutic agent infiltrated at the infusion site.

5. After the _____ puncture, Johnny had to lie down for about an hour.

6. Drinking alcohol, using drugs, and smoking during pregnancy are dangerous to the forming _____.

7. There were _____ all over the child's body, leading to the diagnosis of immune thrombocytopenic purpura (ITP).

8. The _____ of the left kidney was invaded by the tumor.

9. The physical examination of the child with leukemia revealed cervical _____.

10. The tumor was invading the _____, requiring removal of the adjacent hip.

11. Mr. Johnson received medication prior to chemotherapy to prevent _____.

12. If you do not achieve hemostasis during surgery, you can have a serious _____.

Exercise 15.4　　　　　　Pairing Words and Meanings

From this list, locate the term that best matches each of the following definitions. Write the term in the space provided by each definition.

basophil	laparotomy	phagocytosis
ecchymosis	lymphocyte	thrombocytopenia
gallium	necrosis	
hemophilia	orchiectomy	

1. white blood cell _____

2. the process by which certain cells destroy microorganisms _____

3. surgical excision of a testicle _____

4. bruise; purplish spot from accumulation of blood under skin _____

5. a condition with diminished number of platelets, resulting in bleeding and bruising _____

6. a rare metal _____

7. a disorder characterized by excessive bleeding and occurring only in males _____

8. surgical procedure in which an incision is made in abdominal wall _____

9. death of some or all of the cells in a tissue _____

10. leukocytes capable of producing antibodies _____

Exercise 15.5   Creating Terms from Word Forms

Combine prefixes, root words, and suffixes from this list to create medical words that fit the following definitions. Fill in the blanks with the words you construct.

a-, an-	without, no	**basal**	base
cyt/o	cell	**macro**	big
erythr/o	red	**micro**	small
hem/o,	blood	**papilla**	nipple-like
hemat/o		**-logy**	study of
immun/o	safe, protected against	**-oma**	tumor
leuk/o	white	**-osis**	increase or condition
phag/o	eating, swallowing	**-philia**	attraction for
plasm/o	formed; plasma	**-plasia**	growth; formation
reticul/o	net	**-poiesis**	production
thromb/o	clot		

1. no growth _____

2. an immature red cell containing a cytoplasmic network that stains with brilliant cresyl blue _____

3. the production of blood cells _____

4. benign, nipple-like tumor _____

5. fragments of cells that participate in clot formation _____

6. white blood cell that fights bacteria, stains neutral _____

7. study of cells _____

8. ingestion/digestion of cells, bacteria _____

9. study of immune system _____

10. abnormally large cells _____

Exercise 15.6   Proofreading Review

Read the following report excerpt and look for errors in form, meaning, capitalization, word choice, punctuation, and spelling. Mark the corrections on the page and key the excerpt with the errors corrected. Save the document as XXExercise15.06 using your initials in place of *XX* in the file name.

Charlotte is a 30 yr old women who first noted a fullness in the right lower anterior cervical region in the late winter. It had gradually groin in size. In early March she was treated with a one week course of erythromycin with out response. the mass 'bothered" her slightly but it was not painful. Their has been no change in her usually good appetite her weight has remained staple.

The outside radiographic studies were reviewed with the radiologist The chest x-ray reveals a relatively small anterior mediastinal mass (approximately 1/4 of the chest diameter). The chest CT scan conforms the presents of the mediastinal mass, without pulmonary parenchymal involvement.

Exercise 15.7   Thinking Like a Professional

Read this scenario carefully and then select the most appropriate response. Write an explanation for why you think your choice is the best answer.

The physician has dictated a complete History and Physical report to be charted before a scheduled surgical procedure. In the Review of Systems, the physician states the patient is positive for IDDM. Upon review of the report, you note that the only medication included in the report is Nexium and there is no mention of ongoing medical conditions in the Impression. What should you do?

a. Leave the report as dictated, since there is no conflict in the information.
b. Listen again to the Review of Systems and after confirming the correct information was typed, complete the report.
c. Flag the report for physician review.
d. Delete the comment in the Review of Systems and leave the remainder of the report as is.

Best response: _____

Explanation: _____

_____

_____

_____

_____

You will apply the medical specialty and language information you learned in this chapter to transcription work in this section. After you learn the formatting recommendations of the outpatient visit report, you will transcribe eight reports related to seven different patient studies.

Introducing the Outpatient Visit Report

The outpatient visit report (Figure 15.6) is a medical document similar in content to a brief history and physical report.

Required Headings/Content

The report usually begins with the patient's diagnosis and includes a brief history of the illness, the results of a physical examination, results of laboratory tests, the physician's impression, and the treatment plan. The plan may include lab tests scheduled for subsequent visits and referrals to other physicians. The format varies considerably from clinic to clinic. Use the history and physical report as the foundation for the outpatient reports transcribed in this text. If necessary, review page 466 of Appendix A for a list of headings found in the history and physical report.

Turnaround Time

The outpatient visit report is generally transcribed within 48 hours after dictation.

Preparing to Transcribe

To prepare for transcribing dictation, review the common hematology-oncology terms, drugs, and abbreviations presented in this chapter's Terms Bank. Study the format and organization of the model document shown in Figure 15.6, and key the model document, using the history and physical report template on the Dictations and Templates CD as a starting point. Save the document as XXFigure15.06 using your initials in place of XX in the file name. Proofread the document by comparing it with the printed version. Categorize the types of errors you made, and document them on a copy of the Performance Comparison Chart. A template of this chart is available on the Dictations and Templates CD.

Transcribing Reports

Transcribe, edit, and correct each report in the following patient studies. Consult reference books for words or formatting rules that are unfamiliar.

As you work on the transcription assignment for this chapter, fill in the Performance Comparison Chart that you started when you keyed the model document. For at least three of the reports, categorize and document the types of errors you made. Answer the document analysis questions on the bottom of the chart. With continuous practice and assessment, the quality of your work will improve.

PATIENT NAME: Elizabeth Connors
DATE: 01/10/20XX

DIAGNOSIS
Immune thrombocytopenic purpura (ITP).

HISTORY OF PRESENT ILLNESS
The patient was well until 3 weeks ago when she had a viral URI. She had fevers to 101. Yesterday, mother noted a "red rash" on her back and legs and many bruises. She was referred by Dr. Sanderson for evaluation.

PHYSICAL EXAMINATION
GENERAL: The patient appears very well.
VITAL SIGNS: Temperature 98.7, blood pressure 98/56, weight 22 kg.
SKIN: Petechial rash on arms, back, and thighs. Several large ecchymoses over legs, arms, and abdomen.
HEENT: Within normal limits. Fundi within normal limits.
LYMPH NODES: Several small, shotty nodes in submandibular chain.
THORAX AND LUNGS: Clear.
CARDIOVASCULAR: Within normal limits, no murmur.
ABDOMEN: Soft, no palpable masses. Liver not palpable. Spleen not palpable.
EXTREMITIES: Within normal limits.
NEUROLOGIC: Grossly intact.

LABORATORY DATA
WBC 6500, hemoglobin and hematocrit 12.3 and 37.1, platelets 34,000; segs 52, bands 0, eos 3, basos 2, lymphs 43, atypical lymphs 0, ANC 3380.

IMPRESSION
Immune thrombocytopenic purpura.

PLAN
Will repeat counts tomorrow. If platelets are rising, will continue to watch. If decreasing, will hospitalize for a 3-day course of IVIG.
REFERRALS: None at present.
RETURN TO CLINIC: Tomorrow.
LAB/PROCEDURES (NEXT VISIT): Counts.

_____

Sanford J. Arnold, MD
SJA/XX
D: 01/10/20XX
T: 01/12/20XX
cc: Lawrence C. Cohen, MD

Figure 15.6   Outpatient Visit Report Based on History and Physical Template

Elizabeth Connors is a 5-year-old who was well until three weeks ago when she developed a cold with a fever. She recovered in about a week. Yesterday, her mother noticed that her back and legs were covered with tiny red dots that appeared to be a rash. She also had several large bruises on her body. Her mother took Elizabeth to the pediatrician, who sent her to the Hematology Outpatient Clinic.

REPORT 15.1 Outpatient Visit Report

Use the Report1501.mp3 audio file and the history and physical report template (History_and_Physical) when transcribing this outpatient report. Save the document as XXReport15.01, using your initials in place of *XX* in the file name.

Various abbreviations are used in the physical examination and lab data sections. Transcribe abbreviations as dictated, except for "H and H," which should be transcribed as hemoglobin and hematocrit, and otherwise spell out the full word when dictated as such. Some facilities/clients prefer abbreviations be used instead of spelling out the full word in the lab section. Follow the guidelines of the employer.

IVIG is the acronym for intravenous immunoglobulin.

Stephanie Aaron is an 11-year-old who was diagnosed with acute lymphoblastic leukemia (ALL). She completed a 2½-year regimen of chemotherapy and is doing very well off all therapy for 1 year.

REPORT 15.2 Chart Summary

Use the Report1502.mp3 audio file and the chart summary template (Chart_Summary) when transcribing this report. Save the document as XXReport15.02, using your initials in place of *XX* in the file name.

This chart summary report will be set as a narrative report consisting of several paragraphs summarizing the patient's history and treatment. There are no internal headings.

Listen for these terms:
    anaphylactic
    BFM regimen
    cALLa
    FAB L1 morphology
    intrathecal
    methotrexate
    PEG-L-asparaginase
    vincristine

Nettie Brandise is a 24-year-old young woman who was diagnosed with leukemia 5 years ago. She was treated with radiation, chemotherapy, and a bone marrow transplant (BMT) and is doing well off all therapy. She is seen at the Brookfield Oncology Group for followup every 3 months.

REPORT 15.3 Outpatient Visit Report

Use the Report1503.mp3 audio file and the history and physical report template (History_and_Physical) when transcribing this outpatient visit report. Save the document as XXReport15.03, using your initials in place of *XX* in the file name.

Linda Eastman is a 65-year-old woman who had a right radical mastectomy 3 years ago. She presented to urgent care with fever, chills, abdominal pain, and bloody diarrhea, which had been occurring over the previous 2 days. She was transported by ambulance to the hospital for further evaluation and treatment.

REPORT 15.4 History and Physical

Use the Report1504.mp3 audio file and the history and physical report template (History_and_Physical) when transcribing this report. Save the document as XXReport15.04, using your initials in place of *XX* in the file name.

Listen for these terms:
    heme-positive
    nuchal

Charlotte Trent is a 30-year-old woman who noticed that she had a lump on her neck. It caused her no pain so she did not see her physician until it grew bigger. Her internist sent her to the surgeon for a biopsy, which showed Hodgkin disease. She was then referred to the oncologist for further workup and treatment.

REPORT 15.5 Consultation Letter

Use the Report1505.mp3 audio file and the consultation letter template (Consultation_Letter) when transcribing this report. Save the document as XXReport15.05, using your initials in place of *XX* in the file name.

This letter will indicate an enclosure. Do not insert headings within the body of this letter.

Sometimes providers will dictate incorrect words. In this dictation, correct a misstated adjective.

REPORT 15.6 Pathology Report

Use the Report1506.mp3 audio file and the pathology report template (Pathology_Report) when transcribing this report. Save the document as XXReport15.06, using your initials in place of *XX* in the file name. Transcribe the information at the top of the report in the order of the template, not in the order of the dictated content. Use the dictated headings within the transcribed report.

Listen for this cell type name:
   interfollicular
   lacunar
   Reed-Sternberg (cell type name)

Robert Hudson is a 35-year-old man with a history of sickle cell anemia. He has been hospitalized several times to receive intravenous fluids, blood transfusions, and pain medications. Recently, he had a flu-like illness and subsequently presented to the ER with severe pain in the lower left leg.

REPORT 15.7 History and Physical

Use the Report1507.mp3 audio file and the history and physical report template (History_and_Physical) when transcribing this report. Save the document as XXReport15.07, using your initials in place of *XX* in the file name.

In the Physical Examination section, the physician dictates the abbreviation P&A under the lung examination. This acceptable abbreviation stands for percussion and auscultation.

Belinda Kottke is a 57-year-old woman with colorectal cancer that has metastasized to the liver, lung, and brain. She underwent a craniotomy for resection of a brain lesion that was identified on a CT scan.

REPORT 15.8 Discharge Summary

Use the Report1508.mp3 audio file and the discharge summary report template (Discharge_Summary) when transcribing this report. Save the document as XXReport15.08, using your initials in place of *XX* in the file name.

Listen for this drug term:
    Pepcid

This report includes a description of a tapering dose of Decadron. The days and the dosages are dictated in a way that places numbers (for days and dosages) adjacent to each other. When numbers representing two different items are adjacent to each other, spell out one of them to avoid confusion. In this case, spell out the numbers representing the days.

chapter

Sixteen

Immunology

The immune system is a complex system composed of specialized organs, ducts, and cells located throughout the body. It is the body's surveillance system that protects against invading, potentially harmful bacteria, viruses, and parasites, and also threatening cells within the body itself. The area of practice concerned with the functioning of the immune system and the interrelationships between this system and the rest of the body is called immunology. The specialist in the field is called an immunologist. Often the immunologist also specializes in allergy and infectious diseases, as these two specialties relate to the body's immune response to environmental and biological stimuli.

Objectives

» Identify and understand the organs and functions of the immune system.

» Describe concepts in the prevention of infectious disease.

» Describe the major categories of disease that affect the immune system.

» Recognize common microbial pathogens and transcribe them using the correct style and nomenclature.

» Pronounce and correctly spell terminology related to immunology.

» Transcribe dictation related to immunology.

» Describe an autopsy report, including typical content, format, and turnaround time.

With the emergence of acquired immuno-deficiency syndrome (AIDS) in the 1980s, both the medical profession and the public have focused enormous attention on the functioning of the immune system. Breakthroughs in the treatment of immune system disorders are occurring so quickly that medical support personnel, including medical transcriptionists, must make an extra effort to remain knowledgeable about changes and news in this specialty.

Structure and Function

The components of the immune system include the thymus, tonsils, lymph nodes, bone marrow, and spleen, as shown in Figure 16.1. Immunity confers protection from disease from an invading organism. There are two types of immunity: natural, also called innate immunity, which is present at birth, and acquired immunity, which is specific and develops after birth. Acquired immunity develops as a result of exposure to a specific antigen (active acquired immunity) or through immunization (artificially acquired immunity). Immunity may also be acquired through the transfer of antibodies (passive acquired) from a mother's milk to the infant or from the infusion of immunoglobulins (antibodies). The intact skin and mucous membranes are important barriers that enhance the immune system. The hairs in the nose, the cilia of the respiratory tract, the gastric juices, and other internal mechanisms help to protect the internal body from invading pathogens. In order to properly launch an attack against a foreign substance, the body must be able to recognize itself. Human leukocyte antigens (HLA), also called the major histocompatibility complex (MHC), allow the body to distinguish "self" from "non-self."

The immune response begins when the body is invaded by a foreign substance, one that the body does not recognize as "self" (Figure 16.2). Any agent capable of stimulating an immune response is called an antigen. The immune system uses two

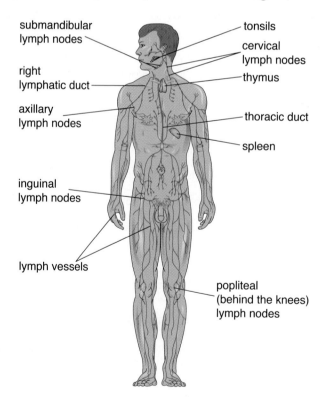

submandibular lymph nodes

tonsils

cervical lymph nodes

right lymphatic duct

thymus

axillary lymph nodes

thoracic duct

spleen

inguinal lymph nodes

lymph vessels

popliteal (behind the knees) lymph nodes

Figure 16.1 Components of the Lymphatic System

different approaches to combating invasion: cellular and humoral. The cellular response includes phagocytosis of the invading organisms by granulocytes and macrophages. Another type of cellular response includes a class of lymphocytes, called T killer cells, which produce cytotoxic substances. Suppressor T cells, on the other hand, down-regulate responses and end an immunological response. The humoral, or antibody, response is carried out by B lymphocytes which manufacture specific antibodies against the invaders. Antibodies are important for "immune memory" and confer specific, long-term protection from infection. Once the body has produced an antibody to a specific antigen, that specific antibody can be "recalled" into action quickly and forestall another infection by the same organism. Vaccination takes advantage of this immunological response by exposing the individual to a harmless form of an invading organism, allowing the body to make antibodies that can be quickly set into motion the next time the body encounters the actual invader.

To enhance the cellular response, the body produces cytokines such as interferon, interleukins, and leukotrienes. These substances, which are released in response to viruses, bacteria, parasites, fungi, neoplastic cells, and transplanted cells (i.e., organ transplants), are called biologic response modifiers (BRMs). Interferon plays an active role in combating viral infections by inhibiting viral proliferation as well as enhancing T-cell function and the phagocytic activity of granulocytes and macrophages. Interferon subclasses are designated with Greek letters (α, alpha; β, beta; γ, gamma; etc.). Many of the symptoms of viral infections (body aches, headache, fever, fatigue) are caused by interferons, not necessarily the viral infection itself. Leukotrienes are another class of BRMs that regulate immune responses. Antileukotriene medications have proven useful in the prevention or moderation of bronchospasm in asthma patients.

Physical Assessment

The physician assesses the immune system by obtaining a complete history, performing a thorough physical examination, and ordering laboratory tests. Frequent illness may suggest that the patient does not have a competent immune system. The very young, the elderly, persons with chronic disease, and persons who are receiving immunosuppressive agents are more susceptible to infection.

The examiner palpates all areas containing superficial lymph nodes. Enlarged lymph nodes, or swollen glands, may indicate an infection. Nodes that have responded to infection or cleared other substances from the body feel spongy, or shotty. Firm, fixed lymph nodes may signal an infection, a serious disorder, or a cancerous node. An enlarged liver or spleen may suggest an abnormality.

Diseases and Conditions

Diseases affecting the immune system can be grouped into several broad categories: infection, allergy, autoimmune disorders, immunodeficiency disorders, immunosuppressive states associated with organ transplant (antirejection medications), and malignancies.

Infectious disease is any disease that is caused by the growth of a pathogenic organism in the body. There are hundreds of organisms capable of causing disease in humans. Table 16.1 lists a few of the most commonly found pathogens. Note that these scientific names for bacteria and fungi include two words. The first is the genus (group) classification, which is always capitalized. The second word is the species within the genus. The species name is never capitalized. When looking up these terms, you may need to first locate the genus name. Species names will be listed beneath the genus name as subentries. Many diseases are contagious, which means that they can be passed to other persons. Sexually transmitted diseases (STDs) are a current health problem in the United States, particularly chlamydial infections and the human immunodeficiency virus (HIV), the causative agent for acquired immunodeficiency syndrome (AIDS).

Infections spread through a series of events that include a causative agent, a reservoir, a portal of exit, a mode of transmission, a mode of entry, and a susceptible host. All of these must be present. If any one element is missing, the series is interrupted and

Table 16.1

Common Pathogens

Genus and Species*	Classification	Associated Condition
Aspergillus fumigatus	fungus	Bronchopulmonary aspergillosis
Campylobacter jejuni	gram-negative rod	Acute gastroenteritis (food poisoning)
Candida albicans	fungus	Normal flora in the GI and GU tract but imbalances lead to thrush (mouth), vaginosis, and rash in intercrural spaces
Clostridium difficile	gram-positive rod	Iatrogenic colitis and diarrhea (following antibiotic use)
Escherichia coli	gram-negative rod	Normal flora in GI and GU tract. May cause infection anywhere, but especially in genitourinary (cystitis) and gastrointestinal tract
Haemophilus influenzae	gram-negative rod	Acute respiratory infections, "pink eye," otitis, and meningitis, especially in infants and children
Helicobacter pylori	gram-negative rod	Gastritis and predominant cause of gastric ulcers
Klebsiella pneumoniae	gram-negative rod	Urinary tract infections and pneumonia, especially in the elderly
Mycobacterium avium-intracellulare complex (MAC)	acid-fast bacilli	Disseminated infection seen in late-stage AIDS
Salmonella typhi	gram-negative rod	Typhoid fever
Salmonella (various species)	gram-negative rod	Acute gastroenteritis (food poisoning)
Pneumocystis jiroveci (formerly carinii)	intracellular organism (exact classification not assigned)	Pneumonia (PCP) in immunocompromised patients, especially AIDS
Staphylococcus aureus	gram-positive cocci	Normal flora but may be pathogenic. Common sites include wounds, hair follicles (furunculosis), skin (cellulitis), and heart (endocarditis); food poisoning (endotoxin) and toxic shock syndrome (exotoxin)
Streptococcus pneumoniae	gram-positive cocci	Sinusitis, meningitis and pneumonia
Neisseria meningitis	gram-negative coccobacilli	Meningococcal septicemia and meningitis, especially in infants and children
Neisseria gonorrhea	gram-negative coccobacilli	Gonorrhea and septic arthritis

*Although reference texts will usually set genus and species names in italic font style, do not use italic for these names in medical transcription.

the spread of infection is halted. The most common method of stopping the spread of infectious agents is to stop the mode of transmission (Figure 16.2). Handwashing is the single most important step to stopping the spread of infection. In addition, immunizations are available to prevent certain diseases from spreading. Smallpox and polio have been virtually eliminated in the United States because of a vigorous immunization program.

Nosocomial infections, those acquired in a hospital setting, are a significant source of morbidity and mortality. Most infections can be treated with antibiotics or antimycotics, but many organisms have become resistant to first-generation antimicrobials and must be treated with second and third-generation medications, which are far more expensive. One of the clinically significant resistant organisms is methicillin-resistant *Staphylococcus aureus* (MRSA, also pronounced "mersa").

Influenza, a viral infection, places an enormous burden on society in both inpatient and outpatient settings. At greatest risk are the youngest and oldest age groups. Today rapid diagnostic tests are approximately 75% sensitive. There are two types of vaccines available in the US: the trivalent inactivated vaccine, which is administered via intramuscular injection; and the live-attenuated vaccine, which is administered as an intranasal spray.

Infants are especially prone to a virus called respiratory syncytial virus (RSV). It often resolves on its own, but in the very young and/or elderly, it can be severe and life-threatening. Today there are several treatments to help prevent high-risk children from the severe complications of this virus.

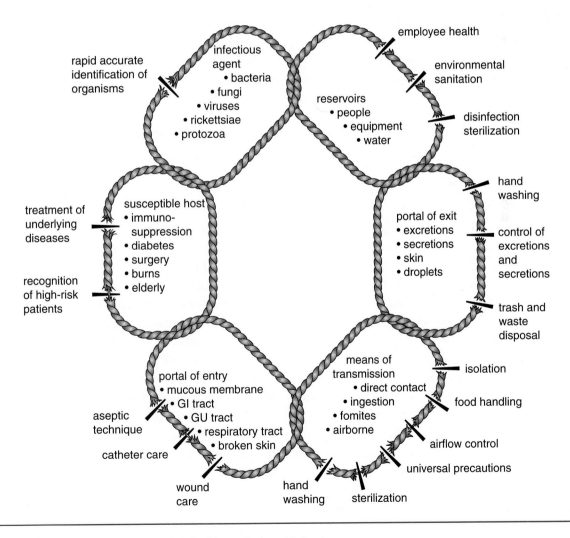

Figure 16.2 Interventions That Halt the Transmission of Infections

Allergic reactions are inappropriate immune responses that range from mild discomfort to life-threatening anaphylactic reactions. Allergens include any antigen that produces an allergic response. Examples include inhalants such as dust, perfumes, and pollens; foods such as chocolate, eggs, wheat, and strawberries; drugs such as antibiotics; and contact substances such as wool, chemicals, animals, and plants. In sensitive individuals, the immune system produces a class of antibodies called IgE that binds to mast cells, causing the release of histamine. The histamine released causes vasodilation and constriction of bronchial smooth muscles. Symptoms of allergy include runny eyes, sneezing, itching, and sometimes a rash. An anaphylactic reaction is a systemic inflammatory reaction that causes a sudden and dramatic drop in blood pressure (from vasodilation). Since allergic responses are marked by the release of histamine, the mainstay of allergy treatment is antihistamines, which block the action of histamine. Desensitization can sometimes be accomplished by exposing the patient to small doses of the antigen repeatedly over time (commonly known as allergy shots).

Autoimmune diseases are disorders resulting from an erroneous response to one's own antigens. Examples of autoimmune diseases include rheumatoid arthritis (RA), multiple sclerosis (MS), myasthenia gravis, Graves disease, and systemic lupus erythematosus (SLE). Rheumatoid arthritis may be diagnosed by the presence of rheumatoid factors (RF) in the patient's serum. Patients with SLE often have antibodies directed against antigens associated with cell nuclei called antinuclear antibodies (ANA). Autoimmune disorders are often genetic; however, some develop after a bacterial or viral infection and are caused by cross-reacting antibodies that are intended to react with a specific foreign antigen but bind with similar "self" antigens by mistake.

Transplanted organs (allografts) carry HLA antigens that are different than the recipient's, thereby eliciting an immune response. To prevent the immune system from destroying the organ graft, transplant patients must take antirejection medications. These medications suppress the immune system in order to prevent organ rejection, but also cause the patient to be susceptible to infection (immunosuppressed).

Immunodeficiency disorders are caused by missing or deficient components of the immune system. The deficiency may be in one of the white blood cell types (e.g., lymphocytes or granulocytes), in a class of immunoglobulins (hypogammaglobulinemia), or in one of the accessory mechanisms such as the complement system. Immunodeficiency syndromes may be inborn or acquired, as in acquired immunodeficiency syndrome (AIDS). HIV, the causative agent of AIDS, primarily infects CD4 cells, also called T helper cells. The reduction of CD4 cells results in a crippling of the cellular immune response. Opportunistic organisms, which are those organisms that do not ordinarily cause disease in healthy individuals, become pathogenic in individuals who are immunocompromised or immunodeficient. Examples of opportunistic organisms include *Pneumocystis jiroveci* (formerly *P carinii*), *Mycobacterium avium-intracellular* complex (MAC), and *Cryptosporidium*.

Common Tests and Procedures

Laboratory tests are most important in diagnosing an immune disorder. Common tests include CBC, ESR (erythrocyte sedimentation rate), and CRP (C-reactive protein), which are nonspecific indicators of inflammation, as well as serological studies, T and B cell counts, and cultures. Serology tests, which evaluate antigen and antibody titers in the serum, are used to evaluate a person with a suspected infection or immune disorder. Table 16.2 shows the symbol and function of immunoglobulins. The name of each immunoglobulin is pronounced as individual letters and written as follows: IgM, IgG, IgA, IgD, and IgE. The presence of specific immunoglobulins (antibodies) in a patient's serum indicates current or past exposure to a particular organism. Since many organisms, especially viruses, cannot be cultured, serological tests are used to detect antigens that are specific for the organism (e.g., HBsAg, which is the hepatitis B virus surface antigen) or antibodies (e.g., HBsAb,

Table 16.2

Immunoglobulins and Their Functions

Ig	Function
IgG	Crosses the placenta and assists with passive and recall immunity
IgA	Found in mucous membranes of the eyes and nose and the gastrointestinal tract; also called secretory immunoglobulin
IgM	Acts as the first line of defense; formed first in response to an antigen
IgD	Acts as the lymphocyte receptor on activated B cells
IgE	Effects the release of histamine from mast cells causing symptoms of allergic reactions such as watery eyes, runny nose, and itching

which is the antibody directed against the surface antigen). The IgM class of antibodies is produced early in an infection and their presence indicates recent or current infection. IgG antibodies appear in the convalescent stage of a disease and become elevated upon subsequent exposure. A common laboratory method for detecting antigens and antibodies is the enzyme-linked immunosorbent assay (ELISA, pronounced ee-**lIz**-a).

It is also possible to test for immune system competency through very sophisticated blood tests that measure lymphocyte subsets, particularly helper (CD4) and suppressor (CD8) lymphocytes, and natural killer cells. AIDS patients are monitored for CD4 levels in order to monitor the efficacy of their treatment.

Allergy testing is a common practice. Scratch tests can determine a person's specific allergies; the radioallergosorbent test (RAST) detects IgE-bound allergens that cause hypersensitivity.

Cultures of urine, blood, sputum, bronchial aspirates, and wounds can help determine the presence of pathogenic organisms. Stool samples can reveal the presence of ova and parasites. After a specimen is collected, it is grown on a culture medium and then tested to determine which antibiotics can kill it. This is known as a culture and sensitivity (C&S).

Terms Bank

These terms and abbreviations provide a foundation for the language and transcription skills you will develop in the following sections of this chapter. Terms marked with » will be included in the reports transcribed in the Building Transcription Skills section.

aerosolized »
(**ayr**-O-sol-Izd) (adj) describing a solution that is dispensed in the form of a mist

allergen
(**al**-er-jen) (n) a substance that produces an allergic reaction

anaphylaxis
(an-a-fl-**lak**-sis) (n) a systemic reaction to an allergen

antibody
(**an**-tee-bod-ee) (n) an immunoglobulin produced as an immune response to a specific antigen

antigen »
(**an**-ti-jen) (n) a substance that causes the formation of an antibody which will react specifically to the antigen to neutralize, destroy, or weaken it

asthma »
(**az**-ma) (n) respiratory disorder with temporary narrowing of the airways, resulting in difficulty in breathing, coughing, gasping, wheezing

atresia »
(a-**tree**-zee-a) (n) congenital absence or closure of a normal body opening or tubular structure

autoimmune disease
(aw-tO-i-**myoon**) (n) any disorder in which the body's immune responses produce antibodies that destroy the body's own tissues

B cell
(n) a type of lymphocyte; produces immunoglobulin antibodies in response to antigens

bronchitis »
(brong-**kI**-tis) (n) inflammation of the bronchi

choana »
(**kO**-an-a) (n) a funnel-shaped opening, especially the posterior opening of the nasal cavity into the nasopharynx

chordae tendineae »
(**kOr**-dee ten-**din**-ee-ay) (n) small tendinous cords (strands) that connect the free edges of the atrioventricular valves to the papillary muscles

coagulopathy »
(kO-ag-yoo-**lop**-a-thee) (n) defect in the blood clotting mechanisms

communicable
(ko-**myoon**-i-ka-bl) (adj) contagious; capable of being spread with direct or indirect contact

complement
(**kom**-ple-ment) (n) a group of proteins that make up a component of the immune system which causes the destruction of foreign cells that have been tagged with complement-fixing antibodies

corticomedullary junction »
(**kOr**-tee-kO-**med**-yoo-lar-ee **jungk**-shun) (n) coming together (junction) of the cortex and medulla of the kidneys

costal
(**kos**-tal) (adj) relating to or located near a rib; the costal margin is the area at the lower end of the rib cage

costophrenic »
(kos-tO-**fren**-ik) (adj) pertaining to the ribs and diaphragm

cytokines
(**sI**-tO-kIns) (n) proteins that are not antibodies but are released on contact with a specific antigen as an immune response

cytomegalovirus
(sI-tO-**meg**-a-lO-**vI**-rus) (n) CMV; one of a group of species-specific herpes viruses which causes infected cells to become enlarged

defervescence »
(def-er-**ves**-ens) (n) time that marks the decline of fever to normal temperature

diverticula »
(dI-ver-**tik**-yoo-la) (n) sacs or pouches in the walls of a canal or organ

duodenum »
(doo-O-**dee**-num / doo-**od**-e-num) (n) first part of the small intestine; it receives material from the stomach and passes it to the jejunum, the medial part of the small intestine

ecchymoses »
(ek-i-**mO**-sees) (n) small, hemorrhagic, discolored, purplish ("black and blue") spots resulting from an accumulation of blood under the skin's surface

empiric
(em-**pir**-ik) (adj) based on practical experience or observation

endocardium »
(en-dO-**kar**-dee-im) (n) serous lining membrane of inner surface and cavities of the heart

enterovirus
(**en**-ter-O-**vI**-rus) (n) a group of viruses that multiply in the gastrointestinal tract but may cause various diseases, such as polio

epicanthic »
(ep-i-**kan**-thik) (adj) pertaining to the vertical fold of skin extending from the root of the nose to the median end of the eyebrow

fibrinopurulent »
(**fI**-bri-nO-**pyoo**-roo-lent) (adj) consisting of pus and fibrin

foramen ovale »
(fO-**ray**-men O-**val**-ay) (n) hole or opening, especially in a bone or membrane; (particularly the opening between the two atria of the fetal heart that closes after birth)

Gram stain
(n) a staining procedure for differentiating bacteria by morphology (rods, cocci) and staining characteristics (gram positive or gram negative)

Graves disease
(n) hyperthyroidism caused by an autoimmune disorder

hematoma »
(hee-ma-**tO**-ma/**hem**-a-tO-ma) (n) a swelling or mass of blood confined to an organ, tissue, or space and caused by a break in a blood vessel

hemophagocytosis »
(hee-mO-**fag**-O-sI-**tO**-sis) (n) ingestion of red blood cells by phagocytes

heparin
(**hep**-a-rin) (n) a naturally occurring anticoagulant (a substance which prevents or slows the clotting of blood)

hepatosplenomegaly »
(**hep**-a-tO-splee-nO-**meg**-a-lee) (n) enlargement of the liver and spleen

histiocyte »
(**his**-tee-O-sIt) (n) a phagocyte present in connective tissue

hypergammaglobulinemia »
(**hI**-per-gam-a-**glob**-yoo-li-**nee**-mee-a) (n) excessive amount of gamma globulins in the blood

iatrogenic
(I-at-rO-**jen**-ik) (adj) relating to a response to medical or surgical treatment; often refers to deleterious side-effects of treatment by a physician

immune system
(i-**myoon**) (n) complex interactions that protect the body from pathogenic organisms and other foreign invaders

immunity
(i-**myoo**-ni-tee) (n) one's resistance to disease

immunodeficiency »
(**im**-yoo-nO-**dee**-fish-en-see) (n) a condition caused by an impaired immune system due to a deficiency or absence of one or more components of the immune system

immunoglobulin »
(im-yoo-nO-**glob**-yoo-lin) (n) antibody protein

immunology
(im-yoo-**nol**-O-jee) (n) study of the body's response to foreign invasion, such as bacteria or viruses, and allergies

immunotherapy
(**im**-yoo-nO-thayr-a-pee) (n) treatment for disease, including cancer, which enhances or manipulates the immune system; may also be called biotherapy

inoculation
(i-nok-yoo-**lay**-shun) (n) the introduction of pathogenic organisms or antigens into the body in order to increase immunity by stimulating the production of antibodies

intercostal »
(in-ter-**kos**-tal) (adj) relating to or located between the ribs

in vitro »
(in **vee**-trO) (adj, adv) literally, in glass; outside the living organism and in an artificial environment, such as a test tube

in vivo
(in **vee**-vO) (adj, adv) literally, in the living body

isoagglutination »
(I-sO-a-gloo-ti-**nay**-shun) (n) process in which antibodies (agglutinins) occurring naturally in blood cause clumping of red blood cells of a different group carrying a corresponding antigen (isoagglutinogen)

Kupffer cells
(**koop**-fer) (n) phagocytes present in the liver

lobule »
(**lob**-yool) (n) a small lobe or primary subdivision of a lobe; typical of pancreas and major salivary glands and may be on the surface by bumps and bulges

lymphocyte »
(**lim**-fO-sIt) (n) a subgroup of white blood cells

lymphopenia
(lim-fO-**pee**-nee-a) (n) a decrease in the number of lymphocytes in the blood

macrophage
(**mak**-rO-fayj) (n) any phagocytic cell, such as histiocytes and Kupffer cells

meatus »
(**mee**-ay-tus) (n) a passage or opening

mesentery »
(**mes**-en-tar-ee) (n) a peritoneal fold encircling the greater part of the small intestines and connecting the intestine to the posterior abdominal wall

neutropenia »
(noo-trO-**pee**-nee-a) (n) a decrease in the number of neutrophils in the blood

neutrophil
(**noo**-trO-fil/**noo**-trO-fIl) (n) the most common type of mature white blood cell; its primary function is phagocytosis; granular leukocyte

nosocomial
(nOs-O-**kO**-mE-al) (adj) relating to a hospital; often used to describe an infection acquired during a hospital stay

opportunistic infection
(n) a disease caused by normally harmless microorganisms when the body's resistance to disease is impaired

otitis
(O-**tI**-tis) (n) inflammation of the ear

parenchyma »
(pa-**reng**-ki-ma) (n) functional part of an organ, apart from supporting or connective tissue

Parvovirus

(**par**-vO-vI-rus) (n) a genus of viruses; strain B19 can cause anemia in humans

pathogen

(**path**-O-jen) (n) any microorganism or substance that can cause a disease

pericardium »

(per-i-**kar**-dee-um) (n) a double-layered sac surrounding the heart and large vessels

petechiae »

(pe-**tee**-kee-ee/pe-**tek**-kee-e/pe-tee-kee-a) (n) minute red spots appearing on the skin as a result of tiny hemorrhages

phagocyte

(**fag**-O-sIt/**fAg**O-sIt) (n) a cell able to engulf and destroy bacteria, foreign particles, cellular debris, and other cells

phagocytosis

(**fag**-O-sI-**tO**-sis) (n) the process in which a cell engulfs and destroys bacteria, foreign particles, cellular debris, and other cells

Pneumocystis jiroveci

(**new**-mO-sist-is yee row **vet** zee eye) (n) an intracellular parasite which causes *Pneumocystis* pneumonia (PCP) in individuals with impaired immune systems

pompholyx

(**pom**-fO-liks) (n) a skin eruption primarily on the hands and feet; may be accompanied by excessive sweating

prophylaxis »

(prO-fi-**lak**-sis) (n) prevention of disease or its spread

protease

(**prO**-tee-ays) an enzyme that breaks down proteins

protease inhibitor

(n) an agent that inhibits (prevents or slows down) the release of protease

pyrexia

(pI-**rek**-see-a) (n) fever

respiratory syncytial virus (RSV)

(sin-**sish**-ul) (n) a highly contagious respiratory illness resembling a moderate to severe cold

retroperitoneal »

(**ret**-rO-per-i-tO-**nee**-al) (adj) located behind the peritoneum outside the peritoneal cavity, such as the kidneys

rheumatoid factors

(roo-**ma**-toyd) (n) antibodies found in the serum of patients with rheumatoid arthritis

serosanguineous »

(**ser**-O-sang-**gwin**-ee-us) (adj) containing or of the nature of serum and blood

sinusitis »

(sI-nu-**sI**-tis) (n) inflammation of the nasal sinuses, occurring as a result of an upper respiratory infection, an allergic response, or a defect of the nose

steroid »

(**steer**-oyd) (n) any of a large number of similar chemical substances, either natural or synthetic; many are hormones; produced mainly in the adrenal cortex and gonads

substernal »

(sub-**ster**-nal) (adj) situated beneath the sternum (breast bone)

systemic lupus erythematosus

(sis-**tem**-ik **loo**-pus er-i-**them**-a-tO-sis/er-i-**thee**-ma-tO-sis) (n) a chronic disease with inflammatory symptoms in various systems of the body; characteristics of the disease and the systems involved may vary widely

T cell

(n) a type of lymphocyte; responsible for cell-mediated immunity

thrombocytopenia »

(**throm**-bO-sI-tO-**pen**-ee-a) (n) abnormal decrease in number of the blood platelets

thrush

(n) infection with the fungus Candida, causing white patches in the mouth and throat

titer »

(**tI**-ter) (n) strength or concentration of a solution; a unit of measurement usually expressed as a ratio that indicates the minimum concentration of an antibody before losing its power to react to a specific antigen

toxoplasmosis

(**tok**-sO-plaz-**mO**-sis) (n) disease caused by a protozoan parasite

tracheoesophageal »

(**tray**-kee-O-e-sof-a-**gee**-al) (adj) pertaining to the trachea and esophagus

urethral »

(yoo-ree-thral) (adj) relating to the urethra, a canal for the discharge of urine from the bladder to the outside of the body

vesicular »

(ve-**sik**-yoo-lar) (adj) pertaining to vesicles or small blisters

virus

(**vI**-rus) (n) an agent that lacks an independent metabolism but infects a host cell, incorporating the virus's genetic material into the host DNA and utilizing the host's cellular components to replicate; not affected by antibiotics

Western blot

(n) a laboratory test to detect the presence of antibodies to specific antigens in the blood

Abbreviations

AFB	acid-fast bacilli
AIDS	acquired immunodeficiency syndrome; caused by HIV
BRM	biologic response modifier
C&S	culture and sensitivity
CBC	complete blood count
CMV	cytomegalovirus; one of a group of large species-specific herpes-type viruses with a wide variety of disease effects
CRP	C-reactive protein
DPT	diphtheria, pertussis, tetanus immunization
EBV	Epstein-Barr virus
ELISA	enzyme-linked immunosorbent assay (test to determine the amount of a given chemical in a mixture); test for AIDS
ESR	erythrocyte sedimentation rate
FUO	fever of unknown origin
GC	gonorrhea
HIV	human immunodeficiency virus; causes deterioration of the immune system
HLA	human leukocyte antigen

HPV	human papillomavirus
MAC	*Mycobacterium avium-intracellular* complex
MHC	major histocompatibility complex
MRSA	methicillin-resistant *Staphylococcus aureus*
MS	multiple sclerosis
PCP	*Pneumocystis* pneumonia
PID	pelvic inflammatory disease
RA	rheumatoid arthritis
RAST	radioallergosorbent test
RF	rheumatoid factor
RSV	respiratory syncytial virus
SLE	systemic lupus erythematosus
STD	sexually transmitted disease
strep	streptococcus
TB	tuberculosis
URI	upper respiratory infection
VD	venereal disease

Building Language Skills

Complete the following exercises, drawing on the information learned in the Exploring Immunology section of this chapter and referencing the Terms Bank.

Exercise 16.1   Matching Sound and Spelling

The numbered list that follows shows the phonetic spelling of hard-to-spell words. Sound out each word and write the correct spelling in the blank space provided. Check your answers in the Terms Bank or other appropriate reference.

1. **noo**-trO-fil _____

2. **path**-O-jen _____

3. prO-fi-**lak**-sis _____

4. **fag**-O-slt _____

5. pl-**rek**-see-a _____

6. ko-**myoon**-i-ka-bl _____

7. i-**myoo**-ni-tee _____

8. nOs-O-**kO**-mee-al _____

9. lim-fO-**pee**-nee-a _____

10. **sef**-a-klor _____

Below is a list of frequently used words that look alike and/or sound alike. Study the meaning and pronunciation of each set of words, read the following sentences carefully, and then circle the word in parentheses that correctly completes the meaning.

accept	(v) to receive, to welcome	**dose**	to give or take a prescribed
except	(v) to eliminate, to exclude		amount of drug
except	(prep) barring, excluding	**doze**	(v) to nap or to snooze
allergen	(n) antigen that causes an allergy	**empiric**	based on experience
antigen	(n) substance causing formation	**enteric**	related to the small bowel
	of antibodies	**Gram**	(capital G) a biological stain used
			in microbiology
anaphylaxis	systemic allergic reaction	**gram**	a unit of weight
prophylaxis	treatment to prevent disease		
coarse	(adj) composed of large particles;	**in vitro**	(adj) in a test tube
	harsh or rough in tone	**in vivo**	(adj) in the living body
course	(n) direction, path	**versus**	against or in contrast to
complement	a component of the immune	**verses**	lines or stanzas in a poem or
	system		song
compliment	an expression of esteem		
complement	to add to, enhance	**wait**	(v) to remain, to stay
		wait	(n) a delay
coastal	(adj) relating to area where land	**weight**	(n) heaviness, load
	and sea meet		
costal	(adj) relating to a rib		

1. The etiology of her bladder infection was not known, but it always responded to (enteric/empiric) antibiotics.

2. The patient tolerated every antibiotic in the treatment regimen (accept/except) Ceclor.

3. After taking her sleep medication, she was able to (dose/doze) intermittently.

4. Tests identified the (allergen/antigen) responsible for his itching, watery eyes.

5. She suffered a minor fracture in the (coastal/costal) area of the upper left quadrant.

6. The patient was unable to (accept/except) the limitations imposed by his illness.

7. The hip is a major (wait-/weight-) bearing joint.

8. The treatment (coarse/course) for non-Hodgkin lymphoma is radiation and chemotherapy.

9. After years of careful research, scientists isolated the pathogen in a (coastal/costal) region of the South.

10. All antirejection drugs (accept/except) one produced severe reactions in the transplant patient.

11. The doctor ordered a culture and (Gram/gram) stain on her urine sample.

12. After the severe (anaphylactic/prophylactic) response, the patient was advised to avoid peanuts.

Exercise 16.3   Choosing Words from Context

When transcribing dictation, the medical transcriptionist frequently needs to consider the situation when determining the word that correctly completes the sentence. From the list below, select the term that meaningfully completes each of the following statements.

aerosolized	immunodeficiency	sinusitis
allergens	in vitro	substernal
antigens	neutrophil count	titer
autoimmune	opportunistic	
costal margin	prophylaxis	

1. It is necessary for children with sickle cell disease to take penicillin daily as _____ against life-threatening infection.

2. When examining the abdomen, the physician percusses and palpates around the _____ for the liver and spleen.

3. New drug therapies are tested _____ in the laboratory before being used in vivo.

4. Mr. Rogers had a severe frontal headache. This is often a sign of an infection called _____.

5. Joanne caught many colds and viruses; therefore, her doctor performed laboratory tests to rule out an/a _____ disorder.

6. When you have a low _____, you may be susceptible to bacterial infections.

7. The varicella _____ was 1:32, indicating a past exposure to chickenpox.

8. Antibodies react specifically with _____ to tag foreign substances for destruction or removal.

9. Whenever John took a deep breath, he had _____ pain.

10. When you have asthma, it is often necessary to have the medications _____ through a nebulizer in order for them to reach deep into the lungs.

11. Rheumatoid arthritis is an/a _____ disease that affects joint tissue.

12. Persons taking immunosuppressing drugs are susceptible to _____ infections.

Exercise 16.4   Pairing Words and Meanings

From this list, locate the term that best matches each of the following definitions. Write the term in the space provided by each definition.

bronchitis	immune system	nadir
cytomegalovirus	immunoglobulins	neutropenia
defervescence	immunology	oral thrush
enterovirus	immunotherapy	
hypergamma- globulinemia		

1. fungal infection of the mouth   _____

2. antibodies produced by B lymphocytes   _____

3. body processes and organs that produce the
    interactions to protect the body from pathogens
    and other invaders   _____

4. inflammation of the mucous membranes of
    the bronchial tubes   _____

5. a virus that multiplies in the intestinal tract   _____

6. abnormally low number of white blood cells
    in the blood   _____

7. study of the body's response to foreign invasion   _____

8. excessive amount of gamma globulins in the blood   _____

9. a herpes-type virus that produces large cells
    and causes illness   _____

10. the lowest point, usually referring to the
    lowest cell count   _____

11. treatment of a disease by enhancing or
    manipulating the immune system   _____

12. the time when body temperature returns to normal   _____

Exercise 16.5   Creating Terms from Word Forms

Combine prefixes, root words, and suffixes from this list to create medical words that fit the following definitions. Fill in the blanks with the words you construct.

anti-	against, antagonistic	path/o	disease
auto-	oneself	phag/o	eating, swallowing
bio-	life	splen/o	spleen
cryo-	cold	globulin	protein
aden/o	gland	macro	large
bacteri/o	bacteria	virus	organism
enter/o	small intestine	-emia	in the blood
hem/o	blood	-genesis	beginning process
immun/o	safe, protected from infection	-ic	of or pertaining to
lymph/o	clear tissue fluid	-itis	inflammation
mening/o	brain and spinal cord membrane	-megaly	oversized
ot/o	ear		

1. protein that precipitates (clumps together) when cold _____

2. protein involved in protecting body _____

3. enlarged spleen _____

4. inflammation of the lymph nodes _____

5. pertaining to a substance that is antagonistic to life _____

6. a virus that infects the small intestine _____

7. bacteria in the blood _____

8. inflammation of the ear _____

9. inflammation of the membrane covering the brain and spinal cord _____

10. large cell capable of eating (engulfing) foreign substances _____

11. the process that initiates a disease _____

12. inflammation of a gland _____

Exercise 16.6   Proofreading Review

Read the following report excerpt and look for errors in form, meaning, capitalization, word choice, punctuation, and spelling. Mark the corrections on this page and key the excerpt with the errors corrected. Save the document as XXExercise16.06 using your initials in place of *XX* in the file name.

HISTORY OF ILLNESS

This is a nown severe asthmatic patient who has been admitted on numerus occasions. She developed her asthma approximately 2 years ago. She was well up until a weak prior to addmission when she developed a cold which caused her to be a short of breath and conjested. The conjestion continued, and he gave herself some infections of Adrenalin.

PHYSICAL EXAM

Physical examination at the time of admission revealed a lady in moderate distress there were wheezes, rails and ronchi throughout all lung fields. Their were some substernal and intracostal retractions. the throat was somwhat inflammed. The rest of the physical examination at the time of admission was entirely within normal limits.

Exercise 16.7   Thinking Like a Professional

Read this scenario carefully and then select the most appropriate response. Write an explanation for why you think your choice is the best answer.

You hear a word that is new to you, so you perform a search on the Internet. The search results show 20 references to the word, mostly from patient advocacy Web sites. What should you do next?

a. Look for the word in a medical dictionary. If not listed in the dictionary, continue the search using a different spelling.

b. Use the word in your document. With 20 references cited, it is reasonable to assume the word is correct.

c. Type the word as spelled on the Web and flag for the dictator to confirm.

d. Check the word using the electronic spell checker and use the spelling since it is recognized by spell check.

Best response: _____

Explanation: _____

_____

_____

_____

You will apply the medical specialty and language information you learned in this chapter to transcription work in this section. After you learn the recommendations for an autopsy report, you will transcribe eight reports related to five different patient studies.

Introducing the Autopsy Report

When a patient dies unexpectedly or if the cause of death is uncertain or needs clarification, the attending physician requests an autopsy. Persons who die at home unexpectedly also will have an autopsy. Often, the findings of the report are summarized in a cover letter (Figure 16.3). The actual autopsy report (Figure 16.4) will vary in length and scope. For example, the report may focus on test results for a single organ. Or, if the autopsy concerns a crime victim, the report may detail the results of an extensive examination and studies of all body systems.

Required Headings/Content

An autopsy report for an autopsy done in a hospital setting will usually include these categories:
- Authorization for the procedure
- Date of examination
- Name of the person performing the autopsy
- Names of the managing and consulting physicians
- Summary of the patient's clinical status and any details known to have contributed to the death
- Description of the body (external examination) and all organs and cavities examined (internal examination)
- Preliminary report based on the gross examination (exam before tissues are removed)
- List of photos and studies completed
- List of microscopic studies
- Diagnosis based on the gross exam and laboratory studies

The report must be signed by the pathologist in compliance with hospital policy and state and federal regulations.

On page 473, Appendix A provides a listing of the headings found in the template for the autopsy report. The template, and the reports transcribed for this chapter, include three levels of headings. The top-level headings are underlined and set in all capital letters. The second-level headings are set in all capital letters and are not underlined. The third-level headings are also set in all capital letters, but they are followed with a colon and run-in text.

Turnaround Time

In a hospital setting, the autopsy report should be completed within 90 days of the patient's death. However, for a criminal investigation, the turnaround time is rapid.

Preparing to Transcribe

To prepare for transcribing dictation, review the common immunology terms, drugs, and abbreviations presented in this chapter's Terms Bank. Study the format and organization of the model documents shown in Figure 16.3 and Figure 16.4, and key the model documents, using the consultation letter and autopsy report templates on the Dictations and Templates CD as a starting point. Save the documents as XXFigure16.03 and XXFigure16.04 using your initials in place of *XX* in the file names. Proofread the documents by comparing them with the printed versions. Categorize the types of errors you made, and document them on a copy of the Performance Comparison Chart. A template of this chart is available on the Dictations and Templates CD.

Transcribing Reports

Transcribe, edit, and correct each report in the following patient studies. Consult reference books for words or formatting rules that are unfamiliar.

As you work on the transcription assignment for this chapter, fill in the Performance Comparison Chart that you started when you keyed the model document. For at least three of the reports, categorize and document the types of errors you made. Answer the document analysis questions on the bottom of the chart. With continuous practice and assessment, the quality of your work will improve.

---

use letter formatting guidelines

December 9, 20XX

Elgar Lewis, MD
Department of Pediatrics
University Medical School
Fort Worth, TX 78095-1509

RE: Rebecca Arnold

Dear Dr. Lewis:

The postmortem examination performed on your patient resulted in the following findings:

I. Acute lymphoblastic leukemia, widely disseminated, including bone marrow, spleen, liver, kidneys, lungs, lymph nodes, and other visceral organs.

II. Hemophagocytosis and intravascular coagulopathy within the bone marrow, spleen, liver, and kidneys.

III. Bleeding diathesis (clinical thrombocytopenia).
A. Massive hemorrhage with hematoma formation in pelvic and lower abdominal retroperitoneal space.
B. Punctate petechiae within the ascending aorta, heart, and gastrointestinal tract.
C. Petechiae, with ecchymoses, both extremities.

Based on the above findings, the cause of death is attributed to massive retroperitoneal bleeding with thrombocytopenia (29,000) arising from intravascular coagulopathy and hemophagocytosis-platelet phagocytosis, in a patient with acute lymphoblastic leukemia.

Marvin L. Smith, MD
Pathologist

MS/XX

Figure 16.3 Autopsy Report (Cover Letter)

AUTOPSY #:   A-4832
PATIENT NAME: Rebecca Arnold
MR #:   0329415
DATE: 12/09/20XX

double-space between sections

This 4-year-old white female was admitted with bruises of a 2-week duration, fever of 1 week, and nose bleeding of 1 day.

On admission, hemoglobin was 5.8, platelets 29,000, WBC 30,200 with 85% lymphoblasts. Acute lymphoblastic leukemia with L1 FAB classification was diagnosed after a bone marrow aspiration and biopsy were performed. She received allopurinol for hyperuricemia with a uric acid of 11.9 mg/dL (normal: 2.6-7.0). She was started on vancomycin for fevers. She was transfused single-donor platelets, but experienced a hypersensitivity reaction with chills, intercostal retractions, and nasal flaring with perioral cyanosis. Although the cyanosis improved and the respiratory distress improved, she developed active bleeding from the bone marrow aspiration site.

Shortly thereafter, the patient passed away, 2 days after her admission.

EXTERNAL EXAMINATION ——— *top-level heading*

The body is that of a well-developed, moderately nourished, pale female child. The body measures 85 cm from crown to heel and weighs 15 kg. The facies are normal. The head is covered by a lot of hair. The eyes are of normal size. There are no epicanthic folds. The external ears show normal cartilaginous development; they are in their normal set location. The external auditory canals are patent. The nasal passages are patent. The posterior choanal canal can be probed. The nasal bridge is normal. The tongue is of normal size, and teeth are present. The tongue is free of ulcers and exudate. The palate is normal. There is no peripheral lymphadenopathy. The chest is symmetrical. The abdomen is slightly distended. Muscle development is normal. The genitalia are those of a normal female child. The urethral meatus is patent. The clitoris is not hypertrophied. The anus is patent. The back shows no scoliosis or kyphosis. There are 5 normally formed digits on the hands and feet, which are free of edema and cyanosis. The palm lines are examined and are not unusual. The nails are developed. The skin shows pallor, petechiae, and ecchymoses.

INTERNAL EXAMINATION

The body is opened through the usual Y-shaped incision. Subcutaneous fat is 0.5 cm thick. The umbilicus is removed en bloc with a wide skin margin.

ABDOMINAL CAVITY ——— *second-level heading*

The peritoneal cavity contains 50 mL of straw-colored, serosanguineous fluid. The abdominal and pelvic organs are in their normal position. The kidneys are normally located.

(continued)

Figure 16.4 Autopsy Report

AUTOPSY REPORT
AUTOPSY #: A-4832
PATIENT NAME: Rebecca Arnold
MR #: 0329415
DATE: 12/09/20XX
Page 2

THORACIC CAVITY
The great veins are flat. Each pleural space contains 20 mL of clear fluid, which is not cultured. No adhesions are found.

PERICARDIAL CAVITY
The pericardium is opened and contains no excess fluid. No adhesions are found. A blood culture is taken.

ORGAN DESCRIPTION   single-space if no text between top- and second-level headings
CARDIOVASCULAR SYSTEM   single-space between subsections
HEART: The apex consists of the right/left ventricles. The aorta and pulmonary artery arise in their normal relation to one another. The pulmonary veins enter the left atrium and no anomalous veins are noted. The heart is opened along the normal blood-flow channels. No abnormal valves are noted. The auricular appendage contains no clots or vegetations. The endocardium of the right atrium is of normal thickness. The septum primum covers the foramen ovale adequately and cannot be probed. The tricuspid valve consists of 3 normal, thin leaflets. The right ventricle shows its usual trabecular muscles: the crista supraventricularis and outflow tract are normal. The pulmonary valve consists of 3 cusps without thickening. The pulmonary artery cannot be opened into the aorta. The main pulmonary artery measures 4.1 cm in circumference. The right and left pulmonary arteries are identified. The left atrium receives 2 pulmonary veins from each lung. The endocardium of the left atrium is thin. The mitral valve contains 2 normal leaflets, inserted by normal, thin chordae tendineae onto the two papillary muscles. The mitral valve is continuous with the aortic valve. The outflow tract of the left ventricle is normal: the aortic valve contains 3 normal cusps. The myocardium of the left ventricle is mildly hypertrophied. The left coronary artery arises from the left coronary cusps, and the right from the right. These pursue their usual course.

double-space above tabular data

MEASUREMENTS		
OPEN CIRCUMFERENCE:	Tricuspid 6.2 cm	Mitral 4.8 cm
	Pulmonic 4.1 cm	Aortic 3.5 cm
THICKNESS:	Right Ventricle 0.25 cm	Left Ventricle 1 cm

double-space below tabular data

AORTA AND GREAT VESSELS: The aorta arises from the left ventricle, gives rise to 3 normal branches, and descends along the left side of the vertebral column.

third-level heading

(continued)

Figure 16.4   Autopsy Report (Continued)

AUTOPSY REPORT
AUTOPSY #: A-4832
PATIENT NAME: Rebecca Arnold
MR #: 0329415
DATE: 12/09/20XX
Page 3

VEINS: The inferior vena cava, superior vena cava, renal veins, and hepatic vein are patent. The splenic vein, inferior mesenteric, superior mesenteric, and portal veins are patent.

RESPIRATORY SYSTEM
The larynx and trachea are free of webs, mucous plugs, foreign bodies, edema, and mucosal ulcerations.
LUNGS: The heart and lungs together weigh 310 g. The pleural surfaces are pale. The bronchial tree is free of mucous plugs and exudate. The pulmonary parenchyma shows consolidation after dissection. The pulmonary arterial tree is free of thromboemboli.

GASTROINTESTINAL SYSTEM
The oral cavity and esophagus are free of fibrinopurulent membranes, vesicular ulcerations, and other lesions. There is no tracheoesophageal fistula, enteric duplication, stenosis, atresia, webs, or diverticula. The stomach is well rugated and free of ulcers. The mesentery is normally rotated. The small intestine is collapsed. The duodenum, jejunum, ileum, and colon are intact and free of serosal and mucosal lesions. The cecum and appendix are in the right lower quadrant. The colon is normally attached to the posterior abdominal wall. No atresias are noted.
LIVER: Weighs 600 g. The capsule is transparent. The liver parenchyma is a normal brown-red and cuts with increased resistance. The lobular pattern is normal.
GALLBLADDER AND BILE DUCTS: The gallbladder contains green bile. Bile stones are absent. The mucosa is green. Bile can be expressed from the gallbladder into the duodenum. The common duct and right and left hepatic ducts are present.
PANCREAS: The pancreas is cut longitudinally and the pancreatic duct is visualized. The lobular pattern is normal. No necrosis is noted.

GENITOURINARY SYSTEM
The kidneys weigh 150 g together and are left attached to the pelvic organs and aorta. The renal veins are opened and contain no thrombi. The renal arteries are normal. The kidneys show normal lobulations. The capsules strip easily, revealing a smooth surface. On cut surface, the corticomedullary junction is sharp. The parenchyma does not bulge from the cut surface. The pyramids and papillae are normal. Pelves are smooth, and ureters arise from these and enter the urinary bladder normally at the trigone. The bladder wall is not hypertrophied. The urethra is opened, and no posterior urethral valves are noted. The uterus is normally formed. The ovaries are unremarkable. The fallopian tubes are of average and uniform width.

(continued)

Figure 16.3 Autopsy Report (Continued)

AUTOPSY REPORT
AUTOPSY #: A-4832
PATIENT NAME: Rebecca Arnold
MR #: 0329415
DATE: 12/09/20XX
Page 4

HEMOLYMPHATIC SYSTEM
SPLEEN: The spleen weighs 145 g. The capsular surface is translucent and contains no wrinkling, exudates, or fibrosis. Cut surface is red and deep purple-brown and consistency is mushy.
LYMPH NODES: The lymph nodes from the cervical, periaortic, peripancreatic, axillary, and inguinal areas are generally swollen.
THYMUS: Weighs 6 g.
BONE MARROW: Red, moist, and ample.

ENDOCRINE SYSTEM
THYROID: The red-brown thyroid is normally placed in relation to the larynx. The weight of the bilateral lobes of thyroid is 4 g.
ADRENALS: The adrenals together weigh 6 g; cut surface shows a normal fetal and adult cortex.

MUSCULOSKELETAL SYSTEM
BONE: Two ribs are taken and bisected. The cartilage, epiphyses, and metaphyses are normal.
SKELETAL MUSCLES: Grossly normal.
JOINTS: Not remarkable.
CRANIAL CAVITY: The reflected scalp shows no evidence of contusion, hematoma, or other lesion. The calvariae and bones at the base of the skull are not remarkable. No fractures or other injuries are present. The dura mater and pia arachnoid and associated spaces are normal in appearance. They are without hemorrhage or evidence of inflammation. The weight of the brain is 1280 g. The cerebral hemispheres are symmetrical and normal in appearance. Cut sections of the brain show symmetry and essentially normal structures throughout. The circle of Willis and other intracranial vessels are normal. The pituitary gland is grossly normal. The pineal gland is present.
SPINAL CORD AND VERTEBRAL COLUMN: Intact.

FINDINGS
I. RESPIRATORY SYSTEM
All lobes of lung show leukemic cell infiltration around the bronchioles or blood vessels. There is edematous fluid accumulated in air spaces of the left lower lobe.

II. CARDIOVASCULAR SYSTEM
Leukemic cell infiltration with scattered aggregates in subepicardial adipose tissue is seen. Myocardium and endocardium are not remarkable.

(continued)

Figure 16.4 Autopsy Report (Continued)

AUTOPSY REPORT
AUTOPSY #: A-4832
PATIENT NAME: Rebecca Arnold
MR #: 0329415
DATE: 12/09/20XX
Page 5

III. GASTROINTESTINAL SYSTEM
LIVER: Shows extensive leukemic cell infiltration within all portal areas, but the hepatic architecture is well preserved. No bile stasis is seen. There was a proliferation of histiocytes with ingested platelets. Red blood cells in dilated sinusoids are seen, which is consistent with hemophagocytic syndrome. Atypical leukemic cells are seen infiltrated in the gastrointestinal mucosa and submucosa.

IV.   GENITOURINARY SYSTEM
KIDNEYS: Bilateral kidneys show leukemic cell infiltration in the interstitium. Hemophagocytic syndrome is seen with erythrophagocytosis or platelet phagocytosis in the renal tubules.
ADNEXA: Adnexa including uterus, ovaries, and fallopian tubes show leukemic cell infiltration. Retroperitoneum and parametrium show hemorrhage admixed with a few atypical cells.
URINARY BLADDER: Shows hematoma formation.

V. HEMATOLOGICAL SYSTEM
SPLEEN: Shows extensive leukemic cell infiltration with congestion and hemorrhage. Hemophagocytosis is seen, also.
BONE MARROW: Shows leukemic cell infiltration with hemophagocytosis.

VI. LYMPHATIC SYSTEM
All lymph nodes reveal atypical leukemic cell infiltration.

VII. ENDOCRINE SYSTEM
Thymus, adrenal glands, thyroid, and pancreas all show leukemic cell infiltration.

_____

Marvin L. Smith, MD

MLS/XX
D: 12/09/20XX
T: 12/13/20XX

Figure 16.3 Autopsy Report (Continued)

June Pringle is a 38-year-old woman who is a severe asthmatic and suffers from chronic sinus problems. She has been to many physicians for treatment of her problems and is on chronic steroid therapy. She is referred to the immunologist for evaluation.

REPORT 16.1 Discharge Summary

Use the Report1601.mp3 audio file and the discharge summary report template (Discharge_Summary) when transcribing this report. Save the document as XXReport16.01, using your initials in place of XX in the file name.

Listen for the following drug terms:

adrenalin

aminophylline (Note that the brand name, Aminophyllin, sounds very similar and is spelled similarly, so you will need to determine if the physician intended to specify the generic or the brand name. In this case, use the generic name.)

prednisone

Solu-Cortef

Transcribe the Physical Examination section in a paragraph, not list format.

REPORT 16.2 Consultation Letter

Use the Report1602.mp3 audio file and the consultation letter template (Consultation_Letter) when transcribing this report. Save the document as XXReport16.02, using your initials in place of XX in the file name.

Listen for the following drug and laboratory terms:

Alupent

immunoglobulins G, A, and M (transcribed as IgG, IgA, and IgM; each is sometimes dictated as the abbreviation)

Transcribe the blood typing terms (anti-A and anti-B) with a lowercase "a" in "anti" and uppercase letters for the antigens A and B.

Riza Prince is a 15-month-old female who was born to a known HIV-positive mother. She has had several admissions to the hospital since birth and has been referred to the Pediatric AIDS Center in Fort Worth for treatment.

REPORT 16.3 Chart Summary

Use the Report1603.mp3 audio file and the chart summary template (Chart_Summary) when transcribing this report. Save the document as XXReport16.03, using your initials in place of *XX* in the file name.

Transcribe the dictated abbreviation FTNSVD as "full-term, normal spontaneous vaginal delivery."

This dictation includes several abbreviations that can be used in the transcribed report. Listen for the following abbreviations:

ANC   absolute neutrophil count
LFTs   liver function tests
LIP   lymphocytic interstitial pneumonitis
PCP   *Pneumocystis jiroveci*

Listen for these drug and disease terms:
Bactrim
hypergammaglobulinemia
pentamidine

As was shown in Chapter 15, some chart summary reports will be set in paragraph style with few internal headings. Set the headings and paragraph breaks dictated by the provider.

This report includes a list of problems, which the dictator has directed to be numbered. Set these numbered subheadings within the Problems section in all capital letters, followed by a colon and run-in text. Because this is a long list, set a blank line space between each numbered subheading. Set runover text flush left. Set the lettered sublist in paragraph style, not list style.

The report will run over onto a second page, so use your judgment as to what the content of the running header should be on the second page.

REPORT 16.4 Consultation Letter

Use the Report1604.mp3 audio file and the consultation letter template (Consultation_Letter) when transcribing this report. Save the document as XXReport16.04, using your initials in place of *XX* in the file name.

Note that data is plural and datum is singular. Today most people use data as a collective term. Use the singular verb as in this report.

Rebecca Arnold is a 4-year-old girl who was admitted to the hospital with a fever, nosebleed, and bruises that had been present for 2 weeks. She was diagnosed with acute lymphoblastic leukemia and was treated with allopurinol, vancomycin and platelet transfusions. Two days after her admission, she died, and an autopsy was performed to confirm the cause of death.

REPORT 16.5 Autopsy Report Cover Letter

Use the Report1605.mp3 audio file and the consultation letter template (Consultation_Letter) when transcribing this report. Save the document as XXReport16.05, using your initials in place of *XX* in the file name.

Set a blank line between each of the numbered findings mentioned in the letter. Do not indent or set a line space between the items in the lettered sublist. Set the sublist in list style.

REPORT 16.6 Autopsy Report

Use the Report1606.mp3 audio file and the autopsy report template (Autopsy_Report) when transcribing this report. Save the document as XXReport16.06, using your initials in place of *XX* in the file name.

As shown in the template, the main section headings are underlined. This is a long report and will require running headers and continued lines. The second-level headings are set in all capital letters followed by a hard return. Third-level headings in the report are set in all capital letters followed by colons and run-in text. The dictator will number the findings, and these should be set as roman numeral second-level headings, each followed with a hard return. Review Figure 16.3 before transcribing this report.

Courtney Baird is a 43-year-old woman with HIV. She reports feeling ill, with a cough and shortness of breath, and presents to her immunologist's office.

REPORT 16.7 History and Physical

Use the Report1607.mp3 audio file and the history and physical report template (History_and_Physical) when transcribing this report. Save the document as XXReport16.07, using your initials in place of *XX* in the file name.

The dictator does not state the physician's name at the top of the report, but use the name indicated in the signature line.

In this report, the word *injection* is used differently than its more common usage. Use your medical dictionary to learn an alternative meaning for this term.

Josh Henry is a 26-year-old man whose 2-year-old daughter was recently diagnosed with chickenpox. Mr. Henry presented to the emergency department with a fever and a vesicular rash covering his body. He was diagnosed with chickenpox, treated with Tylenol and Benadryl, and sent home. However, due to domestic problems, he returned to the hospital and was placed in isolation until the chickenpox lesions crusted.

REPORT 16.8 Discharge Summary

Use the Report1608.mp3 audio file and the discharge summary report template (Discharge_Summary) when transcribing this report. Save the document as XXReport16.08, using your initials in place of XX in the file name.

The Physical Examination section is dictated in paragraph form. Unless otherwise directed by your instructor, transcribe the report using the template's subheadings in list style. Transcribe the dictated aspects of the physical examination in the order of the template's headings.

Medical Report Headings

This appendix lists the main headings found in the various reports transcribed by the medical transcriptionist. A description of the type of information usually found under the report headings is provided where appropriate. These headings correspond with the headings in the templates provided on the Dictations and Templates CD that accompanies this text.

This appendix begins with the history and physical report, but then the reports are presented in the order they are introduced in the specialty chapters in Part 2 of this text. Note that many of the reports will refer back to the history and physical report, as this H&P includes many of the headings used in other reports. Table A.1 lists the reports in alphabetical order, along with the corresponding template file names, where the reports are featured as text figures, and the page number where each report appears in this appendix. In addition to the templates listed in Table A.1, the templates resource also includes a template for a consultation letter, a chart summary, and a neuropsychological evaluation. These are not represented in this appendix because these report types do not contain internal headings.

Standard report headings provide a guide for organizing information consistently across reports. Consistency of heading content and order is important to allow for quick access of information, especially when an electronic medical record is maintained. Templates containing these standard headings are useful tools when transcribing dictated content. (Appendix B explains how to use these templates when transcribing reports.) Organize dictated information under headings and subheadings per the appropriate report's template, but do not force the text to fit a template if conforming to the template would require extensive editing or deconstructing sentences. The order of the template's headings should be maintained, even when information is dictated in a different order than the template.

Reports will usually contain one or two levels of headings within the main body of the report. First-level or main headings within the reports are set without colons, and the text will be keyed on the next line (following a hard return) and flush left with the heading. Second-level subheadings are followed by a colon and will have text keyed one space after the colon, on the same line. Some house styles will request that a line space be set above each heading, no matter the level. However, in this text, our reports are set with no space above subheadings. In the final transcribed report, delete template headings that do not contain dictated content following them.

Reports and letters are set in block style, with all text set flush left and with a ragged right margin. Subsequent paragraphs within report sections are set with a blank line above them and no paragraph indent. Numbered lists are keyed with one space after the period and the runover text flush left. Some styles will direct that a line space should be set between items in a numbered list, but do not set a blank line space between numbered items in reports transcribed for this text. Fonts should be 12-point type, but a slightly smaller font size is acceptable if doing so will allow a report to fit on one page.

Table A.1

Medical Types, Templates, and Resources

Report Title	Template File Name	Text Figure		Appendix A Page Reference
		Figure Number	**Page Reference**	
Autopsy Report	Autopsy_Report	Figure 16.4	456	473
Discharge Summary	Discharge_Summary	Figure 8.3	233	470
Emergency Department Report	Emergency_Dept_Report	Figure 13.7	373	472
History and Physical	History_and_Physical	Figure 12.4	344	466
Labor and Delivery Report	Labor_and_Delivery_Report	Figure 11.6	317	472
Office Note	Office_Note	Figure 5.3	159	469
Operative Report	Operative_Report	Figure 7.6	207	469
Pathology Report	Pathology_Report	Figure 10.7	293	471
Radiology Report	Radiology_Report	Figure 9.6	262	471

History and Physical

CHIEF COMPLAINT

A statement, usually in the patient's words, indicating the patient's primary complaint or reason for seeking care. More than one complaint may be listed.

HISTORY OF PRESENT ILLNESS

A description of the patient's complaint(s) and events leading up to the current encounter. Often, this description begins with a general description of the patient, including the patient's age (e.g., This 36-year-old white female...). Depending on the patient's complaint and the originator's dictation style, the description may be short and succinct or lengthy and intricate.

PAST MEDICAL HISTORY

Past or ongoing medical conditions that may or may not be related to the current illness. This section may also include a list of problems which outlines chronic conditions or unresolved health issues.

SURGICAL HISTORY

A summary of previous surgeries and procedures. Often, surgeries are listed with the date or age of the patient at the time of the listed surgery or procedure. This information may be incorporated into the Past Medical History if not dictated as a separate heading.

SOCIAL HISTORY

Nonmedical information about the patient's lifestyle that may have a bearing on the patient's health. This section may include the patient's occupation, marital status, hobbies, and amount of exercise or physical activity. Habits are usually listed, including tobacco use (including smokeless tobacco), alcohol and/or caffeine consumption, and over-the-counter or illicit drug usage.

FAMILY HISTORY

Pertinent medical facts about the patient's blood relatives (parents, siblings, and children) including hereditary and familial diseases as well as cause of death and age at death.

ALLERGIES

Frank allergies to medications or other items a patient may encounter in a medical setting such as latex or contrast dyes (e.g., barium or iodine). Food, inhalant (e.g., pollens, dust, dander), and contact allergies (e.g., detergents, poison ivy) may also be listed under this heading. Adverse reactions to medications (e.g., nausea, insomnia) are also listed here. Typically, allergies are typed in all caps italic letters to bring added attention to this very important information. Allergies may be formatted as a numbered list when there is more than one allergy dictated.

CURRENT MEDICATIONS

Lists prescription and over-the-counter medications, vitamins, herbs, and other supplements as well as the dose and the regimen. Recently discontinued medications may also be dictated under this section. Medications may be formatted as a numbered list when there is more than one medication dictated.

REVIEW OF SYSTEMS

May be dictated in paragraph form or delineated by body system. Some dictators will merely dictate "noncontributory" or "negative other than those mentioned in the past medical history." The Review of Systems typically includes a list of positive (present) and negative (not present) symptoms and may only include systems that are pertinent to the chief complaint or that correlate with the patient's medical history. This is a list of symptoms *reported by the patient* or *person accompanying the patient* and should not be confused with the Physical Examination, which lists findings *observed by the examiner*. The following gives examples of common terms and typical phrases that might be dictated under the specific subheading. Often there is some overlap (e.g., a rash on the arm might be transcribed under Extremities or Skin). If the dictator does not clearly indicate which subheading, the medical history may give guidance as to which subheading to use when more than one is appropriate (e.g., "change in appetite" might be due to a psychiatric or gastrointestinal disorder).

GENERAL: Fatigue, malaise, change in weight, fever, chills.

SKIN: Rash, pruritus, acne, lesions, scars, tattoos, body piercings, seborrheic keratosis, eczema, psoriasis, hives, hyperpigmentation, boils, pustules, vitiligo, intertrigo, tinea, changes in nails or hair.

HEAD: Headache.

EYES: Itching, excessive tearing, dry eyes, change in vision, blurred vision, use of corrective lenses, diplopia, photophobia, color blindness, night blindness, history of cataracts or glaucoma.

EARS: Pain, discharge, popping, ringing (tinnitus), change in hearing, vertigo, history of PE tubes.

NOSE, SINUSES: Pain, pressure, discharge, itching, sneezing, congestion, difficulty breathing, nosebleeds, mouth breathing, frequent infections, snoring.

MOUTH AND THROAT: Sore throat, dysphagia, hoarseness, postnasal drainage, cold sores, canker sores, ulcers, dysgeusia, bleeding gums, receding gums, bruxism, dentures, TMJ problems, halitosis, dry mouth.

NECK: Stiffness, decreased range of motion, swollen lymph nodes.

BREASTS: Lumps, discharge, pain, tenderness, history of fibrocystic breast disease or cancer.

RESPIRATORY: History of asthma, bronchitis, congestion, cough, hemoptysis, sputum production, wheezing, history of pneumonia or TB, history of COPD.

CARDIAC: Shortness of breath, dyspnea (on exertion or at rest), orthopnea, chest pain, PND, palpitations, "skipped beats," history of murmur or mitral valve prolapse, syncope or near-syncope, cyanosis.

GASTROINTESTINAL: Changes in appetite, nausea, vomiting, abdominal pain, constipation, diarrhea, melena, hematochezia (bright red or dark blood), tarry stools, change in stools (color, smell, or consistency) or change in bowel habits, indigestion, heartburn, reflux, bloating, flatulence, early satiety, belching, hemorrhoids, history of gallstones, jaundice.

GENITOURINARY: Frequency, urgency, incontinence, dribbling, hesitancy, dysuria, hematuria, nocturia, history of urinary stones, erectile dysfunction, flank pain, suprapubic pain.

GYNECOLOGIC: Dysmenorrhea, dyspareunia, discharge, itching, burning, irregular menses, exposure to DES, mittelschmerz.

MUSCULOSKELETAL: Joint pain, joint stiffness, arthritis, back pain, neck pain, muscle aches, decreased range of motion (any joint), warmth or redness in a joint, crepitus, locking, giving way, weakness.

PERIPHERAL VASCULAR: Claudication, lower extremity edema, varicose veins.

NEUROLOGIC: Dysphasia, tremor, tingling, burning, numbness, difficulty with memory, dementia, seizures, ataxia, frequent falls, involuntary movements, clumsiness.

HEMATOLOGIC: Easy bruising or bleeding, history of anemia.

ENDOCRINE: Excessively hot or cold, intolerance to heat or cold, change in weight, change in libido.

PSYCHIATRIC: Anxiety, panic attacks, mood swings, crying spells, depression, suicidal thoughts, hallucinations, delusions, paranoia, change in behavior, obsessive/compulsive behaviors, binge eating, purging, change in libido, insomnia or hypersomnia.

PHYSICAL EXAMINATION

Lists observations made by the examiner. It may be dictated in paragraph form or divided into subheadings. (Use the template's subheadings whenever possible to help organize the information.) The following lists body areas and sample descriptors (keywords) that may be reported under a specific subheading. Often there is some overlap (e.g., arthritis, if not specified, may fall under musculoskeletal or extremities). If the dictator is not clear about which subheading to use, the medical history may give guidance as to which subheading to use (e.g., edema may be attributed to a cardiovascular disorder or listed under musculoskeletal due to an injury).

GENERAL: Age, race, ambulatory status (wheelchair, cane, or walker), nourishment, signs of distress. Keywords: Well nourished, well developed, Caucasian, African American, Asian, Hispanic, no acute distress.

VITAL SIGNS: Keywords: Height, weight, blood pressure, respirations, pulse, temperature, body mass index.

SKIN: Includes pallor, lesions, bruises, moles, rashes in any body area.

HEENT: Head, eyes, ears, nose, and throat. Keywords: Normocephalic, atraumatic, extraocular movements intact or extraocular muscles intact (EOMs), PERRLA, scleral icterus, anicteric sclerae, TMs clear (tympanic membranes), edentulous, nasopharynx clear, moist mucosa, swollen or boggy turbinates.

NECK: Cervical spine and musculature, cervical lymph nodes, carotid arteries. Keywords: Range of motion, stiff, supple, bruits, lymphadenopathy, jugular venous distention (JVD).

LYMPH NODES: Submandibular, cervical chain, axillary, inguinal, popliteal, epitrochlear. Keywords: Shotty, boggy, bulky, lymphadenopathy.

THORAX AND LUNGS: Chest, chest wall, ribs, axillae, lungs, sternum, hilum, bronchi. Keywords: Clear to auscultation and percussion, rales, wheezes, rhonchi, inspiratory, expiratory, costochondral.

CARDIOVASCULAR: Heart and great vessels. Keywords: PMI (point of maximal intensity), rate, rhythm, murmurs, bruits, heaves, thrills.

BREASTS: Specific areas of the breast described relative to an analog clock. Keywords: At the 6 o'clock position, lumps, masses, discharge, pendulous, symmetry, gynecomastia.

ABDOMEN: Right upper quadrant, left upper quadrant, left lower quadrant, right lower quadrant, epigastric, hypogastric, periumbilical. Keywords: Pain or tenderness on palpation, rebound, normal or normoactive, decreased or hyperactive bowel sounds, organomegaly, masses, ascites.

PELVIS: Pelvic and hip bones, inguinal area, internal pelvic organs, and external genitalia. Keywords: Bimanual exam, vulva, vagina, cervix, adnexa, uterus, bladder, perineum, undescended testicles, scrotum, glans penis, shaft.

ANO-RECTAL: Prostate gland, anus, rectum. Keywords: Digital rectal exam (DRE), sphincter tone, internal and external hemorrhoids, vault, guaiac-negative or guaiac-positive stool.

PERIPHERAL VASCULAR: Typically lower extremities, but may also include upper extremities. Keywords: Pulses, pedal pulses, posterior tibial pulses, brachial pulses, varicose veins, capillary refill, Homans sign.

MUSCULOSKELETAL: Back, paravertebral muscles, spine (cervical, thoracic, lumbar, and sacral), joints. Keywords: Flexion, extension, sidebending, rotation, range of motion, weakness, paralysis, kyphosis, lordosis, scoliosis.

EXTREMITIES: Arms, hands, legs, and feet. Keywords: Deep tendon reflexes (DTRs), edema, dependent edema, pitting edema, rubor, shiny skin, decreased hair (especially shins and ankles).

NEUROLOGIC: Cranial nerves, peripheral nerves, reflexes, gait, mentation, memory, speech. Keywords: Grossly intact, Babinski, downgoing.

MENTAL STATUS: Keywords: Affect, oriented, alert, mood, dysthymic, euthymic, appropriate, tangential thoughts, rapid speech.

DIAGNOSTIC STUDIES
Results of imaging studies such as x-ray, MRI, ultrasound, CT scan, and echocardiogram as well as procedures such as colonoscopy, endoscopy, stress test, electromyelogram, nerve conduction study.

LABORATORY DATA
Lists analytical results of blood (serum or plasma), urine, stool, cerebrospinal fluid, other body fluids, and tissue biopsies.

IMPRESSION
May also be dictated as the diagnosis or assessment. Describes the provider's conclusions or working assumptions about the patient's complaints or condition. Often a definitive diagnosis cannot be made until further studies have been completed. The term "rule out" is used to indicate that the disease or condition is highly suspected and that further studies will be ordered to either confirm or disprove the diagnosis. This section may be formatted as a numbered list if the dictator enumerates impressions. Abbreviations representing the diagnosis should not be used in the Impression section. Expand abbreviations when you are certain of their meaning, but leave the abbreviation as dictated when there is any doubt as to its meaning. Non-disease-entity abbreviations may be used (e.g., mg, cm).

PLAN

A list or a paragraph (narrative) of the provider's plan of action to address the items discussed in the impression. May also list clinical reminders, health maintenance reminders, or time interval for followup care. This section may be formatted as a numbered list if the dictator enumerates the plan.

The Impression and Plan sections may be combined and set as a single numbered list with each list item being a separate diagnosis along with the specific plan to address that diagnosis. When dictated together, transcribe under the single section heading: Impression and Plan.

Office Note

This office note template uses the SOAP note format.

SUBJECTIVE

Information gathered from the patient or caregiver including the reason for the visit, symptoms, changes since last visit, and events leading up to the current encounter.

OBJECTIVE

Information obtained by examining the patient or by performing imaging studies or diagnostic tests.

ASSESSMENT

The healthcare provider's conclusions or working assumptions about the patient's complaints or condition. Often a definitive diagnosis cannot be made until further studies have been completed. The term "rule out" is used to indicate the disease or condition is highly suspected and further studies will be ordered to confirm or disprove the diagnosis.

PLAN

See section details in the history and physical report.

Operative Report

PREOPERATIVE DIAGNOSIS

Lists the disease(s) or condition(s) that will be addressed by the operative procedure. If more than one diagnosis, format as a numbered list and change the heading from Diagnosis to Diagnoses. Abbreviations representing the diagnosis should not be used in the Preoperative Diagnosis section. Expand abbreviations when you are certain of their meaning, but leave the abbreviation as dictated when there is any doubt as to its meaning. Non-disease-entity abbreviations may be used (e.g., mg, cm).

POSTOPERATIVE DIAGNOSIS

The disease(s) or condition(s) addressed by the operative procedure. Usually the postoperative diagnosis is the same as the preoperative diagnosis, but the procedure may reveal information that changes the diagnosis. Often, the dictator will simply dictate "same," meaning the preoperative and postoperative diagnoses are the same, but do not transcribe the word "same." Copy and paste the preoperative diagnosis into the postoperative diagnosis. Guidelines pertaining to formatting and use of abbreviations are the same as the Preoperative Diagnosis section.

NAME OF OPERATION

The name of the procedure(s) to be performed. Format as a numbered list if more than one procedure is dictated.

ANESTHESIA

The type of anesthesia to be used (e.g., MAC, general, IV sedation, conscious sedation).

INDICATIONS

The reasons for performing the surgical procedure. May include the patient's clinical history and the rationale for performing the procedure.

INFORMED CONSENT

A statement confirming that consent was given after full disclosure of the risks, benefits, and alternatives of the procedure.

PROCEDURE

A detailed description of the procedure including equipment, instruments, medications, type of wound closure, and medical supplies used during the course of the procedure.

ESTIMATED BLOOD LOSS
An estimate of the amount of blood lost during the course of the procedure.

COMPLICATIONS
A description of any specific complications encountered during the course of the procedure.

SPECIMENS
A list of specimens (e.g., tissue biopsies, fluids, organs) obtained during the procedure and submitted to the laboratory for analysis or diagnostic studies.

Discharge Summary

ADMITTING DIAGNOSIS
One or more diagnosis(es) ascribed to the patient at the time the patient is admitted to the hospital setting. The list may include confirmed diagnoses and/or presumptive (working) diagnoses. If more than one diagnosis is dictated, format as a numbered list and change the heading from Diagnosis to Diagnoses. Abbreviations representing the diagnosis should not be used in the Diagnosis section. Expand abbreviations when you are certain of their meaning, but leave the abbreviation as dictated when there is any doubt as to its meaning. Non-disease-entity abbreviations may be used (e.g., mg, cm).

DISCHARGE DIAGNOSIS
One or more diagnosis(es) ascribed to the patient at the time the patient is discharged from the hospital setting. This list may or may not be the same as the admitting diagnoses. Guidelines pertaining to formatting and use of abbreviations are the same as the Admitting Diagnosis section.

HISTORY OF PRESENT ILLNESS
The symptoms and/or events leading up to the hospital admission.

PAST MEDICAL HISTORY
See history and physical report, page 466.

ALLERGIES
See history and physical report, page 466.

PHYSICAL EXAMINATION
See history and physical report, pages 467–468.
GENERAL:
VITAL SIGNS:
SKIN:
HEENT:
NECK:
LYMPH NODES:
THORAX AND LUNGS:
CARDIOVASCULAR:
BREASTS:
ABDOMEN:
PELVIS:
ANO-RECTAL:
PERIPHERAL VASCULAR:
MUSCULOSKELETAL:
EXTREMITIES:
NEUROLOGIC:
MENTAL STATUS:

DIAGNOSTIC STUDIES
Pertinent tests, procedures, and imaging studies performed during the patient's hospital stay. (Results of tests performed before admission are typically included in the History of Present Illness section.) Results from studies such as x-rays, CT scans, MRI, nuclear imaging, angiography, electrocardiography, and echocardiography. Alternatively, this information may be integrated into the Hospital Course section and not dictated as a separate section.

LABORATORY DATA
A summary of pertinent results obtained through laboratory studies performed on blood, urine, stool, other body fluids, and tissues. Use this heading if these lab results are dictated collectively and not incorporated into Hospital Course section.

HOSPITAL COURSE
A description of pertinent events during the patient's hospital stay. This section may also incorporate diagnostic and laboratory studies. (If dictated together, do not deconstruct sentences in order to separate diagnostic and laboratory data from this section.)

DISPOSITION
Arrangements for the transfer of care following discharge. A patient may be discharged to home or to another healthcare facility such as a skilled nursing facility, nursing home, or rehabilitation facility.

CONDITION ON DISCHARGE
The patient's condition relative to his or her condition on admission (e.g., stable, improved, unimproved).

DISCHARGE INSTRUCTIONS
Instructions the patient and/or caregiver should follow after leaving the hospital such as precautions, instructions for wound care, where to seek additional care, and followup appointment interval.

DISCHARGE MEDICATIONS
All medications and supplements the patient is to take once discharged from the hospital, including medications prescribed before admission that should be continued as well as those added or changed as a result of the hospital stay. Format as a numbered list when more than one medication is dictated.

DISCHARGE DIET
The appropriate diet the patient is to follow once discharged from the hospital such as a liquid diet, liquid progressing to soft solids, ad lib (as desired or tolerated), or diet restrictions such as salt, fat, sugar, or calories.

DISCHARGE PHYSICAL ACTIVITY
Limitations or expectations pertaining to activity levels allowed or encouraged after discharge such as lifting, bending, or squatting, getting in and out of bed, driving, exercising, returning to work, etc.

PLAN
Tests, procedures, appointments, or other activities needed or recommended for followup care after the patient is discharged.

Radiology Report

TEST NAME IN ALL CAPS (e.g., ABDOMINAL MRI)

INDICATION
The patient's diagnosis or a brief description of the patient's clinical history explaining the reason for ordering the imaging study (e.g., status post motor vehicle accident; rule out internal bleeding).

TECHNIQUE
A description of the imaging methods used including the type of equipment, equipment settings (e.g., T2-weighted images), use of contrast media (e.g., iodine, barium), and radioisotopes (e.g., technetium, iodine-131).

FINDINGS
The radiologist's description of the images as well as normal and abnormal findings. Format as a numbered list if the pathologist enumerates the findings.

IMPRESSION
The radiologist's interpretation or conclusions based on the images. The radiologist may recommend further studies, suggest a followup interval, or advise "clinical correlation," meaning the results of the imaging study should be discounted or confirmed in light of the patient's symptoms and clinical history. Format as a numbered list if the radiologist enumerates the impressions. Abbreviations representing the diagnosis should not be used in the Impression section. Expand abbreviations when you are certain of their meaning, but leave the abbreviation as dictated when there is any doubt as to its meaning. Non-disease-entity abbreviations may be used (e.g., mg, cm).

Pathology Report

SPECIMEN
The name of the specimen(s) received (e.g., "lung biopsy," or "amputation, right finger").

PROCEDURE
The name of the procedure performed to obtain the submitted specimen.

CLINICAL HISTORY
The patient's diagnosis or a brief description of the patient's clinical history that is relevant to the submitted specimen (e.g., D&C status post fetal demise; rule out pancreatic cancer). This information is supplied by the provider submitting the specimen and is used to guide the pathologist in the investigation.

GROSS DESCRIPTION
A detailed description of the specimen examined with the naked eye (i.e., no magnification) including number of specimens, dimensions, shape, color, texture, weight, use of fixatives (e.g., formalin), and condition upon receipt by the lab.

MICROSCOPIC DESCRIPTION

A detailed description of the specimen(s) using various staining techniques and microscopy.

DIAGNOSES (GROSS AND MICROSCOPIC)

The pathologist's conclusions or diagnosis(es) based on the gross and microscopic findings. The pathologist may give recommendations for additional studies to confirm or further clarify the diagnosis. The pathologist may also advise "clinical correlation," meaning the results of the pathology study should be confirmed in light of the patient's symptoms and clinical history. Format as a numbered list if the pathologist enumerates the impressions. Abbreviations representing the diagnosis should not be used in the Diagnoses section. Expand abbreviations when you are certain of their meaning, but leave the abbreviation as dictated when there is any doubt as to its meaning. Non-disease-entity abbreviations may be used (e.g., mg, cm).

Labor and Delivery Report

PREOPERATIVE DIAGNOSIS

The diagnosis before delivery. Keywords: Fetal distress, cephalopelvic disproportion, vaginal birth after cesarean. Abbreviations representing the diagnosis should not be used in the Preoperative Diagnosis section. Expand abbreviations when you are certain of their meaning, but leave the abbreviation as dictated when there is any doubt as to its meaning. Non-disease-entity abbreviations may be used (e.g., mg, cm).

POSTOPERATIVE DIAGNOSIS

The diagnosis after delivery, which is usually the same as the preoperative diagnosis, but may change based on the outcome of the delivery. Often, the dictator will simply dictate "same," meaning the preoperative and postoperative diagnoses are the same, but do not transcribe the word "same." Copy and paste the preoperative diagnosis into the postoperative diagnosis. Guidelines pertaining to formatting and use of abbreviations are the same as the Preoperative Diagnosis section.

NAME OF PROCEDURE

Name of surgery or procedure performed.

ANESTHESIA

See operative report, page 469.

INDICATIONS

The reason for performing the procedure or surgery. This section may list a specific diagnosis or briefly describe the patient's clinical history and the rationale for performing the surgery.

INFORMED CONSENT

See operative report, page 469.

PROCEDURE

A detailed description of the course of the procedure including methods, techniques, equipment, instruments, type of wound closure, and supplies used.

ESTIMATED BLOOD LOSS

See operative report, page 470.

COMPLICATIONS

See operative report, page 470.

Emergency Department Report

CHIEF COMPLAINT

The patient's reason for seeking emergency care.

HISTORY OF PRESENT ILLNESS

Describes the patient's symptoms and events leading up to the current encounter. The description is usually limited to information pertinent to the chief complaint.

PAST MEDICAL HISTORY

A summary of pertinent medical events, diseases, or conditions that may have a bearing on the chief complaint.

SURGICAL HISTORY

See history and physical report, page 466.

SOCIAL HISTORY

See history and physical report, page 466.

FAMILY HISTORY

See history and physical report, page 466.

ALLERGIES
See history and physical report, page 466.

CURRENT MEDICATIONS
See history and physical report, page 467.

PHYSICAL EXAMINATION
Details may be limited to areas pertinent to the chief complaint. See history and physical report, pages 467–468.
GENERAL:
VITAL SIGNS:
SKIN:
HEENT:
NECK:
LYMPH NODES:
THORAX AND LUNGS:
CARDIOVASCULAR:
BREASTS:
ABDOMEN:
PELVIS:
ANO-RECTAL:
PERIPHERAL VASCULAR:
MUSCULOSKELETAL:
EXTREMITIES:
NEUROLOGIC:
MENTAL STATUS:

DIAGNOSTIC STUDIES
Pertinent tests, procedures, and imaging studies performed during the patient's encounter in the emergency department (e.g., x-rays, CT scans, MRI, nuclear imaging, angiography, electrocardiography, echocardiography). Alternatively, this information may be incorporated into the following ED Course section.

LABORATORY DATA
A summary of pertinent results obtained through laboratory studies performed on blood, urine, stool, other body fluids, and tissues. Use this heading if these results are not included in the previous Diagnostic Studies section or interspersed in the following ED Course section.

ED COURSE
A description of pertinent events during the patient's encounter in the emergency department. This section may also incorporate diagnostic and laboratory studies if not dictated separately. (If dictated together, do not deconstruct sentences in order to separate diagnostic and laboratory data from ED Course.)

PROCEDURE
Any procedures performed during the course of the patient's encounter in the emergency department (e.g., endoscopy, wound closure, reduction of fractures).

DIAGNOSIS
A final diagnosis, if one has been reached, or a working diagnosis at the time the patient is discharged from the emergency department or transferred to the hospital for continued care. Format as a numbered list if more than one diagnosis is dictated. Abbreviations representing the diagnosis should not be used in the Diagnosis section. Expand abbreviations when you are certain of their meaning, but leave the abbreviation as dictated when there is any doubt as to its meaning. Non-disease-entity abbreviations may be used (e.g., mg, cm).

CONDITION ON DISCHARGE
The condition of the patient at the time of discharge relative to their condition when admitted to the emergency department (e.g., stable, improved, decompensated, compensated expired or deceased).

DISCHARGE MEDICATIONS
A list of medications prescribed for the patient during their emergency department visit. Format as a numbered list if more than one medication is dictated.

PLAN
A list of tests, procedures, appointments, or other activities required or recommended for followup care after discharge. Format as a numbered list if the dictator enumerates the plan.

Autopsy Report

This report contains three levels of headings. The top-level heading in this report is underlined and set in all capital letters format. The second-level heading is set in all capital letters and is not underlined. The third-level heading is set with a colon following and run-in text.

EXTERNAL EXAMINATION

INTERNAL EXAMINATION

ABDOMINAL CAVITY

THORACIC CAVITY

PERICARDIAL CAVITY

ENDOCRINE SYSTEM
THYROID:
PARATHYROIDS:
ADRENALS:

ORGAN DESCRIPTION

CARDIOVASCULAR SYSTEM
HEART:
VEINS:

MUSCULOSKELETAL SYSTEM

CENTRAL NERVOUS SYSTEM

RESPIRATORY SYSTEM
TRACHEA AND BRONCHI:
LUNGS:

INTEGUMENTARY SYSTEM

MICROSCOPIC EXAMINATION

GASTROINTESTINAL SYSTEM
LIVER:
GALLBLADDER AND BILE DUCTS:
PANCREAS:

CARDIOVASCULAR SYSTEM

RESPIRATORY SYSTEM

GENITOURINARY SYSTEM

GASTROINTESTINAL SYSTEM

HEMOLYMPHATIC SYSTEM
SPLEEN:
LYMPH NODES:
THYMUS:
BONE MARROW:

GENITOURINARY SYSTEM

HEMOLYMPHATIC SYSTEM

ENDOCRINE SYSTEM

FINDINGS

How to Use Medical Report Templates

A template is a special type of document that contains standard text and formatting that is used as a framework to create other documents. Template files have .dot or .dotx extensions. When a template file is opened by double clicking on the file name, a document file (.doc or .docx) is created. Editing this opened document does not alter the original template file.

As was explained in Chapter 2 of this text, report templates are valuable productivity tools available to the medical transcriptionist. Templates allow for consistent formatting of reports. The standardization implemented by using report templates makes information easier to find when reports are referenced, increases the MT's productivity, and

improves accuracy. Using templates allows the transcriptionist to focus on the content of the dictation, rather than on the mechanics of the document being created.

Medical Transcription: Techniques, Technologies, and Editing Skills, Third Edition is supported with 12 report templates, each representing the most common report types used in medical transcription. The headings found within these templates correspond with the standard headings defined and described in Appendix A. The templates are available on the Dictations and Templates CD as well as on the Internet Resource Center for this title at www.emcp.net/MedTrans3e. Table B.1 lists the available templates.

Table B.1
Template Names and Chapter References

Template Name	Chapter Featuring This Report Type	Chapters Using This Template
Autopsy_Report.dot	16	16
Chart_Summary.dot	-	6, 7, 15, 16
Consultation_Letter.dot	6	6, 7, 8, 9, 10, 11, 12, 13, 14, 15, 16
Discharge_Summary.dot	8	8, 9, 10, 12, 13, 14, 15, 16
Emergency_Dept_Report.dot	13	13
History_and_Physical.dot	12	9, 12, 13, 14, 15, 16
Labor_and_Delivery_Report.dot	11	11
Neuropsychological_Eval.dot	14	14
Office_Note.dot	5	5, 6, 7, 8
Operative_Report.dot	7	5, 7, 8, 9, 10, 11, 12
Pathology_Report.dot	10	10, 11, 12, 15
Radiology_Report.dot	9	8, 9, 10, 12, 13, 14

If you are using the SNAP document checker program with this textbook, you will need to download the templates for Microsoft Word 2007 from the SNAP Web site. The SNAP-delivered templates will function the same as the templates on the Dictations and Templates CD. However, the CD templates are saved in a format that allows them to be read by earlier versions of Microsoft Word. As a result, they will not work with the document checker software. The SNAP document checker program will only work with Microsoft Word 2007.

Opening and Saving Files Created from Templates

The first thing you should do after opening a document created from a template is to save the file the with the appropriate file name. Throughout this text, you will be directed on the appropriate file name to use with each transcribed report. Follow these instructions, or the instructions of your instructor, and save the files onto your computer's hard drive or removable storage medium (such as a flash drive). Save the file again before printing or closing the file.

Transcribing Using Templates Designed for This Text

The templates created for this text include the appropriate standardized headings for the corresponding reports. The templates include "jump" points. View the jump points by clicking the keys Alt + F9. (Click the Alt key and keep holding it down as you click the F9 key.) A jump point will appear as two braces with two spaces between them. Some jump points may include a description of the type of information to be inserted under that particular heading. When the jump point is selected, it will appear grayed. Press Alt + F9 again to hide the jump points in a document. Transcribe reports with the jump points displayed.

Navigate from jump point to jump point by pressing the F11 key. The F11 key will move the cursor to the next jump point, indicating the next place to begin typing.

The templates also include a programmed field to insert "(continued)" in the documents' running feet as well as subsequent page headers consisting of the report type and page number (presented as a programmed field). The second-page header will also provide jump points for the patient's name and the date of the report. These elements will not appear unless the transcribed document continues onto a second or third page. To open a page's header or footer in Microsoft Word, double click on the header or footer area or use the keyboard shortcut Alt, V, H, pressing the keys sequentially, and releasing them after each click. Once your cursor is in the header or footer, F9 will update the fields with "(continued)" in the footer and the page number(s) in subsequent page headers. Note, in versions prior to 2007, the headers and footers are not visible while the document is displayed in Normal view unless you open the header and footer space using Alt, V, H. To display headers and footers while transcribing, choose Print Layout view (located on the View ribbon) or press Ctrl + Alt + P.

Changing Page and Line Breaks

In addition to font style and line spacing, the document also has "keep with next" formatting applied to all of the major headings in the report. This formatting style will help avoid bad page breaks between an internal heading and the subsequent paragraph. A line of text that has this special pagination format applied to it will have a small black box (■) to the left of it. Formatting symbols are usually hidden, but to reveal them, use the key combination Ctrl + Shift + *. If the formatting symbols are displayed, this key combination will hide the formatting symbols.

Do not force a new page by adding line spaces above headings. If necessary, insert a manual page break using the manual page break command Ctrl + Enter.

Avoid forcing line breaks in the middle of a paragraph by hitting the Enter key or adding spaces within a line to force the line to break at a different place. If you want to avoid a bad line break (such as between a number and unit of measure, like 50 mg), set a nonbreaking space. Insert a nonbreaking space by clicking Ctrl + Shift + Spacebar *instead of* the Spacebar alone. The formatting symbol for a nonbreaking space appears as a degree symbol (°) but this formatting symbol will not print.

There may be times when a line is breaking at a hyphen, and you will want to avoid this situation. Set a nonbreaking hyphen using the Ctrl + Shift + - key combination. The formatting symbol for a nonbreaking hyphen is an en dash (–), but an actual hyphen will print on paper.

Editing Internal Headings

The templates are designed to allow the transcriptionist to edit the standard headings. For example, in the discharge summary report, if there are more than one admitting diagnoses, the template's Admitting Diagnosis heading will need to be revised to read Admitting Diagnos*es*.

If a dictation does not use all of the report template's standardized headings, it is important to delete the heading and the corresponding jump point field from the document. However, do not delete the headings until the completion of the dictation. Sometimes, providers will dictate sections out of order. When using templates, it is important to transcribe the information in the template's order rather than in the dictated order.

Turn Off Automatic Numbered Lists

By default, Microsoft Word will interpret a line that begins with 1 followed by a period and a space as the start of a numbered list and will automatically format the next line of text with a 2. It is important to turn off this feature when transcribing medical documents. Rather than using the automatic numbering and hanging indent format, the numbered lists in reports transcribed for this text should be keyed and set flush left with runover text set flush left (not on a hanging indent). In Microsoft Word, if the automatic numbering feature is turned on, click the AutoCorrectOptions button that appears next to the number. At the drop-down list that displays, click *Stop Automatically Creating Numbered Lists*. To temporarily stop the formatting, click Ctrl + Z immediately after the format change occurs to undo the change.

Creating Templates with Jump Points

Insert a jump point into a document by setting the cursor in the desired location and pressing Ctrl + F9. The field will display when you first enter it, but if you close the document and reopen it, the field will not be displayed. (View jump points using Alt + F9)

You can key reminder text or specific instructions within the jump point field. Key the text in between the two spaces that appear between the two brackets. However, start the text with a \ character. For example, {·\patient name·}. Text keyed within the field will not print or be displayed as part of the final report.

Save a document as a template by selecting the appropriate template format in the *Save as type* option box in the Save as dialog box. In Microsoft Word 2007, you will have to select the *Word 97-2003 Template (*.dot)* option if you want the template to be available to computers running earlier versions of Word.

Managing Files

For information on file management in Windows Vista or Windows XP, go to the Internet Resource Center for this title at www.emcp.net/MedTrans3e. Tutorials are posted under the General Studies Center link.

Editing Speech Recognition Drafts

When a practitioner dictates using speech recognition software, the speech engine produces a text draft of the interpreted audio. Depending on the level of "training" the speech engine has received, the output will be in varying degrees of accuracy. Most speech recognition software requires a minimal training period for the speech engine to produce a draft that is at an acceptable level of accuracy. Studies have shown that if the draft is not at least 85% accurate, it is more efficient to transcribe the entire dictation rather than editing the draft speech recognition output.

There are several ways to train a speech engine. Most speech recognition software requires a minimum amount of speech read into the system using a script. The reading time can vary from 10 to 30 minutes. This dictated text is then a part of the practitioner's dictation profile and used by the speech engine to interpret dictation by that individual.

Another way a speech engine is trained is by editing text. When a medical editor makes a correction on the draft and saves it, the system compares the original with the edited text and adjusts the dictator's profile so it will more accurately interpret future audio files.

Not all dictating practitioners are candidates for speech recognition. Foreign accents and dictations by practitioners who format phrases in ways that are not standard English phraseology can be very difficult for a speech engine to interpret accurately. These dictators may require additional training time, and sometimes are not amenable to using speech recognition. Practitioners who do not dictate in a consistent format make it difficult for a speech engine to "learn" their dictation patterns. In addition, practitioners who dictate very rapidly, in quiet tones, or use a lot of audible pauses (uh, um, ah), contribute to inaccurate interpretations or gaps in the text. Also, background noises (voices, telephones, music, etc.), microphone interference, and telephone line interference will also contribute to poor recognition.

Before working the following exercises, consider these editing tips:

- Punctuation is often not dictated (or is dictated incorrectly), and the medical editor will need to carefully assess each sentence, fragment, and phrase for appropriate punctuation. The medical editor should punctuate based on content, taking into consideration any dictated punctuation.

- The speech recognition software will sometimes misinterpret a medical term that is a homonym; be very critical when editing to make sure that content matches the appropriate definition of the term(s) used.

- Dictation containing a lot of abbreviations or numbers can be challenging for the speech engine to recognize. If the medical editor is unfamiliar with the terminology, even editing will be difficult. Having access to good references will be important. Most speech engines incorporate a medical dictionary and some level of context checking, but this does not negate the need to use references and/or proofing for context.

- Formatting is often templated based on a style guide; however, a practitioner may dictate some formatting as well. The medical editor will need to shape the draft into a properly formatted document. Throughout this textbook there are samples of formatted reports. Use these as a general outline in formatting speech recognized drafts.

- It is very common for dictating providers to number diagnoses. Often after the first one or two, they stop enumerating the diagnoses and simply dictate "next number" or "number next." Be sure to number the diagnoses correctly. When there is more than one diagnosis, it is preferred to change the heading Diagnosis to Diagnoses.

- It is never acceptable to guess if you are not sure about a term or phrase. Do not assume the speech-recognized draft is correct; this portion of the dictation needs to be flagged for the practitioner to resolve.

- Some dictations have a lot of non-word pauses. Practitioners often dictate while reviewing a patient's chart and are forming their thoughts as they speak. These audible pauses can leave holes in the dictation or can cause false interpretation and errors in the draft text.

- Frequently dictators will change their minds mid sentence or refer to a section earlier in the dictation that they would like to edit. It is up to the editor to appropriately alter the text to capture the intent of the dictation.

- Speech recognized text dictated by an individual who speaks very fast is difficult to edit. This is where your experience and access to references are very important. Often speed controls can be used to slow down the dictation to help you hear key sounds that will assist in deciphering a term.

- A practitioner may dictate a number as the first word of a sentence (e.g., "0.25% Marcaine was administered."). It is necessary to reformat the sentence slightly, without changing the meaning or the style of the speaker, so the sentence no longer begins with a number (e.g., "Marcaine 0.25% was administered.").

- At times you will need to add a word (when not stated, but implied) to make a thought complete. This should be done with caution so as not to distort the intended meaning of the original dictation.

- Dictated contractions should always be expanded (e.g., *there's* would be edited to *there is*). A well-programmed speech engine will do this and present it expanded in the draft.

- A common error when beginning transcription is to split combined forms into two words (e.g., normocephalic as normal cephalic). Be sure to check for combined forms.

- When interpreting x-ray results, the radiologist will often compare the current films with previous studies. In the dictation, the previous results may be referred to by the date they were taken. If the dictated date is unclear, it should be confirmed either with the radiologist or the patient's medical record.

- A note to the medical editor is often included in dictated reports. One example would be if results were called to the physician ordering the test at the time of interpretation. Department standards will be used for making notations on the document. It can be a full sentence, or sometimes just a simple notation like "Results called." If a result is called, time is often included.

- Practitioners often dictate using abbreviations for portions of the physical exam; depending on the document type, common abbreviations may be acceptable (e.g., EOMI, PERRLA). However, there are sections of a document where abbreviations are not used; the medical editor will need to assure proper use of abbreviations.

Practice working with draft output created from a speech recognition engine by editing the following excerpts. The draft files (saved in plain-text format) and corresponding audio dictation files (saved as MP3 files) are available on the Dictation and Templates CD that accompanies this textbook. (These electronic resources are found in the folder called Speech_Recognition_Exercises.) Listen to the corresponding dictation file as you edit the draft file on-screen, or mark the text shown on the following pages. Create a final transcription file for each exercise, saving each corrected file using a file name that combines the exercise number and your initials. For example, for the first exercise, name the file XXSR01, replacing *XX* with your initials.

Exercise 1

Dictation File Name: SR01.mp3
Draft File Name: SR01_draft.txt

The 3-year-old child with new-onset bruising and petechiae. He presented to the emergency room on eleven two 2006.

[handwritten: 11 2]

Exercise 2

Dictation File Name: SR02.mp3
Draft File Name: SR02_draft.txt

The patient is a ~~23-year-old with~~ 23-year-old male with a ~~history~~ 24-hour history of diarrhea.

Exercise 3

Dictation File Name: SR03.mp3
Draft File Name: SR03_draft.txt

[handwritten: The] Patient is a 10-year-old Caucasian male with a 3-day history of abdominal pain and diarrhea. ~~and the~~ the patient was ~~sent~~ *[handwritten: brought]* to the emergency room by his parents. He reports ~~that I~~ eating at a ~~as a~~ fast food restaurant approximately 1 week ago. He has also had fevers up to ~~hundred and 2.4~~ *[handwritten: 102.4]*. He complains of diarrhea ~~and that~~ mixed in with ~~that but~~ dark blood.

Exercise 4

Dictation File Name: SR04.mp3
Draft File Name: SR04_draft.txt

Chest xray date 3-13-0 7 *[handwritten: 2007]* time 1625 hours indication fever ap and lateral chest is performed without prior comparison studies there is focal consolidation of the left upper lobe consistent with pneumonia no associated pleural effusion is seen the right lung is clear the paracardiothymic silhouette and osseous structures are unremarkable impression left upper lobe pneumonia results were telephoned to the emergency room at the time of the study.

Exercise 5

Dictation File Name: SR05.mp3
Draft File Name: SR05_draft.txt

~~And~~ his head is atraumatic and normocephalic no eye movements ~~are~~ *[handwritten: were full]* Pupils ~~are~~ equal and reactive to light ~~and~~ ~~is~~ symmetric the tongue was midline on motor examination ~~is normal no of income~~ *[handwritten: he had]* throughout ~~and swollen and~~ and normal reflexes no ataxia.

[handwritten: this, his face was, school, no ataxia, his strength was full, muscle bulk tone + tone]

Exercise 6

Dictation File Name: SR06.mp3
Draft File Name: SR06_draft.txt

[handwritten: 11/22] AP and lateral chest the examination from eleven twenty two 2006 again shows no definite infiltrates cardiothymic image is normal on this limited inspiration theres been no change from previous study impression no interval change and no evidence for acute pleural parenchymal disease.

Exercise 7

Dictation File Name: SR07.mp3
Draft File Name: SR07_draft.txt

[handwritten: 11/12] Examination two views of the chest date three twelve 2007 history testicular mass findings the cardiac pulmonary and mediastinal contours within normal limits there is no effusion a discrete nodule is not appreciated.

Exercise 8

Dictation File Name: SR08.mp3
Draft File Name: SR08_draft.txt

Erect supine abdomen she has left pleural effusion there is no free air or mechanical obstruction conclusion there is stool in the colon conclusion stool-filled colon.

[handwritten: no acute disease]

Exercise 9

Dictation File Name: SR09.mp3
Draft File Name: SR09_draft.txt

Part A is labeled right ovary and tube. The specimen is received fresh and consists of a single fragment of soft tissue grossly consistent with and over the with attached portion of fallopian tube. The ovary measures 2 x 1.5 x 0.9 cm. and a white-tan nodule is identified on the surface measuring 0.5 cm in greatest dimension. Serial sections through the ovary reveal a white-tan heterogeneous cut surface but no other discreet nodules or lesions. The attached fallopian tube measures 4 cm in length with an average diameter of 0.2 cm.

Exercise 10

Dictation File Name: SR10.mp3
Draft File Name: SR10_draft.txt

The external surface of the tube is purple-tan smooth and glistening. Serial sections through the fallopian tube do not reveal any gross lesions. Sections are submitted as follows: entire ovary and representative sections of fallopian tube in A1.

Exercise 11

Dictation File Name: SR11.mp3
Draft File Name: SR11_draft.txt

The bone marrow biopsy is markedly hypercellular with a cellularity of virtually 100%. Diffuse sheets of glass are identified a few scattered thyroid and myeloid cells. Eosinophils are increased. Only a rim rare megacaryocyte is sustained. Special stain for iron shows no stainable marrow iron. Ventricles are satisfactory.

Exercise 12

Dictation File Name: SR12.mp3
Draft File Name: SR12_draft.txt

This is going to be Part D as in David. First diagnosis is going to be gallbladder with extensive mural involvement by well to moderately differentiated adenocarcinoma and focal extension into mucosa. Number two gallbladder mucosa with focal papillary hyperplasia and intestinal metaplasia. Number 3 no definitive vascular invasion is identified. Next diagnosis tumor is present on the serosal surface of the gallbladder. Next diagnosis perineal invasion is identified. Next diagnosis fibroadipose tissue surrounding cystic duct with invasive moderately differentiated carcinoma. (Please see comment)

Exercise 13

Dictation File Name: SR13.mp3
Draft File Name: SR13_draft.txt

Comment the invasive adenocarcinoma involves multiple parts, including the tissue on the bile duct, the portion of the common bile duct, portion of liver and gallbladder. It is felt that the tumor most likely represents a cholangiocarcinoma arising in the liver with extension into adjacent tissue, including gallbladder and common bile duct.

Exercise 14

Dictation File Name: SR14.mp3
Draft File Name: SR14_draft.txt

The lung fields are clear without evidence of pulmonary nodule infiltrate or effusion. Given limitations of lack of intravenous contrast there is no evidence of mediastinal or hilar adenopathy. No axillary adenopathy is seen. Normal thymic tissue is present.

There is no evidence of worrisome lytic or blastic bony lesion.

Impression negative CT of the chest.

Exercise 15

Dictation File Name: SR15.mp3
Draft File Name: SR15_draft.txt

preoperative diagnosis right inguinal hernia postoperative diagnosis right inguinal hernia procedure performed repair of right inguinal hernia ah this patient was born on 10 14 1992 has an asymptomatic right inguinal hernia

Exercise 16

Dictation File Name: SR16.mp3
Draft File Name: SR16_draft.txt

procedure after the patient was identified in the preoperative holding area, procedures were confirmed with the family and the risks were iterated these risks being pain infection bleeding scarring recurrence contra laterality injury to testicular structures testicle vas and vessels and traditional surgery's need for anesthesia which carries along the risks of allergic reaction adverse reactions and anesthetic death he was taken to the operating room placed supine on the operating room table until anesthesia was induced XXX intubated

Exercise 17

Dictation File Name: SR17.mp3
Draft File Name: SR17_draft.txt

the abdomen and genitalia were prepped with betadine and draped in a sterile manner 0.25% Marcaine with epinephrine was used at the level of the anterior superior iliac spine skin and sutures made an inguinal skin crease carried down through skin and subcutaneous tissues through Scarpa fascia external oblique fascia open reduction fibers through the external inguinal ring the cord structures were identified and were mobilized the hernia sac was identified and was mobilized. XXX XXX transected and

the proximal remnant mobilized up to the level of the internal inguinal ring where XXX was doubly placed with 2 o Vicryl suture redundant sac amputated and separated off the operative field

Exercise 18

Dictation File Name: SR18.mp3
Draft File Name: SR18_draft.txt

the distal remnant was removed in its entirety the cord structures were returned to the canal position of the right testicle and the right hemiscrotum was verified the external oblique fascia was reconstituted with 3 o chromic interrupted suture Scarpa's fascia was closed with 3 o chromic interrupted suture the skin was closed with 6 o Monocryl interrupted with subcuticular suture reinforced with Steri-Strips and XXX the patient was awakened in the operating room extubated discharged to the recovery room taking good spontaneous respirations and moving all four extremities the family was notified of the operative findings and status of the conclusion of the procedure.

of patient

Exercise 19

Dictation File Name: SR19.mp3
Draft File Name: SR19_draft.txt

The specimen is submitted fresh label vermiform appendix. The specimen consists of an elongated portion of mucosa, measuring five point seven times one point two centimeter in diameter. 5.7 x 1.2 cm

Exercise 20

Dictation File Name: SR20.mp3
Draft File Name: SR20_draft.txt

Mesoappendix is identified and is congested. A perforation is noted. The tissue surrounding the perforation is ragged and dark red and covered with blood clots. Some purulent material is noted near the tip of the appendix.

Exercise 21

Dictation File Name SR21.mp3
Draft File Name: SR21_draft.txt

The cut surface shows a lumen that contains fecal material and purulent material. No lesions are noted on the wall. The margin is ink black.

Exercise 22

Dictation File Name: SR22.mp3
Draft File Name: SR22_draft.txt

The aspirate smears are cellular and predominately populated by blasts. The blasts are large with finely dispersed cromitin occasionally conspicuous one or more nucleoli sometimes irregular or convoluted nuclei and moderate amounts of bluish cytoplasm. A rare auer rod is identified.

Exercise 23

Dictation File Name: SR23.mp3
Draft File Name: SR23_draft.txt

Myelopoiesis is decreased with decreased and maturation and we will agree to only a rare megakaryocyte is seen. Cytochemical pain stain showed greater than 3% of the blasts are positive for myeloperoxidase however less than 10% of the marrow nucleated elements are promyelocytes or more mature myeloid elements.

Exercise 24

Dictation File Name: SR24.mp3
Draft File Name: SR24_draft.txt

NSE stain shows and if the pain is less than 20% monocytic cells are present in he marrow of satisfactory the differential count is as follows left 7% and 1% erythroids 6% lymphocytes 12% monocytes 1% eosinophils 3%.

Exercise 25

Dictation File Name: SR25.mp3
Draft File Name: SR25_draft.txt

patient is active alert and oriented times three patient follows two and three commands recall is three of three at zero and three of three at five minutes world forward and backwards.

Exercise 26

Dictation File Name: SR26.mp3
Draft File Name: SR26_draft.txt

sensory exam the patient vocalizes appropriately to tactile stimulation coordination is cerebellar finger nose finger nose finger tandem movements tandem walking and gait are normal

Endocrinology Job Simulation

Congratulations! Now that you have developed your medical transcription skills to a high level of competency, you are ready to bring your skills to the marketplace.

You have landed a contract to provide transcription services for a professional association of physicians that specializes in disorders of the endocrine system. You will be expected to be able to recognize the specialized language—terms, abbreviations, tests, and measurements—used by these professionals.

Medical transcription students generally have developed a professional library by the time they are seeking employment or business. You will need to use your knowledge of medical terminology and combine that with reference materials you own or can access on the Internet.

Your contract starts tomorrow! You have a limited time to research a general knowledge of the specific systems, the most common diseases, and the root words and combining forms that will be most useful to you. As always, you will have access to reference material while you work, but for maximum productivity, you should be able to draw upon the resources you carry in your head.

The first day on the job, you may be given the following tasks:

- A pre-employment spelling test, to be administered by the practice's office manager (your instructor).
- Three lists to develop: a) the 25 terms you would anticipate to occur most frequently (base this list on the endocrine disorders with the highest incidence), b) a list of 25 potentially confusing endocrinology terms, and c) the names and reference values of 10 tests of the endocrine system, in table form.
- A number of reports to transcribe. The turnaround time will be determined by the office manager.

Medical Transcriptionist Job Search

Medical transcriptionists should enjoy excellent job prospects, according to the 2006–2007 *Occupational Outlook Handbook*. Propelled by a growing and aging population that will need more healthcare services, employment of medical transcriptionists is projected to grow faster than average for all occupations through 2014.

A wide range of opportunities await the qualified medical transcriptionist. Positions are available not just in hospitals and doctors' offices, but in laboratories and research centers, medical libraries, government medical establishments, rehabilitation facilities, and veterinary clinics. In addition, healthcare associations and insurance companies are places to look for employment.

Individuals can work at home for a medical transcription service, moonlight on the side on short-term projects for extra income, or choose to work part-time. Other options, such as being a supervisor, teaching individuals who want to become medical transcriptionists, or establishing a private business service are also available to a transcriptionist who has had experience in a medical environment.

If you are interested in finding employment, you must be prepared for the job search. Several of the very basic skills you need are ability to learn, accountability for work performed, adaptability to a diversified work environment, and flexibility. In a medical environment, the transcriptionist must have knowledge of medical terminology and must be patient, sympathetic, and a good listener when dealing with patients.

Keep in mind that job responsibilities should be compatible with your abilities and that the job should ultimately lead to upward mobility. This section will help you plan your strategies for the job search.

Defining Your Market

How do you get started? Employers generally prefer individuals who have had work experience and job-specific training rather than a novice. As a candidate for a job, you have to prove that you have the skills and qualities required on the job as well as personal attributes and abilities that other persons lack.

There are various steps you should follow. First, you have to decide what you would really like to do and whether or not your skills, knowledge, and other qualifications meet the requirements of the job. Make a list of your major skills.

Decide where you would like to work—hospital, doctor's office, clinic, walk-in health facility or organization. Then generate a job prospect list that will include the following traditional ways of finding a job. Develop a network of personal contacts—relatives, friends, church officials, etc.—and ask them to keep you in mind if they are aware of job openings. Join professional organizations, attend meetings, and become friendly with individuals in your profession. Make direct contacts with human resources at hospitals or organizations, read newspaper advertisements and journals, apply to temporary agencies, and use private employment agencies.

The Internet is a vast resource for those seeking employment. Internet use has more than doubled since the year 2000. Today over a billion people are on the worldwide web. Individuals are going online to recruit and to search for jobs; therefore, the Internet is *the* marketplace.

The Internet is key to any job search for the following reasons: (1) You can find the hidden job market, which has unadvertised openings; (2) Major corporations list job openings on websites because employers can fill jobs faster and less expensively; (3) Résumés can be sent anywhere in short periods of time; (4) Many categories of jobs can be found; and (5) A search can be done at any time, day or evening.

Creating an Effective Résumé

A résumé is a marketing document by which you hope to make an impression when searching for a job. There are two basic styles of résumés used to get the reader's attention: the chronological and the functional.

The chronological (Figure E.1) résumé lists your work history in reverse chronological order, starting with your present position and working back in time. This type of résumé highlights experience and is most appropriate for someone who has a history of steady, successful work experience in a related field.

The functional résumé (Figure E.2) highlights the skills and accomplishments that make you an ideal candidate for the position for which you are seeking. An employer's attention is drawn to your achievements rather than your employment history. This format is preferred for those new to the job market or switching careers.

Your résumé needs to be easily read and understood by the computer. Many recruiters will ask you to e-mail your résumé to them, and you may also be researching company jobsites and job databases online that will require an electronic résumé. These résumés must be searchable and scannable by the computer. To accomplish this, key words or nouns for database searching must be supplied.

Use your full name as the file name so that your résumé can be easily found.

Often times prospective employers will ask you to e-mail a "plain-text" or a "text" résumé. Plain text refers to a file format that eliminates boldface, italics, and different fonts. Plain text files are thus universal text files that allow recruiters to view all résumés regardless of the software that has been used to create them. Plain text documents have .txt extensions and can be opened in programs such as Notepad. You can create a plain text document from a Microsoft Word file by selecting the *Plain Text (*.txt)* file type option in the Microsoft Word Save As dialog box. However, make sure you test the plain-text file by opening it up in Notepad to make sure the final version is error-free. If further clean-up is needed, make the further edits in Notepad. Additional instructions and helpful tips for creating and e-mailing a plain-text résumé are readily available on the Internet.

Creating an Application Cover Letter

The application cover letter should be included with every résumé you send. This letter is actually the first impression you will make. Therefore, it should state the reason you are looking for a new job, why this job interests you, some aspects of your background, and several important statements that reflect that you are the right person for the position. Indicate where you heard of the opening and how some of your skills and background will show that you are the right person for the job.

In the second paragraph, make a statement focusing on the type of person you are and why you would be an asset to the company. Indicate that the résumé outlines your skills, experience, and education, and stress the qualifications that are right for the job. Be sure to make a very positive statement about the company.

In the closing paragraph, indicate your interest in the job and in working for the company. Request an interview and state that you will call on a particular day and at a particular time to set up an

NAME
Street address
City, State ZIP Code
Telephone
E-mail Address

JOB OBJECTIVE   Statement of objective in sentence form.

WORK EXPERIENCE

Job Title   Employer, Address

Detail your responsibilities, skills used, and on-the-job accomplishments.

(Repeat for all previous jobs)

EDUCATION   Name of College or University
                       Street Address
                       City, State ZIP Code
                       Degree
FIELD OF STUDY   Name of field of study
RELATED COURSES   Name of course
                       _____
                       _____
                       _____

LICENSES AND CERTIFICATIONS

AWARDS

PROFESSIONAL MEMBERSHIPS

This résumé format lists experience in the following order: job objective, experience (starting with present employer and working backwards), education, other credentials.

Figure E.1   Chronological Résumé

NAME
Street Address
City, State ZIP Code
Telephone
E-mail Address

JOB OBJECTIVE   Statement of objective in sentence form.

SPECIAL QUALIFICATIONS
- _____
- _____

WORK EXPERIENCE
       Title_____
       Dates _____
       Duties (use bullets)

       Title_____
       Dates _____

EDUCATION AND TRAINING
       Degree, Major
       College
       Address

LICENSES AND CERTIFICATIONS

AWARDS

PROFESSIONAL MEMBERSHIPS

The functional résumé emphasizes skills and accomplishments.

Figure E.2   Functional Résumé

appointment (be sure to follow through with this). Leave your phone number and/or e-mail address where you can be reached.

Proofread your cover letter carefully. It should reflect well on your competence and editing skills.

Interviewing

The interview is the final and most important step in the job-hunting process. Your performance and responses at the interview will be the final opportunity to demonstrate that you are the best candidate for the job. If you made a good impression, you will get the job offer.

Recently, telephone interviews have become the first contact made with an applicant for a job. A human resource person asks the applicant a few questions that pertain to the job. If the applicant makes a good impression, then a face-to-face interview is scheduled. Before taking the phone interview, find a quiet place to talk where you won't be interrupted. Have a pen and paper ready to take notes. Be sure to have a copy of your résumé and information on the company you are interviewing with handy, so that you can refer to it during the call. It may be helpful to practice by having a friend call and run through a mock interview with you.

A computerized interview is also used by many companies. In this situation, the computer asks questions about the background, skills, and previous work experience of the applicant. Good and appropriate responses might lead to a face-to-face interview. Prepare yourself for the next interview by carrying out the following procedures:

- Research the company and gather information about its product, services, growth, culture, and employee/employer relations.
- Consider each interview you have as a learning situation.
- Determine the good points you made at the interview and those that were not so favorable. Study them and prepare yourself for the next interview.
- Make a list of the most frequently asked questions and think about your responses.
- Evaluate yourself, your behavior, your likes and dislikes, previous accomplishments that demonstrate your marketable skills, and your motivation. This will give you the self-confidence you need when responding to questions.
- Be prompt, be cordial, watch your body language, dress conservatively, and keep cell phones turned off.

Abbreviations and Acronyms

A

A&P	auscultation and percussion
a.c.	before meals
a.m.	morning
AB, Ab	abortion
ABG	arterial blood gas (gases)
AC	air conduction
ACC	accommodation
ACE	angiotensin converting enzyme
ACG	angiocardiography
ACL	anterior cruciate ligament
ACS	American Cancer Society
ACTH	adrenocorticotropic hormone
AD	right ear (auris dextra)
ADH	antidiuretic hormone
ADLs	activities of daily living
ad lib.	as needed
AE	above-elbow (amputation)
AF or A fib	atrial fibrillation
AFB	acid-fast bacilli
AFP	alpha fetoprotein
A/G	albumin/globulin ratio
AGN	acute glomerulonephritis
AHF	antihemophilic factor VIII
AHG	antihemophilic globulin factor VIII
AICA	anterior inferior communicating artery
AIDS	acquired immunodeficiency syndrome
AK	above-knee (amputation)
ALL	acute lymphocytic leukemia (lymphoblastic)
ALS	amyotrophic lateral sclerosis
ALT	alanine aminotransferase
AMA	American Medical Association
AML	acute myeloid leukemia
ANC	absolute neutrophil count
ANLL	acute nonlymphoblastic leukemia
ANS	autonomic nervous system
AOM	acute otitis media
AP	anterior posterior/anteroposterior
APL or APML	acute promyelocytic leukemia
ARDS	acute respiratory distress syndrome
AROM	active range of motion
AS	left ear (auris sinistra)/ aortic stenosis
ASD	atrio septal defect
ASHD	arteriosclerotic heart disease
AST	aspartate aminotransferase
ATN	acute tubular necrosis
AUB	abnormal uterine bleeding
AV	atrioventricular

B

BaE or BE	barium enema
baso	basophil
BBB	bundle-branch block
BBT	basal body temperature
BCC	basal cell carcinoma
BCE	basal cell epithelioma
BCM	below costal margin
BCP	birth control pill(s)
BE	below the elbow (amputation)
BFM	Berlin-Frankfurt-Munster; bicep femoral muscle
b.i.d.	twice a day
BiPAP	bilevel positive airway pressure
BK	below the knee (amputation)
BM	bowel movement/bone marrow
BMA	bone marrow aspiration
BMP	basic metabolic profile or panel
BMR	basal metabolic rate
BMT	bone marrow transplant
BNP	brain natriuretic peptide
BOM	bilateral otitis media
BOOP	bronchiolitis obliterans with organizing pneumonia
BP	blood pressure
BPH	benign prostatic hypertrophy
BRM	biological response modifier
BSE	breast self-exam
BSO	bilateral salpingo oophorectomy
BTL	bilateral tubal ligation
BUN	blood urea nitrogen (lab test)
Bx, BX, bx	biopsy

C

C	celsius or centigrade
C&S	culture and sensitivity
C1, etc.	cervical vertebrae
CA	cancer, carcinoma
CA-125	ovarian carcinoma antigen
Ca^+	calcium
CABG	coronary artery bypass grafting
CAD	coronary artery disease
CALLA	common acute lymphocytic leukemia antigen
cap	capsule

CAT scan	computerized axial tomograpy scan		DHEAS	dehydroepiandrosterone sulfate
CBC	complete blood count		DI	diabetes insipidus
CC	cardiac catheterization		DIC	disseminated intravascular coagulation
cc	cubic centimeter		diff	differential
CCU	coronary care unit		DIP joint	distal interphalangeal joint
CDH	congenital dislocation of the hip		DJD	degenerative joint disease
CEA	carcinoembryonic antigen		DM	diabetes mellitus
CF	circumflex (artery)		DNA	deoxyribonucleic acid
cGy	centigray		DNR	do not resuscitate
CHF	congestive heart failure		DO	Doctor of Osteopathy
CIN	cervical intraepithelial neoplasia		DOA	date of admission; dead on arrival
CK	creatine kinase		DOB	date of birth
CK-MB	creatine kinase myocardial band		DOS	date of service
Cl	chloride		DPT	diphtheria, pertussis, tetanus immunization
CLL	chronic lymphocytic leukemia			
cm	centimeter		DRE	digital rectal exam
CMG	cystometrogram		DSM-IV	*Diagnostic and Statistical Manual of Mental Disorders, Fourth Edition*
CML	chronic myelocytic leukemia			
CMV	cytomegalovirus		DTR	deep tendon reflex
CN	cranial nerves		DUB	dysfunctional uterine bleeding
CNS	central nervous system		DVT	deep vein thrombosis
c/o	complained of		DVT	deep venous thrombosis
CO_2	carbon dioxide		DX, Dx	diagnosis
COLD	chronic obstructive lung disease			
contra	against			

E

COPD	chronic obstructive pulmonary disease		EAC	external auditory canal
			EBV	Epstein-Barr virus
CP	chest pain		ECCE	extracapsular cataract extraction
CPAP	continuous positive airway pressure		ECG or EKG	electrocardiogram
CPD	cephalopelvic disproportion		ECT	electroconvulsive therapy
CPR	cardiopulmonary resuscitation		EDC	estimated date of confinement
CRC	colorectal cancer		EEG	electroencephalogram or electroencephalography
CRP	C-reactive protein			
CS, C-section	cesarean section		EENT	eye, ear, nose, and throat
CSF	cerebrospinal fluid		EF	ejection fraction
CT	computed tomography		EGD	esophagogastroduodenoscopy
CTS	carpal tunnel syndrome		ELISA	enzyme linked immunosorbent assay
CV	cardiovascular			
CVA	cerebrovascular accident/costovertebral angle		Em	emmetropia
			EMG	electromyography
			ENG	electronystagmography
CXR	chest x-ray		ENT	ear, nose, and throat
cysto	cystoscopy		EOM	extraocular muscles; extraocular movements

D

d	day		EOMI	extraocular muscle intact
D	diopter		eos	eosinophil
D&C	dilatation and curettage		ER	emergency room
D&E	dilation and evacuation		ERCP	endoscopic retrograde
dB	decibel		ERG	electroretinography
dbHL	decibel hearing level		ESR	erythrocyte sedimentation rate
DC	discharge		EST	electric shock therapy
DCBE	double (air) contrast barium enema		ESRD	end-stage renal disease
DCR	dacryocystorhinostomy		ESWL	extracorporeal shock-wave lithotripsy
DDD	degenerative disk disease		EtOH	ethanol (ethyl alcohol)
DDS	Doctor of Dental Surgery		et al.	and others
derm.	dermatology		EXT, ext	extremities
DES	diethylstilbestrol			

F

F	Fahrenheit
FAAP	Fellow of the Academy of Pediatrics
FAB	French-American-British Level 1 (classification system for leukemia)
FACP	Fellow of the American College of Physicians
FACS	Fellow of the American College of Surgeons
FAP	familial adenomatous polyposis
FBS	fasting blood sugar
FDA	Food and Drug Administration
FDG	^{18}F-fluoro-2-deoxyglucose fluorodeoxyglucose
FEF	forced expiratory flow
FEF_{25-75}	forced midexpiratory flow during the middle half of the FVC
FEKG	fetal electrocardiogram
FEV	forced expiratory volume
FEV_1	forced expiratory volume in one second
FEV_3	forced expiratory volume in three seconds
FH	family history
FHR	fetal heart rate
FHT	fetal heart tones
FIO_2	fractional inspired oxygen concentration
FOBT	fecal occult blood test
FROJM	full range of joint motion
FROM	full range of motion
FS	frozen section
FSH	follicle-stimulating hormone
FSIQ	full scale intelligence quotient
FTI	free thyroxine index
FTND	full term, normal delivery
FTNSVD	full term, normal spontaneous vaginal delivery
FUO	fever of unknown origin
FVC	forced vital capacity
FVL	flow volume loop
fx	fracture

G

g	gram
G6PD	glucose-6-phosphate dehydrogenase
GABHS	group A beta-hemolytic *streptococcus*
GAD	generalized anxiety disorder
GB	gallbladder
GC	gonococcus (gonorrhea)
GE	gastroesophageal
GERD	gastroesophageal reflux disease
GFR	glomerular filtration rate
GGT	gamma-glutamyl transferase
GI	gastrointestinal
gr	grain
GTT	glucose tolerance test
gtt, gtts	drop or drops

GU	genitourinary
Gy	gray
GYN	gynecology

H

h	hour
H&E	hematoxylin and eosin (stains for specimens on microscopic slides)
H/O	history of
HAL	hyperalimentation
HAV	hepatitis A virus
HBV	hepatitis B virus
hCG	human chorionic gonadotropin
HCl	hydrochloric acid
HCT, Hct	hematocrit
HCV	hepatitis C virus
HD	hip disarticulation/Hodgkin disease (Hodgkin lymphoma)
HDL	high density lipoprotein
HEENT	head, ears, eyes, nose, throat
HF	heart failure
Hg	mercury
HGB, Hgb	hemoglobin
HCG, hCG	human chorionic gonadotropin
HIV	human immunodeficiency virus
HLA	human leukocyte antigen
HNP	herniated nucleus pulposus
HNPCC	hereditary nonpolyposis colon cancer (Lynch Syndrome)
HP	hemipelvectomy
HPI	history of present illness
hpf	high-power field
HPV	human papillomavirus
HRT	hormone replacement therapy
hsCRP	highly sensitive C-reactive protein
h.s.	hour of sleep
HSG	hysterosalpingography
HSV-1	herpes simplex virus type 1
HSV-2	herpes simplex virus type 2
HTN	hypertension

I

I&D	incision and drainage
I&O	intake and output
IBD	inflammatory bowel disease
IBS	irritable bowel syndrome
ICA	internal carotid artery
ICCE	intracapsular cataract extraction
ICP	intracranial pressure
ICU	intensive care unit
ID	internal development (ortho)
Ig	immunoglobulin
IICP	increased intracranial pressure
IM	intramuscular
IMA	internal mammary artery
INR	international normalized ratio

IOL	intraocular lens
IOP	intraocular pressure
IPPB	intermittent positive pressure breathing
IQ	intelligence quotient
IS	incentive spirometry
IS	intracostal space
ITP	immune (idiopathic) thrombocytopenic purpura
IUD	intrauterine device
IV	intravenous
IVC	intravenous cholangiography
IVDA	intravenous drug abuser
IVIG	intravenous immunoglobulin
IVP	intravenous pyelogram

J

JVD	jugular venous distention

K

K	potassium
K+	potassium
kg	kilogram
KD	knee disarticulation
KOH	potassium hydroxide
KUB	kidneys, ureters, bladder (x-ray)

L

L	liter
L&A	light and accommodation
L1, etc.	lumbar vertebrae
LAD	left anterior descending coronary artery
LASIK	laser assisted in-situ keratomileusis
lb	pound
LAT	lateral
LCA	left coronary artery
LCF	left circumflex
LDH	lactate dehydrogenase
LDL	low density lipoprotein
LE	left eye
LEEP	loop electrosurgical excision procedure
LES	lower esophageal sphincter
LESI	lumbar epidural steroid injection
leuk	leukocytes
LH	luteinizing hormone
LIMA	left internal mammary artery
LLQ	left lower quadrant
LMCA	left main coronary artery
LMP	last menstrual period
LOC	loss of consciousness
LP	lumbar puncture
LPA	left pulmonary artery
LPN	Licensed Practical Nurse
LRQ	lower right quadrant
LUQ	left upper quadrant
lymphs	lymphocytes

M

m	meter
mcg	microgram
MAB	monoclonal antibody
MAC	*Mycobacterium avium-intracellular* complex
MAOI	monoamine oxidase inhibitor
MCH	mean corpuscular hemoglobin
MCHC	mean corpuscular hemoglobin concentration
MCL	midclavicular line
MCP joint	metacarpophalangeal joint
MCV	mean corpuscular volume
MD, M.D.	Medical Doctor or Doctor of Medicine
MDI	metered dose inhaler
mEq	millequivalents
mets	metastases
METs	metabolic equivalent of tasks
mg	milligram
MHC	major histocompatibility complex
MI	myocardial infarction
mm	millimeter
mn or m	minum
MMPI-2	Minnesota Multiphasic Personality Inventory-2
mono	monocyte
MPA	main pulmonary artery
MR	mitral regurgitation
MRA	magnetic resonance angiography
MRI	magnetic resonance imaging
MRSA	methicillin-resistant *Staphylococcus aureus*
MS	mitral stenosis
MS	multiple sclerosis
MTP joint	metatarsophalangeal joint
MUGA	multiple gated acquisition (scan)
MVP	mitral valve prolapse
MYOP or my	myopia

N

n.p.o.	nothing by mouth
Na+	sodium
NAD	no acute distress
NB	newborn, note well
NCV	nerve conduction velocity
neuts	neutrophils
NG	nasogastric
NKDA	no known drug allergy
NL	normal limits
NPH	neutral protamine Hegedron
NSAID	nonsteroidal anti inflammatory drug

O

O_2	oxygen
OA	osteoarthritis
OB	obstetrics

OCD	obsessive-compulsive disorder	PMN	polymorphonuclear leukocyte
OD	right eye (oculus dexter)/doctor of optometry/(drug) overdose	PMP	previous menstrual period
		PND	paroxysmal nocturnal dyspnea
OM	obtuse marginal (coronary artery)	PNH	paroxysmal nocturnal hematuria
OR	operating room	PNS	peripheral nervous system
ORIF	open reduction and internal fixation	polys	polymorphonuclear neutrophils
ortho	orthopedics	PPVT-III	Peabody Picture Vocabulary Test, Third Edition
os	mouth		
OS	left eye (oculus sinister)	PRK	photorefractive keratectomy
OTC	over the counter	PROM	passive range of motion
Oto	otology	PSA	prostate specific antigen
OU	both eyes (oculus uterque)	PT	prothrombin time; physical therapy
oz	ounce	PTA	prior to admission
		PTC	percutaneous transhepatic cholangiography

P

p.c.	after meals	PTH	parathyroid hormone
p.m.	afternoon, evening	PTSD	posttraumatic stress disorder
p.p.	postprandial (after eating)	PTT	partial thromboplastin time
p	pulse	PUD	peptic ulcer disease
P&A	percussion and auscultation	PVC	premature ventricular contraction
PA	posterior anterior; physician's assistant		
PAM	potential acuity meter		

Q

PAN	periodic alternating nystagmus	q.h.	every hour
PAP	positive airway pressure	q.2h	every 2 hour
Pap	Papanicolaou	q.i.d.	four times a day
PAT	paroxysmal atrial tachycardia	q.n.s.	quantity not sufficient
Path	pathology	q.o.d.	every other day
PBI	protein bound iodine		

R

PCI	percutaneous coronary intervention	R	respiration
PCOS	polycystic ovary syndrome	R/O	rule out
PCP	*pneumocystis* pneumonia/*pneumocystis jiroveci*	RA	rheumatoid arthritis
		rad	radiation dose
PCV	packed cell volume	RAD	reactive airway disease
PD	peritoneal dialysis	RAI	radiation iodine
PD	Parkinson disease	RAO	right anterior oblique (view)
PDA	posterior descending artery; patent ductus arteriosus	RAST	radioallergosorbent test
		RBC	red blood cell
PE	physical exam	RCA	right coronary artery
PE tubes	pressure-equalizing tubes	RDS	respiratory distress syndrome
PEEP	positive end expiratory pressure	RE	right eye
PEF	peak expiratory flow	REM	rapid eye movement
per	through, by	RF	rheumatoid factor
PERLA	pupils equal, reactive to light and accommodation	Rh	rhesus factor
		RICE	rest, ice, compression, and elevation
PERRLA	pupils equal, round, reactive to light and accommodation	RLQ	right lower quadrant
		RN, R.N.	Registered Nurse
PET	positron emission tomography	RNA	ribonucleic acid
pH	hydrogen ion concentration	ROJM	range of joint motion
PICA	posterior inferior communicating artery	ROM	range of motion
		ROP	retinopathy of prematurity
PID	pelvic inflammatory disease	RP	retrograde pyelogram
PIP joint	proximal interphalangeal joint	RPA	right pulmonary artery
PKU	phenylketonuria	RRR	regular rate and rhythm
plts or PLT	platelets	RSV	respiratory syncytial virus
PMD	primary medical doctor	RT	radiation therapy
PMH	past medical history		
PMI	point of maximal impulse		

RUQ	right upper quadrant
Rx, RX	prescription

S

S aureus	*staphylococcus aureus*
S1, etc.	sacral vertebrae
SA	sinoatrial node
SAR	seasonal allergic rhinitis
SBFT	small-bowel follow-through
SCC	squamous cell carcinoma
SD	shoulder disarticulation
sed rate	sedimentation rate (erythrocyte sedimentation rate)
segs	segmented neutrophils
SFA	superficial femoral artery
SIDS	sudden infant death syndrome
SL	semilunar
SLE	systemic lupus erythematosus
SMR	submucosal resection
SNS	somatic nervous system
SOB	shortness of breath
SOM	serous otitis media
Sp.gr.	specific gravity
SPECT	single photon emission computed tomography
SSRI	selective serotonin reuptake inhibitor
ST	esotropia
staph	*staphylococcus*
Stat	immediately
STD	sexually transmitted disease
strep	*streptococcus*

T

T	temperature
T&A	tonsillectomy and adenoidectomy
T1, etc.	thoracic vertebrae
tab	tablet
TAH	total abdominal hysterectomy
TAH/BSO	total abdominal hysterectomy with bilateral salpingo-oophorectomy
TAT	Thematic Apperception Test
TB	tuberculosis
tbs, tblsp	tablespoonful
TBS	The Bethesda System
TEE	transesophageal echocardiogram
TENS	transcutaneous electric nerve stimulation
THA	total hip arthroplasty
TIA	transient ischemic attack
t.i.d.	three times a day
TM	tympanic membrane
TMJ	temporomandibular joint
TNM	tumor, nodes, metastasis (refers to tumor staging)
TPN	total parenteral nutrition
TPR	temperature, pulse, respiration

TSH	thyroid stimulating hormone
tsp	teaspoonful
TTH	thyrotrophic hormone
TUR	transurethral resection (bladder or prostate)
TURP	transurethral resection of the prostate
Tx	treatment

U

UA or U/A	urinalysis
UC	uterine contractions
UGI	upper gastrointestinal
ULQ	upper left quadrant
ung.	ointment
UPJ	ureteropelvic junction
UPPP	uvulopalatopharyngoplasty
URI	upper respiratory infection
URQ	upper right quadrant
USP	United States Pharmacopeia
UTI	urinary tract infection
UV	ultraviolet
UVJ	ureterovesical junction

V

V/Q	ventilation/perfusion
VA	visual acuity
VBAC	vaginal birth after cesarean section
VC	vital capacity
VCUG	voiding cystourethrogram
VD	venereal disease
VHD	ventricular heart disease
VDRL	Venereal Disease Research Laboratory
VF	visual field
VH	vaginal hysterectomy
VLDL	very low density lipoprotein
VSD	ventricular septal defect

W

WAIS	Wechsler Adult Intelligence Scale
WBC	white blood cell
WDWN	well developed, well nourished
Wgt, wt	weight
WNL, W.N.L.	within normal limits
WMS-III	Wechsler Memory Scale, Third Edition

X

x	by (size, 5 x 5 inches)
XT	exotropia
XRT	x-ray therapy, radiation therapy
XX	female sex chromosomes
XY	male sex chromosomes

Glossary

A

abdomen
(ab-**dO**-men/**ab**-dO-men) (n) that part of the body between the chest and the pelvis (the lower part of the trunk of the body)

abduction
(ab-**duk**-shun) (n) the lateral movement of a limb away from the median plane of the body

abrasion
(a-**bray**-zhun) (n) scraping away of skin or mucous membrane by friction

abscess
(**ab**-ses) (n) a pus-filled cavity, usually because of a localized infection

accommodation
(ah-kom-o-**day**-shun) (n) the eye's ability to focus or see

achalasia
(ak-e-**lay**-zha) (n) failure to relax, especially a sphincter

acne
(**ak**-nee) (n) an eruption of papules or pustules on the skin, involving the oil glands

acyanotic
(ay-sI-a-**not**-ik) (adj) pertaining to the absence of cyanosis (slightly bluish, grayish, slatelike, or dark purple discoloration of the skin due to a reduction of oxygenated blood

additive
(**ad**-i-tiv) (n) a substance which is added in small quantities to improve the qualities of the original

adduction
(ad-**duk**-shun) (n) movement of a leg or arm toward the middle of the body

adenitis
(ad-e-**nI**-tis) (n) inflammation of a lymph node or gland

adenocarcinoma
(ad-en-O-**kar**-si-nO-ma) (n) malignant tumor of epithelial cells arising from the glandular structures which are a part of most organs of the body

adenoidectomy
(ad-e-noy-**dek**-tO-mee) (n) surgical removal of the adenoids from the nasopharynx

adenopathy
(ad-e-**nop**-a-thee) (n) swelling or enlargement of any gland, especially the lymph nodes

adenosis
(ad-e-**nO**-sis) (n) any disease of a gland, especially of a lymphatic gland

adhesion
(ad-**hee**-zhun) (n) the union of opposing surfaces, especially opposing surfaces of a wound in the abdominal cavity

adipose
(**ad**-i-pOz) (adj) containing fat

adjuvant
(**ad**-joo-vant) (n) therapy given to enhance another therapy's effect such as giving chemotherapy before surgical therapy

adnexal
(ad-**nek**-sal) (adj) relating to appendages or accessory parts of an organ

adrenarche
(**ad**-ren-ar-kee) (n) the beginning of hormonal activity that leads up to puberty and the associated sexual development

aerosol
(**ayr**-O-sol) (n) a liquid or solution dispensed as a fine mist or a product dispensed from a pressurized container as a fine mist

aerosolized
(**ayr**-O-sol-Izd) (adj) describing a solution that is dispensed in the form of a mist

afebrile
(ay-**feb**-rIl) (adj) without fever

afferent
(**af**-er-ent) (adj) inward or toward a center, as a nerve; carrying a sensory impulse

agglutination
(a-gloo-ti-**nay**-shun) (n) the process in which cells group or clump together, especially as a response to a specific antibody; commonly used in blood typing

agnosia
(ag-**nO**-see-a) (n) unable to perceive or recognize sensory stimuli

agraphia
(a-**graf**-ee-a) (n) impairment of the ability to write

akinesis

(ay-kI-**nee**-sis) (n) an extrapyramidal disorder causing a loss of power to perform voluntary movements

ala nasi

(**a**-la **nay**-sI) (adj) the outer flare of each nostril; alae nasi (a-lee) (pl)

albinism

(**al**-bi-nizm/al-**bin**-izm) (n) a congenital lack of melanin in the skin, hair, and eyes

albumin

(al-**byoo**-min) (n) a type of simple protein, varieties of which are widely distributed throughout the tissues and fluids

albuterol

(al-**byoo**-ter-ol) (n) bronchodilator available in oral and inhalent forms to be used in asthma, emphysema, and other lung conditions

alimentary canal

(al-i-**men**-ter-ee ka-**nal**) (n) gastrointestinal tract; tubelike structure through which food passes and is digested and absorbed

allergen

(**al**-er-jen) (n) a substance that produces an allergic reaction

allogeneic

(al-O-je-**ne**-ik) (adj) describing tissues or cell types that are from different individuals belonging to the same species; describing individuals of the same species

alopecia

(al-O-**pee**-shee-a) (n) partial or total loss of hair

alopecic

(al-O-**pee**-sik) (adj) relating to alopecia

alpha fetoprotein

(al-fa fee-tO-**prO**-teen) (n) a protein normally produced during the 12th to 15th week of gestation and may also appear in the serum of patients with embryonal carcinomas or carcinoma of the GI tract (stomach, colon, pancreas) or the lung

alveolus

(al-**vee**-O-lus) (n) tiny chambers of the lungs where the exchange of oxygen and carbon dioxide takes place; alveoli (al-vee-O-lI) (pl)

amblyopia

(am-blee-**O**-pee-a) (n) decreased vision in one or both eyes; not correctable

ambulation

(am-byoo-**lay**-shun) (n) walking or moving about

amenorrhea

(a-men-O-**ree**-a) (n) stoppage or absence of menses

amnesia

(am-**nee**-zee-a) (n) a disturbance of long-term memory; total or partial inability to recall past experiences

amniocentesis

(**am**-nee-O-sen-**tee**-sis) (n) taking a sample of amniotic fluid

amnion

(**am**-nee-on) (n) the inner of the fetal membranes; a thin transparent sac that holds the fetus

amphotericin

(**am**-fO-tear-a-sin) (n) a toxic antibiotic reserved for use in serious, potentially fatal infections of fungi and protozoa; amphotericin B

amplitude

(**am**-pli-tood) (n) the extent of a vibrating or alternating movement or wave from the average to the extreme; a louder sound has a greater amplitude

Amsler test

(**ahm**-zler) (n) used to evaluate visual field defects

anagen

(**an**-a-jen) (n) the actively growing phase of the hair growth cycle

anaphylactic

(**an**-a-fi-**lak**-tik) (adj) describing an allergic hypersensitivity reaction of the body to a substance

anaphylaxis

(an-a-fl-**lak**-sis) (n) a systemic reaction to an allergen

anastomosis

(a-**nas**-tO-mO-sis) (n) a natural or surgical connection between two blood vessels, spaces, or organs

anesthesia

(an-es-**thee**-zee-a) (n) absence of sensation, especially pain; usually applied to the medical technique of reducing or eliminating a person's sensation of pain to enable surgery to be performed

anesthetic

(**an**-es-**thet**-ik) (n) the medications used to produce anesthesia

aneurysm

(**an**-yoo-rizm) (n) bulging out of an arterial wall due to a weakness in the wall

angina pectoris

(**an**-ji-na/an-**jI**-na **pek**-tO-ris) (n) an attack of intense chest pain; also known as stenocardia

angiodysplasia

(**an**-jee-O-dis-**play**-zee-a) (n) degenerative stretching or enlarging of the blood vessels in an organ

angioedema

(an-jee-O-e-**dee**-ma) (n) periodically recurring episodes of noninflammatory swelling

angiography

(an-jee-**og**-ra-fee) (n) x-ray of blood vessels, usually after injecting a radiopaque substance

angioma

(an-jee-**O**-ma) (n) a swelling or tumor composed primarily of blood vessels; spider, strawberry, cherry angiomas

anhidrosis

(an-hI-**drO**-sis) (n) the suppression or absence of perspiration

anicteric

(an-ik-**ter**-ik) (adj) without jaundice or icterus (a yellowing of the skin and whites of the eyes)

ankylosis

(ang-ki-**lO**-sis) (n) stiffening or rigidity of a joint either as a result of a disease process or from surgery

ankylotic
(ang-ki-**lot**-ik) (adj) relating to or having ankylosis

annulus
(**an**-yoo-lus) (n) a circular structure or opening

anorexia
(an-O-**rek**-see-a) (n) diminished appetite; aversion to food

anosmia
(an-**ahz**-mee-a) (n) inability to smell

anovulation
(an-ov-yoo-**lay**-shun) (n) absence of egg production or release from the ovary

anovulatory
(an-**ov**-yoo-la-tOr-ee) (adj) not accompanied by production of or discharge of an ovum (egg) or suppressing ovulation

antecubital
(an-te-**kyoo**-bi-tal) (adj) front of the elbow; often the site for drawing blood

anteflexion
(an-te-**flek**-shun) (n) the abnormal position of an organ that is bent forward over itself

anterior
(an-**teer**-ee-or) (adj) front of a part, organ, or structure

antibody
(**an**-tee-bod-ee) (n) an immunoglobulin produced as an immune response to a specific antigen

anticholinergic
(an-tI-kO-lin-**er**-jik) (n) acting against an acetylcholine receptor; a class of drugs used to treat nausea

anticonvulsant
(**an**-tee-kon-**vul**-sant) (n) a therapeutic agent that prevents seizures

antiemetic
(**an**-ti-ee-**met**-ik) (n) pharmacologic agent used to decrease nausea and/or vomiting

antigen
(**an**-ti-jen) (n) a substance that causes the formation of an antibody which will react specifically to the antigen to neutralize, destroy, or weaken it

antiplatelet therapy
(anti-**playt**-let) (n) medications used to decrease platelet activity, reducing the likelihood of clot formation, especially in patients at risk for myocardial infarction

Antivert
(**an**-ti-vert) brand name for meclizine; used to treat vertigo

aorta
(ay-**Or**-ta) (n) the main artery leaving the heart

aortic root
(ay-**Or**-tik) (n) the opening of the aorta in the left ventricle of the heart

aortogram
(ay-**Or**-tO-gram) (n) x-ray of the aorta after injection of a radiopaque substance

Apgar score
(n) scoring system to assess newborn's physical condition

aphagia
(a-**fay**-jee-a) (n) inability to swallow

aphasia
(a-**fay**-zee-a) (n) difficulty with using and understanding words

aphonia
(a-**fO**-nee-a) (n) loss of the voice as a result of disease or injury

aphthous stomatitis
(**af**-thus stO-ma-**tI**-tis) (n) small ulcers of the mucous membrane of the mouth

apocrine
(**ap**-O-krin) (adj) relating to sweat glands

apophyseal
(a-pO-**fiz**-ee-al) (adj) relating to or having an apophysis

apophysis
(a-**pof**-i-sis) (n) a projection or outgrowth of a bone

apoptosis
(ap-O-**tO**-sis / **ap**-op-**tO**-sis) (n) a cell fragmenting into pieces which are phagocytosed by other cells; programmed cell death

aqueous humor
(**ak**-wee-us **hu**-mer) (n) the watery fluid that fills the anterior and posterior chambers of the eye

arachnoid
(a-**rak**-noyd) (n) the middle of the three membranes covering the brain; it is a delicate fibrous membrane, resembling a cobweb

arrhythmia
(a-**rith**-mee-a) (n) disturbance of normal rhythm; irregular heartbeat

arteriosclerosis
(ar-**teer**-ee-O-skler-**O**-sis) (n) hardening of the arteries

arteritis
(ar-tur-**I**-tis) (n) inflammation of one or more arteries

artery
(**ar**-ter-ee) (n) a vessel that carries blood away from the heart to other tissues throughout the body

arthralgia
(ar-**thral**-jee-a) (n) joint pain

arthritis
(ar-**thrI**-tis) (n) inflammation of one or more joints

arthroplasty
(**ar**-thrO-plas-tee) (n) surgical repair of a joint; creation of a new joint

articulation
(ar-tik-yoo-**lay**-shun) (n) the connecting of bones as a joint

arytenoid
(ar-i-**tee**-noid) (adj) resembling a ladle or pitcher mouth; (n) the muscle and cartilage of the larynx

arytenoid
(ar-i-**tee**-noyd) (n) cartilage and muscles of the larynx

ascending aorta
(n) the beginning section of the aorta, rising from the left ventricle of the heart to the arch

ascites
(a-**sI**-teez) (n) accumulation of fluid in the peritoneal cavity

asepsis
(a-**sep**-sis) (n) lack of germs; a state of sterility; methods used to create or maintain a sterile environment

aseptic
(a-**sep**-tik/ay-**sep**-tik) (adj) sterile; being without infection or contamination

asparaginase
(as-**par**-a-ji-nays) (n) an antineoplastic agent derived from the bacterium Escherichium coli

assessment
(as-**ses**-ment) (n) a complete evaluation of the patient; diagnosis

astereognosis
(a-**steer**-ee-og-**nO**-sis) (n) loss of the ability to judge the form of an object by touch

asthma
(**az**-ma) (n) respiratory disorder with temporary narrowing of the airways, resulting in difficulty in breathing, coughing, gasping, wheezing

astigmatism
(a-**stig**-ma-tizm) (n) visual condition in which light rays entering the eye are bent unequally, preventing a sharp focus point on the retina

asymmetry
(ay-**sim**-e-tree) (n) lack of symmetry of parts or organs on opposite sides of body

asymptomatic
(ay-simp-tO-**mat**-ik) (adj) without symptoms

ataxia
(a-**tak**-see-a) (n) muscular incoordination

atelectasis
(at-e-**lek**-ta-sis) (n) incomplete expansion of the lungs at birth or collapse of the adult lung

atherosclerosis
(**ath**-er-O-skler-**O**-sis) (n) buildup of fatty plaques inside arteries; a type of arteriosclerosis

atraumatic
(ay-traw-**mat**-ik) (adj) without injury or trauma

atresia
(a-**tree**-zee-a) (n) congenital absence or closure of a normal body opening or tubular structure

atrial
(**ay**-tree-al) (adj) relating to the atrium

atrioventricular
(**ay**-tree-O-ven-**trik**-yoo-lar) (adj) relating to both the atria (upper chambers) and the ventricles (lower chambers) in the heart, or blood flow between them

atrioventricular groove
(n) a groove visible on the outside of the heart between the atria and the ventricles

atrium
(**ay**-tree-um) (n) one of the two upper chambers of the heart

atrophy
(**at**-rO-fee) (n) a decrease in size of a part or organ; a wasting away of tissue as a result of disuse, radiation therapy, surgery, disease

attenuation
(a-ten-yoo-**ay**-shun) (n) process of weakening, such as the potency of a drug or the virulence of a disease-causing germ

audiologic
(aw-dee-O-**loj**-ik) (adj) pertaining to hearing disorders or loss

audiometry
(aw-dee-**om**-e-tree) (n) test used to measure hearing (using an audiometer)

aura
(**aw**-ra) (n) a sensation, as of light or warmth, that may precede an attack of migraine or a seizure

aural
(**aw**-ral) (adj) relating to the ear

auricle
(**aw**-ri-kl) (n) external ear; pinna

auscultation
(aws-kul-**tay**-shun) (n) process of listening through a stethoscope for sounds produced in some of the body cavities, especially chest and abdomen, in order to detect abnormal conditions

autoimmune disease
(aw-tO-i-**myoon**) (n) any disorder in which the body's immune responses produce antibodies that destroy the body's own tissues

autologous
(aw-**tol**-O-gus) (adj) indicating something that has its origin within an individual, especially a factor present in tissues or fluids

axial
(**ak**-see-al) (adj) situated in or relating to an axis

axilla
(**ak**-sil-a) (n) the armpit

axillary node
(**ak**-sil-ayr-ee nOd) (n) any of the lymph glands of the armpit that help to fight infection in the neck, chest, and arm area

B

B cell
(n) a type of lymphocyte; produces immunoglobulin antibodies in response to antigens

Babinski reflex
(bab-**in**-skeez **ree**-fleks) (n) an extension or moving of the big toe upward or toward the head, with the other toes fanned out and extended when the sole of the foot is stimulated

bacteremia
(bak-ter-**ee**-mee-a) (n) the presence of bacteria in the blood

Bactrim
(**back**-trim) (n) brand name for co-trimoxazole, a sulfonamide antibiotic

barotrauma
(bair-O-trah-ma) (n) injury caused by increased pressure

Barrett esophagus
(**bair**-it ee-**sof**-a gus) (n) chronic peptic ulceration of the lower esophagus

bedsore
(**bed**-sor) (n) an infected wound on the skin that occurs at pressure points in patients confined to bed

benign
(bee-**nIn**) (adj) describing a mild illness or a nonmalignant tumor

bibasilar
(bI-**bays**-i-lar) (adj) occurring in both bases

bifurcation
(bI-fer-**kay**-shun) (n) forking into two branches

bilateral
(bI-**lat**-er-al) (adj) affecting or relating to two sides

bile
(bIl) (n) a thick, yellow-green-brown fluid secreted by the liver

biliary
(**bil**-ee-ayr-ee) (adj) relating to bile or the gallbladder and its ducts

bilirubin
(bil-i-**roo**-bin) (n) a red bile pigment, formed from hemoglobin during normal and abnormal destruction of erythrocytes

biopsy
(**bI**-op-see) (n) removal of a small amount of tissue and/or fluid from the body for microscopic examination; the specimen obtained

bleomycin
(blee-O-**mI**-sin) (n) antitumor agents

blepharectomy
(blef-ar-**ek**-tO-mee) (n) excision of a lesion of the eyelid

blepharitis
(blef-a-**rI**-tis) (n) inflammation of the eyelid

bolus
(**bO**-lus) (n) a mass of something such as masticated (chewed) food or substance that is ready to be swallowed; an amount of medication

Botox
(**bO**-tawks) (n) Clostridium botulinum toxin A, injected into the skin around the eyes, forehead, and lips to remove facial lines

Bovie
(**bO**-vee) (n) an instrument used for electrocautery

brachial
(**bray**-kee-al) (adj) pertaining to the arm

Braxton Hicks sign
(n) irregular contractions of the uterus after the first trimester of pregnancy

BRCA 1 and 2 genes
("braka 1" and "braka 2") (n) acronym for two genes associated with increased risk of breast and ovarian cancer

breech presentation
(n) fetal position in which the feet or buttocks appear first in the birth canal

bronchial
(**brong**-kee-al) (adj) relating to the bronchi

bronchiectasis
(brong-kee-**ek**-ta-sis) (n) persistent, abnormal widening of the bronchi, with an associated cough and spitting up of mucus

bronchiole
(**brong**-kee-Ol) (n) one of the smaller subdivisions of the bronchi

bronchitis
(brong-**kI**-tis) (n) inflammation of the bronchi

bronchovesicular
(**brong**-kO-ve-**sik**-yoo-lar) (adj) relating to the bronchioles and alveoli in the lungs

bronchus
(**brong**-kus) (n) the divisions of the trachea leading to the lungs; bronchi (brong-kI) (pl)

Brudzinski sign
(n) in meningitis, if a leg is passively flexed, a similar movement occurs in the other leg; if the neck is passively flexed, the legs also flex

bruit
(**broo**-ee/broot) (n) an adventitious sound of venous or arterial origin heard on auscultation

buccal
(**buk**-al) (adj) relating to the area inside the cheek

bulbar
(**bul**-bar) (adj) bulb-shaped or relating to the medulla oblongata in the brain

bulimia
(boo-**lim**-ee-a) (n) a chronic disorder involving repeated and secretive bouts of binge eating followed by self-induced vomiting, use of laxatives, or vigorous exercise in order to prevent weight gain

bulla
(**bul**-a) (n) large bleb in the skin that contains fluid; bullae (pl)

bullae
(**bul**-ee) (n, pl) blisters of the skin containing clear fluid

C

cachexia
(ka-**kek**-see-a) (n) a general weight loss and wasting occurring in the course of a chronic disease or emotional disturbance

café-au-lait spots
(kaf-ay-O-**lay** spots) (n) light brown spots of patchy pigmentation of the skin

calcaneus
(kal-**kay**-nee-us) (n) heel bone; calcanei (kal-kay-nee-I) (pl)

calcification
(**kal**-si-fi-**kay**-shun) (n) a hardening of tissue resulting from the formation of calcium salts within it

calculus
(**kal**-kyoo-lus) (n) stone; a hard stone-like mass formed in the body; calculi (pl)

caliber
(**kal**-i-ber) (n) diameter of a tube or vessel; e.g., a blood vessel

callous
(**kal**-us) (adj) being hardened and thickened, having calluses; also feeling no emotion or sympathy

callus
(**kal**-us) (n) thickened skin that develops at points of pressure or friction; the bony deposit which develops around the broken ends of bone during healing

candidal rash
(**kan**-di-dal rash) (n) a rash which usually includes itching, a white discharge, peeling, and easy bleeding; caused by the yeastlike fungus Candida; common examples are diaper rash, thrush, and vaginitis

cannula
(**kan**-yoo-la) (n) a tube for insertion into a duct or cavity to allow the escape of fluid

cannulate
(**kan**-yoo-layt) (v) to introduce a cannula through a passageway

capillary
(**kap**-i-layr-ee) (n) smallest type of blood vessels connecting arterioles and venules

capillary fragility
(**kap**-i-layr-ee) (n) used in a test to determine the presence of vitamin C deficiency or thrombocytopenia; pressure is applied to the arm, and then the number of petechiae (representing broken capillaries) in a small area are counted

capnography
(cap-**nog**-ra-phy) (n) measurement of exhaled carbon dioxide via a capnogram which produces a visual display of the exhaled carbon dioxide

capsular
(**cap**-soo-lar) (adj) pertaining to a sheath of continuous enclosure around an organ or structure

carbuncle
(**kar**-bung-kl) (n) subcutaneous, pus-filled interconnecting pockets, caused by staphylococcal infection; eventually discharges through an opening in the skin

carcinoma
(kar-si-**nO**-ma) (n) malignant growth of epithelial cells that occurs in the linings of the body parts and in glands

cardiac tamponade
(**kar**-dee-ak tam-po-**nayd**) (n) compression of the venous return to the heart by fluid or blood in the pericardium

cardiomyopathy
(**kar**-dee-O-mI-**op**-a-thee) (n) disease of the heart muscle

cardioversion
(**kar**-dee-O-ver-zhun) (n) the conversion of an abnormal cardiac rhythm to a normal cardiac rhythm

carotid
(ka-**rot**-id) (n) paired arteries (right and left) that arise from the aorta and provide the principal blood supply to the head and neck

carpal
(**car**-pal) (adj) relating to a carpus, a bone in the wrist

carpal tunnel
(**kar**-pul **tun**-nul) (n) where the median nerve and flexor tendons pass through the wrist

caruncle
(**kar**-ung-kl) (n) small, fleshy outgrowth

cataract
(**kat**-a-rakt) (n) clouding of the lens of the eye, resulting in loss of transparency

catheter
(**kath**-e-ter) (n) a tube inserted into the body for removing or instilling fluids for diagnostic or therapeutic purposes

catheterization
(**kath**-e-ter-I-**zay**-shun) (n) the insertion of a catheter

causalgia
(kaw-**zal**-jee-a) (n) burning pain, usually associated with peripheral nerve damage

cauterization
(kaw-ter-i-**zay**-shun) (n) destroying tissue by burning for medical reasons

cautery
(**kaw**-ter-ee) (n) a means of destroying tissue by electricity, freezing, heat, or corrosive chemicals

cavernous sinus thrombosis
(**kav**-er-nus **sI**-nus throm-**bO**-sis) (n) a group of symptoms caused by an obstruction in the cavernous intracranial sinus

cecum
(**see**-kum) (n) any part ending in a cul-de-sac; specifically the closed, pocket-like beginning of the large intestine in the lower right part of the abdomen

ceftazidime
(sef-**taz**-i-deem) (n) antibiotic used in the treatment of moderate to severe infections

cellular
(**sel**-yoo-lar) (adj) composed of or derived from cells

cellular immunity
(n) immunity which is based on the T cells recognizing the antigen itself, rather than the presence of an antibody; cell-mediated immunity

cellulitis
(sel-yoo-**lI**-tis) (n) inflammation of the connective tissue caused by infection

centimeter
(**sen**-ti-mee-ter) (n) unit of measurement; one hundredth of a meter; approximately 0.4 inches

central nervous system (CNS)
(n) portion of the nervous system consisting of the brain and spinal cord

cephalad
(**sef**-a-lad) (adv) toward the head

cephalalgia
(**sef**-al-**al**-jee-a) (n) headache

cephalocaudal
(**sef**-a-lO-**caw**-dal) (adj) relating to the axis of the body from the head to the base of the spine

cerclage
(sair-**klazh**) (n) procedure to encircle tissues with a ligature, wire, or loop

cerebellar
(ser-e-**bel**-ar) (adj) relating to the cerebellum, the part of the brain concerned with the coordination and control of voluntary muscular activity

cerebrospinal
(**ser**-a-brO-**spI**-nal, se-**ree**-brO-**spI**-nal) (adj) referring to the brain and spinal cord

cerebrovascular
(ser-e-brO-**vas**-kyoo-lar) (adj) relating to the blood vessels of the brain, especially to pathological changes

cerumen
(se-**roo**-men) (n) earwax

cervical
(**ser**-vi-kal) (adj) relating to a neck, or cervix, especially the neck (cervix) of the uterus

cervix

(**ser**-viks) (n) the neck or part of an organ resembling a neck, such as the cervix of the uterus

chalazion

(ka-**lay**-zee-on) (n) a chronic inflammatory granuloma of the meibomian gland

chancre

(**shang**-ker) (n) hard sore; the sore that develops at the site of entry of a pathogen

chemosis

(kee-**mO**-sis) (n) an accumulation of fluid in the eye, causing swelling around the cornea

chemotherapy

(kem-O-**thayr**-a-pee / **keem**-O-thayr-a-pee) (n) treatment of disease with drugs

chloasma

(klO-**as**-ma) (n) light brown patches on the face and elsewhere; commonly associated with pregnancy

choana

(kO-an-a) (n) a funnel-shaped opening, especially the posterior opening of the nasal cavity into the nasopharynx

cholangiography

(kO-lan-jee-**og**-ra-fee) (n) x-ray examination of the bile ducts

cholecystectomy

(**kO**-lee-sis-**tek**-tO-mee) (n) excision of the gallbladder

cholecystitis

(**kO**-lee-sis-tI-tis) (n) inflammation or irritation of gallbladder, usually caused by the presence of gallstones

choledocholithiasis

(kO-**led**-O-kO-lith-I-a-sis) (n) presence of calculi (stones) in the common bile duct

cholelithiasis

(kO-lee-lith-I-a-sis) (n) formation or presence of gallstones in the gallbladder which may not cause any symptoms or perhaps only vague abdominal discomfort and intolerance to certain foods

cholesteatoma

(kO-les-tee-a-**tO**-ma) (n) a tumor-like mass of scaly epithelium and cholesterol in the middle ear

chondral

(**kon**-drul) (adj) relating to cartilage

chondritis

(kon-**drI**-tis) (n) inflammation of cartilage

chondromalacia

(**kon**-drO-ma-**lay**-shee-a) (n) softening of cartilage

chordae tendineae

(**kOr**-dee ten-**din**-ee-ay) (n) small tendinous cords (strands) that connect the free edges of the atrio-ventricular valves to the papillary muscles

choroid

(**kO**-royd) (n) a vascular membrane surrounding the eyeball, between the retina and sclera

chromosome

(**krO**-mO-sOm) (n) the structure in the cell nucleus that transmits genetic information; consists of a double strand of DNA in the form of a helix; there are normally 46 in humans

Chvostek sign

(**khvosh**-teks) (n) an abnormal spasm of facial muscles when the facial nerve is tapped lightly

cicatrix

(**sik**-a-triks) (n) scar

ciliary action

(**sil**-ee-ar-ee) (n) the lashing movement of a group of cilia, which can produce a current of movement in a fluid

cilium

(**sil**-ee-um) (n) a short hairlike extension of a cell surface, capable of lashlike movement, which aids in the movement of unicellular organisms and in the movement of fluids in higher organisms; eyelash; cilia (pl)

circumflex

(**ser**-kum-fleks) (adj) bending around; describes anatomical structures that are shaped like an arc of a circle

circumscribed

(**ser**-kum-skrIbd) (adj) having a boundary; confined

cirrhosis

(sir-**rO**-sis) (n) a degenerative liver disease characterized by damaged cell function and impaired blood flow

cirrhotic

(sir-**rot**-ik) (adj) affected with cirrhosis

claudication

(klaw-di-**ka**-shun) (n) limping; painful cramps in calf of leg due to poor blood circulation

clavicle

(**klav**-i-kl) (n) clavicula; collar bone

clavicula

(kla-**vik**-yoo-la) (n) clavicle; collar bone

clavicular

(kla-**vik**-yoo-lar) (adj) pertains to the clavicle, or collarbone

clonus

(**klO**-nus) (n) abnormal condition in which a skeletal muscle alternately contracts and relaxes

clubbing

(**klub**-ing) (n) condition of the fingers and toes in which their ends become wide and thickened; often a sign of disease, especially heart or lung disease

coagulation

(kO-ag-yoo-**lay**-shun) (n) process of blood clotting

coagulopathy

(kO-ag-yoo-**lop**-a thee) (n) a disorder affecting the blood's ability to clot correctly

cochlea

(**kok**-lee-a) (n) a spiral-shaped cavity in the internal ear

collagen

(**kol**-le-jen) (n) the gelatin or sticky substance of skin, bone, cartilage, ligaments, and connective tissue

collaterals

(ko-**lat**-er-als) (n) accompanying, as side by side; blood vessels that branch from larger vessels

colonic
(ko-**lon**-ic) (adj) pertaining to the colon

colostomy
(kO-**los**-to-mee) (n) surgical creation of an opening in the abdominal wall to allow material to pass from the bowel through that opening rather than through the anus

colostrum
(kO-**los**-trum) (n) the first milk secreted after childbirth

colposcopy
(kol-**pos**-ko-pee) (n) examination of the tissues of the vagina and cervix with a lighted instrument that magnifies the cells

comedo
(**kom**-i-dO) (n) in a hair follicle or oil gland, a plug of dead cells and oily secretions; blackhead; comedones (com-i-dO-neez) (pl)

communicable
(ko-**myoon**-i-ka-bl) (adj) contagious; capable of being spread with direct or indirect contact

complement
(**kom**-ple-ment) (n) a group of proteins that make up a component of the immune system which causes the destruction of foreign cells that have been tagged with complement-fixing antibodies

compressible
(kom-**pres**-i-bl) (adj) pressed together; made more compact by or as by pressure

concha
(**kon**-ka) (n) a shell-shaped anatomical structure, such as the auricle of the ear; conchae (pl)

concussion
(kon-**kush**-un) (n) an injury resulting from violent striking or shaking, especially an injury to the brain

conductive deafness
(n) hearing impairment due to obstruction of sound waves; the sound waves are not passed on to the inner ear

condyle
(**kon**-dil) (n) the rounded projecting end of a bone where ligaments are attached

condyloma
(kon-di-**lO**-ma) (n) warty growth in the genital area

confluent
(**kon**-floo-ent) (adj) merging together; connecting

congenital
(kon-**jen**-I-tal) (adj) present at birth

congestive heart failure
(CHF) (kon-**jes**-tiv) (n) condition in which the heart is unable to pump adequate blood to the tissues and organs, often due to myocardial infarction

conjunctiva
(kon-junk-**ti**-va) (n) the mucous membrane covering the front of the eyeball and inside the eyelids; conjunctivae (pl)

conjunctival
(kon-junk-**tI**-val) (n) pertaining to the mucous membrane that lines eyelids and is reflected onto eyeball

conjunctivitis
(kon-junk-ti-**vI**-tis) (n) inflammation of the conjunctiva

consolidation
(kon-sol-i-**day**-shun (n) solidification into a firm, dense mass

contusion
(kon-**too**-zhun) (n) a bruise

coprolalia
(kOp-rO-**lay**-lee-a) (n) involuntary utterance of obscene words, often seen in Tourette syndrome

cornea
(**kor**-nee-a) (n) the outer, transparent portion of the eye through which light passes to the retina

corneal
(**kor**-nee-al) (adj) the clear, transparent, anterior portion of the fibrous coat of the eye composing about one-sixth of its surface

cornual
(kor-noo-al) (adj) relating to a horn-shaped structure, as in the cornual area of the uterus

coronal
(ka-**rO**-nal) (adj) pertaining to a corona, a structure resembling a crown

coronary bypass surgery
(**kOr**-o-nayr-ee) (n) vein grafts or other surgical methods are used to carry blood from the aorta to branches of the coronary arteries in order to increase the flow beyond a local obstruction

coronary cusp
(n) one of the triangular parts of a heart valve

cor pulmonale
(kore pool-mO-**nah**-ly) (n) pulmonary disease which causes backward pressure on heart and resulting heart damage due to resistance to blood flow through the lung tissue

cortex
(**kor**-tex) (n) the outer layer of an organ, such as the kidney, as distinguished from the inner portion, or medulla

cortical
(**kOr**-ti-kal) (adj) relating to a cortex

corticomedullary junction
(**kOr**-tee-kO-**med**-yoo-lar-ee **jungk**-shun) (n) coming together (junction) of the cortex and medulla of the kidneys

coryza
(ko-**rI**-za) (n) acute rhinitis; acute head cold; inflammation of the mucous membrane of the nose with sneezing, tearing, and watery nasal discharge

costal
(**kos**-tal) (adj) relating to or located near a rib; the costal margin is the area at the lower end of the rib cage

costophrenic
(kos-tO-**fren**-ik) (adj) pertaining to the ribs and diaphragm

Coumadin
(**coo**-mah-din) (n) Brand name for warfarin, an agent to prevent blood clots

COX-2 inhibitor
(KOX too in-**hi**-bi-tor) (n) an agent which inhibits production of cyclo-oxygenase-2; a class of drugs used to treat pain, especially arthritis

craniotomy
(cray-nee-**ot**-O-mee) (n) surgical opening into the skull, performed to control bleeding, remove tumors, relieve pressure inside the cranium, or insert electrodes for diagnosis

cranium
(**kray**-nee-um) (n) the bony skull that holds the brain

crepitus
(**krep**-i-tus) (n) grating sound or vibration made by movement of fractured bones (bone fragments); crepitation

cribriform
(**krib**-ri-form) (adj) perforated with small holes of uniform size; (n) a polyporous structure

cricoid cartilage
(**krI**-koyd) (n) a ring-shaped cartilage in the lower part of the larynx

Crohn disease
(krOn) (n) chronic inflammatory condition affecting the colon and/or terminal part of the small intestine and producing frequent episodes of diarrhea, abdominal pain, nausea, fever, weakness, and weight loss

cryosurgery
(**krI**-O-ser-jer-ee) (n) the use of extreme cold to destroy tissue

cryptitis
(crip-**tI**-tis) (n) inflammation of a crypt or follicle

cul-de-sac
(kool-de-**sak**) (n) a blind pouch

culdoscopy
(kool-**dos**-kO-pee) (n) introduction of an endoscope through the posterior vaginal wall

culture
(**kul**-chur) (n) propagation of microorganisms in a solid or liquid medium

cupping
(**cup**-ping) (n) formation of a hollow or cup-shaped excavation

curettage
(koo-re-**tahzh**) (n) scraping of an interior of a cavity, usually to remove growths or tissue

cutaneous
(koo-**tay**-nee-us) (adj) pertaining to the skin

cuticle
(**kyoo**-ti-kl) (n) the edge of thickened skin around the bed of a nail; the sheath surrounding the base of a hair follicle

cyanosis
(sI-a-**nO**-sis) (n) bluish discoloration of the skin and/or mucous membranes, occurring when the oxygen in the blood is sharply diminished, as in carbon monoxide poisoning

cyanotic
(sI-a-**not**-ik) (adj) pertaining to cyanosis

cyclooxygenase-2
(sI-**klO**-oks-i-jen-**ays**) (n) a prostaglandin produced by the body which promotes pain and inflammation.

cyst
(sist) (n) a bladder or an abnormal sac containing gas, fluid, or a semi-solid material

cystic
(**sis**-tik) (adj) relating to a cyst

cystic duct
(n) the duct of the gallbladder which unites with the hepatic duct from the liver to form the common bile duct

cystic fibrosis
(**sis**-tik fI-**brO**-sis) (n) an inherited disease in which the mucus-producing glands become clogged with thick mucus; digestion and respiration are affected

cystitis
(sis-**tI**-tis) (n) inflammation of the urinary bladder

cystoscopy
(sis-**tos**-ko-pee) (n) examination of the inside of the urinary bladder with a lighted instrument inserted through the urethra

cystostomy
(sis-**tos**-tO-mee) (n) surgical creation of an opening in the bladder

cytokines
(**sI**-tO-kIns) (n) proteins that are not antibodies but are released on contact with a specific antigen as an immune response

cytomegalovirus
(sI-tO-**meg**-a-lO-**vI**-rus) (n) CMV; one of a group of species-specific herpes viruses which causes infected cells to become enlarged

D

dacryocystorhinostomy
(**dak**-ree-O-sis-tO-rI-**nos**-tO-mee) (n) a surgical opening to provide drainage between the tear duct and the nasal mucosa

dactylomegaly
(dak-til-O-**meg**-a-lee) (n) abnormal enlargement of one or more fingers or toes

debride
(da-**breed**/dee-**brId**) (v) to remove unhealthy tissue and foreign material to prevent infection and permit healing

debulking
(n) a surgical procedure to remove part of a tumor which otherwise cannot be completely excised

decelerations
(dee-cel-er-**ay**-shunz) (n) decreases in speed or rate (of contractions)

decompression
(**dee**-kom-presh-un) (n) removal of bone to relieve pressure

deep vein (or venous) thrombosis
(deep vayn throm-**bO**-sis) (n) a clump of various blood components in a blood vessel, forming an obstruction

defervescence
(def-er-**ves**-ens) (n) time that marks the decline of fever to normal temperature

defibrillator
(dee-**fib**-ri-lay-ter) (n) an agent, measure, or machine, e.g., an electric shock, that stops fibrillation of the ventricular muscle and restores the normal beat

degenerative
(di-**jen**-er-a-tiv) (adj) relating to or causing deterioration or worsening of a condition

dehydration
(dee-hI-**dray**-shun) (n) extreme loss of water from the body tissues

delusion
(dee-**loo**-zhun) (n) belief in something in spite of incontrovertible evidence

dementia
(dee-**men**-shee-a) (n) a general mental deterioration due to organic or psychological factors

Demerol
(**dem**-err-all) (n) brand name for meperidine, a narcotic analgesic

dermabrasion
(**der**-ma-bray-zhun) (n) peeling of skin done by a mechanical device with sandpaper or wire brushes

dermatitis
(der-ma-**tI**-tis) (n) inflammation of skin often evidenced by itching, redness, and lesions

dermatitis medicamentosum
(der-ma-**tI**-tis med-i-ka-men-**tO**-sa) (n) a skin eruption caused by ingestion, injection, or inhalation of a drug

dermatology
(der-ma-**tol**-o-jee) (n) the study of the skin, hair, and nails

dermatophyte
(**der**-ma-tO-flt) (n) a parasitic fungus that causes skin disease

desiccate
(**des**-i-kayt) (v) to dry out

Dexedrine
(**dex**-a-dreen) (n) brand name for dextroamphetamine, a CNS stimulant

diabetes insipidus
(dI-a-**bee**-tez in-**sip**-i-doos) (n and adj) disease caused by insufficient secretion of antidiuretic hormone (AHD) from the posterior pituitary gland

diagnosis
(dI-ag-**nO**-sis) (n) deciding the nature of a medical condition by examination of the symptoms; diagnoses (pl)

diaphoresis
(**dI**-a-fO-**ree**-sis) (n) profuse perspiration or sweating

diaphoresis
(**dI**-a-fO-**ree**-sis) (n) profuse perspiration or sweating

diaphragm
(**dI**-a-fram) (n) the muscle that separates the thoracic (chest) and abdominal cavities

diaphysis
(dI-**af**-i-sis) (n) shaft of a long bone

diathesis
(dI-a-**thee**-sis) (n) unusual predisposition to certain disease conditions

diffuse
(di-**fyoos**) (adj) spreading, scattered

digital
(**dij**-i-tal) (adj) relating to or resembling a finger or toe

digoxin
(di-**jok**-sin) (n) a heart stimulant

Dilantin
(dill-**ann**-tin) (n) brand name for phenytoin, used for the prevention and management of seizures

dilatation
(dil-a-**tay**-shun) (n) stretching or enlarging; dilation

dilation
(dI-**lay**-shun) (n) expansion of an organ or vessel

diltiazem
(dil-**tie**-a-zem) (n) a generic calcium channel blocker, used for hypertension

diplopia
(di-**plO**-pee-a) (n) double vision

discrete
(dis-**kreet**) (adj) separate; distinct

distal
(**dis**-tal) (adj) away from a center or point of reference; toward the far end of something

distally
(**dis**-ta-lee) (adv) occurring farthest from the center, from a medial line, or from the trunk

distention
(dis-**ten**-shun) (n) the state of being stretched out or inflated

distraction
(dis-**trak**-shun) (n) a force applied to body parts to separate bony fragments or joint surfaces

distress
(n) trouble; mental or physical suffering

diuretic
(dI-yoo-**ret**-ik) (n) an agent that increases the excretion of urine

diverticula
(dI-ver-**tik**-yoo-la) (n) sacs or pouches in the walls of a canal or organ

diverticulosis
(**dI**-ver-tik-yoo-**lO**-sis) (n) presence of diverticula (pouches) in the intestinal tract

Doppler
(**dop**-ler) (n) a diagnostic instrument that emits an ultrasonic beam into the body

dorsal
(**dor**-sal) (adj) relating to the back; posterior

dorsum
(**dOr**-sum) (n) the back or posterior surface of a part

ductus arteriosus
(**duk**-tus ar-ter-ee-**O**-sus) (n) blood vessel in the fetus connecting the pulmonary artery directly to the ascending aorta, thus bypassing the pulmonary circulation

duodenum
(doo-O-**dee**-num / doo-**od**-e-num) (n) first part of the small intestine; it receives material from the stomach and passes it to the jejunum, the medial part of the small intestine

dural
(**doo**-ral) (adj) pertaining to the dura mater, the outer membrane covering the spinal cord and brain

dura mater
(**doo**-ra **may**-ter / **mah**-ter) (n) the outermost of the three membranes surrounding the brain and spinal cord; it is tough and fibrous

dyseidetic
(dis-I-**det**-ik) (adj) inability to visualize and recall objects (words) previously seen

dysfunction
(dis-**funk**-shun) (n) abnormal or impaired function

dysgerminoma
(dis-jer-mi-**nO**-ma) (n) a rare cancerous ovarian tumor

dysgeusia
(dis-**goo**-see-a) (n) dysfunctional sense of taste

dyslexia
(dis-**lek**-see-a) (n) impairment of ability to read in which letters and words are reversed

dyslipidemia
(dis-lip-i-**dee**-mee-a)(n) abnormal ratios of high density lipoproteins (HDL), low density lipoproteins (LDL) and very low density lipoproteins (VLDL) in the blood

dysmenorrhea
(dis-men-Or-**ee**-a) (n) painful menstruation

dyspareunia
(dis-pa-**roo**-nee-a) (n) painful sexual intercourse

dyspepsia
(dis-**pep**-see-a) (n) imperfect digestion; epigastric discomfort

dysphagia
(dis-**fay**-jee-a) (n) difficulty swallowing

dysphonetic
(dis-fO-**net**-ik) (adj) inability to connect sounds to objects (words)

dysphoria
(dis-**fOr**-ee-a) (n) mood characterized by anxiety, depression, discontent

dyspnea
(disp-**nee**-a) (n) shortness of breath; difficulty in breathing

dysuria
(dis-**yoo**-ree-a) (n) painful or difficult urination, symptomatic of numerous conditions (e.g., cystitis; urethritis; infection in urinary tract)

E

ecchymosis
(ek-i-**mO**-sees) (n) small, hemorrhagic, discolored, purplish ("black and blue") spots resulting from an accumulation of blood under the skin's surface; ecchymoses (pl)

eccrine
(**ek**-rin) (adj) relating to sweat glands

echocardiogram
(ek-O-**kar**-dee-O-gram) (n) a sound-wave image of the heart's size, position, and motion

echolalia
(ek-O-**lay**-lee-a) (n) involuntary repetition of a word or sentence just spoken by another person

ectopic pregnancy
(ek-**top**-ik) (n) pregnancy in which a fertilized ovum is implanted outside the uterus, often in a fallopian tube

eczema
(**ek**-si-ma / **eg**-ze-ma) (n) inflammatory condition of the skin characterized by blisters, redness, and itching

edema
(e-**dee**-ma) (n) excessive accumulation of fluid in tissues, especially just under the skin or in a given cavity

edematous
(e-**dem**-a-tus) (adj) having edema

effacement
(ee-**fays**-ment) (n) thinning of the cervix just before or during labor

effusion
(e-**fyoo**-zhun) (n) escape of fluid into a cavity or tissues; the fluid itself

egophony
(ee-**gof**-O-nee) (n) an abnormal voice sound, like the bleating of a goat

ejection fraction
(e-**jec**-shun **frak**-shun) (n) the fraction of blood expelled from the ventricle after contraction, normally 50–60%

electrocardiogram
(ee-**lek**-trO-**kar**-dee-**O**-gram) (n) a graphic record of electrical waves within the heart

electrocautery
(ee-**lek**-trO-**caw**-ter-ee) (n) application of a needle or snare heated by an electric current to destroy tissue

electrodesiccation
(el-ek-trO-de-si-**kay**-shun) (n) destruction of tissue by the use of electrical current; fulguration

electrolysis
(el-ek-**trol**-i-sis) (n) destruction of a hair follicle by passing an electrical current through it

electrolyte
(ee-**lek**-trO-lIt) (n) an ionized chemical capable of conducting an electric current; the body contains many different electrolytes in specific amounts to keep it functioning properly

electron
(ee-**lek**-tron) (n) a subatomic particle with a negative charge

electrophoresis
(ee-**lek**-trO-fO-**ree**-sis) (n) the movement of charged suspended particles through a liquid medium in response to changes in an electric field; for example, a hemoglobin electrophoresis measures the types of hemoglobin in the blood

ellipse
(el-**lipz**) (n) a conic section taken either parallel to an element or parallel to the axis of the intersected cone; an oval

elute
(ee-**loot**) to remove from a solid by gradually dissolving in fluid

embolism
(**em**-bO-lizm) (n) blockage of a blood vessel by an abnormal object, such as a clot

embryo
(**em**-bree-O) (n) in humans, the developing prenatal child from conception to the end of the second month

embryonal
(**em**-bree-O-nal) (adj) relating to an embryo; in an early stage of development

emesis
(**em**-e-sis) (n) vomiting; may be of gastric, systemic, nervous, or reflex origin

emetic
(e-**met**-ik) (n) pharmacologic agent used to induce vomiting and eliminate toxic substances

empiric
(em-**pir**-ik) (adj) based on practical experience or observation

en bloc
(ahn blok) (adj) as a whole, in one piece

encephalopathy
(en-**sef**-a-**lop**-a-thee) (n) disease or dysfunction of the brain

encopresis
(en-cO-**pree**-sis) (n) inability to control bowel movements, fecal incontinence

endocapillary
(en-dO-**cap**-i-layr-ee) (n) within one of the tiny blood vessels

endocarditis
(**en**-dO-kar-**dI**-tis) (n) inflammation of the endocardium and/or the heart valves

endocardium
(en-dO-**kar**-dee-im) (n) serous lining membrane of inner surface and cavities of the heart

endocervical
(en-dO-**ser**-va-cal) (adj) pertaining to the lining of the canal of the cervix uteri

endometrial
(en-do-**mee**-tree-al) (adj) pertaining to the mucous membrane lining of the uterus

endometrium
(**en**-dO-**mee**-tree-um) (n) lining of the womb, composed of three layers and shed during menstruation

endoscope
(**en**-dO-skOp) (n) a lighted instrument for examining the inside of a body cavity or organ

endotracheal tube
(en-dO-**tray**-kee-al toob) (n) a catheter inserted through the mouth or nose into the trachea to maintain an open airway to deliver oxygen to permit suctioning of mucus or to prevent aspiration of foreign materials

engorged
(en-**gorjd**) (adj) filled to the limit of expansion

enteral
(**en**-ter-al) (adj) into or by way of the intestine

enterovirus
(**en**-ter-O-**vI**-rus) (n) a group of viruses that multiply in the gastrointestinal tract but may cause various diseases, such as polio

enucleation
(ee-noo-klee-**ay**-shun) (n) removal of a tumor or structure as a whole, as in removal of the eyeball

enuresis
(en-yoo-**ree**-sis) (n) bed-wetting; involuntary urination, especially at night in bed

eosinophil
(ee-O-**sin**-O-fil) (n) a type of white blood cell readily stained with eosin

ephelides
(ef-**ee**-lI-deez) (n, pl) freckles

epicanthic
(ep-i-**kan**-thik) (adj) pertaining to the vertical fold of skin extending from the root of the nose to the median end of the eyebrow

epidermis
(ep-i-**der**-mis) (n) the top or outer layer of the skin

epididymis
(ep-i-**did**-i-mis) (n) one of a pair of long, coiled ducts in the scrotum; they carry and store spermatozoa between the testes and ductus deferens

epidural
(ep-i-**doo**-ral) (adj) located over or under the dura

epigastric
(ep-i-**gas**-trik) (adj) related to or describing the area between the costal margins and the subcostal plane (top center of the abdomen)

epiglottis
(**ep**-i-**glot**-is) (n) flap of elastic cartilage at the back of the mouth that covers the opening to the windpipe during swallowing, thereby preventing choking.

epiglottitis
(ep-i-glot-**tI**-tis) (n) inflammation of the epiglottis, causing potentially fatal airway obstruction, especially in small children

epilepsy
(**ep**-i-lep-see) (n) convulsive disorder

epileptiform
(ep-i-**lep**-ti-fOrm) (adj) having the form of epilepsy

epinephrine
(ep-I-**nef**-rin) (n) a hormone of the adrenal medulla that acts as a strong stimulant and blood vessel constrictor

epiphora
(ee-**pif**-O-ra) (n) overflow of tears

epiphyseal
(ep-i-**fiz**-ee-al) (adj) relating to an epiphysis

epiphysis
(e-**pif**-i-sis) (n) end of a long bone, separated by cartilage from the shaft until the bone stops growing when the shaft and end are joined

epiploic
(**ep**-i-**plO**-ik) (adj) relating to the omentum, a fold of peritoneum attached to the stomach and connecting it with the adjacent organs

episiotomy
(e-peez-ee-**ot**-O-mee) (n) incision of perineum to facilitate delivery and prevent laceration (jagged tear)

epispadias
(ep-i-**spay**-dee-as) a malformation in which the urinary meatus is on the upper surface of the penis

epistaxis
(**ep**-i-**stak**-sis) (n) nosebleed

epithelial
(ep-i-**thee**-lee-al) (adj) composed of epithelium, cell layers covering the outside body surface as well as forming the lining of hollow organs and the passages of the respiratory, digestive, and urinary tracts

epithelium
(ep-i-**thee**-lee-um) (n) cell layers covering the outside body surfaces as well as forming the lining of hollow organs (e.g., the bladder) and the passages of the respiratory, digestive, and urinary tracts

eructation
(ee-ruk-**tay**-shun) (n) belching

erythema
(er-i-**thee**-ma) (n) redness of the skin resulting from dilation of the capillaries, as occurs in sunburn

erythema infectiosum
(er-i-**thee**-ma in-fek-shee-**O**-sum) (n) a mild, infectious disease characterized by an erythematous rash; also called fifth disease

erythematous
(er-i-**them**-a-tus/er-i-**thee**-ma-tus) (adj) relating to or having erythema; reddened; inflamed

erythrocyte
(e-**rith**-rO-sIt) (n) mature red blood cell

erythroderma
(e-**rith**-rO-**der**-ma) (n) any skin condition associated with unusual redness of the skin

erythromycin
(**ee**-rith-rO-**mI**-sin) (n) antibiotic used to treat infections caused by a wide variety of bacteria and other microorganisms

esophageal varices
(ee-**sof**-i-**jee**-al **vair**-i-seez) (n) bulging, tortuous veins in the lower esophagus which are prone to ulceration and massive bleeding; caused by hypertension in the portal circulation.

esophagus
(ee-**sof**-a-gus) (n) the muscular canal that connects the pharynx and stomach

esotropia
(es-O-**trO**-pee-a) (n) a condition in which one or both eyes appear to turn inward; cross eye(s)

estradiol
(es-tra-**dI**-ol) (n) a hormone produced by the ovary; often used to treat menopausal symptoms

ethmoidal
(eth-**moy**-dal) (adj) relating to the ethmoid bone or ethmoid sinus

eustachian tube
(yoo-**stay**-shun / yoo-**stay**-kee-an) (n) a tube leading from the middle ear to the nasopharynx; thus air pressure is equalized on both sides of the tympanic membrane

euthymic
(yoo-**thI**-mik) (adj) characterized by moderation of mood

eversion
(ee-**vur**-zhun) (n) turning out or inside out

exacerbation
(eg-zas-er-**bay**-shun) (n) aggravation of symptoms or increase in the severity of a disease

exanthema
(eg-zan-**thee**-ma) (n) a disease, such as measles or chickenpox, accompanied by a general rash on the skin, which may have particular characteristics specific to the disease

excision
(ek-**si**-zhun) (n) cutting out; surgical removal of all or part of a lesion, structure, or organ

excisional biopsy
(ek-**sizh**-un-al bI-op-see) (n) surgical removal of a tissue for microscopic examination

excoriation
(eks-kO-ree-**ay**-shun) (n) a scratching or scraping injury to the skin

excrescence
(eks-**kres**-ens) (n) abnormal projection or outgrowth; such as a wart

exophthalmos
(ek-sof-**thal**-mos) (n) protrusion of the eyeball(s)

exotropia
(ek-sO-**trO**-pee-a) (n) outward turning of one eye relative to the other

expectoration
(ek-spek-tO-**ray**-shun) (n) expelling by mouth; spitting

expiratory
(ek-**spI**-ra-**tO**-ree) (adj) relating to expiration, or breathing out air from the lungs

extension
(eks-**ten**-shun) (n) a motion of an extremity which reduces the angle of the joint (straightening)

extensor
(eks-**ten**-ser, eks-**ten**-sOr) (n) muscle that, when flexed, causes extension of a joint or straightening of an arm or leg

extrahepatic
(eks-tra-he-**pat**-ik) (adj) unrelated to or located outside the liver

extraocular
(eks-tra-**ok**-yoo-lar) (adj) outside the eye

extravasation
(eks-**trav**-a-**say**-shun) (n) a leakage of fluid (e.g., blood) to the tissues outside the vessel normally containing it, which may occur in injuries, burns, and allergic reactions

exudate
(**eks**-oo-dayt) (n) any fluid that has oozed out of a tissue, usually due to inflammation or injury

exudated
(eks-yoo-**day**-ted) (adj) pertaining to any fluid that has exuded out of a tissue or its capillaries

exudates
(**eks**-oo-daytz) (n) accumulations of fluid in a cavity; matter that penetrates through vessel walls into adjoining tissues

exudative
(**eks**-oo-dayt-iv) (adj) relating to exudate

F

facial
(**fay**-shul) (adj) relating to the face

fallopian tubes
(fa-**lO**-pee-an) (n) passageways from ovaries to uterus

familial
(fa-**mi**-lee-al) (adj) pertaining to a disease or characteristic that is present in some families

fascia
(**fash**-ee-a) (n) fibrous connective tissue that supports soft organs and encloses structures such as muscles; fasciae (pl)

fascial
(**fash**-ee-al) (adj) relating to fascia

fasciitis
(fa-see-**I**-tis) (n) inflammation of the fascia

fecalith
(**fee**-ka-lith) (n) a hard mass consisting of impacted feces

femoral
(**fem**-o-ral) (adj) relating to the thigh artery or bone, the femur

femoralis
(fem-or-**awl**-is) (adj) pertaining to the femur, the longest and strongest bone in body, going from hip to knee

fenestra ovalis
(fe-**nes**-tra O-**val**-is) (n) an oval opening between the middle ear and the vestibule; closed by the base of the stapes

fetal distress
(**fee**-tal) (n) life-threatening condition affecting the fetus

fetoprotein
(fee-tO-**prO**-teen) (n) antigen (substance or organism that produces an antibody) naturally present in the fetus and sometimes present in adults with certain cancers

fibrinogen
(fi-**brin**-O-jen) (n) a substance in the blood plasma that can be converted into fibrin to produce blood clotting

fibrinopurulent
(**fI**-bri-nO-**pyoo**-roo-lent) (adj) consisting of pus and fibrin

fibrinous
(**fI**-brin-us) (adj) pertaining to, of the nature of, or containing fibrin (a whitish filamentous protein)

fibroid
(**fI**-broyd) (adj) composed of fibers or fibrous tissue

fibrosis
(fI-**brO**-sis) (n) a condition marked by thickening and scarring of connective tissue

fifth disease
(n) erythema infectiosum; a mild, infectious disease characterized by an erythematous rash

fissure
(**fish**-ur) (n) a deep furrow, cleft, or slit; e.g., in the liver, lungs, ligaments, brain, or teeth

fistula
(**fis**-tyoo-la) (n) abnormal opening or channel connecting two internal organs or leading from an internal organ to the outside. They are due to ulceration, a wound that does not heal, injury, or tumor

fixation
(fik-**say**-shun) (n) process of securing a part, as by suturing

flank
(flaynk) (n) the fleshy part of the side between the ribs and the hip bone

flaring
(**flayr**-ing) (adj) widening of an area, as the nostrils; a spreading area of redness around a lesion

flatulence
(**flat**-yoo-lens) (n) presence of an excessive amount of gas in the stomach and intestines

flexion
(**flek**-shun) (n) the act of bending or the condition of being bent, in contrast to extending

flexor
(**flek**-ser, **flek**-sOr) (n) muscle that bends a joint

flexure
(**flek**-sher) (n) a bend, as in an organ or structure

floater
(**flO**-ter) (n) spot in the visual screen when one stares at a blank wall; caused by bits of protein and other debris moving in front of the retina

fluorescein
(**floor**-ess-scene) (n) a yellow dye which glows in visible light

follicle
(**fol**-i-kl) (n) pouch-like cavity, such as a hair follicle in the skin enclosing a hair, or a graafian follicle

follicular
(fo-**lik**-yoo-lar) (adj) pertaining to a follicle or follicles (a small secretory sac or cavity [pouchlike cavity, as that in the skin enclosing a hair])

folliculitis
(fol-i-kyoo-**lI**-tis) (n) inflammation of the hair follicles

foramen
(fO-**ray**-men) (n) hole or opening, especially in a bone or membrane

foramen ovale
(fO-**ray**-men O-val-ay) (n) hole or opening, especially in a bone or membrane; (particularly the opening between the two atria of the fetal heart that closes after birth)

foramina
(for-**ray**-mi-na) (n) apertures or perforations through a bone or a membrane structure; plural of foramen

fossa
(**fos**-a) (n) channel or shallow depression; fossae (pl)

fracture
(**frak**-chur) (v) to break; (n) a broken bone

fremitus
(**frem**-i-tus) (n) a vibration that can be felt by the hand on the chest

fulguration
(ful-gyoo-**ra**-shun) (n) destruction of tissue by the use of electrical current; electrodessication

fundus
(**fun**-dus) (n) that part of the interior of the eyeball exposed to view through an ophthalmoscope; lowest part; fundi (pl)

funduscopic
(fun-dus-**kop**-ik) (adj) pertaining to examination of the fundus of the eye by an ophthalmoscope

funduscopy
(fun-dus-**kop**-ee) (n) examination of the fundus of the eye using a funduscope; ophthalmoscopy

fungal
(**fung**-gal) (adj) caused by fungus or pertaining to fungus

fungating
(**fung**-gayt-ing) (adj) growing rapidly like a fungus, applied to certain tumors

furuncle
(**fyoo**-rung-kl) (n) a localized, pus-forming infection in a hair follicle or gland

G

gadolinium
(gad-O-**lin**-ee-um) (n) a rare earth metallic element

gallbladder
(**gawl**-**blad**-er) (n) pear-shaped organ that is located on the lower surface of the liver and is a reservoir for bile until discharged through the cystic duct

gallium
(**gal**-ee-um) (n) a rare metal; a gallium scan after an infusion of gallium provides a better view of lymphatic tissue

ganglion
(**gang**-glee-on) (n) a group of nerve cell bodies located in the peripheral nervous system

gangrene
(**gang**-green) (n) death of cells or tissue due to obstruction of blood supply

gastritis
(gas-**trI**-tis) (n) inflammation of the gastric (stomach) mucosa

gastroenteritis
(**gas**-trO-en-ter-**I**-tis) (n) inflammation of the gastric mucosa and intestine

gastroesophageal
(**gas**-trO-ee-soph-a-**jee**-al) (adj) related to both stomach and esophagus

Gastrografin
(Gas-tro-**graf**-in) (n) brand name for an oral contrast medium used for radiographic examination of the alimentary tract

gastroparesis
(gas-**trO**-pa-**ree**-sis) (n) weakness of gastric peristalsis causing delayed emptying of the stomach

genital
(**jen**-i-tal) (adj) relating to reproduction or the organs of reproduction

genitalia
(**jen**-i-**tay**-lee-a) (n) the genitals; male or female reproductive organs, especially the external ones

gestation
(jes-**tay**-shun) (n) the intrauterine development of an infant; pregnancy

gestational age
(ges-**tay**-shun-al aj) (n) age of a fetus or newborn, usually expressed in weeks since the onset of the mother's last menstrual period

gingiva
(**jin**-ji-va) (n) the gum; the tissue that attaches the teeth to the jaws

gingival
(**jin**-ji-val) (adj) relating to the gums

girdle
(**ger**-dl) (n) a zone or belt

gland
(n) organ that secretes one or more substances not needed by the organ itself

glans
(n) the head of the penis; "glans penis"

Glasgow coma scale
(**glas**-gO / **glaz**-gO) (n) a clinical scale to assess impaired consciousness; assessment includes motor responsiveness, verbal performance, and eye opening

glaucoma
(glaw-**kO**-ma) (n) disease of the eye in which intraocular pressure increases, damaging the optic nerve; can lead to blindness

glial cells
(**glee**-al sels) (n) cells of the nervous system with functions other than transmitting signals

glomerulus
(glO-**mayr**-yoo-lus) (n) a cluster of capillaries at the beginning of each nephron (the functional unit of the kidney); glomeruli (pl)

glossopharyngeal neuralgia
(**glos**-O-fa-**rin**-jee-al noo-ral-jee-a) (n) a condition of sharp spasmic pain in the throat or palate

glove-stocking anesthesia
(**an**-es-**thee**-see-a) (n) glove or gauntlet anesthesia is loss of sensation in the hand; stocking anesthesia is loss of sensation in the area covered by a stocking

grand mal (seizure)
(grahn mal) (n) generalized tonic-clonic seizure

Goldmann perimeter screen test
(n) assesses patient response when a light comes into view

gonioplasty
(gO-ni-O-**plas**-tee) (n) procedure that contracts the peripheral iris to eliminate contact with the trabecular meshwork

gonioscopy
(gO-ni-O-**skOp**-ee) (n) procedure that allows viewing of the anterior chamber angle

gonorrhea
(gon-O-**ree**-a) a contagious disease usually affecting the genitourinary tract; transmitted chiefly by sexual intercourse; caused by Neisseria gonorrhea

graafian follicle
(**graf**-ee-an) (n) a mature follicle on the ovary in which an oocyte matures and is released at ovulation

Gram stain
(n) a staining procedure for differentiating bacteria by morphology (rods, cocci) and staining characteristics (gram positive or gram negative)

granuloma
(gran-yoo-**lO**-ma) (n) a mass of tissue consisting of many newly growing capillaries formed during the healing process; growth may be due to injury, infection, or inflammation

Graves disease
(n) hyperthyroidism caused by an autoimmune disorder

gravida
(**grav**-i-da) (n) a pregnant woman; may be used in combination with a number or prefix to indicate the number of pregnancies and their outcome

gross
(grOs) (adj) visible to the naked eye

guaiac
(**gwI**-ak) (n) reagent used to test for occult blood

guttural
(**gut**-er-al) (adj) relating to the throat, or guttur

H

H2 receptor antagonist
(an-**tag**-on-ist) (n) a class of drugs which blocks the action of histamine on H2 receptors, preventing the release of hydrochloric acid. Cimetidine and ranitidine (Zantac) are the most common drug in this class.

hallucination
(ha-**loo**-si-**nay**-shun) (n) the sensory perception (see, hear, smell, or taste) of something that does not actually exist or has not actually occurred

heart failure
(n) a cardiac syndrome resulting in a change of cardiac structure and function leading to a decrease in the ventricles' ability to properly fill or eject blood.

helix
(**hee**-liks) (n) the folded edge of the external ear

hemangioma
(he-**man**-jee-**O**-ma) (n) a congenital benign tumor consisting of a mass of blood vessels

hemarthrosis
(**hee**-mar-**thrO**-sis / **hem**-ar-**thrO**-sis) (n) accumulation of blood in a joint

hematemesis
(hee-ma-**tem**-e-sis) (n) vomiting of blood

hematochezia
(hee-ma-tO-**kee**-zee-a) (n) passage of bloody stools

hematocrit
(**hee**-ma-tO-krit / **hem**-a-tO-krit) (n) centrifuge for separating solids from plasma in the blood; measure of the volume of red blood cells as a percentage of the total blood volume

hematology
(hee-ma-**tol**-o-jee) (n) the study of blood

hematoma
(hee-ma-**tO**-ma) (n) a tumor or swelling that contains blood

hematopoiesis
(**hee**-ma-tO-poi-**ee**-sis) (n) the process by which red and white blood cells and platelets are formed

hematuria
(hee-ma-**too**-ree-a) (n) presence of blood in the urine

hemifocal
(hem-i-**fO**-kal) (adj) refers to half of the body; usually a type of seizure

hemiparesis
(hem-ee-pa-**ree**-sis, hem-ee-**par**-e-sis) (n) muscular weakness of one half of the body

hemodynamic
(**hee**-mO-dI-**nam**-ik) (adj) relating to the mechanics of blood circulation

hemoglobin
(hee-mO-**glO**-bin) (n) the iron-containing pigment of the red blood cells

hemoglobinopathy
(**hee**-mO-glO-bi-**nop**-a-thee) (n) a hereditary disorder characterized by the synthesis of abnormal hemoglobin molecules

hemolysis
(hee-**mol**-i-sis) (n) the destruction of red blood cells which leads to the release of hemoglobin

hemophagocytosis
(hee-mO-**fag**-O-sI-**tO**-sis) (n) ingestion of red blood cells by phagocytes

hemophilia
(hee-mO-**fil**-ee-a) (n) a hereditary disorder caused by a deficiency of one or more clotting factors causing increased tendency to hemorrhage

hemoptysis
(hee-**mop**-ti-sis) (n) expectoration of blood; spitting or coughing up blood

hemorrhage
(**hem**-o-rij) (n) loss of a large amount of blood quickly, either externally or internally

hemorrhagic
(hem-O-**raj**-ik) (adj) relating to or experiencing a hemorrhage

hemorrhoid
(**hem**-a-royd) (n) varicose vein of anal opening

hemosiderin
(hee-mO-**sid**-er-in) (n) an iron-containing pigment derived from hemoglobin when red blood cells disintegrate

hemosiderosis
(hee-mO-sid-er-**O**-sis) (n) an accumulation of hemosiderin in the tissues

hemostasis
(**hee**-mO-stay-sis / hee-**mos**-ta-sis) (n) cessation of bleeding either naturally through the blood coagulation process, mechanically (with surgical clamps), or chemically (with drugs)

hemostatic
(hee-mO-**stat**-ik) (adj) relating to procedure, device, or substance that stops flow of blood

hemothorax
(hee-mO-**thor**-aks) (n) blood in the chest cavity

heparin
(**hep**-a-rin) (n) a naturally occurring anticoagulant (a substance which prevents or slows the clotting of blood)

hepatic
(he-**pat**-ik) (adj) pertaining to the liver

hepatitis
(hep-a-**tI**-tis) (n) acute or chronic inflammation of the liver

hepatoduodenal
(**hep**-at-O-doo-O-**dee**-nal) (adj) referring to the portion of the lesser omentum (fold of peritoneal tissue attaching and supporting the stomach and adjacent organs) between the liver and the duodenum

hepatomegaly
(**hep**-a-tO-**meg**-a-lee) (n) enlargement of the liver

hepatosplenomegaly
(**hep**-a-tO-splee-nO-**meg**-a-lee) (n) enlargement of the liver and spleen

hernia
(**her**-nee-a) (n) protrusion of an organ or part of an organ or other structure through the muscle wall of the cavity that normally contains it

herpes zoster
(**her**-peez **zos**-ter) (n) a viral infection causing inflammation along the path of nerve with associated painful vesicles (blisters) on the skin above; shingles

hiatal
(hI-**ay**-tal) (adj) pertaining to a hernia of part of the stomach into the opening in the diaphragm, through which the esophagus passes

hilar
(**hI**-lar) (adj) pertaining to a hilum, the part of an organ where the nerves and vessels enter and leave

hippocampus
(hip-O-**kam**-pus) (n) structure within the brain

hirsutism
(**hur**-soot-izm) (n) excessive body hair

histiocyte
(**hiss**-tee-O-cyte) (n) a cell that participates in the body's reaction to infection or injury; found in connective tissue

histology
(his-**tol**-O-jee) (n) a science of tissues, including their cellular composition and organization

homeostasis
(**hO**-mee-O-**stay**-sis) (n) equilibrium in the body with respect to various functions (e.g., temperature, heart rate) and to the chemical compositions of the fluids and tissues

homocysteine
(ho-mO-**sis**-te-een) (n) a sulfur-containing amino acid homologous with cysteine; elevated levels in the blood are an independent risk factor for cardiovascular disease (cf homocystine)

hordeolum
(hor-**dee**-O-lum) (n) a stye; a suppurative inflammation of a gland of the eyelid

humeral
(**hyoo**-mer-al) (adj) pertaining to the humerus, the upper bone of arm extending from the elbow to the shoulder joint where it articulates with the scapula

humerus
(**hyoo**-mer-us) (n) the long bone of the upper arm

hydrocephalic
(hI-drO-se-**fal**-ik) (adj) relating to or having hydrocephalus

hydrocephalus
(hI-drO-**sef**-a-lus) (n) increased accumulation of cerebrospinal fluid within the ventricles of the brain

hydrocephaly
(hI-drO-**sef**-a-lee) (n) the condition of having hydrocephalus

hyperdiploid
(**hI**-per-**dip**-loyd) (n) an individual organism or cell that has one or more extra chromosomes; (adj) relating to such an individual or cell

hyperemesis
(hI-per-**em**-e-sis) (n) excessive vomiting

hyperemia
(hI-per-**ee**-mee-a) (n) increased blood in part of the body, caused by inflammatory response or blockage of blood outflow

hyperemic
(hI-per-**ee**-mik) (adj) showing hyperemia

hyperesthetic
(hI-per-es-thet-ik) (adj) characterized by acute sensitivity to pain or other stimuli

hypergammaglobulinemia
(**hI**-per-gam-a-**glob**-yoo-li-**nee**-mee-a) (n) excessive amount of gamma globulins in the blood

hyperglycemic
(**hI**-per-glI-**see**-mic) (adj) pertaining to or characterized by hyperglycemia, an abnormally large concentration of glucose in the circulating blood

hyperlipidemia
(hI-per-lip-i-**dee**-mee-a) (n) presence of excess lipids, especially cholesterol, in the blood

hypermenorrhea
(**hI**-per-men-O-**ree**-a) (n) lengthy or heavy menses; menorrhagia

hyperopia
(hI-per-**O**-pee-a) (n) farsightedness

hyperpigmentation
(hI-per-pig-men-**tay**-shun) (n) darkening of the skin due to excessive pigment in the skin

hyperplasia
(hI-per-**play**-see-a) (n) increase in size of a tissue or organ due to an increase in the number of cells (not including tumor formation)

hyperplastic
(hI-per-**plas**-tik) (adj) relating to hyperplasia

hyperreflexia
(**hI**-per-ree-**flek**-see-a) (n) a condition marked by exaggerated deep tendon reflexes

hypertrophy

(hI-**per**-trO-fee) (n) increase in size

hypertropia

(hI-per-**trO**-pee-a) (n) a type of squint in which the eye looks upward

hyphae

(**hI**-fay) (n) cells forming the filaments of mold

hypnotic

(hip-**not**-ik) (n) an agent which brings on sleep

hypokinesis

(**hI**-pO-ki-**nee**-sis) (n) decreased or slow motor reaction to stimulus

hypomenorrhea

(**hI**-pO-men-O-**ree**-a) (n) decreased menses

hypometabolism

(**hI**-pO-me-**tab**-O-lizm) (n) lowered metabolism

hypoperfusion

(**hI**-pO-per-**fyoo**-zhun) (n) lower-than-normal passage of a liquid through an organ or body part

hypospadias

(**hI**-pO-**spay**-dee-as) (n) a malformation in which the urinary meatus is on the ventral side of the penis, proximal to its normal glanular position

hypotropia

(**hI**-pO-**trO**-pee-a) (n) a type of squint in which the eye looks downward

hysterectomy

(his-ter-**ek**-tO-mee) (n) surgical removal of the uterus

I

iatrogenic

(I-at-rO-**jen**-ik) (adj) relating to a response to medical or surgical treatment; often refers to deleterious side-effects of treatment by a physician

ichthyosis

(ik-thee-**O**-sis) (n) condition in which the skin is dry and scaly, resembling fish skin

ictal

(**ik**-tal) (adj) referring to the onset of a seizure

icteric

(ik-**ter**-ik) (adj) related to or affected with jaundice

idiopathic

(**id**-ee-O-**path**-ik) (adj) of unknown cause; describes a disease for which no identifiable cause can be determined

idiopathy

(id-ee-**op**-a-thee) (n) any disease of unknown cause

ileitis

(il-ee-**I**-tis) (n) inflammation of the ileum (lower-three-fifths of the small intestines)

ileostomy

(**il**-ee-**os**-tO-mee) (n) surgical formation of an opening of the ileum (distal portion of the small intestine) onto the abdominal wall through which feces pass

ileum

(**il**-ee-um) (n) the third portion of the small intestine, about 12 feet in length, extending from the junction with the jejunum to the ileocecal opening

ileus

(**il**-ee-us) (n) obstruction of the intestines

ilium

(**il**-ee-um) (n) the broad, flaring portion of the hip bone

immune system

(i-**myoon**) (n) complex interactions that protect the body from pathogenic organisms and other foreign invaders

immunity

(i-**myoo**-ni-tee) (n) one's resistance to disease

immunodeficiency

(**im**-yoo-nO-**dee**-fish-en-see) (n) a condition caused by an impaired immune system due to a deficiency or absence of one or more components of the immune system

immunoglobulin

(im-yoo-nO-**glob**-yoo-lin) (n) antibody protein

immunohistochemistry

(**im**-yoo-nO-**his**-tO-**kem**-is-tree) (n) special techniques used on cells to identify certain characteristics, especially the presence of specific antigens

immunology

(im-yoo-**nol**-O-jee) (n) study of the body's response to foreign invasion, such as bacteria or viruses, and allergies

immunotherapy

(**im**-yoo-nO-thayr-a-pee) (n) treatment for disease, including cancer, which enhances or manipulates the immune system; may also be called biotherapy

impetigo

(im-pe-**tI**-gO) (n) a streptococcal or staphylococcal infection of the skin characterized by lesions, usually on the face, which rupture and become covered with a thick yellow crust; highly contagious

incised

(in-**sIzd**) (adj) cut with a knife

incisional biopsy

(in-**si**-zhun-al **bI**-op-see) (n) removal of part of a lesion for microscopic examination

incision and drainage

(n) commonly dictated "I and D"; procedure of cutting through an infected lesion and allowing it to drain

incus

(**ing**-kus) (n) the anvil-shaped bone in the middle ear

Indocin

(in-**doe**-sin) (n) brand name for indomethacin, an analgesic nonsteroidal anti-inflammatory drug

infarction

(in-**fark**-shun) (n) formation of dead tissue as a result of diminished or stopped blood flow to the tissue area

inferior

(in-**fee**-ree-Or) (adj) lower; below; of lesser value

infiltrate

(in-**fil**-trayt) (v) to pass into or through a substance or a space

infraumbilical
(**in**-fra-um-**bil**-i-kal) (adj) below the umbilicus (navel)

infundibulopelvic
(in-fun-**dib**-yoo-lO-**pel**-vik) (adj) relating to or located in the infundibulum (the end of the fallopian tube farthest from the uterus) and the pelvis

infundibulum
(in-fun-**dib**-yoo-lum) (n) a funnel-shaped opening

inguinal
(**ing**-gwin-al) (adj) pertaining to the region of the groin

inoculation
(i-nok-yoo-**lay**-shun) (n) the introduction of pathogenic organisms or antigens into the body in order to increase immunity by stimulating the production of antibodies

in situ
(in **sI**-too) (adj, adv) in position; at the original location, or site

inspiratory
(in-**spI**-ra-tO-ree) (adj) relating to inhalation, drawing air into the lungs

integumentary
(in-teg-yoo-**men**-ta-ree) (adj) relating to the skin

intercostal
(in-ter-**kos**-tal) (adj) relating to or located between the ribs

interictal
(in-ter-**ik**-tal) (adj) between seizures

interstitial
(in-ter-**stish**-al) (adj) relating to or located in the space between tissues, such as interstitial fluid

intertriginous
(in-ter-**trij**-i-nus) (adj) characterized by intertrigo

intertrigo
(in-ter-**trI**-gO) (n) irritation (dermatitis) of juxtaposed surfaces of skin such as between the thighs, folds of skin, or under pendulous breasts caused by retained sweat, moisture, friction, and concomitant overgrowth of microorganisms such as Candida species

intestine
(in-**tes**-tin) (n) the portion of the alimentary canal extending from the pyloric opening of the stomach to the anus (opening of the rectum)

intimal
(**in**-ti-mal) (adj) relating to the innermost lining of a part, especially of a blood vessel; (n) intima

intraductal
(adj) inside a duct

intrahepatic
(**in**-tra-he-**pat**-ik) (adj) within the liver

intramural
(in-tra-**myoo**-ral) (adj) within the wall of a cavity

intraocular pressure
(in-tra-**ok**-yoo-lar **presh**-er) (n) the pressure of the fluid within the eye

intrauterine
(in-tra-**yoo**-ter-in) (adj) within the uterus

intravenous
(IV) (**in**-tra-**vee**-nus) (adj) within or by way of a vein

introitus
(in-**trO**-i-tus) (n) an opening or entrance into a canal or cavity, such as the vagina

intussusception
(**in**-tus-su-**sep**-shun) (n) taking up or receiving one part within another, especially the infolding of one segment of the intestine within another

inversion
(in-**vur**-shun) (n) reversal of position, as upside down or inside out

in vitro
(in **vee**-trO) (adj, adv) literally, in glass; outside the living organism and in an artificial environment, such as a test tube

in vivo
(in **vee**-vO) (adj, adv) literally, in the living body

iris
(**I**-ris) (n) colored portion of the eye that regulates the amount of light entering through the pupil; irides (ir-i-deez) (pl)

ischemia
(is-**kee**-mee-a) (n) decreased blood supply due to obstruction, such as narrowing of the blood vessels

ischium
(**is**-kee-um / **ish**-ee-um) (n) bone upon which body rests when sitting; fuses with the ilium and pubis to form the pelvis; ischia (is-kee-a) (pl)

isoagglutination
(I-sO-a-gloo-ti-**nay**-shun) (n) process in which antibodies (agglutinins) occurring naturally in blood cause clumping of red blood cells of a different group carrying a corresponding antigen (isoagglutinogen)

J

jaundice
(**jawn**-dis) (n) yellowish skin and whites of the eyes

jugular
(jug-**yoo**-lar) (adj) relating to the throat or neck

K

karyotype
(**kar**-ee-O-tIp) (n) chromosomal makeup of a cell; often displayed as chromosome pairs arranged by size

keloid
(**kee**-loyd) (n) a mass of scar tissue

keratin
(**ker**-a-tin) (n) a tough, fibrous protein in skin, hair, and nails

keratoplasty
(**ker**-a-tO-**plas**-tee) (n) surgery on the cornea, especially transplant of a cornea

keratosis
(ker-a-**tO**-sis) (n) a condition in which the skin thickens and builds up with excessive keratin

keratotic
(ker-a-**tot**-ik) (adj) relating to keratosis

kidneys
(**kid**-neez) (n) a pair of bean-shaped organs near the spinal column that filter blood and produce urine

knuckle
(**nuk**-l) (n) a finger joint; an abnormal kink or loop

Kupffer cells
(**koop**-fer) (n) phagocytes present in the liver

kyphosis
(kI-**fO**-sis) (n) abnormal curving of the spine causing a hunchback

L

labial
(**lay**-bee-al) (adj) relating to the lips

labyrinth
(**lab**-i-rinth) (n) an anatomical structure made up of a complex of cavities, such as the inner ear

labyrinthitis
(**lab**-i-rin-**thI**-tis) (n) inflammation of the inner ear (labyrinth) or ethmoidal labyrinth (nose)

lacrimation
(**lak**-ri-**may**-shun) (n) secretion of tears

lamina
(**lam**-i-na) (n) thin membrane or plate-like structure, such as the two parts of a vertebra that join to hold the spinous process of the vertebra over the spinal cord (pl laminae)

laminar
(**lam**-i-nar) (adj) relating to lamina

laparoscope
(**lap**-a-rO-skOp) (n) a device for observing the inside of an organ or cavity

laparotomy
(lap-a-**rot**-O-mee) (n) a surgical incision made into the abdominal wall

laryngectomy
(**lar**-in-**jek**-tO-mee) (n) surgical removal of the larynx

laryngostomy
(**lar**-ing-**gos**-tO-mee) (n) surgically creating an opening into the larynx

larynx
(**lar**-ingks) (n) the voice box, located between the pharynx and the trachea

laser iridotomy
(ir-i-**dot**-O-mee) (n) cutting some of the fibers of the iris with a laser

LASIK
(**lay**-sik) (n) acronym for laser-assisted in-situ keratomileusis

lateral
(**lat**-er-al) (adj) relating to a side, away from the center plane; e.g., cheeks are lateral to the nose

latissimus
(la-**tis**-i-mus) (n) denoting a broad anatomical structure, such as a muscle

Le Fort
(n) classification system for facial fractures

leiomyoma
(lI-O-mI-**O**-ma) (n) benign tumor arising from smooth muscle

lesion
(**lee**-zhun) (n) general term for any visible, circumscribed injury to the skin; such as, a wound, sore, rash, or mass

lethargy
(**leth**-ar-jee) (n) state of sluggishness, stupor, unresponsiveness

leukemia
(loo-**kee**-mee-a) (n) production of abnormal white blood cells; a type of cancer of the blood

leukocyte
(**loo**-kO-sIt) (n) white blood cell

leukoplakia
(loo-kO-**play**-kee-a) (n) a precancerous change in a mucous membrane, such as the mouth or tongue

leukotrienes
(loo-kO-**trI**-eens) (n) mediators of inflammation

levator
(le-**vay**-ter/le-**vay**-tOr) (n) muscle that lifts or raises the body part to which it is attached

ligament
(**lig**-a-ment) (n) band of fibrous connective tissue that binds joints together and connects bones and cartilage

linear
(**lin**-ee-ar) (adj) pertaining to or resembling a line

lipping
(**lip**-ing) (n) excessive growth in a liplike shape at the edge of a bone

lithotomy
(li-**thot**-O-mee) (n) surgical removal of a stone, especially from the urinary tract

lithotripsy
(**lith**-O-trip-see) (n) procedure using a laser to break apart stones (calculi)

lobe
(lOb) (n) rounded part of an organ, separated from other parts of the organ by connective tissue or fissures

lobectomy
(lO-**bek**-tO-mee) (n) surgical procedure in which a lobe is removed (thyroid, brain, liver, and lungs are divided into lobes)

lobule
(**lob**-yool) (n) a small lobe or primary subdivision of a lobe; typical of pancreas and major salivary glands and may be on the surface by bumps and bulges

lochia
(**lO**-kee-a) (n) vaginal discharge occurring after childbirth

loop
(n) a curve or bend forming a complete or almost complete oval or circle

lordosis
(lOr-**dO**-sis) (n) abnormal curving of the spine causing a swayback

loupe
(loop) (n) a magnifying lens

lucency
(**loo**-sen-see) (n) the quality or state of being lucent

lucent
(**loo**-sent) (adj) bright, clear, allowing light to pass

lumbar
(**lum**-bar) (adj) pertaining to the part of the back between the thorax and pelvis

lumen
(**loo**-men) (n) cavity, canal, or channel within an organ or tube; lumina or lumens (pl)

luminal
(**loo**-min-al) (adj) related to the lumen of a tubular structure, such as a blood vessel

lymph
(limf) (n) a thin fluid that bathes the tissues of the body, circulates through lymph vessels, is filtered in lymph nodes, and enters the blood stream through the thoracic duct

lymphadenitis
(**lim**-fad-e-**nI**-tis) (n) inflammation of one or more lymph nodes

lymphadenopathy
(lim-fad-e-**nop**-a-thee) (n) any disorder of lymph nodes or of the lymphatic system

lymphatic
(lim-**fat**-ik) (adj) relating to or resembling lymph or lymph nodes

lymphoblastic
(lim-fO-**blas**-tik) (adj) relating to or resembling lymphoblasts, immature white blood cells

lymphocyte
(lim-**fO**-sIt) (n) a subgroup of white blood cells produced in lymphatic tissue. Lymphocytes normally make up 22-28% of peripheral white cells.

lymphocytic
(lim-fO-**sit**-ik) (adj) relating to or characteristic of lymphocytes

lymphoid
(**lim**-foyd) (adj) resembling lymph or relating to the lymphatic system

lymphoma
(lim-**fO**-ma) (n) a general term for various types of tumors of the lymphatic system

lymphopenia
(lim-fO-**pee**-nee-a) (n) a decrease in the number of lymphocytes in the blood

lytic
(**lit**-ik) (adj) pertaining to lysis, a gradual subsidence of the symptoms of an acute disease

M

macrophage
(**mak**-ro-fayj) (n) a large scavenger cell (phagocyte) that digests micro-organisms and cell debris

macula
(**mak**-yoo-la) (n) small discolored spot on the retina

macule
(**mak**-yool) (n) a small discolored spot on the skin

maculopapular
(mak-yoo-lO-**pap**-yoo-lar) (adj) describing skin lesions that are raised in the center

malaise
(ma-**layz**) (n) a feeling of general discomfort or uneasiness, often the first indication of an infection or other disease

malformation
(mal-for-**may**-shun) (n) abnormal development or structure of the body or a part

malignancy
(ma-**lig**-nan-see) (n) a cancer that is invasive and spreading

malleolus
(ma-**lee**-O-lus) (n) either of the two bumplike projections on each side of the ankle; malleoli (pl)

malleus
(**mal**-ee-us) (n) the largest of the three inner ear bones; club-shaped; attached to the tympanic membrane

mammary
(**mam**-a-ree) (adj) relating to the breast

mammogram
(**mam**-O-gram) (n) x-ray of the breast

mandibular
(man-**dib**-yoo-lar) (adj) relating to the lower jaw

mania
(**may**-nee-a) (n) a psychiatric disorder characterized by restlessness, euphoria, grandiosity, and poor judgment with symptoms of insomnia, rapid speech, and distractibility

mastication
(mas-ti-**kay**-shun) (n) process of chewing food

mastoiditis
(mas-toy-**dI**-tis) (n) inflammation of the mastoid process (part of the temporal bone behind the ear)

maxilla
(mak-**sil**-a) (n) the upper jaw

maxillary sinus
(**mak**-si-layr-ee **sI**-nus) (n) an air cavity in the body of the upper jaw bone; connects with the middle passage (meatus) of the nose

meatus
(mee-**ay**-tus) (n) a passage or channel, especially with an external opening

meconium
(mee-**kO**-nee-um) (n) first bowel movement of a newborn, which are thick, sticky, greenish to black and composed of bile pigments and gland secretions

mediastinal
(**mee**-dee-as-**tI**-nal) (adj) relating to the space in the chest cavity between the lungs that contains the heart, aorta, esophagus, trachea, and thymus

mediolateral
(**mee**-dee-O-**lat**-er-al) (adj) relating to the middle and side of a structure

medulla oblongata
(me-**dool**-a ob-long-**gah**-ta) (n) the lowest part of the brain, connecting to the spinal cord; contains the cardiac, vasomotor, and respiratory centers of the brain

melanin
(**mel**-a-nin) (n) naturally-occurring dark brown or black pigment found in the hair, skin, and eyes

melanocyte
(**mel**-an-O-sIt) (n) a cell that produces melanin

melanocytic
(mel-a-nO-**sit**-ik) (adj) pertaining to or composed of melanocytes

melena
(me-**lee**-na) (n) passage of dark, tarry stool

melitis
(mee-**ll**-tis) (n) inflammation of the cheek

menarche
(me-**nar**-kee) (n) the initial menstrual period

Ménière disease
(mayn-**yairz**) (n) a disease of the inner ear with attacks of dizziness, nausea, ringing in the ear, and increasing deafness

meninges
(me-**nin**-jeez) (n) membranes covering the brain and spinal cord

meningitis
(men-in-**jI**-tis) (n) inflammation of the membranes of the brain or spinal cord

meningocele
(me-**ning**-gO-seel) (n) protrusion of the brain or spinal cord through a defect in the skull or spinal column

menometrorrhagia
(**men**-O-mee-trO-**ray**-jee-a) (n) excessive menstrual bleeding or bleeding between menstrual periods

menopause
(**men**-O-pawz) (n) the end of a woman's reproductive period of life and cessation of menses

menorrhagia
(men-O-**ray**-jee-a) (n) prolonged or heavy menses; hypermenorrhea

menorrhalgia
(men-O-**ral**-jee-a) (n) painful menstruation or pelvic pain accompanying menstruation

menses
(**men**-seez) (n) monthly flow of bloody fluid from the uterus

menstruation
(men-stroo-**ay**-shun) (n) the discharge of a bloody fluid from the uterus at regular intervals during the life of a woman from puberty to menopause

mesentery
(**mes**-en-tar-ee) (n) a peritoneal fold encircling the greater part of the small intestines and connecting the intestine to the posterior abdominal wall

mesial
(**mee**-zee-al; **mes**-ee-al) (adj) situated toward the midline of the body or the central part of an organ or tissue (also called medial)

mesosalpinx
(**mez**-O-**sal**-pinks) (n) free end of the broad ligament which supports the fallopian tubes

metaphyseal
(met-a-**fiz**-ee-al) (adj) relating to a metaphysic

metaphysis
(me-**taf**-i-sis) (n) a conical section of bone between the epiphysis and diaphysis of long bones

metaplasia
(me-ta-**play**-zee-a) (n) conversion of a tissue into a form that is not normal for that tissue

metastasis
(me-**tas**-ta-sis) (n) the shifting of a disease from one part of the body to another, especially in cancer; metastases (pl)

metastatic
(met-a-**stat**-ic) (n) pertaining to metastasis (movement of cells, especially cancer cells, from one part of the body to another)

metatarsal
(met-a-**tar**-sal) (adj) relating to a metatarsus; (n) a metatarsal bone

metatarsus
(met-a-**tar**-sus) (n) any of the five long bones of the foot between the ankle and the toes

metrorrhagia
(mee-trO-**ray**-jee-a) (n) bleeding from the uterus between menstrual periods

microscopy
(mI-**kros**-kO-pee) (n) use of a microscope to magnify and examine objects

micturition
(mik-choo-**rish**-un) (n) urination

milia
(**mil**-ee-a) (n, pl) whiteheads, due to obstruction of the outlet of hair follicles or sweat glands

miliaria
(mil-ee-**ay**-ree-a) (n) a skin eruption of small vesicles and papules; heat rash

millicuries
(**mil**-i-**kyoo**-rees) (n) a unit of radioactivity, abbreviated mCi

mitotic
(mI-**tot**-ik) (adj) pertaining to mitosis, a type of cell division in which a cell divides into two genetically identical daughter cells

mitral
(**mI**-tral) (adj) relating to the bicuspid or mitral valve of the heart, between the atrium and the ventricle on the left side of the heart

monoclonal antibody
(mon-O-**klO**-nal **an**-tee-bod-ee) (n) an antibody produced by a cloned cell that is biologically engineered to create a specific antibody directed against a particular antigen

morphology
(mOr-**fol**-O-jee) (n) the shape and structure of an organism or body part

motility
(mO-**til**-i-tee) (n) ability to move spontaneously

mucoperiosteum
(**myoo**-kO-per-ee-os-tee-um) (n) the mucous membrane covering the hard palate at the front of the roof of the mouth

mucosa
(myoo-**kO**-sa) (n) mucous membrane

mucosal
(myoo-**kO**-sal) (adj) concerning any mucous membrane

mucous
(**myoo**-kus) (adj) having the nature of or resembling mucus

mucus
(**myoo**-kus) (n) viscous (sticky, gummy) secretions of mucous membranes and glands

multinucleated
(mul-ti-**noo**-klee-ay-ted) (adj) possessing several nuclei

multipara
(mul-**tip**-a-ra) (n) a woman who has given birth to two or more children

murmur
(**mer**-mer) (n) abnormal heart sound

myasthenia gravis
(mI-as-**thee**-nee-a **grav**-is) (n) a chronic progressive muscular weakness, beginning usually in the face and throat, due to a defect in the conduction of nerve impulses

mycosis
(mI-**kO**-sis) (n) disease caused by a fungus

mydriatic
(mi-dree-**at**-ik) (n) pharmaceutical agent which dilates pupil

myelocyte
(**my**-e-lo-cyte) (n) immature granulocytic leukocyte normally found in bone marrow and present in the circulatory blood in certain diseases, e.g., myelocytic leukemia

myocardial
(mI-O-**kar**-dee-al) (adj) relating to the myocardium, the heart muscle

myopia
(mI-**O**-pee-a) (n) nearsightedness; visual defect in which parallel rays come to a focus

myringitis
(mir-in-**jI**-tis) (n) inflammation of the tympanic membrane; tympanitis

myringoplasty
(mi-**ring**-gO-**plas**-tee) (n) surgical repair of the eardrum

myringotomy
(mir-ing-**got**-o-mee) (n) surgical incision into the tympanic membrane

N

nafcillin
(naf-**sill**-in) (n) an antibiotic; one of the varieties of penicillin

naris
(**nay**-ris) (n) nostril; nares (nay-rees) (pl)

nasopharynx
(**nay**-zO-far-ingks) (n) open chamber behind the nose and above the palate

nausea
(**naw**-zee-a, **naw**-zha) (n) an inclination to vomit

nauseous
(**naw**-zee-us; **naw**-shus) (adj) causing nausea or feeling nausea

nebulization
(**neb**-yoo-li-**zay**-shun) (n) production of fine particles, such as a spray or mist, from liquid

necrosis
(ne-**crO**-sis) (n) dead areas of tissue or bone surrounded by healthy parts

necrotic
(ne-**krot**-ik) (adj) relating to or undergoing necrosis

neoadjuvant
(nee-O-**ad**-joo-vant) (adj) used in conjunction with other types of therapy

neoplasm
(**nee**-O-plazm) (n) any abnormal growth of tissue, usually malignant; tumor

neoplastic
(nee-O-**plas**-tik) (adj) pertaining to the nature of new, abnormal tissue formation; usually refers to cancer

nephrectomy
(ne-**frek**-tO-mee) (n) surgical removal of a kidney

nephrolithiasis
(**nef**-rO-li-**thI**-a-sis) (n) presence of stones (calculi) in the kidney(s)

nephrolithotomy
(**nef**-rO-li-**thot**-O-mee) (n) surgical incision into a kidney to remove stones (calculi)

nephron
(**nef**-ron) (n) the functional unit of the kidney that filters the blood

nephrostomy
(ne-**fros**-tO-mee) (n) surgical creation of an opening in the kidney for drainage

neural
(**noo**-ral) (adj) relating to nerves or the nervous system

neuralgia
(noo-**ral**-jee-a) (n) pain of a severe, throbbing, or stabbing character along the course of a nerve

neurapraxia
(noor-a-**prak**-see-a) (n) loss of conduction in a nerve without structural degeneration

neurasthenia
(noor-as-**thee**-nee-a) (n) a condition, commonly accompanying or following depression, characterized by fatigue believed to be brought on by psychological factors

neurilemma
(noor-i-**lem**-a) (n) a cell that enfolds one or more axons of the peripheral nervous system

neuroblastoma
(**noor**-O-blas-**tO**-ma) (n) malignant (cancerous) tumor containing embryonic nerve cells

neuroectodermal
(**noo**-rO-ek-tO-**der**-mal) (adj) embryonic tissue that gives rise to nerve tissue

neuromuscular
(noor-O-**mus**-kyoo-lar) (adj) pertains to the muscles and nerves

neuron
(**noor**-on) (n) nerve cell; the morphological and functional unit of the nervous system, consisting of the nerve cell body, the dendrites, and the axon

neuropathy
(noo-**rop**-a-thee) (n) disorder affecting the cranial or spinal nerves

neutropenia
(noo-trO-**pee**-nee-a) (n) a decrease in the number of neutrophils in the blood

neutrophil
(**noo**-trO-fil / **noo**-trO-fIl) (n) the most common type of mature white blood cell; its primary function is phagocytosis; granular leukocyte

nevus
(**nee**-vus) (n) congenital discoloration of the skin; birthmark or mole; nevi (pl)

nocturia
(nok-**too**-ree-a) (n) frequent urination during the night

node
(nOd) (n) a small knot of tissue, distinct from surrounding tissue; a lymph node

nodular
(**nod**-yoo-lar) (adj) containing or resembling nodules; having small, firm, knotty masses

nodule
(**nod**-yool) (n) a small mass, distinct from surrounding tissue

nosocomial
(nOs-O-**kO**-mE-al) (adj) relating to a hospital; often used to describe an infection acquired during a hospital stay

nuchal
(**noo**-kal) (adj) pertaining to the neck, or nucha (nape of neck)

nulligravida
(nul-i-**grav**-i-da) (n) a woman who has never been pregnant

nulliparous
(nul-**ip**-a-rus) (adj) a woman who has not had a child

nystagmus
(nis-**tag**-mus) (n) involuntary, rhythmic oscillation of the eyeballs

O

obese
(o-**bees**) (adj) very fat

oblique
(ob-**leek**) (adj) slanting

obturator
(**ob**-too-ray-tor) (n) device or body structure that closes up or covers an opening

obtuse
(ob-**toos**) (adj) dull or blunt; not pointed or acute

obstipation
(ob-sti-**pay**-shun) (n) severe constipation

occiput
(**ok**-si-put) (n) the back part of the skull

occlusion
(o-**kloo**-zhun) (n) blockage, such as coronary occlusion

occult blood
(ok-**ult**) (n) blood in the stool in amounts too small to be seen but detectable with laboratory tests

ocular
(**ok**-yoo-lar) (adj) concerning the eye or vision

odontoid process
(O-**don**-toyd **pros**-es) (n) the toothlike projection from the upper surface of the second cervical vertebra on which the head rotates

oligohydramnios
(**ol**-i-gO-hI-**dram**-nee-os) (n) abnormally small amount of amniotic fluid

oligomenorrhea
(**ol**-i-gO-men-O-**ree**-a) (n) infrequent or very light menstrual bleeding

omental
(O-**men**-tal) (adj) relating to the omentum

omentum
(O-**men**-tum) (n) fold of peritoneal tissue attaching to and supporting the stomach and intestines

onycholysis
(on-ee-**kol**-i-sis) (n) loosening of the nails from their beds

oophorectomy
(O-of-Or-**ek**-tO-mee) (n) surgical removal of one or both ovaries

opacification
(O-**pas**-i-fi-kay-shun) (n) clouding or loss of transparency, especially of the cornea or lens of the eye

opacity
(O-**pas**-i-tee) (n) state of being opaque, impenetrable by visible light rays or by forms of radiant energy, such as x-rays

ophthalmologist
(of-thal-**mol**-o-jist) (n) a physician specializing in diseases of the eye

ophthalmoscopy
(of-thal-**mos**-ko-pee) (n) procedure used to examine the optic nerve head for color, shape, and vascularization

ophthalmus
(of-**thal**-mus) (n) the eye

opportunistic infection
(n) a disease caused by normally harmless microorganisms when the body's resistance to disease is impaired

optic
(**op**-tik) (adj) pertaining to the eye or sight

optic chiasm
(**op**-tik **kI**-azm) (n) the point of crossing of the optic nerves

optometrist
(op-**tom**-e-trist) (n) a professional who tests visual acuity and prescribes corrective lenses

orbital cellulitis
(**or**-bit-al sel-yoo-**lI**-tis) (n) inflammation of tissue around or behind the eye

orchidopexy
(Or-ki-**dop**-eks-ee) (n) surgical procedure in which an undescended testicle is sutured into place; also orchiopexy

orchiectomy
(Or-kee-**ek**-tO-mee) (n) surgical removal of one or both testes

orchiocele
(Or-kee-O-seel) (n) scrotal hernia; tumor of a testis

organism
(**or**-ga-nizm) (n) a living plant, animal, or microorganism

organomegaly
(Or-ga-nO-**meg**-a-lee) (n) abnormal enlargement of an organ, particularly an organ of the abdominal cavity, such as the liver or spleen

orifice
(**or**-i-fis) (n) mouth, entrance, or outlet of any aperture

orthopnea
(Or-thop-**nee**-a) (n) difficulty in breathing when lying down

oscilloscope
(o-**sil**-O-scOp) (n) an instrument which displays electrical oscillations (waves) on a screen

osseous
(**os**-ee-us) (adj) bony; resembling bone; osteal

ossicles
(os-i-kls) (n) small bones, such as the auditory ossicles (the three bones of the inner ear)

osteal
(**os**-tee-ul) (adj) bony; resembling bone; osseous

ostealgia
(os-tee-**al**-jee-a) (n) pain in a bone

ostectomy
(os-**tek**-tO-mee) (n) surgical removal of all or part of a bone

osteophyte
(**os**-tee-O-fIt) (n) a bony outgrowth; projection or bone spur

osteoporosis
(os-tee-O-pO-**rO**-sis) (n) abnormal loss of bone tissue, causing fragile bones that fracture easily

osteosarcoma
(os-tee-O-sar-**ko**-ma) (n) a tumor of the bone, usually highly malignant

ostial
(**os**-tee-ul) (adj) relating to any opening (ostium)

otalgia
(O-**tal**-jee-a) (n) earache

otitis
(O-**tI**-tis) (n) inflammation of the ear

otitis externa
(O-**tI**-tis eks-**ter**-na) (n) inflammation of the external ear

otitis media
(O-**tI**-tis **mee**-dee-a) (n) inflammation of the middle ear

otorhinolaryngology
(O-tO-**rI**-nO-lar-in-**gol**-o-jee) (n) study of the ears, nose, and throat

otosclerosis
(O-tO-sklee-**rO**-sis) (n) a growth of sponge-like bone in the inner ear, eventually leading to deafness

otoscope
(**O**-tO-skOp) (n) an instrument for examining the eardrum

otoscopy
(O-**tos**-kO-pee) (n) visual examination of the ear with an otoscope

ototoxic
(O-to-**tok**-sic) (adj) harmful to the organs of hearing or auditory nerve

oximetry
(ok-**sim**-i-tree) (n) a method of measuring the amount of oxygen combined with the hemoglobin in a blood sample

P

palate
(**pal**-at) (n) the roof of one's mouth, composed of the hard palate (front) and the soft palate (back)

palliative
(**pal**-ee-a-tiv) (adj) describes a treatment that minimizes symptoms but does not cure the disease

pallor
(**pal**-or) (n) abnormal paleness of the skin; deficiency of color

palpable
(**pal**-pa-bl) (adj) able to be identified by touch

palpate
(**pal**-payt) (v) to examine by touch; to feel

palpation
(pal-**pay**-shun) (n) technique of examination in which the examiner feels the firmness, texture, size, shape, or location of body parts

palpitations
(pal-pi-**tay**-shuns) (n) stronger and more rapid heartbeats as felt by the patient; pounding or throbbing of the heart

palsy
(**pawl**-zee) (n) an abnormal condition characterized by partial paralysis

pancreas
(**pan**-kree-as) (n) gland lying behind the stomach that produces and secretes insulin, glucagon, and digestive enzymes

pancrelipase
(pan-kree-**lip**-ase) (n) standardized preparation of enzymes with amylase and protease, obtained from the pancreas of hogs

papilledema
(**pap**-ill-e-**dee**-ma) (n) edema and inflammation of the optic nerve at its point of entrance into the eyeball

papillopathy
(pap-i-**lop**-a-thee) (n) the blood supply to the optic disk and retina is obstructed; often producing low-tension glaucoma

papule
(**pap**-yool) (n) a small, solid, raised skin lesion, as in chickenpox

para
(**par**-a) (n) a woman who has given birth to one or more children; the term may be used in combination with a number or prefix to indicate how many times a woman has given birth

paracentesis
(pair-a-sen-**tee**-sis) (n) a procedure for withdrawing fluid from a body cavity, often referring to removal of fluid from the peritoneal cavity

paraplegia
(par-a-**plee**-jee-a) (n) paralysis of the lower portion of the body and of both legs

parasite
(**par**-a-sIt) (n) an organism that lives on or in another and draws its nourishment therefrom

parenchyma
(pa-**reng**-ki-ma) (n) the functional or specific tissue of an organ, not including supporting or connective tissue

parenchymal
(pa-**reng**-ki-mal) (adj) pertaining to the distinguishing or specific cells of a gland or organ contained in and supported by the connective tissue framework

parenteral
(pa-**ren**-ter-al) (adj) not through the digestive system, such as introduction of nutrients into the veins or under the skin

paresthesia
(par-es-**thee**-zee-a) (n) an abnormal sensation of tingling, prickling, burning

parietal
(pa-**ree**-e-tal) (adj) pertaining to the inner walls of a body cavity

paronychia
(par-O-**nik**-ee-a) (n) infected skin around the nail

paroxysmal
(par-ok-**siz**-mal) (adj) relating to or recurring in paroxysms (sudden, severe attacks of symptoms or convulsions)

Parvovirus
(**par**-vO-vI-rus) (n) a genus of viruses; strain B19 can cause anemia in humans

patent
(**pa**-tent) (adj) open; unblocked

pathogen
(**path**-O-jen) (n) any microorganism or substance that can cause a disease

pathologic
(path-O-**loj**-ik) (adj) pertaining to pathology, the medical science concerned with all aspects of disease, especially with the structural and functional changes caused by disease

pectoriloquy
(pek-tO-**ril**-O-kwee) (n) voice sounds transmitted through the pulmonary structures, clearly audible on auscultation

pectus carinatum
(**pek**-tus kar-i-**nay**-tum) (n) forward protusion of the sternum; pigeon breast

pectus excavatum
(**pek**-tus eks-ka-**vay**-tum) (n) markedly sunken sternum; funnel breast

pedal
(**ped**-al or **pEd**al) (adj) relating to the foot

pedicle
(**ped**-i-kl) (n) the stem that attaches a new growth

pedunculated
(pee-**dung**-Q-late-ed) (adj) possessing a stalk

pelvic
(**pel**-vik) (adj) relating to or located near the pelvis

pelvis
(**pel**-vis) (n) the bones in the lower portion of the trunk of the body; the bones between the spine and legs

pemphigus
(**pem**-fi-gus) (n) a distinctive group of diseases marked by successive crops of bullae

pendulous
(**pen**-ju-lus) (adj) loosely hanging

percussion
(per-**kush**-un) (n) a technique of physical examination in which the sound of fingers or a small tool tapping parts of the body is used to determine position and size of internal organs and to detect the presence of fluid

percutaneous
(per-kyoo-**tay**-nee-us) (adj) through the skin

perforation
(per-fO-**ray**-shun) (n) abnormal opening or hole in a hollow organ

perfusion
(per-**fyoo**-zhun) (n) passing of a fluid through spaces

periauricular
(**per**-ee-aw-**rik**-yoo-lar) (adj) around the ear

pericardial
(per-i-**kar**-dee-al) (adj) surrounding the heart; relating to the pericardium

pericardial effusion
(per-i-**kar**-dee-al e-**fyoo**-zhun) (n) increased fluid in the pericardial sac

pericarditis
(per-i-kar-**dI**-tis) (n) an inflammatory disease of the pericardium (tough outer layer of the heart wall and lining of the pericardial sac that surrounds the heart)

pericardium
(per-i-**kar**-dee-um) (n) a double-layered sac surrounding the heart and large vessels

pericolonic
(per-ee-ko-**lon**-ik) (adj) pertaining to the region around the colon

perihilar
(per-i-**hI**-lar) (adj) occurring near the hilum, the part of an organ where the nerves and vessels enter and leave

perineum
(**per**-i-**nee**-um) (n) the external region between the urethral opening and the anus, including the skin and underlying tissues

peripheral iridectomy
(per-**if**-er-al ir-i-**dek**-tO-mee) (n) procedure that creates a hole in the iris; used to relieve high intraocular pressure

peripheral nervous system
(per-**if**-er-al) (n) portion of nervous system that connects the CNS to other body parts

peripheral vascular disease
(pe-**rif**-e-ral **vas**-kyoo-lar)(n) any disorder affecting the blood circulatory system, except the heart

peristalsis
(per-i-**stal**-sis) (n) the movement of the intestine or other tubular structure, characterized by waves of alternate circular contraction and relaxation of the tube by which the contents are propelled onward

peritoneal
(per-i-tO-**nee**-al) (adj) relating to the peritoneum

peritoneum
(per-i-tO-**nee**-um) (n) lining of the abdominal cavity

perseveration
(per-sev-er-**ay**-shun) (n) an uncontrollable, persistent thought

petechia
(pe-**tee**-kee-a/pe-**tek**-ee-a) (n, sing.) tiny reddish or purplish flat spot on the skin as a result of a tiny hemorrhage within the skin (usually used in the plural form, petechiae)

petechiae
(pe-**tee**-kee-ee/pe-**tek**-kee-e/pe-tee-kee-a) (n) minute red spots appearing on the skin as a result of tiny hemorrhages

petechial
(pee-**tee**-kee-al/pee-**tek**-ee-al) (adj) relating to or having petechiae, tiny reddish or purplish spots on the skin from broken capillaries

petit mal
(pe-**tee** mahl) (n) a type of seizure characterized by a brief blackout of consciousness with minor rhythmic movements, seen especially in children

Pfannenstiel incision
(**fahn**-in-shteel) (n) a transverse incision made just above the pubes

phacoemulsification
(fak-O-ee-mul-si-fi-**kay**-shun) (n) process that disintegrates a cataract using ultrasonic waves

phagocyte
(**fag**-O-sIt/**fAg**O-sIt) (n) a cell able to engulf and destroy bacteria, foreign particles, cellular debris, and other cells

phagocytosis
(**fag**-O-sI-**tO**-sis) (n) the process in which a cell engulfs and destroys bacteria, foreign particles, cellular debris, and other cells

pharyngitis
(far-in-jI-tis) (n) inflammation of the pharynx

pharynx
(**far**-ingks) (n) throat; passageway for air from nasal cavity or larynx, and food from mouth to esophagus

phasic
(**fay**-sic) (adj) pertaining to a phase, a stage of development

phlebitis
(fle-bI-tis) (n) inflammation of a vein

phlebotomy
(fle-**bot**-O-mee) (n) incision into a vein for drawing blood

phobia
(**fO**-bee-a) (n) an unfounded fear that invokes a state of panic

phonation
(fO-**nay**-shun) (n) process of uttering vocal sounds

photon
(**fO**-ton) (n) a unit of radiant energy or light intensity

photophobia
(fO-tO-**fO**-bee-a) (n) marked intolerance to light

pia mater
(**pI**-a **may**-ter/**pee**-a **mah**-ter) (n) the innermost of the three membranes surrounding the brain and spinal cord; it carries a rich supply of blood vessels

pigment
(**pig**-ment) (n) any organic coloring substance in the body

pigmented
(**pig**-men-ted) (v) colored by a pigment

pilocarpine
(pI-lO-**kar**-peen) (n) a parasympathomimetic agent used to treat glaucoma

pineal gland
(**pin**-ee-al) (n) small, cone-shaped gland in the brain thought to secrete melatonin

pinna
(**pin**-a) (n) the external ear; auricle; pinnae (pin-ee) (pl)

Pitocin
(pi-**tO**-sin) (n) brand name for oxytocin, a synthetically produced, naturally-occurring hormone

pituitary gland
(pi-**too**-i-tayr-ee) (n) gland suspended from the base of the hypothalamus

plantar
(**plan**-tar) (adj) relating to the undersurface (sole) of the foot; a reflex

platelet
(**playt**-let) (n) disc-shaped, small cellular element in the blood that is essential for blood clotting

pleura
(**ploor**-a) (n) membrane lining the chest cavity and covering the lungs

pleural
(**ploo**-ral) (adj) concerning the pleura (serous membrane that enfolds both lungs and is reflected upon the walls of the thorax and diaphragm)

pleurisy
(**ploor**-i-see) (n) inflammation of the pleura; pleuritis

plexus
(**plek**-sus) (n) a network of intersecting nerves and blood vessels or of lymphatic vessels

pluripotential
(**ploo**-ree-pO-**ten**-shal) (adj) not having a fixed or defined potential development. White blood cells are developed from a single pluripotential cell which is capable of differentiating into the various types of white cells

Pneumocystis jiroveci
(**new**-mO-sist-is yee row **vet** zee eye) (n) an intracellular parasite which causes *Pneumocystis pneumonia* (PCP) in individuals with impaired immune systems

pneumonia
(noo-**mO**-nee-a) (n) inflammation and congestion of the lung, usually due to infection by bacteria or viruses

pneumonitis
(noo-mO-**nI**-tis) (n) inflammation of the lungs

pneumoperitoneum
(**noo**-mO-per-i-ton-**ee**-um) (n) condition in which air or gas is collected in the peritoneal cavity

pneumothorax
(noo-mO-**thor**-aks) (n) abnormal presence of air or gas in the chest cavity

poikilocytosis
(**poy**-ki-lO-sI-**tO**-sis) (n) having poikilocytes (abnormal and irregularly shaped red blood cells) in the blood

polycystic
(pol-ee-**sis**-tik) (adj) having or consisting of many cysts

polydipsia
(pol-ee-dip-**see**-a) (n) excessive thirst

polyneuropathy
(**pol**-ee-noo-**rop**-a-thee) (n) a disorder involving two or more peripheral nerves

polyp

(**pol**-ip) (n) a general descriptive term used with reference to any mass of tissue that bulges or projects outward or upward from the normal surface level

polyphagia

(pol-ee-**fay**-jee-a) (n) eating abnormally large amounts of food at a meal

polyuria

(pol-ee-**yoo**-ree-a) (n) excessive urinary output

pompholyx

(**pom**-fO-liks) (n) a skin eruption primarily on the hands and feet; may be accompanied by excessive sweating

popliteal

(pop-**lit**-ee-al) (adj) concerning the posterior surface of the knee

porphyrins

(**pOr**-fi-rinz) (n) a group of pigmented compounds essential to life; for example, hemoglobin contains the heme porphyrin

postictal

(pOst-**ik**-tal) (adj) relating to the period following a seizure

precordial

(pree-**kor**-dee-al) (adj) pertaining to the precordium (region of the chest over the heart)

preeclampsia

(pree-ee-**klamp**-see-a) (n) development of hypertension, proteinuria and/or edema during pregnancy

presbycusis

(**prez**-bee-**koo**-sis) (n) the loss of hearing acuity due to aging

presbyopia

(prez-bee-**O**-pee-a) (n) farsightedness associated with aging

presents

(pre-**sents**) (v) appears; shows; displays; the symptoms displayed are the presenting symptoms

Prilosec

(**pry**-low-sec) (n) brand name for omeprazole, a gastric acid secretion inhibitor

primipara

(prE-**mip**-ah-ra) (n) a woman who has had one pregnancy that produced a living infant

prognosis

(prog-**nO**-sis) (n) the expected outcome of a disease

prolapse

(prO-**laps**) (n) dropping of an organ from its normal position, a sinking down

pronator

(**prO**-nay-ter, **prO**-nay-tOr) (n) muscle that moves a part into the prone position

prophylaxis

(prO-fi-**lak**-sis) (n) prevention of disease or its spread

proprioception

(**prO**-pree-O-**sep**-shun) (n) sensation due to receiving stimuli from muscles, tendons, or other internal tissues which provides a sense of movement and position of the body

prostate gland

(**pros**-tayt) (n) a gland located at the base of the bladder and surrounding the beginning of the urethra in the male

prostatic

(pros-**tat**-ik) (adj) relating to the prostate gland

prosthesis

(pros-**thee**-sis) (n) artificial replacement for a diseased or missing part of the body, such as artificial limbs; prostheses (pl)

protease

(**prO**-tee-ays) an enzyme that breaks down proteins

protease inhibitor

(n) an agent that inhibits (prevents or slows down) the release of protease

proteinaceous

(**prO**-tee-**nay**-shus/**prO**-tee-i-**nay**-shus) (adj) relating to or resembling proteins

proteinuria

(prO-tee-**noo**-ree-a) (n) presence of abnormally large amounts of protein in the urine

proton

(**prO**-ton) (n) a positively charged particle that is a fundamental component of the nucleus of all atoms; used in radiotherapy

proton pump inhibitor

(**prO**-ton) (n) a class of drugs which prevents the release of hydrochloric acid in the stomach; used to treat symptoms of hyperacidity (GERD, peptic ulcer disease)

protuberant

(prO-**too**-ber-ant) (adj) pertaining to a part that is prominent beyond a surface, like a knob

proximal

(**prok**-si-mal) (adj) nearest the point of attachment, center of the body, or point of reference

proximally

(**prok**-si-mal-lee) (adv) occurring nearest to the point of attachment, center of the body, or point of reference

pruritic

(pru-**ri**-tic) (adj) itching

pruritus

(proo-**rI**-tus) (n) itching skin condition

pseudoephedrine

(soo-dO-i-**fed**-rin) (n) a generic drug; decongestant

Pseudomonas

(soo-dO-**mO**-nas) (n) a genus of gram-negative rods, which is a significant human pathogen

psoriasis

(sO-**rI**-a-sis) (n) chronic skin disease in which reddish scaly patches develop

psychosomatic

(**sI**-kO-sO-mat-ik) (adj) relating to the influence of the mind upon the functions of the body

pterygium

(ter-**ij**-ee-um) (n) web eye; an outward growth of tissue of the eye

pterygoid plate

(**ter**-i-goyd) (n) wing-shaped bones at the back of the nasal cavity

ptosis
(**tO**-sis) (n) sagging of the upper eyelid

punch biopsy
(punch **bI**-op-see) (n) a special instrument is used to take a small cylindrical piece of tissue for microscopic examination

pupil
(**pyoo**-pil) (n) the round opening in the center of the iris which opens or closes to adjust to light

pupillary
(**pyoo**-pi-layr-ee) (adj) relating to the pupil of the eye

purpura
(**pur**-poo-ra) (n) any of several bleeding disorders in which the escape of blood into tissues below the skin causes reddish or purplish spots

purulent
(**pyoor**-u-lent) (adj) relating to, containing, or forming pus

pustular
(**pus**-choo-lar) (adj) relating to or having pustules

pustule
(**pus**-chool) (n) small pus-containing elevation on the skin

pyelogram
(**pI**-el-O-gram) (n) x-ray of the kidney and ureters; usually a radiopaque dye is injected into the patient to show the outline of the kidney and associated structures

pyrexia
(pI-**rek**-see-a) (n) fever

pyrosis
(pI-**rO**-sis) (n) heartburn

Q

quadriceps
(kwah-dri-seps) (adj) four-headed, as a quadriceps muscle; one of the extensor muscles of the legs

quadriparesis
(kwod-ri-pa-ree-sis) (n) paralysis of both arms and both legs

R

radial keratotomy
(**ray**-dee-al ker-ah-**tot**-O-mee) (n) incision(s) in the cornea radiating out from the center

radiculopathy
(ra-**dik**-yoo-**lop**-a-thee) (n) disease of the spinal nerve roots

radiograph
(**ray**-dee-O-graf) (n) a negative image in photographic film made by exposure to x-rays or gamma rays that have passed through matter or tissue

radiology
(rA-dE-**ol**-O-jE) (n) the field of study involving ionizing radiation, ultrasound, nuclear imaging techniques, and radioisotopes to create medical images for the diagnosis and treatment of disease

radiopaque
(ray-dee-O-**payk**) (adj) opaque to x-rays or other radiation; an injection of a radiopaque dye or substance may be used to visualize areas of the body by x-ray

radiotherapy
(ray-dee-O-**thayr**-a-pee) (n) the treatment of disease by application of radium, ultraviolet, and other types of radiation

rales
(rahls) (n) abnormal sounds, such as rattling or bubbling, heard on auscultation of the lungs

ramus
(**ray**-mus) (n) branch, especially of a nerve or blood vessel

recession
(ree-**sesh**-un) (n) the withdrawal of a part from its normal position

rectal
(**rek**-tal) (adj) relating to the rectum, the lower part of the large intestine

rectovaginal
(**rek**-tO-**vaj**-i-nal) (adj) relating or located near the rectum and vagina

rectus
(**rec**-tus) (adj) relating to the rectus muscle of the eye

referral
(ree-**fer**-al) (n) a physician's sending of a patient to another physician

reflex
(**ree**-fleks) (n) an involuntary response to a stimulus

reflux
(**ree**-fluks) (n) abnormal backflow, as sometimes occurs with fluids in the esophagus or other body parts

refractory
(ree-**frak**-tO-ree) (adj) obstinate, stubborn; resistant to ordinary treatment

regimen
(**rej**-i-men) (n) plan of therapy, including drugs

regression
(ree-**gresh**-un) (n) returning to an earlier condition

regurgitation
(ree-**ger**-ji-**tay**-shun) (n) a backward flowing, as a backflow of blood through a defective heart valve or the bringing up of gas or undigested food from the stomach

renal
(**ree**-nal) (adj) related to the kidney

renal failure
(**ree**-nal) (n) inability of the kidneys to function

resection
(ree-**sek**-shun) (n) surgical removal of a portion of a structure or organ

residual
(re-**zid**-yoo-al) (adj) related to a residue which is left behind

respiration
(res-pi-**ray**-shun) (n) inhalation and exhalation; the exchange of gases—oxygen and carbon dioxide—between an organism and the environment

respiratory
(**res**-per-a-tOr-ee) (adj) relating to respiration

respiratory distress syndrome
(**res**-pi-ra-tOr-ee dis-**tres** sin-drOm) (n) acute lung disease, especially in premature newborn babies, caused by a lack of surfactant in the lung tissue

respiratory syncytial virus (RSV)
(sin-**sish**-ul) (n) a highly contagious respiratory illness resembling a moderate to severe cold

Restylane
(**res**-sti-layn) (n) an injection of hyaluronic acid used to decrease the appearance of facial lines

reticulocyte
(re-**tik**-yoo-lO-sIt) (n) a red blood cell containing a network of granules representing an immature stage in development

retina
(**ret**-i-na) (n) innermost layer of the eyeball that receives images formed by the lens and transmits visual impulses through the optic nerve to the brain; composed of light-sensitive nerves

retinal hemorrhage
(**ret**-i-nal **hem**-or-age) hemorrhage of the retina

retinitis pigmentosa
(ret-in-**I**-tis pig-men-**toe**-saw) (n) an inflammation of the retina with pigment changes, eventually leading to blindness

retinoblastoma
(**ret**-i-nO-blas-**tO**-ma) (n) malignant sarcoma or neoplasm of the retina; hereditary and generally occurring in young children

retinopathy
(ret-i-**nop**-a-thee) (n) any disorder of the retina without inflammation

retinoscopy
(ret-i-**nos**-ko-pee) (n) light beam test used to detect refractive errors

retraction
(ree-**trak**-shun) (n) the act of pulling back

retrograde
(**ret**-rO-grayd) (adj) moving or going backward

retroperitoneal
(ret-rO-per-i-tO-**nee**-al) (adj) located behind the peritoneum outside the peritoneal cavity, such as the kidneys

rhabdomyosarcoma
(**rab**-dO-**mI**-O-sar-**kO**-ma) (n) highly malignant tumor developing from striated muscle cells

rheumatic fever
(roo-**mat**-ik **fee**-ver) (n) fever following infection with Streptococcus bacteria; may affect the joints, skin, and heart

rheumatoid
(**roo**-ma-toyd) (adj) resembling rheumatism, with pain, inflammation, and deformity of the joints

rheumatoid factors
(roo-**ma**-toyd) (n) antibodies found in the serum of patients with rheumatoid arthritis

rhinitis
(rI-**nI**-tis) (n) inflammation of the mucous membrane of the nose

rhinophyma
(rI-nO-**fI**-ma) (n) enlargement of the nose from severe rosacea

rhinoplasty
(**rI**-nO-plas-tee) (n) surgery to correct a defect in the nose or to change its shape

rhinorrhea
(rI-nO-**ree**-a) (n) a watery discharge from the nose

rhonchus
(**rong**-kus) (n) abnormal sound heard on auscultation of the chest, usually during expiration; rhonchi (pl)

rigidity
(ri-**jid**-i-tee) (n) stiffness; inflexibility

Rinne test
(**rin**-ne) (n) also Rinne's (rin-ez); a hearing test comparing perception of air and bone conduction in one ear with a tuning fork; normally air conduction is more acute

Romberg
(**rom**-berg) (n) a simple test to assess for loss of proprioception wherein the patient stands with feet apart and then closes their eyes

rubella
(roo-**bel**-a) (n) a contagious viral disease with fever and a red rash; German measles

S

sac
(sak) (n) pouch

sagittal
(**saj**-i-tal) (adj) relating to a line from front to back in the middle of an organ or the body

salivary gland
(**sal**-i-vayr-ee) (n) a gland that secretes saliva into the mouth

Salter-Harris
(**sawl**-ter **har**-is) (n) classification system for epiphysial plate injuries

saphenous vein
(sa-**fee**-nus vayn) (n) either of two main veins in the leg that drain blood from the foot

sarcoidosis
(**sar**-koid-O-sis) (n) a systemic disease of unknown cause resulting in interstitial fibrosis involving the lungs, lymph nodes, skin, liver, spleen, eyes, phalangeal bones, and parotid glands

scabies
(**skay**-beez) (n) contagious rash with intense itching; caused by mites

scan
(n) scanning a tissue, organ, or system using a special apparatus that displays and records its image, such as computer tomography (CAT scan); the image so obtained

scapula
(**skap**-yoo-la) (n) a large, triangular, flattened bone lying over the ribs

sciatica
(sI-**at**-i-ka) (n) pain in the lower back and hip radiating down the back of the thigh into the leg, usually due to herniated lumbar disk

scirrhous
(**skir**-us) (adj) describing or resembling a hard, fibrous, malignant tumor

sclera
(**skleer**-a) (n) a fibrous coat that covers approximately five-sixths of the outer tunic of the eye; sclerae (pl)

sclerosis
(sklee-**rO**-sis) (n) hardening or induration of an organ or tissue, especially that due to excessive growth of fibrous tissue

sclerostomy
(skle-**ros**-tO-mee) (n) surgical formation of an opening in the sclera

sclerotic
(sklee-**rot**-ic) (adj) pertaining to or affected with sclerosis, a condition that shows hardness of tissue resulting from inflammation, mineral deposits, or other causes

scoliosis
(skO-lee-**O**-sis) (n) abnormal curvature of the spine to one side

scotoma
(skO-**tO**-ma) (n) a blind spot; a small area of defective vision

scrotal
(**skrO**-tal) (adj) relating to the scrotum

scrotum
(**skrO**-tum) (n) the pouch of skin containing the testes

sebaceous
(see-**bay**-shus) (adj) relating to sebum

seborrhea
(seb-O-**ree**-a) (n) overactivity of the oil glands of the skin

sebum
(**see**-bum) (n) an oily secretion of the oil glands of the skin

seed
(n) as related to oncology, it is the beginning of a tumor

seeding
(n) the local spreading of immature tumor cells

semicircular canals
(**sem**-ee-sir-kyoo-lar ka-**nals**) (n) three fluid-filled loops in the labyrinth of the inner ear, associated with the body's sense of balance

sensorineural deafness
(**sen**-sOr-i-**noor**-al) (n) hearing impairment due to nerve disturbance

sentinel node
(**sen**-ti-nal nOd) (n) an enlarged, supraclavicular lymph node infiltrated with cancer cells that have metastasized from an obscurely located primary cancer

septal
(**sep**-tal) (adj) pertaining to a dividing partition

septum
(**sep**-tum) (n) division between two cavities or two masses of tissue, e.g., nasal septum; septa (pl)

sequela
(see-**kwel**-a) (n) an abnormal condition resulting from a disease; sequelae (see-**kwel**-ee) (pl)

serosanguineous
(**ser**-o-san-**gwin**-ee-us) (adj) characterized by blood and serum

serous
(**seer**-us) (adj) relating to or having a watery consistency

serous otitis media
(**seer**-us O-**tI**-tis **mee**-dee-a) (n) inflammation of the middle ear accompanied by production of a watery fluid (serum)

sessile
(**sess**-il) (adj) attached directly at the base; not on a stalk

Seton procedure
(n) placing of a tube in the anterior chamber to drain fluid and decrease the intraocular pressure

sheath
(n) structure surrounding an organ, body part, or object

shotty
(**shot**-ee) (adj) resembling shot (hard pellets) to the touch; as shotty nodes

shunt
(shunt) (v) to turn away from; to divert

sickle cell anemia
(**sik**-l sel a-**nee**-mee-a) (n) hereditary blood disease in which abnormal hemoglobin causes red blood cells to become sickle-shaped, fragile and nonfunctional, leading to many acute and chronic complications

sigmoid colon
(**sig**-moyd **kO**-lon) (n) that part of the colon extending from the end of the descending colon to the rectum

sigmoidoscopy
(**sig**-moy-**dos**-ko-pee) (n) the inspection of the rectum and colon via endoscope

singultus
(sin-**gul**-tus) (n) hiccups

sinus
(**sI**-nus) (n) a passageway or hollow in a bone or other tissue

sinus rhythm
(**si**-nus **rith**-um) (n) normal cardiac rhythm

sinusitis
(sI-nu-**sI**-tis) (n) inflammation of the nasal sinuses, occurring as a result of an upper respiratory infection, an allergic response, or a defect of the nose

situs
(**sI**-tus) (n) a position

sitz bath
(sitz) (n) immersion of only the peritoneum and buttocks

sleep apnea syndrome
(**ap**-nee-a) (n) breathing stops, briefly and periodically, due to partial upper airway obstruction during sleep

slit lamp
(n) instrument consisting of a microscope and a thin, bright beam of light; used to examine the eye

somatization
(**sO**-mat-I-**zay**-shun) (n) a condition in which a person expresses psychological needs through physical symptoms

sonography
(so-**nog**-ra-fi) (n) ultrasonography; use of high-frequency sound waves to produce an image of an organ or tissue

sonometer
(**son**-O-mee-ter) (n) a bell-shaped instrument used to measure hearing

speculum
(**spek**-yoo-lum) (n) an instrument used for examining the interior of a cavity

sphenoidal

(sfee-**noy**-dal) (adj) concerning the sphenoid bone

sphenoidal sinus

(sfee-**noy**-dal) (n) one of two sinuses in the sphenoid bone opening to the nasal cavity

sphincter

(**sfingk**-ter) (n) a muscle that encircles a duct, tube, or opening in such a way that its contraction constricts the opening

sphincter of Oddi

(**sfingk**-ter of Od-**I**) (n) the sphincter which controls secretions from the liver, pancreas and gallbladder into the duodenum

sphincterotomy

(sfink-tur-**ot**-O-mee) (n) procedure that produces cuts in the iris sphincter muscle to allow pupillary enlargement

spinous

(**spI**-nus) (adj) pertaining to or resembling a spine, a short, sharp process of bone

splenectomy

(sple-**nek**-tO-mee) (n) surgical removal of the spleen

splenic

(**splen**-ik) (adj) referring to the spleen

splenomegaly

(sple-nO-**meg**-a-lee) (adj) enlargement of the spleen

spondylitis

(spon-di-**lI**-tis) (n) inflammation of one or more vertebrae

sporadic

(spO-**rad**-ik) (adj) occurring occasionally or in isolated situations

sprain

(n) injury to a joint by overstretching the ligaments; (v) to injure a joint and sometimes the nearby ligaments or tendons

sputum

(**spyoo**-tum) (n) spit; expectorated material

squamous

(**skway**-mus) (adj) covered with scale-like cells

stapes

(**stay**-peez) (n) the smallest and innermost of the three auditory bones in the inner ear; stirrup

staphylococcemia

(staf-i-lO-kok-**see**-mee-a) (n) the presence of staphylococci (bacterial microorganisms) in the blood

Staphylococcus aureus

(staf-il-O-**kok**-us **awr**-ee-us) (n) a common species of Staphylococcus (a bacteria), present on nasal mucous membranes and skin that causes pus-producing infections

station

(**stay**-shun) (n) the degree of descent of the presenting part of the fetus, measured in relation to the ischial spines of the maternal pelvis and reported in negative to positive numbers

steatorrhea

(stee-**a**-tO-**ree**-a) (n) presence of large amounts of fat in the stool caused by a failure to digest and absorb fat

stenocardia

(sten-O-**kar**-dee-a) (n) an attack of intense chest pain; also called angina pectoris

stenosis

(ste-**nO**-sis) (n) narrowing or constriction of a passageway or opening, such as a blood vessel

sterile

(**ster**-il) (adj) free from living microorganisms

sternocleidomastoid

(**ster**-nO-**klI**-dO-**mas**-toyd) (n) one of two muscles arising from the sternum and the inner part of the clavicle

sternum

(**ster**-num) (n) the breast bone

steroid

(**steer**-oyd) (n) any of a large number of similar chemical substances, either natural or synthetic; many are hormones; produced mainly in the adrenal cortex and gonads

strabismus

(stra-**biz**-mus) (n) improper alignment of eyes; crossed eye(s)

strain

(n) injury, usually to muscle, caused by overstretching or overuse; (v) to injure muscles by overstretching or overuse

strep

(n) short form of Streptococcus, a genus of bacteria; many species cause disease in humans

Streptococcus

(strep-tO-**kok**-us) (n) a genus of bacteria; many species cause disease in humans

stress incontinence

(stres in-**kon**-ti-nens) (n) inability to retain urine under tension, such as sneezing or coughing

sty

(stI) (n) an infection of a marginal gland of the eyelid; stye

subcutaneous

(sub-kyoo-**tay**-nee-us) (adj) under the skin

subcuticular

(sub-kyoo-**tik**-yoo-lar) (adj) beneath the cuticle of epidermis

subdural hematoma

(sub-**doo**-ral hee-ma-**tO**-ma / hem-a-**tO**-ma) (n) an accumulation of blood under the dura mater surrounding the brain

subjective data

(sub-**jek**-tiv **day**-tah) (n) information revealed by the patient to the health care provider

sublingual

(sub-**ling**-gwahl) (adj) beneath the tongue

subluxation

(n) (sub-luk-**sA**-shun) incomplete dislocation of a joint

submandibular

(sub-man-**dib**-yoo-lar) (adj) under the lower jaw

substernal

(sub-**ster**-nal) (adj) situated beneath the sternum (breast bone)

subxiphoid
(sub-**zif**-oyd) (adj) below a sword-shaped structure, as the xiphoid process, a structure beneath the lowest portion of the sternum

supine
(soo-**pIn**) (adj) lying on the back

suppuration
(**sup**-yu-**ray**-shun) (n) the production or discharge of pus

supraglottic
(soo-pra-**glot**-ik) (adj) located above the glottis, the sound-producing apparatus of the larynx

suprapubic
(soo-pra-**pyoo**-bik) (adj) above the pubic bones

supratentorial
(**soo**-pra-ten-**tO**-ree-al) (adj) located above the tentorium, a tentlike structure

suture
(**soo**-chur) (n and v) natural seam, border in the skull formed by the close joining of bony surfaces; closing a wound with a sterile needle and thread

symphysis
(**sim**-fi-sis) (n) joint in which fibrocartilage firmly unites the bones

syncopal
(**sin**-kO-pal) (adj) relating to fainting

syncope
(**sin**-ko-pee) (n) fainting

syndrome
(**sin**-drOm) (n) the signs and symptoms that constitute a specific disease

synovial fluid
(si-**nO**-vee-al **floo**-id) (n) protective lubricating fluid around joints

systemic lupus erythematosus
(sis-**tem**-ik **loo**-pus er-i-**them**-a-tO-sis/er-i-**thee**-ma-tO-sis) (n) a chronic disease with inflammatory symptoms in various systems of the body; characteristics of the disease and the systems involved may vary widely

systolic
(sis-**tol**-ik) (adj) pertaining to systole, the part of the heart cycle in which the heart is in contraction

T

T cell
(n) a type of lymphocyte; responsible for cell-mediated immunity

tachycardia
(**tak**-e-**kar**-dee-a) (n) an abnormally rapid heart rate

tachycardiac
(**tak**-e-**kar**-dee-ak) (adj) relating to or suffering from an abnormally rapid heart rate

tachycardic
(**tak**-e-**kar**-dik) (adj) relating to or suffering from an abnormally rapid heart rate

tachypnea
(**tak**-ip-**nee**-a) (n) rapid rate of breathing

tangent screen test
(n) maps the field of vision using a marker

Tanner staging
(n) method of indicating the sexual development of a child or adolescent

tarsal
(**tar**-sal) (adj) relating to a tarsus, a bone in the midfoot

telogen
(**tel**-O-jen) (n) the resting phase of the hair growth cycle

temporal
(**tem**-po-ral) (adj) pertaining to the temple of the head or the corresponding lobe of the brain

tenesmus
(te-**nez**-mus) (n) involuntary straining and the urge to defecate with little or no passage of stool

testicular
(tes-**tik**-yoo-lar) (adj) related to the testes, a pair of male gonads or sex glands that produce sperm and secretes androgens

texture
(**teks**-chur) (n) character, structure, and feel of parts of the body

thalassemia
(thal-a-**see**-mee-a) (n) an inherited disorder characterized by abnormal synthesis of one or both of the globin chains that combine to form hemoglobin

thecal
(**thee**-kal) (adj) referring to a covering or enclosure

thelarche
(thee-**lar**-kee) (n) the beginning of breast development in girls

theophylline
(thee-**off**-i-lin) (n) a drug used in chronic obstructive lung disease

thermodilution
(**ther**-mO-di-**loo**-shun) (n) method of determining cardiac output; involves injecting a cold liquid into the bloodstream and measuring the temperature change downstream

thoracoscopy
(thor-a-**kos**-kO-pee) (n) diagnostic examination of the pleural cavity with an endoscope

thoracotomy
(thor-a-**kot**-O-mee) (n) surgical incision of the chest wall

thorax
(**thor**-aks) (n) the chest

thrombocytopenia
(**throm**-bO-sI-tO-**pee**-nee-a) (n) an abnormal decrease in platelets in the blood, resulting in bleeding and easy bruising

thrombocytopenic
(**throm**-bO-sI-tO-**pee**-nik) (adj) relating to thrombocytopenia

thrombophlebitis
(**throm**-bO-fle-**bI**-tis) (n) inflammation of a vein with clot formation (thrombus)

thrombosis
(throm-**bO**-sis) (n) the formation, development, or existence of a blood clot, or thrombus, within the vascular system

thrombus
(**throm**-bus) (n) blood clot attached to the interior wall of a vein or artery

thrush
(n) infection with the fungus Candida, causing white patches in the mouth and throat

thyroid
(**thI**-royd) (n) a gland in the neck that secretes thyroid hormone

thyromegaly

(thI-rO-**meg**-a-lee) (n) enlargement of the thyroid gland

tibia

(**tib**-ee-a) (n) inner and thicker of the two bones of the human leg between the knee and the ankle; shinbone

tibial

(**tib**-ee-al) (adj) relating to the tibia

tinea

(**tin**-ee-a) (n) fungal infection; such as tinea pedis or athlete's foot

tinnitus

(ti-**nI**-tus) (n) noise, such as ringing, in the ears

titer

(**tI**-ter) (n) strength or concentration of a solution; a unit of measurement usually expressed as a ratio that indicates the minimum concentration of an antibody before losing its power to react to a specific antigen

tobramycin

(tO-bra-**mI**-sin) (n) an antibiotic drug

tomographic

(tO-**mog**-ra-feek) (adj) referring to an x-ray technique which displays an organ or tissue at a particular depth

tonometry

(tO-**nom**-et-ree) (n) a test that measures intraocular pressure

tonsils

(**ton**-silz) (n) lymphoid tissue structures in the oropharynx

TORCH

acronym for toxoplasmosis, other infections, rubella, cytomegalovirus infection, and herpes simplex. A TORCH titer is performed on pregnant women to assess their immune status.

torso

(**tor**-sO) (n) trunk of the body

toxoplasmosis

(**tok**-sO-plaz-**mO**-sis) (n) disease caused by a protozoan parasite

trabeculectomy

(tra-bek-yoo-**lek**-tO-mee) (n) surgical removal of a section of the cornea to decrease intraocular pressure in patients with severe glaucoma

trabeculoplasty

(tra-**bek**-yoo-lO-**plas**-tee) (n) surgical procedure that decreases intraocular pressure in open-angle glaucoma

trachea

(**tray**-kee-a) (n) the windpipe

tracheoesophageal

(**tray**-kee-O-e-sof-a-**gee**-al) (adj) pertaining to the trachea and esophagus

tracheostomy

(tray-kee-**os**-tO-mee) (n) a surgically created opening into the trachea (windpipe)

tracheotomy

(**tray**-kee-**ot**-O-mee) (n) the surgical procedure in which a tracheostomy is created

tragus

(**tray**-gus) (n) the small projection of cartilage in front of the external opening to the ear canal

transaminase

(trans-**am**-i-nays) (n) an enzyme that catalyzes transamination, the transfer of an animo group from one compound to another or the transposition of an animo group within a single compound

transesophageal

(tranz-ee-sof-a-**jee**-al) (adj) pertaining to an abnormal opening between the trachea and esophagus

transmural

(trans-**myoo**-ral) (adj) relating to the entire thickness of the wall of an organ

transperineal

(trans-per-i-**nee**-al) (adj) across or through the perineal region between the urethral opening and the anus, including the skin and underlying tissues

transurethral

(trans-yoo-**ree**-thral) (adj) through the urethra, such as a surgical procedure

transverse

(trans-**vers**) (adj) lying at right angles to the long axis of the body; crosswise

trocar

(**trO**-kar) (n) sharply pointed surgical instrument used for aspiration or removal of fluids from cavities

trochanter

(trO-**kan**-ter) (n) one of the projections at the upper end of the femur (thigh bone)

trochanteric

(trO-kan-**ter**-ik) (adj) related to a trochanter, either of the two bony processes below the neck of the femur)

tumor

(**too**-mor) (n) abnormal mass of tissue; neoplasm

turbinate

(**ter**-bi-nayt) (n) one of several thin, spongy, bony plates within the walls of the nasal cavity

turgor

(**ter**-gOr) (n) normal tension in a cell; swelling

tympanic

(tim-**pan**-ik) (adj) pertaining to the middle ear or tympanic cavity

tympanic membrane

(tim-**pan**-ik) (n) eardrum

tympanometric

(**tim**-pa-nO-**met**-rik) (adj) pertaining to tympanometry, a procedure for evaluation of motility of eardrum and middle ear disorders

tympanoplasty

(**tim**-pa-nO-**plas**-tee) (n) surgical repair of the middle ear

Tzanck smear

(tsangk smeer) (n) a method to help diagnose skin lesions by the miscroscopic examination of material from them

U

ulcer
(**ul**-ser) (n) a break in skin or mucosal surface with erosion, loss of tissue, and accompanying inflammation

ulcerative colitis
(**ul**-ser-a-tiv kO-**lI**-tis) (n) a chronic disease characterized by ulcers in the colon and rectum

ultrasound
(**ul**-tra-sownd) (n) sound waves at very high frequencies used in the technique of obtaining images for diagnostic purposes

umbo
(**um**-bO) (n) the inner surface of the tympanic membrane where it connects with the malleus in the middle ear

unilateral
(yoo-ni-**lat**-e-ral) (adj) affecting or occurring on only one side

unremarkable
(adj) nothing unusual is noted

upper respiratory infection (URI)
(n) an infection of the upper respiratory tract such as the common cold, laryngitis, sinusitis, and tonsillitis

ureter
(yoo-**ree**-ter/**yoo**-ree-ter) (n) either of a pair of tubes that carry urine from the kidney to the urinary bladder

ureteral
(yoo-**ree**-te-ral) (adj) relating to the ureters

ureteroscopy
(n) procedure to pass a ureteroscope up through the bladder into the ureter to inspect the ureteral lumen

urethra
(yoo-**ree**-thra) (n) a tube that drains urine from the bladder to the outside

urethral
(yoo-**ree**-thral) (adj) relating to the urethra, a canal for the discharge of urine from the bladder to the outside of the body

urethroscopy
(yoo-ree-**thros**-ko-pee) (n) an examination of the inside of the urethra with a urethroscope, a lighted instrument

urticaria
(er-ti-**kar**-ee-a) (n) hives; an eruption of itching red, raised lesions

urticarial
(er-ti-**kar**-ee-al) (adj) relating to or having urticaria

uterine
(**yoo**-ter-in/**yoo**-ter-In) (adj) relating to the uterus (the female reproductive organ where the fertilized egg develops before birth; the womb)

uveitis
(yoo-vee-**I**-tis) (n) inflammation of the uvea, including the choroid and the iris

uvula
(**yoo**-vyoo-la) (n) small, fleshy mass hanging from the soft palate in the mouth

uvulitis
(yoo-vyoo-**lI**-tis) (n) inflammation of the uvula

uvulopalatopharyngoplasty
(**yoo**-vyoo-lO-**pal**-a-tO-fa-**rin**-gO-plas-tee) (n) UPPP for short; a surgical treatment for sleep apnea for patients who cannot tolerate or respond to medical therapies

V

varicella
(var-i-**sel**-a) (n) chickenpox; a highly contagious viral disease

varices (plural of varix)
(**vair**-i-seez) (n) dilated, enlarged or tortuous veins

varicose veins
(var-I-kOs vaynz) (n) veins that become distended, swollen, knotted, tortuous, and painful because of poor valvular function

vascular
(**vas**-kyoo-lar) (adj) relating to the blood vessels

vascularity
(vas-kyoo-**lar**-i-tee) (n) the blood vessels in a part of the body

vasectomy
(va-**sek**-tO-mee) (n) excision of a portion of the vas deferens, in association with prostatectomy or to produce sterility

vena cava
(**vee**-na **kav**-a) (n) one of the largest veins of the body; venae cavae (pl)

veno-occlusive
(**vee**-nO O-**kloo**-siv) (adj) concerning obstruction of veins

venous
(**vee**-nus) (adj) relating to a vein or veins

ventricle
(**ven**-tri-kl) (n) either of the two lower chambers of the heart; areas of the brain that produce and drain cerebrospinal fluid (csf)

ventriculogram
(ven-**trik**-yoo-lO-gram) (n) an x-ray of the ventricles

ventriculography
(ven-trik-yoo-**log**-ra-fee) (n) x-ray visualization of heart ventricles after injection of a radiopaque substance

vertebral
(ver-**tee**-bral) (adj) relating to a vertebra or the vertebrae

vertex
(**ver**-teks) (n) the crown or top of the head

vertigo
(**ver**-tig-O) (n) dizziness

vesical
(**ves**-i-kul) (adj) referring to the bladder or gallbladder

vesicle
(**ves**-i-kl) (n) blister; small, raised skin lesion containing clear fluid

vesicouterine
(**ves**-i-kO-**yoo**-ter-in) (adj) pertaining to the urinary bladder and uterus

vesicular
(ve-**sik**-yoo-lar) (adj) pertaining to vesicles or small blisters

vesiculopustular

(ves-**ick**-you-low-**pus**-to-ler) (adj) characterized by vesicles and pustules

vestibulum

(ves-**tib**-yoo-lum) (n) the central cavity of the labyrinth in the inner ear, between the cochlea and the semicircular canals

viable

(**vI**-a-bl) (adj) capable of surviving; living

vibrissae

(vI-**bris**-a) (n) nose hairs

villi

(**vil**-I) (n) many tiny projections, occurring over the mucous membrane of the small intestine that accomplish the absorption of nutrients and fluids; villus (sing)

villous

(**vil**-us) (adj) relating to villi

vincristine

(vin-**kris**-teen) (n) an antineoplastic drug that disrupts cell division and is used to treat many cancers, especially those of the lymphatic system.

virus

(**vI**-rus) (n) an agent that lacks an independent metabolism but infects a host cell, incorporating the virus's genetic material into the host DNA and utilizing the host's cellular components to replicate; not affected by antibiotics

viscera

(**vis**-er-a) (n) main internal organs within the trunk of the body, especially those in the abdominal cavity

visceral

(**vis**-er-al) (adj) relating to or located near the viscera

visceromegaly

(**vis**-er-O-**meg**-a-lee) (n) generalized enlargement of the abdominal organs

Vistaril

(**viss**-ta-rill) (n) brand name for hydroxyzine, used for the treatment of anxiety and nausea

visualization

(**vich**-oo-al-I-**zay**-shun) (n) the act of viewing an object, especially the picture of a body structure as obtained by x-ray study

vitiligo

(vi-ti-**lee**-gO) (n) white patches, due to loss of pigment, appearing on the skin

vitreous

(**vit**-ree-us) (adj) resembling glass

vitreous humor

(**vit**-ree-us **hyoo**-mer) (adj) glassy; gelatin-like substance within the eyeball

vortex

(**vor**-teks) (n) whirlpool; resembling a whirlpool

vulva

(**vul**-va) (n) external female genital organs; vulvae (pl)

vulvar

(**vul**-var) (adj) relating to the vulva

W

Weber test

(**web**-er) (n) a hearing test performed with a tuning fork placed at points in the middle of the skull to determine where the vibration is heard (not where it is felt)

Western blot

(n) a laboratory test to detect the presence of antibodies to specific antigens in the blood

wheal

(hweel) (n) a raised, red circumscribed lesion usually due to an allergic reaction; usually accompanied by intense itching; welt

wheezing

(**hweez**-ing) (n) breathing with difficulty and with a whistling sound; can be heard aloud and/or on auscultation

Wright peak flow

(n) maximum flow of expired air as measured by the Wright flowmeter

X

Xalatan

(**zal**-a-tan) (n) eyedrops used to treat glaucoma by increasing drainage of aqueous humor.

xanthoma

(zan-**thO**-mah) (n) yellowish nodules in or under the skin, especially in the eyelids

xanthopsia

(zan-**thop**-see-a) (n) yellow vision; a condition in which everything seen appears yellowish

xeromammogram

(zeer-O-**mam**-o-gram) (n) type of x-ray of the breast

xerosis

(zer-**O**-sis/zee-r**O**-sis) (n) dry skin

xerostomia

(zeer-O-**stO**-mee-a) (n) dryness of the mouth

xiphoid

(**zif**-oyd) (adj) referring to the xiphoid process, the cartilage at the lower end of the sternum (breast bone); also spelled xyphoid

Xylocaine

(**zI**-lO-kayn) (n) trade name for lidocaine hydrochloride

Y

yolk sac

(**yOk** sak) (n) a membranous sac surrounding the food yolk in the embryo

Index

Foot pedal, 36
Forceps, *98*
Formatting document, 46, *47*
For the Record
    Web site for, 21
Fractions
    use of figures in, 125
Fracture, 361, *361*
Fragments, sentences, 100, 101
Frontal plane, 86
FTP software, 57
Fundus, 300, *300*

G

Gallbladder, *270*, *271*, *272*
Gallstones, *274*, *275*
Gastroenterologist, 269
Gastroenterology, 269–291
    abbreviations, 284
    anatomic structure and function
        of, 270–271, *270–273*
    defined, 269
    diseases and conditions, *274*,
        274–277, *275*
    physical assessment, 271–272
    tests and surgical procedures,
        277–278
Gastroesophageal reflux disease
    (GERD), 274
Gastroscopy, 277
Genitalia
    female, 300–301, *300–302*
    male, *327*, *328*
Glasgow coma scale, 384
Glaucoma, 170
Glomerulonephritis, 328
Glomerulus, 326, *327*
Gonioscopy, 171
Gonorrhea, 303
Graafian follicle, 301
Graves disease, 442
Gray, *92*
Gynecologist, 299
Gynecology. *See also* Obstetrics/
    gynecology
    defined, 299

H

Haemophilus influenza, 195, 218
Hair, 143
Hair follicle, 143
Handwashing, 441
Headset, 36

Health Insurance Portability and
    Accountability Act (HIPAA)
    confidentiality and privacy, 24, 27
Health Level Seven (HL7)
    standards for medical reports, 22
Hearing loss, 194
Heart, 241–260
    anatomic structure and function
        of, 242–244, *242–244*
    blood flow in, *243*
    diseases and conditions, 245–246
    electrical current flow in, *244*
    internal structures of, *243*
    physical assessment, 244
    position of heart in thoracic
        cavity, *242*
    tests and surgical procedures,
        246–248
Heart attack, 245
Heartburn, 274, *274*, *275*
Heart failure, 245
Helicobacter pylori, 274–275
Hematologist-oncologist, 411
Hematology/oncology, 411–429
    abbreviations, 423
    anatomic structure and function,
        412–415, 412–416
    blood clotting cascade, 414, *415*,
        416
    blood types and transfusions,
        414, *415*
    blood typing based on principle
        of agglutination, 414, *414*
    components of blood, 412, *413*
    defined, 411
    diseases and conditions, 416–418
    phases of blood cell differentia-
        tion, *412*
    physical assessment, 416
    tests and surgical procedures,
        418–419, *419*
Hematopoiesis, 412
Hemoglobin, 416–417
Hemophilia, 414
Hemorrhoids, *274*, *275*
Henle, loop of, *326*, *327*
Hepatitis, 276–277
Herniated intervertebral disk, 361
Herpes, 303
Herpes zoster, 143
Hiatal hernia, *274*, *275*
Histology, 79
History and physical report
    description of, 24

history section, 341
impressions and plan section, 342
main headings, 466–469
physical examination, 342
required headings/content, 341
review of systems section, 342
samples of, *25*, *26*
transcription skills practice,
    343–345
turnaround time, 342–343
Hordeolum, 170
Horizontal plane, 86, *86*
Hormone therapy, 418
Hospital chart, 24, 27
Human immunodeficiency virus
    (HIV), 303, 439
Human papillomavirus (HPV), 303
Hypercoagulation disorder, 417
Hyperplasia, 95
Hypertensive heart disease, 245–246
Hypertrophy, 95
Hypertropia, 170
Hyphens
    compound adjectives, 132–134
    general rule for use of, 132
    other uses of, 136
    prefixes, 134–135
    suffixes, 134–135
    suspended, 135
Hypogastric region, 81, *81*
Hysterectomy, 304

I

Icons, *40*
IgA, 442–443, *443*
IgD, 442–443, *443*
IgE, 442–443, *443*
IgG, 442–443, *443*
IgM, 442–443, *443*
Immune thrombocytopenic purpura
    (ITP), 417
Immunity
    acquired, 438
    natural, 438
Immunoglobulins, 442–443, *443*
Immunologist, 437
Immunology, 437–453
    abbreviations, 447
    anatomic structure and function,
        438, *438–439*
    common pathogens, *440*
    components of lymph system,
        438

diseases and conditions, 439–442, *440, 441*
  immunoglobulins and function of, 442–443, *443*
  interventions that halt transmission of infection, 439, 441, *441*
  physical assessment, 439
  tests and procedures, 442–443
Incus, 190, *190*
Independent contractor, *29*
Index counters, *37*
Infections
  common pathogens for, *440*
  of heart, 246
  interventions that halt transmission of, 439, 441, *441*
Inferior, *84–85, 86, 86*
Influenza, 441
Informed consent, *29*
Injury prevention, 61–63
Institute of Safe Medication Practices (ISMP), 118
Internal rotation, *86*
Internet
  browser, 54
  connection to, 54
  online references, 20–21
Intestine
  large, *270, 271, 273*
  small, *270, 271*
Invasion of the right of privacy, *29*
Inversion, *86, 87*
Inverted sentences, 108
Iris, 168, *168*
Irritable colon, *274, 275*
Ischemic heart disease, 245

J

Jargon
  dealing with, 14
Joint Commission
  standards for medical reports, 21
Joints, *356, 360*
Jump macro, 52, 476

K

Keloid, *144*
Keratin, 142
Keratitis, 170
Keratoconus, 170
Keyboard
  basic conventions for, 42–43
  shortcut keys, *44*

Kidneys, 326–327, *326–327*
Kidney stones, 328–329
Klebsiella pneumoniae, 218

L

Labor and delivery report
  main headings, 472
  required headings/content, 316
  transcription skills practice, 316–318
  turnaround time, 316
Laboratory word book, 18
Labyrinth, 190, *191*
Labyrinthitis, 194
Larynx, 192, *193*
Lateral, *84–85*
Lateral decubitus, *93*
Left hypochondriac region, 81, *81*
Left lower quadrant (LLQ), 81, *81, 273*
Left lumbar region, 81, *81*
Left upper quadrant (LUQ), 81, *81, 273*
Legal issues, 24, 27–28, *29*
Legal terms, *29*
Leiomyomas, 303
Lens, 168, *168*
Leuk/o, *87*
Levels of organization, 77–79
  body systems, 79
  cells, 78–79
  organs, 79
  tissue, 79
Libel, *29*
Lichenification, *144*
Ligaments, 356
Lingual tonsils, 192, *193*
Lipase, 271
Lithotripsy, 329
Liver, *270, 271*
Lumbar puncture (LP), 388
Lumbar vertebrae, 80, *82*
Lungs. *See also* Pulmonology
  anatomic structure and function of, *216,* 216–217
Luteal phase, 301
Luteinizing hormone (LH), 300
Lymphangiograph, *92*
Lymph nodes, 438, *438*
Lymph system, 414

M

Macros, 52
Macular degeneration, 171
Macule, *144*
Magnetic resonance imaging (MRI), 388
  process of, 90
  terms associated with, *92–93*
Malleus, 190, *190*
Malpractice, *29*
Malware, 59
Mammogram, 304
Mandible, 192
Mastectomy, 304
Mathematical expressions
  use of figures in, 124
Maxilla, 192
Maximize, *40*
Measles, 143
Measurements
  abbreviations for units of, 129
  use of figures in, 124
Medial, *84–85*
Mediastinum, 242
Medical dictionary, 17
Medical equipment book, 18
Medical glossary, 17
Medical imaging, 88–93
  computed tomography, 89–90
  diagnostic procedure terminology, *92–93*
  fluoroscopy, 89
  magnetic resonance imaging, 90
  nuclear medicine, 91
  radiology, 89
  sonography, 89
Medical phrase index, 18
Medical records, 21–29. *See also* Medical reports
  confidentiality, 24, 27–28
  hospital charts, 24, *27*
  legal issues, 24, 27–28, *29*
  legal terms, *29*
  medical report as, components of, 23–24
  narrative-style charting, 23
  ownership of document and content, 28
  problem-oriented medical record, 22
  release of information, 28
  retention of, 28
  SOAP note format, 23

Mouse
    Ctrl + drag, 42
    double click, 41
    drag, 41
    drag and drop, 41
    using, 39, 41–42
Mouth, 270
Movement terms, 86, *86*
Multiple sclerosis (MS), 442
Murmurs, 244
Muscles
    cardiac, *356*
    function of, *356*
    musculoskeletal system, *357–358*
    skeletal, *356, 360*
    smooth, *356*
Muscle tissue, 79
Musculoskeletal system, 356,
    357–360
Myasthenia gravis, 442
Myelograph, *92*
Myelography, 388
Myocarditis, 246
Myocardium, 242

N

Nails, 143
Narrative-style charting, 23
Nasopharynx, 192
National Committee for Quality
    Assurance (NCQA)
    standards for medical reports, 22
Natural immunity, 438
Needle, *98*
Nephrologist, 325
Nephrology. *See also* Urology/
    nephrology
    defined, 325
Nephron, *326, 327*
Nephrotic syndrome, 328
Nerve conduction velocity (NCV),
    388
Nerve tissue, 79
Nervous system
    anatomic structure and function,
        380, *381–384*
Networks, computer, 54
Neuroendocrine system, 380
Neuroglia, 380
Neurologist, 379
Neurology
    abbreviations, 393
    anatomic structure and function,
        380, *381–384*

defined, 379
    diseases and conditions, 385–386
    physical assessment, 382,
        384–385
    tests and surgical procedures,
        387, 387–388
Neuron, 380, *384*
Neuropsychological evaluation
    required headings/content, 402
    transcription skills practice,
        402–405
    turnaround time, 402
Neurosurgeon, 379
Neurotransmitters, 380
Nodule, *144*
Nonprivileged information, *29*
Norepinephrine, 380, *382*
Nose, 189–213
    anatomic structure and function
        of, 190–192, *190–193*
    diseases and conditions, 194–195
    physical assessment, 192, 194
    tests and surgical procedures, 195
Nosocomial infection, 441
Notification area, *40*
Nouns
    collective, 104
    proper, 116–118
    subject-verb agreement, 102–104
Nuclear medicine
    process of, 91
    terms associated with, *92–93*
Nucleus, 78, *78*
Numbers
    age, 123
    basic rule for using numbers in
        word or figure form, 122–123
    dates, 123
    decimals, 125
    fractions, 125
    measurements, mathematical
        expressions and symbols, 124
    money, 124
    numeric ranges, 125
    plurals, 116
    time, 123–124
    vertebrae, 124–125
Numeric ranges, 125

O

Object
    pronoun as, 106
Objective
    in SOAP note format, 23

Objective information
    in history and physical, 24
Obstetrician, 299
Obstetrics/gynecology, 299–315
    abbreviations, 309
    anatomic structure and function,
        300–301, *300–302*
    bimanual method of palpating
        internal genitalia, *302*
    defined, 299
    diseases and conditions, 303
    external female genitalia, *302*
    internal female genitalia, *300*
    physical assessment, 301–302,
        301–302
    structure of female breast, *301*
    tests and surgical procedures,
        304
Occupational Safety and Health
    Administration
    ergonomic workstations, 62
Office note, 158–165
    main headings, 469
Oncology. *See also* Hematology/
    oncology
    defined, 411
OneLook
    Web site for, 21
Oocyte, 301
Operative report, 23
    required headings/content, 206
    transcription skills practice,
        206–208
    turnaround time, 206
Ophthalmologist, 167
Ophthalmology, 167–188
    abbreviations, 175
    anatomic structure and function
        of, 168, *168*
    defined, 168
    diseases and conditions, 169–171
    physical assessment, 168–169
    tests and surgical procedures, 171
Ophthalmoscope, 169, *169*, 171
Optometrist, 167
Orchidopexy, 329
Organelles, 78, *78*
Organs, 79
Oropharynx, 192
Orthopedics, 355–371
    abbreviations, 365
    anatomic structure and function,
        356, *357–360*
    defined, 355–371